Modern Management
of Endometriosis

Modern Management of Endometriosis

Edited by

Professor Christopher Sutton
Professor of Gynaecological Surgery
University of Surrey Post-Graduate Medical School and
Consultant Gynaecologist
Royal Surrey County Hospital
Guildford,
UK

Kevin Jones
Consultant Obstetrician and Gynaecologist
Great Western and Ridgeway Hospitals
Swindon
UK

G. David Adamson
Director of Fertility Physicians of Northern California
Palo Alto, CA
USA

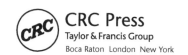

CRC Press
Taylor & Francis Group
Boca Raton London New York

CRC Press is an imprint of the
Taylor & Francis Group, an **informa** business

CRC Press
Taylor & Francis Group
6000 Broken Sound Parkway NW, Suite 300
Boca Raton, FL 33487-2742

First issued in paperback 2019

© 2011 by Taylor & Francis Group, LLC
CRC Press is an imprint of Taylor & Francis Group, an Informa business

No claim to original U.S. Government works

ISBN-13: 978-1-84214-276-9 (hbk)
ISBN-13: 978-0-367-39166-9 (pbk)

A CIP record for this book is available from the British Library.

Library of Congress Cataloging-in-Publication Data available on application

**Visit the Taylor & Francis Web site at
http://www.taylorandfrancis.com**

**and the CRC Press Web site at
http://www.crcpress.com**

Dedication

From Christopher Sutton:
I would like to dedicate this book to my wife, children and grandchild

From Kevin Jones:
I would like to dedicate this book to my parents and my wife and children who have always supported me throughout my career

From David Adamson:
Dedicated to my wife, Rosemary,
And my children, Stephanie, Rebecca and Eric
Who give me reason to do the best I can
For each and every patient
With much gratitude for all their
Understanding, patience, and support

Contents

Contributors

Jason Abbott MD PhD FRCOG FRANZCOG
School of Women & Infants Health
University of Western Australia
King Edward Memorial Hospital
Subiaco, Australia

G. David Adamson MD FRCSC FACOG FACS
Director of Fertility Physicians of
Northern California
Palo Alto and San Jose
CA, USA

Abdul Aziz Al-Shahrani MD
Fellow of Reproductive Endocrinology and
Infertility
McGill University Department of Obstetrics &
Gynecology
Montreal, Canada

Saikat Banerjee MRCOG
Clinical Fellow in Minimal Access Surgery
Ashford & St Peter's NHS Trust
St Peter's Hospital
Chertsey
Surrey, UK

Agneta Bergqvist MD PhD
Associate Professor, Senior Lecturer
Karolinska Institutet
Department of Obstetrics and Gynaecology
Danderyds Hospital
Stockholm, Sweden

Bruno Borghese MD
Assistance Publique – Hospitaux de Paris (AP-HP)
Service de Gynécologie Obstétrique II
Unité de Chirurgie Gynécologique
Paris, France

Revaz Botroschivili MD
Département de Gynécologie Obstétrique et
Reproduction Humaine et Laboratoire de Biologie
de la Reproduction et du Développement
Centre hospitalier universitaire et Université
d'Auvergne
Clermont-Ferrand, France

Jan Brosens MD PhD
Institute of Reproductive and
Developmental Biology
Wolfson and Weston Research Centre for Family
Health
Imperial College London
Hammersmith Hospital
London, UK

Ivo Brosens MD PhD
Leuven Institute for Fertility and Embryology
Leuven
Belgium

Mauro Busacca MD
Professor and Head of Obstetrics and Gynecology
University of Milan
Macedonio Melloni Hospital
Milan, Italy

Michel Canis MD
Département de Gynécologie Obstétrique et
Reproduction Humaine et Laboratoire de Biologie
de la Reproduction et du Développement
Centre hospitalier universitaire et Université
d'Auvergne
Clermont-Ferrand, France

Charles Chapron MD
Professor, Paris V Descartes University
Assistance Publique – Hospitaux de Paris (AP-HP)
Service de Gynécologie Obstétrique II
Unité de Chirurgie Gynécologique
Paris, France

Nicolas Chopin MD
Assistance Publique – Hopitaux de Paris (AP-HP)
Service de Gynécologie Obstétrique II
Unité de Chirurgie Gynécologique
Paris, France

Thomas M D'Hooghe MD PhD
Coordinator Leuven University Fertility Center
Department of Obstetrics & Gynaecology
University Hospital Gasthuisberg
Leuven, Belgium

Michael P Diamond, MD FACOG
Kamran S. Moghissi Professor and Associate
Chair of Obstetrics and Gynaecology and
Director, Division of Reproductive
Endocrinology and Infertility
Wayne State University
MI, USA

Jacques Donnez MD PhD FRCOG (ad eundem)
Department of Gynecology
Catholic University of Louvain
Cliniques Universitaires St-Luc
Brussels, Belgium

Cindy Farquhar MBChB MD FRCOG FRANZCOG CREIMPH
Postgraduate Professor of Obstetrics and
Gynaecology
University of Auckland
Auckland, New Zealand

Jean-Michel Foidart MD PhD
Department of Obstetrics and Gynecology
Laboratory of Tumor and Development Biology
University of Liege
Liège, Belgium

Hervé Foulot MD
Assistance Publique – Hopitaux de Paris (AP-HP)
Service de Gynécologie Obstétrique II
Unité de Chirurgie Gynécologique
Paris, France

Ian S Fraser MD FRANZCOG FRCOG
Professor in Reproductive Medicine
Department of Obstetrics and Gynaecology
University of Sydney
Sydney, Australia

Ray Garry MD FRCOG FRANZCOG
Professor in Gynaecology
School of Women & Infants Health
University of Western Australia
King Edward Memorial Hospital
Subiaco, Australia

Anu Goswami MD MRCOG
Associate Professor
Department of Obstetrics and Gynaecology
BP Koirala Institute of Health Sciences
Dharan, Nepal

Pat Haines BSC RGN MBAcC
Clinical Nurse Practitioner
Acupuncture Practitioner
The Royal Surrey County Hospital
Dept of Obstetrics and Gynaecology
Guildford, UK

Roger Hart MD FRCOG
Professor in Gynaecology
School of Women & Infants Health
University of Western Australia
King Edward Memorial Hospital
Subiaco, Australia

Pascale Jadoul MD
Department of Gynecology
Catholic University of Louvain
Cliniques Universitaires St-Luc
Brussels, Belgium

Laurent Janny MD
Département de Gynécologie Obstétrique et
Reproduction Humaine et Laboratoire de Biologie
de la Reproduction et du Développement
Centre hospitalier universitaire et Université
d'Auvergne, Clermont-Ferrand, France

Kevin Jones BSc MB ChB MSc MD MRCOG
Consultant Obstetrician and Gynaecologist
Great Western and Ridgeway Hospitals
Swindon, UK

Meenal Kamble MD
Département de Gynécologie Obstétrique et
Reproduction Humaine et Laboratoire de Biologie
de la Reproduction et du Développement
Centre hospitalier universitaire et Université
d'Auvergne, Clermont-Ferrand, France

Jöerg Keckstein MD
Professor in Gynaecology
University of Ulm
Chief of Department of Gynaecology
and Obstetrics
Landeskrankenhaus Villach
Villach, Austria

Stephen Kennedy MD
Clinical Reader/Hon Consultant
Nuffield Department of Obstetrics & Gynaecology
University of Oxford
John Radcliffe Hospital
Oxford, UK

Karen Kinkel MD PhD
Institute of Radiology and Foundation des
Grangettes
Clinique des Grangettes
Canton of Geneva, Switzerland

Philippe R Koninckx MD PhD
Department Obstetrics and Gynaecology
University Hospital Gasthuisberg
Catholic University Leuven (K.U.Leuven)
Leuven, Belgium

Cleophas M Kyama MD
Leuven University Fertility Centre
Department of Obstetrics & Gynaecology
University Hospital Gasthuisberg
Leuven, Belgium

Georgine Lamvu MD MPH
Division of Advanced Laparoscopy and
Pelvic Pain
University of North Carolina at Chapel Hill
Chapel Hill, NC, USA

B Victor Lewis MD FRCS FRCOG
Consultant Gynecologist
BUPA Hospital
Bushey, UK

Steven R Lindheim MD
Associate Professor
The Division of Reproductive Endocrinology and
Infertility
Department of Obstetrics and Gynecology
University of Wisconsin School of Medicine
Madison, WI, USA

Enda McVeigh MD FRCOG
Nuffield Department of Obstetrics and
Gynaecology
University of Oxford
John Radcliffe Hospital
Oxford, UK

Peter J Maher MD MB BS FRCOG FRANZCOG
Director, Endosurgery Unit
Associate Professor
Department of Obstetrics & Gynaecology
University of Melbourne
Mercy Hospital for Women
Melbourne, Australia

Cécile Malartic MD
Assistance Publique – Hospitaux de Paris (AP-HP)
Service de Gynécologie Obstétrique II
Unité de Chirurgie Gynécologique
Paris, France

Dan C Martin MD
Clinical Professor
Department of Obstetrics and Gynecology
University of Tennessee Health Sciences Center
Memphis, TN
USA

Charles E Miller MD FACOG
Clinical Associate Professor
Department Obstetrics and Gynecology
University of Illinois at Chicago
Arlington Heights
IL, USA

Jason M Mwenda MD
Division of Reproductive Biology
Institute of Primate Research
Karen
Nairobi, Kenya

Michelle Nisolle MD PhD
Department of Obstetrics and Gynecology
University of Liege
Liège, Belgium

David L Olive MD
Professor
The Division of Reproductive Endocrinology and
Infertility
Department of Obstetrics and Gynecology
University of Wisconsin School of Medicine
Madison
WI, USA

David H Oram FRCOG
St Bartholomew's Hospital
London, UK

Stefano Palomba MD
Assistant Professor of Obstetrics & Gynecology
University 'Magna Graecia' of Catanzaro
Catanzaro, Italy

Rusudan Piekrischvili MD
Département de Gynécologie Obstétrique et
Reproduction Humaine et Laboratoire de Biologie
de la Reproduction et du Développement
Centre hospitalier universitaire et Université
d'Auvergne
Clermont-Ferrand, France

Mark Possover MD PhD
Chief of the Department of Gynecology &
Obstetrics & Neuro-Functional Pelvic Surgery
Training Center of the ISPS
St. Elizabeth Hospital
Cologne, Germany

Jean Luc Pouly MD
Département de Gynécologie Obstétrique et
Reproduction Humaine et Laboratoire de Biologie
de la Reproduction et du Développement
Centre hospitalier universitaire et Université
d'Auvergne
Clermont-Ferrand, France

Elizabeth A Pritts MD
Assistant Professor
The Division of Reproductive Endocrinology and
Infertility
Department of Obstetrics and Gynecology
University of Wisconsin School of Medicine
Madison
WI, USA

Timothy Rockall MD FRCS
Minimal Access Therapy Training Unit (MATTU),
Royal Surrey County Hospital
Guildford, UK

Barnaby D Rufford MB BS MRCOG
Department of Gynaecological Oncology
St Bartholomew's Hospital
London, UK

Vikas Sachar MD FACOG
Wayne State University – Medicine
Obstetrics–Gynecology
Hutzel Hospital,
MI, USA

Benoît Schubert MD
Département de Gynécologie Obstétrique et
Reproduction Humaine et Laboratoire de Biologie
de la Reproduction et du Développement
Centre hospitalier universitaire et Université
d'Auvergne
Clermont-Ferrand, France

Angela J Skull MS FRCS
Minimal Access Therapy Training Unit (MATTU),
Royal Surrey County Hospital
Guildford, UK

Mireille Smets MD PhD
Department of Gynecology
Catholic University of Louvain
Cliniques Universitaires St-Luc
Brussels, Belgium

Jean Squifflet MD
Department of Gynecology
Catholic University of Louvain
Cliniques Universitaires St-Luc
Brussels, Belgium

John F Steege MD
Professor and Director
Division of Advanced Laparoscopy and
Pelvic Pain
University of North Carolina at Chapel Hill
Chapel Hill, NC, USA

Lisa Story MB BS MRCOG
Nuffield Department of Obstetrics & Gynaecology
University of Oxford, Oxford, UK

Christopher Sutton MA MB BCH FRCOG
Professor of Gynaecological Surgery
University of Surrey Post-Graduate Medical
School
and
Consultant Gynaecologist
Royal Surrey County Hospital
Guildford, UK

Rose CY Tse MD MRCOG FHKAM
Department of Obstetrics and Gynaecology
Queen Elizabeth Hospital, Hong Kong

Togas Tulandi MD MHCM
Professor of Obstetrics and Gynecology and
Milton Leong Chair in Reproductive Medicine
McGill University
Montreal, Canada

Michele Vignali MD
Assistant Professor of Obstetrics and Gynecology
University of Milan
Macedonio Melloni Hospital
Milan, Italy

Hubert Wiesinger MD
Chief of Department of Surgery
Landeskrankenhaus Villach
Nikolaigasse
Villach, Austria

Jeremy T Wright FRCOG
Consultant Gynaecologist
Ashford & St Peter's NHS Trust
St Peter's Hospital
Chertsey, Surrey, UK

Denniz Zolnoun MD MPH
Division of Advanced Laparoscopy and
Pelvic Pain
University of North Carolina at Chapel Hill
Chapel Hill, NC, USA

Fulvio Zullo MD
Chief of the Department of Obstetrics &
Gynecology
University 'Magna Graecia' of Catanzaro
Catanzaro, Italy

Acknowledgments

From Christopher Sutton:
I would also like to acknowledge the huge amount of work and effort put in by my personal assistant Lynda Moorby, because most of the editing and correcting came via our office.

I would also like to acknowledge the debt that the Minimal Access Surgery Department of the Royal Surrey County Hospital owes to Gilly Ross and her team of fund raisers who have worked tirelessly for the charity, The Guildford Laser Appeal, and subsequently BLASER (British Laser Appeal for Surgical Equipment and Research) which has over the years provided us with all the equipment and lasers for advanced operative laparoscopy and without their help we would never have achieved the results that have gone into this book.

From David Adamson:
I would like to thank Christopher Sutton, Kevin Jones, and Nick Dunton for asking me to participate in this project, and acknowledge the commitment to excellence of all the authors and professionals who made publication of this textbook possible.

SECTION I
General Background

1 The history of endometriosis

Christopher Sutton

Although shrouded in the mists of antiquity, descriptions of most gynecologic diseases can be recognized in the writings of Hippocrates (Figure 1.1), Soranus of Ephesus, or followers of the Roman god of healing Asclepios (Latin Aesculapius) (Figure 1.2), or the Hebrew Talmud, but this is not the case with endometriosis. There is no reference to it in any medical historical encyclopedias, such as the *Cambridge World History of Human Disease*, edited for the Cambridge University Press in 1993 by Kenneth Kiple.[1] Even the *Encyclopaedia of Medical History* by Roderick McGrew[2] published in 1985 and the extensive study by the television historian Roy Porter, entitled *The Greatest Benefit to Mankind*,[3] published in 1997, does not mention endometriosis at all.

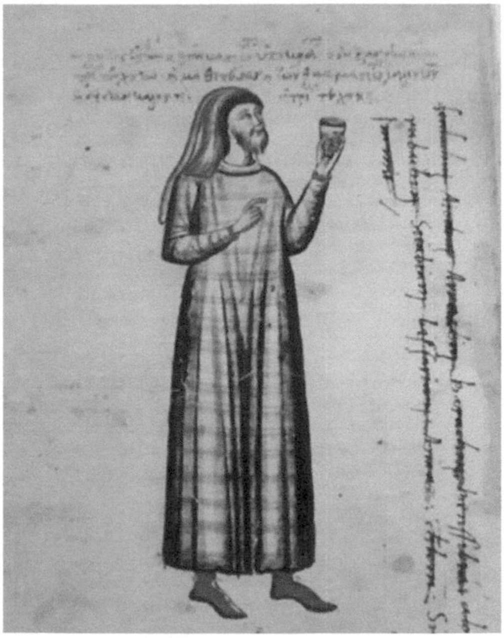

The earliest reference I can find is that by the German physician Daniel Shroen, published in 1690, some 24 years after the Great Fire of London, in his book *Disputatio Inauguralis Medica de Ulceritus Ulceri*.[4] In that volume he minutely describes ulcers that in their primary form were distributed throughout the 'stomach' (the peritoneum) and were located just as prominently in the bladder, the intestines, the broad ligament, and the outside of the uterus and cervix. He was sufficiently perspicacious to state categorically, 'this is

Figure 1.1 Hippocrates (c. 460–377 BC) as depicted in a 14th-century miniature. He is shown inspecting urine, a procedure which epitomizes the doctor's examination of his patient at this period. (National Library, Paris, France)

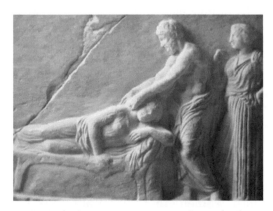

Figure 1.2 Asclepios treats a young patient who has an injured shoulder. The subject is a classical one and is typical of numerous votive stelae from the Greek world. (Museum of Piraeus, Athens, Greece.)

a female disorder, characteristic of those who are sexually maturing'. Although it was referred to by several authors in the 17th and 18th centuries,[5] a graphic description of the disease appeared in the book by the Scottish obstetricians Balfour and Smellie published in Edinburgh in 1776, entitled *Dissertatio Medica Inauguralis de Utero Inflammatione Ejusdem*, in which the authors describe the disease as 'an affliction that permeated the whole female system ... producing morbid symptoms that manifestly changed the disposition of the entire body'.[6] Those of us that have spent most of our working lives looking after women with this unpleasant disease will surely recognize this description.

It is nevertheless interesting that in spite of these very dramatic accounts of the symptomatology by physicians in the 17th and 18th century, who clearly were unaware of the pathogenesis, there are no accounts of the disease in ancient times. I have a theory about this, but I have to admit that it is purely conjectural. Professor Jacques Donnez and Professor Michelle Nisolle, when they were working together at the Catholic University Hospital of Louvain in Brussels, came up with the idea that endometriosis is in fact three completely separate conditions: namely, superficial peritoneal endometriosis, ovarian endometriomas, and deep infiltrating disease of the rectovaginal septum and the uterosacral complex which is in reality adenomyosis.[7] If one accepts the premise that retrograde menstruation is the main cause of superficial peritoneal endometriosis, then one would expect to find the disease more often in women with an increased exposure to menstruation. Such increases are inherent in the modern tendency for women to delay childbearing until their late 30s or early 40s. In ancient Roman times, however, a young girl would typically marry at the age of 14 years old, sometimes earlier, and normally would be expected to become pregnant within a few months of marriage. In the absence of any reliable contraception, she would continue to have pregnancies, only delayed by breastfeeding, which usually would create a postpartum amenorrheic state. Since the average age of death in those times was 35 years old, the number of exposures of a woman of those times to retrograde flow of endometrial tissue was minimal compared to her modern-day counterpart. It is probably for this reason that endometriosis was regarded as an affliction of modern times and, until recently, was considered to be a disease of more affluent Western women. In recent years, however, this trend has become less evident and, with the worldwide increase in the use of laparoscopy to diagnose the condition, it is becoming all too obvious that endometriosis is not merely a disease of

'well-to-do ladies of European extraction' but it poses a significant health problem in other countries with increasing medical and technological development such as Singapore, Malaysia, India, China and particularly Japan, which may have the highest incidence in the world.[8]

A review of the relevant literature suggests that Belgium has the highest incidence of the disease in Europe. According to a report from the World Health Organisation,[9] the highest concentrations of dioxin in breast milk in the world are in Belgium and, interestingly, the highest concentration of cases is reputedly in the main industrial corridor running along the south of the country.[10] Philippe Koninckx and his colleagues have suggested that dioxin and polychlorinated biphenyl pollution is a possible cofactor in the initiation and/or development of deep infiltrating endometriosis[11] and this has resulted in a steadily increasing proportion of hysterectomies performed in Belgium for this type of disease (from 10% in 1965 to over 18% in 1984[12,13]) and this has continued to rise since then.

Dioxin has immunosuppressive activities and is a potent inhibitor of T-lymphocyte function.[14,15] A group of rhesus monkeys which were chronically exposed to dioxin for a period of 4 years and followed by serial laparoscopies were found to have developed endometriosis 7 years after the termination of dioxin exposure and in the majority of these cases it was of the deeply infiltrating adenomyotic variety.[16] Dioxin is a potentially harmful byproduct of the chlorine bleaching process used in the wood pulp industry, which includes the manufacture of feminine hygiene products such as tampons. It is therefore of some concern that young girls are increasingly being encouraged to use tampons and therefore may possibly be exposing the tissues of the rectovaginal septum and posterior vaginal fornix to the chronic exposure from a known immunosuppressant from a very early age. It has been suggested that a woman may use as many as 11 000 tampons in her lifetime, and this represents a worrying level of dioxin exposure to the delicate vaginal tissue in the posterior fornix, which could result in deep infiltrating endometriosis and could explain the increasing incidence of this condition in young women. It would also explain the rising incidence of this particular type of disease and the fact that it was virtually unknown in ancient times and can genuinely be considered a new disease that has resulted from industrial or commercial pollutants. The fact that dioxins are released into the atmosphere as part of the incineration of domestic waste is an added cause for concern.

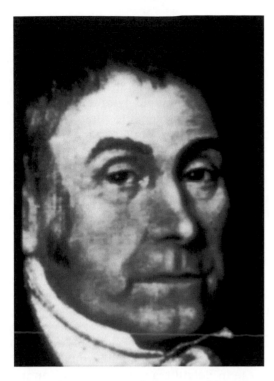

Figure 1.3 Ephraim McDowell was a Scottish surgeon, trained in Edinburgh, who performed the first abdominal operation for a massive ovarian cyst on Christmas Day 1809 in Danville, Kentucky, USA.

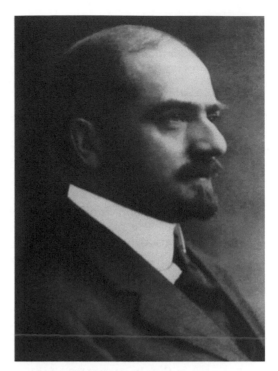

Figure 1.4 Thomas Stephen Cullen.

The third type of endometriosis, ovarian endometriomas (chocolate cysts), would only have been discovered at laparotomy. Since the first laparotomy was performed by Ephraim McDowell (Figure 1.3) on Christmas Day 1809 in Danville, Kentucky,[17] it can be seen that surgery is a relatively modern intervention in historical terms and explains why this disease is absent from ancient historical texts.

Theories of origin

Von Recklinghausen first named the condition as endometriosis in 1885[18] and he suggested that it developed from tissue of Wolffian origin. The first detailed pathologic description of the disease was by Carl von Rokitansky,[19] a Czech research pathologist working in Vienna, who also, with others, described the condition of vaginal atresia known as the Rokitansky–Küstner–Hauser syndrome. In the following year, he described the condition of ovarian endometriosis, which was described by him as cystosarcoma adenidese ovarii uterinum.[20] In 1896 Thomas Cullen described adenomyoma of the round ligaments, which he asserted was tissue of Müllerian origin.[21] Two years later, Iwanhoff[22] advocated the theory of serosal metaplasia and the following year Russell, also writing in the *Johns*

Hopkins Hospital Bulletin described aberrant portions of the Müllerian duct found in an ovary.[23] Further ideas on the pathogenesis were put forward during the late 19th century and developed in the early part of the last century.

In 1919 Thomas Cullen (Figure 1.4) described the adenoma of the rectovaginal septum in an address to the Western Surgical Association in Kansas City, which was published in the *Archives of Surgery* the following year.[24] He described tumours of non-striped muscle, with islands of uterine mucosa scattered throughout them, that arise from behind the cervix and that spread laterally to blend with the anterior wall of the rectum and the uterosacral ligaments. He also mentioned that these may also invade the broad ligaments, encircle the ureter, and break through into the vagina. At the end of his address he said to the rather astounded audience:

> Many of you have undoubtedly seen them, but may not have recognised them. They are of unusual importance and, if overlooked, will in time cause the patient to become a chronic invalid, and in some instances will undoubtedly lead to her death.

One cannot but feel that he then got rather carried away by saying:

In less than 10 years I feel sure the surgeon will recognise and operate on these 'adenomyomas of the rectovaginal septum' long before the wall of the rectum or the broad ligament have been involved.

Some 86 years later very few gynecologists, certainly in this country, seem able to recognize this disease and appreciate the clinical importance of the findings, let alone operate decisively to cure the patient.

In 1921 Dr John Albertson Sampson (Figure 1.5), who practiced in Albany, New York State, began a series of reports starting with a description of ovarian endometriomas, which he described as 'perforating haemorrhagic (chocolate) cysts of the ovary.'[25] Once his interest had been fired he began to publish a series of reports on endometriosis, including the possibility of malignant development[26,27] and during the following years, his theory of retrograde menstruation as the main etiologic factor in the development of this disease was published in a series of articles.[28,29] His explanation seemed eminently logical because he surmised that the actual implantation of fragments of the shed endometrium that had been regurgitated from the fimbrial ends of the tubes explained the origin of the disease. This seemed justified by the observation of menstrual blood in the cul-de-sac at the time of laparotomy, and also that the sites of implantation most frequently seen are in the pouch of Douglas and the ovary closely adjacent to the tubal fimbriae and that these viable fragments would be expected to gravitate to these sites and implant and grow to produce the characteristic lesions.

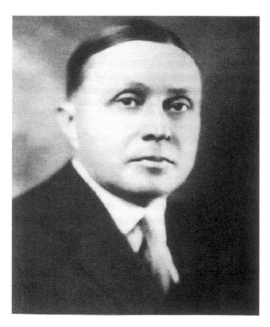

Figure 1.5 John Albertson Sampson.

After its publication, the Sampson theory gave rise to much debate and still does to this day.[30] The main objection to Sampson's theory of retrograde menstruation was the frequent observations of endometriosis occurring at distant sites, such as the umbilicus, inguinal lymph nodes, the dome of the diaphragm, and the pleura, and this was explained by the theory of celomic metaplasia described by Iwanhoff[22] and Meyer.[31] Other theories were put forward to explain the spread of endometriosis to distant sites and the theory of endolymphatic spread was first proposed by Halban.[32] Sampson also demonstrated metastatic or embolic endometriosis in the venous circulation, suggesting that hematogenous dissemination of the disease was a possibility.[33] The first report of urinary tract involvement was by Judd in 1921.[34] There is almost certainly an element of truth in all of these theories and the etiology and pathogenesis of endometriosis are eloquently described in the relevant chapters in this book by Michelle Nisolle and her team from the University of Liege in Belgium and by Stephen Kennedy and Lisa Story from the University of Oxford in England.

The era of laparoscopy and laparoscopic surgery

The main reason that endometriosis can claim to be a modern disease is that it has only been fully appreciated since the invention of laparoscopy. Since ancient times, it would appear that *Homo sapiens* has always had an irrepressible desire to peer inside the body cavities, and the rectal speculum (used by the Kos School led by Hippocrates (460–375 BC)) is remarkably similar to the instrument that we would recognize today.[35] A modern gynecologist would equally have no difficulty in recognizing and using the bivalve speculum that was buried in AD 70 during the colossal eruption of Vesuvius that buried the city of Pompeii and can be seen in the Institute Rizzoli in Bologna (Figure 1.6).

The claim to be the father of modern endoscopy should go to Bozzini,[36] an Italian who described a technique of examining the interior of the urethra in 1805 employing reflected light from a candle with a mirror directing the rays along a metal tube. In spite of his pioneering work, the poor man was censured by the Medical Faculty of Vienna for 'undue curiosity'. It was not for another 50 years that Desormeaux[37] described a workable cystoscope (Figure 1.7) that incorporated a lamp burning alcohol and turpentine with a chimney to enhance the flame; for this, he was awarded a share of the Argenteuil prize, awarded by the Academie Imperiale de Medicine de Paris in 1865.

Probably the first endoscopic examination of the abdominal cavity was performed in 1901 by von Ott[38] from St Petersburg, who examined the abdominal cavity of a pregnant woman through a culdoscopic incision using a head mirror to reflect the light. The credit for the first true laparoscopy on a human must go to Jacobaeus of Stockholm,[39] who in 1910 described inspection of the peritoneal, thoracic, and pericardial cavities. Just 1 month later, Kelling reported on 45 laparoscopies that he had performed; he described the appearance of the normal liver and also the livers of those with tumors and tuberculosis. Many years before this, in 1902, Kelling,[40] who was the Professor of Medicine in Dresden, described to the German Biological and Medical Society in Hamburg the examination of the human esophagus and stomach with a cystoscope, which he also used to examine the abdominal cavity of a dog. He used air filtered through cotton wool to produce the pneumoperitoneum. Sadly he and his wife died in the dreadful air raid of Dresden in 1945 and his house together with all his records were completely destroyed. According to Gordon and Taylor,[35] Kelling, von Ott, and Jacobaeus should be looked upon as the fathers of laparoscopy.

The development of operative laparoscopy

Although we tend to think of Raoul Palmer (Figure 1.8) and Kurt Semm (Figure 1.9) as the fathers of operative laparoscopy, the first person to perform an operative procedure was Kalk,[41] who began to perform liver biopsies through a second puncture under laparoscopic control in 1929. In 1933, Fervers[42] designed instruments with which intra-abdominal adhesions could be divided by electrosurgery. I was alarmed to discover that he actually used pure oxygen as the insufflating gas and apparently experienced 'great concern' at the audible explosions and flashes of light produced by the combination of oxygen and high-frequency electric current within the abdominal cavity when he described the first case of laparoscopic adhesiolysis. A year later, John C Ruddock[43] designed a single-puncture operating laparoscope that allowed both biopsy and coagulation to achieve hemostasis. It became increasingly obvious that female sterilization could be achieved by fulgurating the tube with electrocautery and, although this was suggested by Bosch[44] in Switzerland in 1936 and by Anderson[45] the following year in the United States, the first surgeons

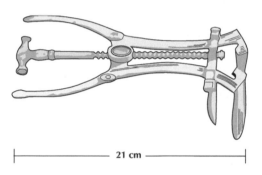

Figure 1.6 Three-bladed vaginal speculum discovered in Pompeii in AD 70.

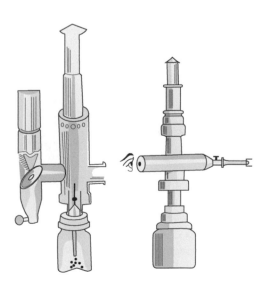

Figure 1.7 The endoscope designed by Desormeaux incorporated a lamp fueled by alcohol and turpentine and a separate viewing channel.

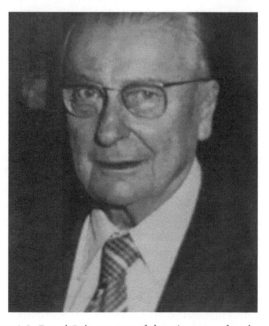

Figure 1.8 Raoul Palmer, one of the pioneers of early operative laparoscopy in Paris, France.

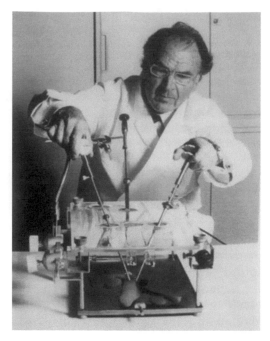

Figure 1.9 Kurt Semm, Professor of Obstetrics and Gynecology in Kiel University, Germany. He was a trained bioengineer and one of the great pioneers and inventors of equipment and operations in operative laparoscopy.

to have reported actual sterilization were Power and Barnes[46] in the United States in 1941. The first report of the use of laparoscopy to diagnose an ectopic pregnancy was by Hope in 1937, who also came from the United States.

It is interesting that in spite of all this activity from the United States, laparoscopy was virtually abandoned in North America and replaced by culdoscopy in many centers;[47] nevertheless, laparoscopy continued to develop in Europe under the influence of Raoul Palmer from Paris[48] and later Hans Frangenheim from Konstanz in Germany. Presumably, the Second World War presented difficulties in communication and exchange of ideas between the two continents and it was not until Patrick Steptoe (Figure 1.10) visited Raoul Palmer in Paris and subsequently described the technique of laparoscopy that the first book in the English language was published in 1967. In that volume, Steptoe described several laparoscopic operations, including aspiration of ovarian cysts and simple ovarian cystectomy, as well as laparoscopic ventrosuspension, which is rarely practiced nowadays. As is well known, Steptoe continued his interest in laparoscopy and many surgeons from the United Kingdom visited him to learn this new technique, even though it meant journeying to Oldham, an industrial town in Lancashire, in the North of England. In spite of the drabness of the surroundings, work of univer-

sal importance was taking place with the collaboration of the physiologist and embryologist Robert Edwards from the Cambridge University's. Department of Physiology, which eventually resulted in the first baby produced by in vitro fertilization in the world: Louise Brown was born in Oldham at nearly midnight on the 25th July 1978.

Initial problems with power sources

It was obvious by the 1970s that the dawn of laparoscopic surgery had arrived, but clearly there were difficulties in the initial instrumentation and particularly in the energy needed to provide hemostasis or to occlude the fallopian tubes. Although the experience of Fervers described above did not result in any injury, others were not so fortunate. One of the first large audits of laparoscopic sterilization using electrosurgery in the UK[49] conducted a nationwide survey of the mortality and morbidity associated with laparoscopic sterilization in the 1970s and were horrified to find that there were a large number of accidents from the stray radiofrequency energy of monopolar electrosurgery. In 1972, Frangenheim[50] in Europe and in 1974 Rioux and Cloutier[51] in North America introduced electrocoagulation both for sterilization and for controlling bleeding. In those

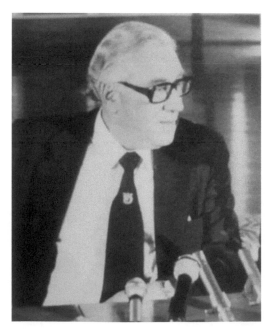

Figure 1.10 Patrick Christopher Steptoe (1913–1988) learnt operative laparoscopy with Raoul Palmer and wrote the first textbook on laparoscopy in the English language. Subsequently, in collaboration with Robert Edwards, a physiologist and embryologist from Cambridge University, resulted in the first successful pregnancy with in-vitro fertilization.

days electrosurgery did not have the same safeguards to prevent burns from insulation failure or capacitative coupling incorporated in modern electrosurgical generators and there was sufficient concern over the incidence of electrosurgical injuries that it was banned in Germany. Professor Kurt Semm from Kiel introduced endocoagulation, whereby the tissue was heated slowly to 120°C to denature protein and cause hemostasis and occlusion of the tubes without any electric current passing through the body. Semm can be considered one of the great pioneers of operative laparoscopy, because he was not only a very gifted surgeon but also a trained medical engineer. He introduced safer systems for insufflating CO_2 to achieve a pneumoperitoneum at a set pressure and also devised various instruments; he was the first to perform many advanced laparoscopic procedures such as appendicectomy and his own version of the subtotal intrafascial hysterectomy.[52]

The evolution of the laparoscopic appearances of endometriosis

When he was describing the appearances of endometriosis at laparotomy, Sampson used terms such as red raspberries, purple raspberries, blueberries, blebs, and peritoneal pockets in his original series of articles.[25,26,29] Subsequent articles tended to emphasize the blue or black classical 'powder-burn' appearance of endometriosis and, certainly, when I started doing laparoscopies in the 1970s this was considered the hallmark of the diagnosis of endometriosis to the extent that this was called a typical lesion. This attitude changed completely with the publication of the seminal paper by Jansen and Russell, entitled 'Non-pigmented endometriosis: clinical, laparoscopic and pathological definition', which described a whole range of different appearances such as white opacified peritoneum resembling vesicles or 'sago-grains', red flame-like telangiectatic lesions, and glandular lesions resembling endometrium at hysteroscopy.[53] Jansen and Russell showed that many of these macroscopic appearances are associated with active endometriosis by demonstrating endometrial glands and stroma on histologic inspection of peritoneal biopsies in 67–81% of cases. Other lesions such as subovarian adhesions, yellow-brown peritoneal patches, and circular peritoneal defects had endometriosis in 50% of the biopsies. In fact, although Sampson had mentioned peritoneal pouches in his original description, they later became associated with two gynecologists from the Southern United States, Allen and Masters.[54] These Southern gentlemen suggested that these lesions, which were particularly common in the black population, were due to

childbirth trauma or possibly damage from vigorous sexual intercourse, but it was later found out that biopsy of the base of these peritoneal defects virtually always revealed endometriosis and a causal relationship was postulated.[55] It is my belief that they represent the early stage of cul-de-sac obliteration, which later develops into deep infiltrating endometriosis. Redwine[56] suggested that there appeared to be a relationship between the color and the age of the endometrial implants and, indeed, even with the age of the patient; the non-hemorrhagic lesions are more usually found in young women and the black deposits laden with hemosiderin are more common in older patients.

Martin et al pioneered excisional techniques using CO_2 laser laparoscopically for the treatment of abnormal-appearing peritoneum,[57] provided the basis for extensive histologic studies of abnormal peritoneum, and, in a subsequent study, used up to 20 descriptive terms to characterize the appearance of endometriosis.

In a 3-year prospective study of 643 consecutive laparoscopies in the early 1990s, Koninckx et al demonstrated a highly significant correlation between pain and the depth of the endometriotic implant and showed that deeply infiltrating endometriosis was found primarily in the retroperitoneal areas in the rectovaginal septum, the uterosacral ligaments, and, occasionally, in the pelvic sidewall around the ureter and the uterovesical fold.[58] These sclerotic lesions with considerable fibromuscular hyperplasia can often be palpated rather than seen and are best diagnosed by a clinical examination, preferably performed during menstruation.

As the 1990s slowly turned into the new millennium, it became increasingly obvious that most tertiary referral centers dealing with a large volume of patients with endometriosis were increasingly seeing patients with deep infiltrating disease. Many of these patients had such obvious large painful nodules in the vaginal fornices that it is difficult for me to believe that this disease existed to the same extent 20 years ago. I am strongly of the opinion that it is a new disease that is increasingly presenting and not due to the fact that we did not recognize it in the past.

Classification

As with other complex disease entities, a grading system was found necessary but, unfortunately with endometriosis, this is particularly difficult because there is no direct correlation between the volume of endometriotic tissue and the severity of symptoms with regard either to pain or to infertility. The different appearances of endometriosis at laparoscopic inspection referred to in the above section and the different histologic characteristics of the lesions make classification and staging of endometriosis particularly difficult. Nevertheless, there have been numerous attempts at classification, frequently devised by pathologists and physiologists. Indeed, the first descriptive classification was that of Sampson, when he described hemorrhagic cysts in the ovaries of 14 young women and subsequently staged endometrial hematomas by their histologic appearance.[59] The various classifications of endometriosis have been the subject of a comprehensive review by Groff.[60] He lists 14 different classifications of endometriosis, the most useful of which were those produced by Acosta et al,[61] Kistner et al,[62] Buttram,[63] and, finally, the American Fertility Society (AFS)[64] classification of 1975, which was revised in 1985 and is the most frequently used classification in modern times. All of these classification systems have their failings, because they attempt to correlate increasing disease severity with subsequent fertility outcome: the disease score from stage I to stage IV increases with the involvement of the ovaries and with the amount of adhesions present. Although this does serve as a basis for comparison of different treatment regimens, and although the revised AFS classification is the best we have to date, it does not take into account the fact that most patients present with pain symptoms. It is well known that some patients can have severe pain from even minimal endometriosis, due to the activity of even small implants that produce a large amount of prostanoids and other pain-mediating substances. By contrast, other patients have stage IV disease with ovarian endometriomas and a fixed pelvis due to dense adhesions, where the pathology of endometriosis is only discovered as a result of investigation of a pelvic mass when the patient has complained of no pain symptoms at all. Additionally, the revised AFS scoring system does not take into account deep retroperitoneal endometriosis, where the pain is directly related to the depth of the lesions.[65] In some of these situations the woman can be complaining of severe dyspareunia, dysmenorrhea, and dyschezia, and yet laparoscopic inspection might only reveal a small dimple of retraction between the rectum and the vagina with nodular disease palpable but out of sight of laparoscopic inspection, in which case the AFS score would be zero.

In order to overcome these problems, Professor Ray Garry of the University of Western Australia in Perth has suggested a much more logical and commonsense approach, which he outlines fully in Chapter 5 on outcome measures. He points out that in the clinical setting there are two distinct phenotypes, which can be defined by the presence or absence of palpable nodules in the deep pelvis. Patients with such nodules, with or without ovarian endometriomas, usually have severe symptoms and a definite risk of bowel and urinary tract involvement and even a small risk of malignant progression. The predominant histologic feature of this group of patients is extensive fibromuscular hyperplasia similar to adenomyomas of the uterine musculature. These patients will usually need extensive surgical intervention in a tertiary referral center that is staffed with an adequate number of highly skilled surgeons, not only laparoscopic gynecologic surgeons but also those colorectal and urologic surgeons who have also developed laparoscopic skills for this very difficult type of surgery. Professor Garry has suggested that this group of patients should be classified under the heading of Cullen's syndrome, the eponym being derived from Thomas Cullen's original descriptions of adenomyomas behind the cervix and in the rectovaginal septum. The other group of patients who have the typical red and black lesions with the characteristic histologic feature of endometrial-like glands and stroma with no palpable nodules in the deep pelvis could be classified as Sampson's syndrome, since he initially described retrograde menstruation as the likely etiology for these superficial implants on the peritoneal surface. Furthermore, this group of patients can usually be treated by a combination of medical and surgical treatment, which would not be beyond the skill of a laparoscopic gynecologic surgeon in any district hospital.[66]

The development of medical treatment

The first attempt at hormonal therapy to treat endometriosis was the introduction of a high-dose estrogen (stilbestrol regimen) by Karnaky in 1948,[67] but many patients found this treatment unacceptable due to side effects. Before the widespread adoption of laparoscopy to diagnose endometriosis, there were reports of using methyl-testosterone as a therapeutic trial because it was often very effective at alleviating the pain associated with endometriosis but did not appear to enhance fertility.[68]

'Pseudo-pregnancy' therapy was introduced by Robert Kistner in 1958[69] based on Sampson's observation that pregnancy had a beneficial effect on patients with endometriosis. With this regimen, there was an initial decidualization of the deposits followed after several months by atrophy of the endometriotic implants.[70] This pseudo-pregnancy treatment remained popular throughout the 1970s and was effective with both oral and injectable progesterones. Later, a similar effect was obtained with the combined oral contraceptive pill taken continuously. The first drug to be approved for the treatment of endometriosis was danazol, an isoxazole derivative of 17-alpha-ethinyl-testosterone originally produced from the Mexican yam. This was introduced by Greenblatt et al in 1971;[71] it was originally thought to produce a pseudo menopause but, subsequently, was found to act primarily by diminishing the mid-cycle luteinizing hormone (LH) surge, producing a chronic anovulatory state. The actual action of this drug was found to be much more complicated. It also caused elevation of estrogen and androgen levels and altered steroidogenesis in the ovary and the adrenal glands and, although causing atrophy of endometriotic implants, was, not surprisingly, accompanied by unpleasant side effects such as acne, seborrhea, hirsutism, and, more rarely, irreversible deepening of the voice and clitoral hypertrophy. In view of its expense, multiple side effects, and adverse effect on the lipid profile, the drug could not be given long term. A seminal study by Evers,[72] which took two groups of women on a 6-month course of danazol, and performed a second-look laparoscopy in the last treatment month in one group and 2 months after cessation of treatment in the other group, found that in the latter group there was significant recurrence of the disease.

The next approach was that of medical oophorectomy using gonadotropin releasing hormone agonists (GnRH-a) first reported by Meldrum et al in 1982.[73] This continuous stimulation caused 'down-regulation' with desensitization of the pituitary gland receptors, resulting in a hypogonadal state that could last some 50 days after the administration of the last injection. The predictable menopausal side effects, such as hot flashes, headache, and vaginal dryness, could be ameliorated by add-back therapy with estrogen, but again this new group of drugs did not hold the initial promise because the disease appeared to be reactivated in a large percentage of patients after therapy was discontinued. Nevertheless these drugs, together with danazol and newer compounds such as immunomodulators, GnRH antagonists, aromatase inhibitors, tumor necrosis factor-alpha (TNF-α) inhibitors, angiogenesis inhibitors, and matrix metalloproteinase (MMP) inhibitors, together with the levonorgestrel-producing intrauterine device, have a role to play, either pre-operatively or postoperatively or when surgery

has failed, and this whole area of modern medical treatment is ably reviewed in Chapter 6 on the medical treatment of endometriosis by David Olive.

The development of power sources for the laparoscopic treatment of endometriosis

When we first started using the CO_2 laser down the laparoscope in 1982, the equipment needed for laparoscopic surgery was still in its infancy; all devices were reusable and most of them were fairly primitive. We had scissors that were not self-sharpening and very quickly became blunt, bipolar diathermy that often failed to function. Monopolar electrosurgery had been banned in Germany and there was still considerable concern about its safety and in order to achieve hemostasis from a bleeding vessel, we had to resort to Kurt Semm's endocoagulator, which slowly heated tissue to 120°C and slowly cooled down, which was extremely time-consuming. When I was appointed as a consultant at Guildford, a university town about 50 km south west of London, in an extremely affluent part of the south east of England, I was impressed by the number of cases of endometriosis that we diagnosed by laparoscopy. Drug treatment at that time was generally unsatisfactory and expensive, with considerable side effects and a high incidence of recurrence after cessation of therapy. We were therefore looking for an energy source that would allow us to safely ablate the endometriotic implants at the same time as we made the diagnosis. Having had considerable experience using the CO_2 laser in the treatment of cervical intraepithelial neoplasia, we decided to adopt that as our power source. Thinking we were the first center in the world to do this, we designed our own instruments, comprising a simple cannula that was attached to the laser arm by a fixed focused lens coming to a sharp focus 20 mm beyond the end of the cannula. We also designed two other probes: one with a mirror to allow the beam to be used at 45° to the axis of the cannula and another one with a backstop to prevent onward transmission of the beam for the treatment of adhesions. Our initial concern was about the safety of this new procedure, but having punctured total colectomy specimens bathed in an atmosphere of CO_2 and finding that there were no methane explosions, we regarded this as the worst-case scenario and also felt that it was highly unlikely that one would perforate the bowel since the laser was only activated when the helium–neon aiming beam was in a safe area.

We rapidly became experienced in laser tissue interaction and performed studies on the healing of laser wounds, as described in Chapter 12. We were extremely impressed with the almost perfect healing, with a complete absence of any contracture or scar formation, which had been our experience using electrosurgery. We therefore thought this was possibly the ideal energy source to use for the ablation of endometriosis and, after we had safely performed 100 cases with 6 months follow-up,[74] we tried to publish our results in the *British Journal of Obstetrics and Gynaecology*. However, the editor at that time, a true academic, pointed out that he wouldn't dream of publishing details of a completely new technique unless we followed the patients for 5 years. This we eventually did.[75] After the first 6 months of using what we thought was a new technique, I saw an article by Dr James Daniel from Nashville, Tennessee, describing his initial experience, and it was obvious that we had independently started at almost the same time. In his article there was a further reference to a French team at Clermont-Ferrand led by Professor Maurice Bruhat who had presented an abstract at the Fourth Congress of the International Society for Laser Surgery held in Tokyo in 1979, and therefore historical credit for the first use of the CO_2 laser went to Maurice Bruhat and his team from France.[76] They had used instrumentation designed by Yoni Tadir for the Sharplan Laser Company, which unfortunately was much more cumbersome and difficult to use than the simple second puncture cannula that we had devised. Gradually the French team changed from employing the CO_2 laser to electrosurgery, which in the intervening years had become considerably safer.

During the 1980s there were many reports of laser surgery from the United States and Europe.[77–81]

One of the disadvantages of the CO_2 laser delivery system is that the beam has to be transmitted by a series of mirrors down hollow tubes from the generator to the patient and it is easy for the mirrors to go out of alignment, especially if the laser is pushed from one part of the hospital to another. This is less of a problem nowadays, with the new carbon fiber arms, which are much more robust, but, nevertheless, the flexible fiber lasers had the advantage of being able to aim the laser beam to get to areas of difficult access. The argon laser was developed by Budd Keye[82] and his colleagues at the University of Utah, and the KTP/532 laser was initially evaluated for the treatment of endometriosis, and particularly endometriomas, by Daniell.[83] Both these lasers operate in the visible light portion of the electromagnetic spectrum; the argon laser produces blue light and the KTP/532 laser, which is produced by passing Nd:YAG laser energy through a potassium titanyl phosphate crystal (which halves the wavelength and doubles the frequency), produces emerald green light. Both these lasers can be used in the presence of blood and other fluids and do not penetrate as deeply as the Nd:YAG laser, which was introduced by Lomano.[84] The Nd:YAG is an invisible light laser, with a long wavelength of 1064 nm, that penetrates deeply into tissues, so that it is difficult to know quite how far the zone of irreversible tissue necrosis is going. Although this made it an excellent laser for initial studies on endometrial ablation, it was not safe to use in the bare fiber mode within the peritoneal cavity. In order to get round this problem, laser manufacturers introduced sculpted quartz or artificial sapphire tips which effectively concentrated the energy of the beam as it leaves the tip. The advent of these probes resulted in the production of laser scalpels that restored a tactile sense to what was previously 'no touch' surgery. Unfortunately, these fibers are now single use and extremely expensive, so add considerably to the cost of laser surgery. Experiments have shown that these devices do not work until they are contaminated with tissue debris, which ignites, causing the temperature of the tip to rise to as high as 600°C. Cutting is achieved by a purely thermal effect that could be achieved much more simply with an electrosurgical needle at a fraction of the cost.[85]

With the increasing safety of electrosurgery in recent years and the development of the ultrasonic scalpel,[85] many laparoscopic surgeons have abandoned these various lasers, although the KTP/532 laser still gives excellent results for the photocoagulation of ovarian endometriomas.[86] Although many of the leading endometriosis surgeons still use the CO_2 laser, because of its precision and the almost bloodless and rapid vaporization which can be accomplished with very few complications, other surgeons have tended to use fine electrosurgical needles or scissors and the harmonic scalpel, which uses ultrasound energy to vibrate the scalpel blade at 55 000 vibrations a second by cutting tissue with minimal smoke production, is increasingly popular. These extremely fast vibrations generate low heat at the incision site, but the combination of this heat and the rapid vibration causes proteins to denature, forming a coagulum that seals small vessels and results in minimal bleeding and tissue blanching without charring. Although there is no smoke production, there is a mist of fine fatty droplets from the incised tissue, which can interfere with visualization and can at times be as big a nuisance as smoke production with lasers and electrosurgery. Although the ultrasonic scalpel is much cheaper in terms of capital expenditure than the CO_2 laser, the latter has no ongoing costs except for annual maintenance, whereas the vibrating element of the ultrasonic scalpel is disposable and quite expensive.[85] Other devices such as the Helica thermal coagulator and the cold plasma coagulator are only really useful for dealing with superficial peritoneal endometriosis because of a limited depth of penetration. They are really no use at all for dealing with deep infiltrating disease, although the manufacturers of Helica have introduced a cutting probe that appears promising. There is much controversy about the best power sources to use for laparoscopic surgery of endometriosis. In the final analysis, it is the surgeon's own skill and experience, together with personal preference of the technique employed and careful patient selection that plays a much more important role than the energy source employed in terms of the clinical outcome of laparoscopic surgery.[87]

Evidence-based surgery

Looking back on the development of laparoscopic surgery in the past 25 years, it is a great shame that all the initial studies were entirely retrospective in nature and therefore not acceptable by the rigorous criteria of evidence-based medicine. Randomized, prospective, double-blind controlled studies have for a long time been part of the rigorous control needed for the introduction of new drugs. Until 1994, there had been no such trials in the laparoscopic surgical treatment of endometriosis, whereas there had been numerous studies comparing different drugs and different drug regimens with placebo in a controlled prospective fashion. It was not therefore surprising that we, as laparoscopic surgeons, were regarded with disdain by academic colleagues, and I think this failing on our part hindered the widespread acceptance of laparoscopic surgery. Our surgical colleagues did not appear to have the same problem because, although there were no really well-conducted randomized controlled trials (RCTs) during the development of laparoscopic cholecystectomy, it became obvious that this was the best surgical treatment for this disease and that it was considered unnecessary. I suppose if one looks at all the various organs of the body that require removal, the gallbladder is the most obvious choice where minimal access surgery with its small scars, short hospital stay, and rapid recovery has almost completely replaced an operation that was extremely painful and required quite a long convalescence.

In order to address this problem, our department at the Royal Surrey County Hospital in Guildford published the first prospective, double-blind RCT of laser laparoscopy in the treatment of pelvic pain associated with minimal, mild, and moderate endometriosis.[88] The conclusion of this study was that laser laparoscopy was a safe, simple, and effective treatment in alleviating pain symptoms in women with stage I, II, and III endometriosis compared with those in the sham arm of the study who had had a diagnostic laparoscopy alone and no treatment apart from aspiration of the serosanguinous fluid in the posterior cul-de-sac. This study and the various problems associated with it are discussed in detail in Chapter 12. One of the major criticisms was that we had included laparoscopic uterine nerve ablation as part of our protocol for treating the endometriotic implants with the CO_2 laser, which raised the question of whether the excellent results in terms of pain relief were due to the ablation of the implants or whether it was the division of the nerves that was responsible. We therefore conducted a similar double-blind, prospective, RCT comparing ablation of endometriotic implants alone with ablation of the endometriotic implants plus uterine nerve ablation. We found that the nerve ablation did not add anything to the pain relief. The results in terms of pain relief were the same in both arms of the trial and also the same as they had been in the initial study.[89] Interestingly, an independent RCT by Paolo Vercellini et al from Milan came to the same conclusion.[90] Their study was not double-blind, but did have more patients than ours and a slightly longer follow-up of 9 months. The outcome of this study was a surprise to me, because I was under the impression that uterine nerve ablation was effective in the treatment of pelvic pain and particularly dysmenorrhea. However when I looked at some of the laparoscopic laser uterine nerve ablation (LUNA) second-look laparoscopies that we had conducted over the years, it occurred to me that there was an enormous volume of the uterosacral ligament complex removed and I have an idea that we were removing a lot of deep infiltrating endometriosis, which is known to be a highly effective treatment for deep dyspareunia and dysmenorrhea.[39]

Currently, surgery seems to be the best option for relieving pain due to endometriosis and also, particularly if adhesions or ovarian endometriomas are present, for improving prospects for fertility. The real problem we have still to grapple with is to try and stop recurrence. Enormous strides have been made in unravelling the pathogenesis of this obscure disease. These are covered in detail in various chapters of this book. It is becoming obvious that there is a very definite role for adjuvant postoperative medical therapy and an exciting future lies ahead with the development of some of these new drugs, particularly non-hormonal compounds such as immunomodulators.

REFERENCES

1. Kiple K, ed. The Cambridge world history of human disease. Cambridge: Cambridge University Press; 1993.
2. McGrew R. Encyclopaedia of medical history. New York: McGraw-Hill; 1985.
3. Porter R. The greatest benefit to mankind: a medical history of humanity. London: Norton; 1997.
4. Shroen D. Disputatio inauguralis medica de ulceritus ulceri. Jena, German Democratic Republic: Krebs; 1690: 6–17.
5. Knapp VJ. How old is endometriosis? Late 17th and 18th century European descriptions of the disease. Fertil Steril 1999; 72:(1): 10–14.
6. Smellie W. In: Balfour and Smellie, eds. Dissertatio medica inauguralis de utero inflammatione ejusdem. Edinburgh: Edinburgh University Press; 1776: 16–22.
7. Nisolle M, Donnez J. Peritoneal endometriosis, ovarian endometriosis and adenomyotic nodules of the rectovaginal septum are three different entities. Fertil Steril 1997; 68(4): 585–596.
8. Miyazawa K. Incidence of endometriosis among Japanese women. Obstet Gynecol 1976; 48: 407–409
9. World Health Organisation (WHO). Level of PCB's, PCDD's and PCDF's in breast milk. Result of WHO coordinated inter laboratory quality control studies and analytical field studies. WHO Environmental Health Series; 1989
10. Donnez J. Personal communication; 2000
11. Koninckx PR, Braet P, Kennedy S, et al. Dioxin pollution and endometriosis in Belgium. Hum Reprod 1994; 9: 1001–1002.
12. National Center for Health Statistics. Hysterectomies in the United States 1965–84. Hyattsville, Maryland. 1986: 145–156.
13. National Center for Health Statistics. Vital and health statistics. Data from the National Health Survey; Series 3, No. 92. DHSS Publ (PHS) 1987; 88–175.
14. Holsapple MP, Snyder NK, Wood SC, et al. A review of two, three, seven, eight – tetrachlorodibenzo-P-dioxin-induced changes in immuno competence. Toxicology 1991; 69: 219–255.
15. Neubert R, Jacob-Muller U, Stahlmann R, et al. Polyhalogenated dibenzo-p-dioxins and dibenzofurans and the immune system. Arch Toxicol 1991; 65(3): 213–219.
16. Rier SE, Martin DC, Bowman RE, et al. Endometriosis in rhesus monkeys (*Macaca mulatta*) following chronic exposure to 2,3,7,8-tretrachlorodibenzo-p-dioxin. Fundam Appl Toxicol 1993; 21: 433–414.
17. Sutton CJG. RCOG Historical Lecture 1993: 150 years of hysterectomy; from Charles Clay to laparoscopic hysterectomy. The Year Book of the Royal College of Obstetricians and Gynaecologists. London: RCOG Press; 1994; 3: 29–40.
18. Von Recklinghausen F. Veber die venose embolic und den regrograden transport in den venen und in den lymphgefasse. Virchows Arch 1885, 100: 503–509.
19. Von Rokitansky C. Weber Uterusdrusen-Neubildung in Uterus und Tubenwandung. Zkk Gesellsch d Aerz te zu Wien 1860; 37: 577–579.
20. Ricci JV. One hundred years of gynaecology 1800–1900. Philadelphia: The Blakiston Company; 1945: 110, 157, 163, 491.
21. Cullen TS. Adenomyoma of the round ligament. Johns Hopkins Hosp Bull 1896; 7: 112–113.
22. Iwanhoff NS. Monatts Geburtsch Gynakol 1898; 7: 195–198.
23. Russell WW. Aberrant portions of the Mullerian duct found in an ovary. Johns Hopkins Hospital Bull 1899; 10: 8–9.
24. Cullen TS. The distribution of adenomyomas containing uterine mucosa. Arch Surg 1920; 1: 215–283.
25. Sampson JA. Perforating haemorrhagic (chocolate) cysts of the ovary. Their importance and especially their relation to pelvic adenomas of endometriotic type ('adenomyoma' of the uterus, rectovaginal septum, sigmoid etc.). Arch Surg 1921; 3: 245–322.
26. Sampson JA. Benign and malignant endometrial implants in the peritoneal cavity and their relation to certain ovarian tumours. Surg Gynecol Obstet 1924; 38: 287–311.
27. Sampson JA. Endometrial carcinoma of the ovary arising in endometrial tissue in that organ. Arch Surgery 1924; 10: 1–72.
28. Sampson JA. Heterotopic or misplaced endometrial tissue. Am J Obstet Gynecol 1925; 10: 649–664.
29. Sampson JA. Peritoneal endometriosis due to the menstrual dissemination of endometrial tissue into the peritoneal cavity. Am J Obstet Gynecol 1927; 14: 422–469.
30. Redwine DB. Was Sampson wrong? In: Redwine DB, ed. Surgical management of endometriosis. London: Martin Dunitz; 2004: 1–11.
31. Meyer R. Ubber eine adenomatose. Wuchurng der serosa in eine bauchnabe. Z Geburts Gynakol 1903; 49: 32–45.
32. Halban J. Histeroadenosis metastatic. Wien Klin Wchnschr 1924; 37: 1205.
33. Sampson JA. Metastatic or embolic endometriosis due to menstrual dissemination of endometrial tissue into the venous circulation. Am J Pathol 1927; 3: 93–151.
34. Judd ES. Adenomyomata presenting as a tumour of the bladder. Surg Clin North Am 1921; 1: 1271–1273.
35. Gordon AG, Taylor PJ. History and development of endoscopic surgery. In: Sutton C, Diamond M, eds. Endoscopic surgery for gynaecologists, 2nd edn. London: WB Saunders; 1998: 1–8.
36. Bozzini P. Der lichtleiter odere beschreibung einer eingachen vorrichtung und ihrer anwendung zur erleuchung innerer hohlen und zwischeraume deslebenden animaleschen corpses. Weimer: Landes-Industrie-Comptoi; 1805.
37. Desormeaux AJ. De l'endoscopie et de ses applications au diagnostic et au traitment des affections de l'uretre et de la vessie. Paris: Baillière; 1865.

38. von Ott D. Ventroscopic illumination of the abdominal cavity in pregnancy. Zhurnal Akrestierstova 1 Zhenskikh Boloznei 1901; 15: 7–8.

39. Jacobaeus HC. Uber due Moglichkeil die Zystoskopie bei Untersuchlung seroser Hohlungen anzerwerden. Munchener Medizinische Wochenschrift 1910; 57: 2090–2092.

40. Kelling G. Uber Oesophagoskopie, Gastroskopie und Koelioskopie. Munchner Medizinische Wochenschrift 1902; 49 (1): 22–24.

41. Kalk H. Erfahrungen mit der Laparoskopie. Zeitschrift fur Kliniche Medezin 1929; 111: 303–348.

42. Fervers C. Die laparoskopie mit dem Cystoskope. Ein Beitrag zur Vereinfachung der Technik und zur endoskopichen Strangdurchtrennung in der Bauchole. Mediziniche Klinik 1933; 29: 1042–1045.

43. Ruddock JC. Peritoneoscopy. Western J Surg 1934; 42: 392–405.

44. Bosch PF. Laparoskopiche sterilization. Schweizerische Zeitschrift fur Krankenhaus und Anstaltswesen 1936.

45. Anderson ET. Peritoneoscopy. Am J Surg 1937; 35: 136–139.

46. Power FH. Barnes AC. Sterilization by means of peritoneoscopic fulguration: a preliminary report. Am J Obst Gynecol 1941; 41: 1038–1043.

47. Decker A. Culdoscopy: its diagnostic value in pelvic disease. JAMA 1949; 140: 378–385.

48. Palmer R. La coelioscopie. Bruxelles Med 1948; 28: 305–312.

49. Chamberlain GVP, Carron-Brown JC. Gynaecological laparoscopy. The report of the Working Party of the Confidential Enquiry into Gynaecological Laparoscopy London: RCOG; 1978.

50. Frangenheim H. Laparoscopy and culdoscopy in gynaecology. London: Butterworth; 1972.

51. Rioux JE. Cloutier D. A new bipolar instrument for laparoscopic tubal sterilization. Am J Obstet Gynecol 1974; 119: 737–739.

52. Semm K. Atlas of laparoscopy and hysteroscopy. Philadelphia: WB Saunders; 1977.

53. Jansen RPS, Russell P. Non-pigmented endometriosis: clinical, laparoscopic and pathological definition. Am J Obstet Gynecol 1986; 155: 115–159.

54. Allen WM, Masters WH. Traumatic laceration of uterine support. Am J Obstet Gynecol 1995; 70: 500–513.

55. Chatman DL. Pelvic peritoneal defects in endometrosis: Alan-Master's Syndrome revisited. Fertil Steril 1981; 36: 751–754.

56. Redwine DB. Age related evolution in colour appearance of endometriosis. Fertil Steril 1987; 48(6): 1062–1063.

57. Martin DC, Hubert GD, Vander Zwaag R, et al. Laparoscopic appearances of peritoneal endometriosis. Fertil Steril 1989; 51: 63–67.

58. Koninckx PR, Meuleman C, Demeyere S, et al. Suggestive evidence that pelvic endometriosis is a progressive disease, whereas deeply infiltrating endometriosis is associated with pelvic pain. Fertil Steril 1991; 55: 759–765.

59. Sampson JA. The life history of ovarian haematomas (haemorrhagic cysts) of endometrial (Mullerian) type. Am J Obstet Gynaecol 1922; 4(4): 451–512.

60. Groff TR. The classification of endometriosis: a comprehensive review In: Thomas E, Rock J, eds. Modern approaches to endometriosis. Dordrecht: Kluwer; 1991: 131–150.

61. Acosta AA. Buttram DC Jr, Besch PK, et al. A proposed classification of endometriosis. Obstet Gynaecol 1973; 42: 19–25.

62. Kistner RW, Siegel AM, Behrman SJ. Suggestive classification for endometriosis and relationship to infertility. Fertil Steril 1977; 78, 1008–1010.

63. Buttram VC Jr. An expanded classification of endometriosis. Fertil Steril 1978; 30: 240–242.

64. Revised American Fertility Society classification of endometriosis. Fertil Steril 1985; 43: 351–352.

65. Cornillie FJ, Oosterlynck D, Lauweryns JM, et al. Deeply infiltrating pelvic endometriosis: histology and clinical significance. Fertil Steril 1990; 53: 978–983.

66. Garry R. Quality of life outcome following laparoscopic surgery for endometriosis related pain. B J Obstet Gynaecol 1999; 107: 44–54.

67. Karnaky KJ. The use of Stilboestrol for endometriosis. South Med J 1948; 41: 1109–1112.

68. Hamblen EC. Androgen treatment of women. South Med J 1957; 50: 743–745.

69. Kistner RW. The use of newer progestins in the treatment of endometriosis. Am J Obstet Gynecol 1958; 75: 264–278.

70. Andrews MC, Andrews WC, Strauss AF. Effects of progestin-induced pseudo pregnancy on endometriosis: clinical and microscopic studies. Am J Obstet Gynecol 1959; 78: 776.

71. Greenblatt RB, Dmowski LP, Mahesh U, et al. Clinical studies with an antigonadotrophin – Danazol. Fertil Steril 1971; 22: 102–103.

72. Evers JH. The second look laparoscopy for evaluation of the result of medical treatment of endometriosis should not be performed during ovarian suppression. Fertil Steril 1987; 47: 502–504.

73. Meldrum DR, Chang RJ, Lou J, et al. "Medical oophorectomy" using a long-acting GnRH agonist – a possible new approach to the treatment of endometriosis. J Clin Endocrinol Metab 1982; 54: 1081–1083.

74. Sutton C. Initial experience with carbon dioxide laser laparoscopy. Lasers MedSci 1986; 1: 25–31.

75. Sutton C, Hill D. Laser laparoscopy in the treatment of endometriosis: a five year study. Br J Obstet Gynaecol 1990; 97: 181–185.

76. Bruhat M, Mages C, Manhes M. Use of carbon dioxide laser via laparoscopy. In: Kaplan I, ed Laser surgery III. Proceedings of the 3rd Congress for the International Society for Laser Surgery. International Society for Laser Surgery, Tel Aviv, 1979; 275–282.

77. Daniell JF. Operative laparoscopy for endometriosis. Semin Reprod Endocrinol 1985; 3(4): 353–359.

78. Feste JR. Laser laparoscopy: a new modality. J Reprod Med 1985; 30: 413–418.

79. Davis GD. Management of endometriosis and its

associated adhesions with the CO_2 laser laparoscope. Obstet Gynaecol 1986; 68: 422–425.

80. Nezhat C, Crogey SR, Garrison CP. Surgical treatment of endometriosis via laser laparoscopy. Fertil Steril 1986; 45: 778–783.

81. Donnez J. Carbon dioxide laser laparoscopy in infertile women with adhesions or endometriosis. Fertil Steril 1987; 48: 390–394.

82. Keye WR, Matson GA, Dixon J. The use of the argon laser in the treatment of experimental endometriosis. Fertil Steril 1983; 39: 26–31.

83. Daniell JF. Laparoscopic evaluation of the KTP/532 laser for treating endometriosis – initial report. Fertil Steril 1986; 46: 373–377.

84. Lomano JM. Laparoscopic ablation of endometriosis with the YAG laser. Lasers SurgMed 1983; 3: 179–183.

85. Sutton C. Power sources in endoscopic surgery. Curr Opin Obstet Gynaecol 1995; 7: 248–256.

86. Sutton CJG. Endometriosis: the ovarian endometrioma. In: Phipps J, ed. Adnexal masses. Infertility and Reproductive Medicine Clinics of North America 1995; 6(3): 591–613.

87. Tulandi T, Bugnah M. Operative laparoscopy: surgical modalities. Fertil Steril 1995; 63: 237–245.

88. Sutton CJG, Ewen SP, Whitelaw N, et al. Prospective, randomised, double-blind controlled trial of laser laparoscopy in the treatment of pelvic pain associated with minimal, mild and moderate endometriosis. Fertil Steril 1994; 62: 696–700.

89. Sutton CJG, Dover RW, Pooley A, et al. Prospective, randomised, double-blind controlled trial of laparoscopic laser uterine nerve ablation in the treatment of pelvic pain associated with endometriosis. Gynecol Endosc 2001; 10: 217–222.

90. Vercellini P, Aimi G, Busacca M, et al. Laparoscopic uterosacral ligament resection for dysmenorrhoea associated with endometriosis: results of a randomised controlled trial. Fertil Steril 1997; 68: 3–5.

2 Etiology of endometriosis

Lisa Story and Stephen Kennedy

Introduction

Endometriosis is an important gynecologic disease that is characterized by the presence of endometrial-like tissue in sites outside the uterine cavity. The prevalence is unknown because of the need for a surgical procedure to determine who is affected, but it has been estimated that up to 10% of all premenopausal women are affected.[1]

The etiology and pathogenesis have not been fully elucidated. Many theories have been proposed, but no single theory sufficiently accounts for all aspects of this enigmatic disease, which makes it likely that several mechanisms are involved.[2] An alternative explanation is that endometriosis is a heterogeneous rather than a single disease: in other words, peritoneal, deeply infiltrating, ovarian, and extrapelvic endometriosis are manifestations of different disease processes, each with their own etiology.[3]

This chapter is not intended to be a systematic review of the extensive literature on the subject, particularly as some excellent reviews have appeared in 2003–4 dealing with specific fields such as animal models,[4] cell adhesion,[5] genetics,[6] genomics,[7] immunology,[8] matrix metalloproteinases,[9] and neoplastic processes.[10] We have simply outlined the principal theories that fit these approaches to understanding the etiology of the separate disease types and referred to some of the key supporting papers.

Peritoneal endometriosis

'Peritoneal' endometriosis comprises superficial lesions scattered over the peritoneal, serosal, and ovarian surfaces. They were typically described as superficial 'powder-burn' or 'gunshot' lesions until atypical or 'subtle' lesions were recognized in the 1980s,[11] including red implants (petechial, vesicular, polypoid, hemorrhagic, red flame-like) and serous or clear vesicles which may represent earlier, functionally more active forms of the disease or, alternatively, transient physiologic variants without any pathologic significance.[12]

Such lesions may be explained in part by Sampson's theory of retrograde menstruation, first proposed in 1927, in which he suggested that menstrual effluent is transported into the peritoneal cavity in a retrograde direction along the fallopian tubes.[13] Thereafter, the refluxed endometrial tissue implants onto the surface of exposed tissues, principally the peritoneum.

Since first proposed, the theory has been supported by a number of observations. For example, Halme et al demonstrated that blood was present in the peritoneal fluid of 90% of women with patent fallopian tubes undergoing laparoscopy in the premenstrual period but, if the tubes were occluded, only 15% had evidence of blood in the pelvis.[14] The anatomic distribution of disease provides further evidence: Jenkins et al showed that endometriotic lesions occur predominantly in dependent areas of the pelvis, where pooling of menstrual effluent is expected to occur.[15] There are also animal studies which support the theory. Te Linde and Scott inverted the cervices of 10 rhesus monkeys, resulting in menstruation into the peritoneal cavity: 50% of the animals developed evidence of endometriosis as well as extensive adhesions.[16]

There is therefore clear evidence supporting retrograde menstruation and subsequent implantation as likely mechanisms to explain how peritoneal endometriosis develops. However, most women do not develop endometriosis even though retrograde menstruation is a common occurrence. Several explanations have been put forward to account for this paradox.

First, the amount of menstrual effluent present in the peritoneal cavity may be an important factor influencing the likelihood of endometriosis developing. Not surprisingly, studies have demonstrated a higher incidence of endometriosis in women with increased menstrual exposure due to:

- obstructed outflow associated with Müllerian anomalies, such as congenital absence of the cervix[17]
- short menstrual cycles, increased duration of bleeding and decreased parity.[1]

Secondly, factors affecting the adherence, implantation, and proliferation of endometriotic tissue within the peritoneal cavity may vary between women, as may clearance of endometrial cells from the pelvis.

Cell adhesion

Cell adhesion molecules have been suggested as mediators in the initial attachment of endometrial tissue to the peritoneal surface, via both intracellular and cell matrix adhesion processes, although the precise nature of these processes remains to be determined. At present, the evidence indicates that many of the mechanisms involved in attachment and early invasion are functioning aberrantly in endometriosis.

For example, integrins – cell surface glycoproteins which attach cells to the extracellular matrix (ECM) – are expressed differently in eutopic endometrium and endometriotic tissue.[18,19] More specifically, α_3 and α_6 integrin subunits have been shown to have aberrant expression in endometriotic tissue.[20] Similarly, expression of epithelial (E) cadherin, a calcium-dependent cell–cell adhesion molecule which acts as a tumor suppressor in

malignant tissues,[21] is decreased in endometriotic tissue compared to eutopic endometrium.[22] In-vitro studies support these findings, as invasive endometrial tissue has decreased levels of E-cadherin.[23] Thus, the increased invasiveness of endometriotic tissue may be mediated by decreased expression of E-cadherin, possibly through the action of a presently unknown heat-stable protein in peritoneal fluid.[24]

Intercellular adhesion molecule 1 (ICAM-1) may also play a role in the pathogenesis of endometriosis. ICAM-1 is a cell surface glycoprotein that promotes adhesion in immunologic and inflammatory reactions. Levels are high in the peritoneal fluid of women with endometriosis and are lowered by medical treatment.[25] ICAM-1 is thought to impair the activity of natural killer (NK) cells[26] which may affect the clearance of menstrual debris (see below). Lastly, an increased frequency of a polymorphism in the *ICAM-1* gene, the G/R241 allele, has been reported in women with severe endometriosis, although the variant's functional significance is still unknown.[27] Thus, it is conceivable that the way in which adhesion molecules are expressed on endometrial and other cells in the peritoneal cavity may influence the ability of the tissue to attach to peritoneal surfaces.

Invasion

Once adhesion has occurred, local degradation of the ECM, by proteolytic digestion, is required for successful implantation. Two groups of proteolytic enzymes are thought to be responsible for breaking down the ECM, which consists of collagens and glycoproteins such as fibronectin and laminin: serine proteases and matrix metalloproteinases (MMPs). Metalloproteinase expression is highly up-regulated in eutopic endometrium during menstruation,[28] which may contribute to the invasive potential of shed cells. MMP1 is also expressed in red endometriotic lesions independent of the stage of the menstrual cycle,[29] which may mean that such enzymes are important in facilitating the invasive properties of endometriotic tissue once established within the peritoneum.

MMPs are controlled by a number of factors, including specific tissue inhibitors of metalloproteinases (TIMPs), inflammatory mediators, and hormones. For example, in a nude mouse model of endometriosis created using human endometrium, treatment with progesterone decreased MMP production, resulting in reduced implantation, whereas estrogen maintained MMP production, leading to increased implantation of the transplanted tissue.[30] The inhibitory action of progesterone can be opposed by interleukin 1α (IL-1α), which has been shown to stimulate MMP3 and MMP7 expression in the secretory phase.[28]

Immunosurveillance

It has been suggested that defects in the normal immunologic mechanisms responsible for the clearance of menstrual effluent from the peritoneal cavity may increase the likelihood of endometrial cells implanting.[31] For example, Oosterlynk et al demonstrated that there is decreased cytotoxicity to endometrial cells in women with endometriosis because of (1) a defect in NK activity and (2) partial resistance of the endometrium to NK cytotoxicity.[32] However, it remains unclear whether such immune system abnormalities are truly a cause or a result of the disease.

The role of immune cells and their secretory products in peritoneal fluid, peripheral blood, and endometriotic tissue has been extensively investigated. Increased concentrations of peritoneal fluid leukocytes are found in endometriosis, particularly in women with stage I–II disease.[33] Levels of macrophages, helper T lymphocytes, and natural killer (NK) cells are elevated compared to those in fertile controls, although similar findings occur in women with unexplained infertility.[33] Macrophages are found at greater levels in the peritoneal fluid of women with endometriosis than any other cell type, probably as a result of increased levels of chemotactic agents such as monocyte chemotactic protein 1 (MCP1) and RANTES (before regulated upon activation, normal T-cell expressed and secreted).[31]

Although cell numbers are increased, this does not appear to facilitate clearing of ectopic tissue from the peritoneal cavity; rather, secretion of substances by macrophages probably contributes to the survival of the ectopic endometrium. These factors include cytokines such as IL-1, IL-6, IL-8, IL-10, tumor necrosis factor alpha (TNF-α), and various other growth and angiogenic factors.[34] The endometriotic implants themselves can be induced to secrete substances, such as IL-6 and vascular endothelial growth factor (VEGF), that promote their own survival by generating and maintaining an extensive blood supply both within and around the ectopic tissue.[35] Other sources of VEGF include peritoneal fluid macrophages and eutopic endometrium.[35]

This relationship between the immune system and endometrial viability may be mediated by proteins such as ICAM-1, acting as a ligand for leukocyte integrins. Ectopic endometrium expresses higher levels of both the cell-bound and soluble form of ICAM-1 (sICAM-1), and sICAM-1 can interfere with ICAM-1-mediated immune function, which may explain how ectopic endometrial cells escape immune surveillance.[36]

An alternative hypothesis involves the Fas-Fas ligand (FasL) expression system. Cells expressing FasL induce apoptosis when bound to Fas-bearing immune cells. FasL expression by endometrial cells in vitro can be induced in macrophage-conditioned media. This up-regulation of expression is thought to be due to the production of macrophage-derived growth factors, in particular platelet-derived growth factor (PDGF) and transforming growth factor (TGF)-β_1.[37] It is possible a similar process occurs in vivo, i.e. the pro-inflammatory peritoneal fluid of women with endometriosis induces Fas-mediated apoptosis of activated immune cells via increased FasL expression on endometrial cells. This could be a mechanism for endometrial cells to escape immune surveillance, and subsequently implant and proliferate within the peritoneal cavity.

Changes in systemic humoral immunity have been implicated, as there are numerous reports of altered B-cell function and antibody production.[38] Women with endometriosis also appear to have a higher incidence of some autoimmune diseases, such as rheumatoid arthritis, systemic lupus erythematosus, and Sjögren's syndrome.[39] However, it is uncertain to what extent these findings indicate that endometriosis itself is an autoimmune disease.

Ovarian endometriomas

The pathogenesis of ovarian endometriomas is controversial and three hypotheses have been proposed to account for such disease. The first hypothesis suggests that superficial lesions on the ovarian cortex become inverted and invaginated; the other hypotheses are that endometriomas are derived from functional ovarian cysts or metaplasia of the coelomic epithelium covering the ovary.

Hughesdon proposed the first hypothesis in 1957.[40] After performing serial sections of ovaries containing endometriomas, he concluded that the cysts were formed by invagination of the cortex after menstrual debris from superficial endometriotic lesions (resulting from regurgitated endometrial tissue) had accumulated on the surface of the ovary. Evidence to support this theory comes from the work of Brosens et al, who used ovarioscopy to inspect and biopsy the inner aspects of ovarian endometriomas.[41] Their studies confirmed that in most cases the endometriomas were formed by invagination of the cortex and that active implants were located at the site of invagination.

The theory is also consistent with the finding of lateral asymmetry of ovarian endometriomas: the cysts occur more frequently on the left than the right[42] which, in turn, is consistent with the anatomy of the region. The colon impinges on the left fallopian tube and ovary and is often fixed to the pelvis by adhesions, which creates a disruption of flow of regurgitated material that makes cells more prone to adherence, implantation, and proliferation within the hemi pelvis. This idea is supported by the finding that non-endometriotic, ovarian cysts occur with the same frequency in the left and right ovaries.[43]

However, the rare finding of an endometrioma in a patient with Rokitansky–Küster–Hauser syndrome,[44] is entirely inconsistent with Hughesdon's theory and that of Sampson, given that a woman without a uterus cannot have retrograde menstruation. Interestingly, it was Sampson who first suggested a role for follicles in the pathogenesis of ovarian endometriomas in 1921[45] (the second theory) and, in a retrospective study, Jain and Dalton claimed to have proven the theory by monitoring ovarian follicles serially using transvaginal ultrasound scanning before they became laparoscopically confirmed endometriomas.[46]

The third theory states that the mesothelium overlying the ovary invaginates to form mesothelial inclusions; a metaplastic process then occurs, resulting in the formation of endometriomas, for which a number of supporting arguments are presented in a recent review.[47] It is certainly feasible that these invaginations could form intraovarian endometriomas through a metaplastic process, not too dissimilar from the one first proposed by Meyer in 1919.[48] Some of the observations that support the theory are that the mesothelium covering the ovary has been shown to invaginate into the cortex;[49] epithelial invaginations are in continuum with the endometriotic tissue,[50] and the walls of endometriomas can invaginate 'secondarily' into the ovarian cortex.[3]

Although generally acknowledged as a benign disease, endometriomas have many features in common with neoplasia such as clonal proliferation.[51–54] The disease has also been associated clinically with subtypes of ovarian malignancy, in particular endometrioid and clear cell carcinoma.[55] Genetic alterations in endometriotic tissue have been described in loss of heterozygosity (LOH) studies,[50–59] and using comparative genomic hybridization (CGH) and fluorescence in situ hybridization (FISH),[60–62] particularly involving chromosomal regions containing known or putative tumor suppressor genes (TSGs) previously implicated in ovarian cancer such as 1q21, 9p21 and 17p13.1. These data led a number of groups to suggest that ovarian and probably deeply infiltrating endometriosis both develop like a tumor and that identifying the genes responsible might be important in understanding the initiation of endometrioid and clear cell ovarian carcinomas. More recently, however, using laser capture microdissection to isolate endometriotic from normal tissue and more reliable methodology, other groups have questioned whether endometriomas are truly monoclonal[51] and whether they demonstrate LOH at TSG loci[63].

Deeply infiltrating disease

Deeply infiltrating disease of the rectovaginal septum was first described by Sampson in 1922.[64] Since then, three hypotheses have been proposed to explain the occurrence of this variety of endometriosis. The first two hypotheses suggest that such lesions originate from secondary infiltration of (1) peritoneal endometriosis or (2) uterine adenomyosis; the third hypothesis postulates that they arise as a result of a metaplastic process.

Cullen first suggested that rectovaginal disease occurs as a result of direct extension of lower uterine adenomyosis into the rectovaginal septum.[65] However, Brosens has argued there is no evidence that adenomyotic lesions will progress to or acquire an invasive phenotype. Although there is in-vitro evidence that endometriotic cells have invasive potential, endometriosis does not invade the ovarian stroma or fat in the retroperitoneal space in vivo.[66] On the other hand, Vercellini et al concluded, on the basis of finding that pouch of Douglas depth and volume are reduced in women with deeply infiltrating endometriosis, that such lesions develop not in the rectovaginal septum but intraperitoneally, and that anterior rectal wall adhesions produce a false bottom, which creates an erroneous impression of extraperitoneal origin.[67]

Donnez et al compared the histologic appearance of endometriotic nodules taken from the rectovaginal septum with black peritoneal lesions.[68] The nodules were composed of smooth muscle, endometrial glands, and scanty stroma, which implied that stroma is not required in such lesions for glandular epithelium to have invasive potential. They concluded that rectovaginal nodules should therefore be considered adenomyomas, i.e. well-circumscribed nodular aggregates of hyperplastic smooth muscle and glandular elements, and that such nodules are a different entity to peritoneal lesions as they probably arise from metaplasia of müllerian rests.

Lastly, Koninckx and Martin have suggested that deep endometriosis should be divided into three types.[69] They hypothesised that:

- type I (conical lesions with the largest area exposed to the peritoneal cavity) results from infiltration of superficial endometriosis
- type II (adhesions covering deep lesions) is caused by retraction
- type III (the largest area being under the peritoneal cavity) is due to local metaplasia.

Genetic factors

There is increasing evidence that genetic factors are implicated in the pathogenesis of endometriosis.[70] The clinical evidence was confined initially to case control studies showing that endometriosis occurs 6–9 times more commonly in the first-degree relatives of affected women compared to controls,[71–73] with some suggestion, using magnetic resonance imaging (MRI) as the diagnostic test, that this effect may be more pronounced in the relatives of women with severe disease.[74]

Subsequently, compelling evidence has emerged from the analysis of over 3000 monozygotic and dizygotic twin pairs on the Australian National Health and Medical Research Council Twin Register, suggesting that 51% of the variance of the latent liability to the disease may be attributable to additive genetic influences.[75]

The heritability of endometriosis is also apparent in non-human primates, which develop the disease spontaneously. Over a 20-year period, at the Wisconsin National Primate Research Center, 142 rhesus macaques with disease have been identified principally from necropsy records, giving a prevalence of 31.4%.[76] All the cases have been used to construct an extended, multigenerational pedigree and 9 nuclear families consisting of 1602 females in total. A high degree of heritability is suggested by a significantly higher mean kinship coefficient among affected compared with unaffected animals, and a higher recurrence risk for full-sibs compared to paternal and maternal half-sibs.

The data imply that endometriosis is inherited as a complex genetic trait like diabetes or asthma, which means that a number of genes interact with each other to confer disease susceptibility but the phenotype only emerges in the presence of environmental risk factors. Dioxin is an industrial pollutant that has particularly been implicated,[77] although in a critical appraisal of all the human and non-human primate evidence, Guo recently concluded that there was insufficient evidence to support the theory.[78]

The attempt to identify disease predisposing genes currently involves two main approaches:

- hypothesis-free linkage analysis
- hypothesis-driven study of 'functional' candidate genes (i.e. those genes that have biologic plausibility or have previously been implicated in disease-associated mechanisms).

The latter approach involves comparing the frequency of single nucleotide polymorphisms (SNPs) or mutations in functional candidates amongst cases and controls in association studies.

The 'functional' candidate genes studied to date fall into four broad mechanistic systems:

- retrograde menstruation
- the differential growth and differentiation of endometriotic cells
- hormonal pathways
- detoxification mechanisms.

It has been argued that findings have been inconsistent because for one reason most studies have used inappropriate controls.[79] However, confusion is also created by underpowered studies and/or investigating genes involved in mechanisms without sufficient evidence to support their biologic plausibility. The subject has been extensively reviewed,[70] and up-to-date information about all relevant studies is maintained on a genetic epidemiology website.[80]

The alternative approach which is being undertaken by a number of research groups around the world is linkage analysis. This entails a genome-wide screen with approximately 400 evenly spaced microsatellite markers followed by further fine mapping and association studies with 'positional' candidates in linked regions. The largest of such endeavors is known as the International

Endogene Study – a collaboration between the University of Oxford and the Australian Cooperative Research Centre for Discovery of Genes for Common Human Diseases (Gene CRC), and their respective commercial partners. Their two projects – the OXEGENE (Oxford Endometriosis Gene) Study and the Genes Behind Endometriosis Study – started independently in 1995 based upon previous research.[75,81,82] Both groups have mainly collected affected sister-pairs using similar recruitment methods.[83] The combined data set consists of over 2500 families.[83,84] Although suggestive linkage has been reported for one chromosomal locus based upon the analysis of marker data (400 markers at ~10 cM) generated for a total of 289 families from the complete data set, containing 374 sister-pairs plus other affected relatives, the results of the full genome-wide scan of all the collected families have not yet been published.

Conclusion

At least three different forms of endometriosis have been characterized and it is likely that each is derived by separate mechanisms. Peritoneal endometriosis can be explained in part by the theory of retrograde menstruation and implantation. However, certain aspects, such as why not all women with retrograde menstruation develop the disease, have yet to be elucidated. Rectovaginal nodules and ovarian endometriomas are both probably derived by a process of metaplasia. However, in deeply infiltrating disease, this may occur in Müllerian remnants within the rectovaginal septum, whereas in the case of endometriomas it may occur within invaginated epithelial inclusion cysts. Having said that, the factors initiating these metaplastic processes remain to be characterized, although it is hoped that the genetic dissection of these various phenotypes will provide an explanation.

REFERENCES

1. Eskenazi B, Warner ML. Epidemiology of endometriosis. Obstet Gynecol Clin North Am 1997; 24(2): 235–258.

2. Giudice LC, Kao LC. Endometriosis. Lancet 2004; 364(9447): 1789–1799.

3. Nisolle M, Donnez J. Peritoneal endometriosis, ovarian endometriosis, and adenomyotic nodules of the rectovaginal septum are three different entities. Fertil Steril 1997; 68(4): 585–596.

4. Story L, Kennedy S. Animal studies in endometriosis: a review. ILAR J 2004; 45(2): 132–138.

5. Witz CA. Cell adhesion molecules and endometriosis. Semin Reprod Med 2003; 21(2): 173–182.

6. Bischoff F, Simpson JL. Genetics of endometriosis: heritability and candidate genes. Best Pract Res Clin Obstet Gynaecol 2004; 18(2): 219–232.

7. Giudice LC. Genomics' role in understanding the pathogenesis of endometriosis. Semin Reprod Med 2003; 21(2): 119–124.

8. Seli E, Arici A. Endometriosis: interaction of immune and endocrine systems. Semin Reprod Med 2003; 21(2): 135–144.

9. Osteen KG, Igarashi TM, Yeaman GR, et al. Steroid and cytokine regulation of matrix metalloproteinases and the pathophysiology of endometriosis. Gynecol Obstet Invest 2004; 57(1): 53–54.

10. Varma R, Rollason T, Gupta JK, et al. Endometriosis and the neoplastic process. Reproduction 2004; 127(3): 293–304.

11. Jansen RP, Russell P. Nonpigmented endometriosis: clinical, laparoscopic, and pathologic definition. Am J Obstet Gynecol 1986; 155(6): 1154–1159.

12. Koninckx PR, Oosterlynck D, D'Hooghe T, et al. Deeply infiltrating endometriosis is a disease whereas mild endometriosis could be considered a non-disease. Ann N Y Acad Sci 1994; 734: 333–341.

13. Sampson JA. Peritoneal endometriosis due to the menstrual dissemination of endometrial tissue into the peritoneal cavity. Am J Obstet Gynecol 1927; 14: 422–469.

14. Halme J, Hammond MG, Hulka JF, et al. Retrograde menstruation in healthy women and in patients with endometriosis. Obstet Gynecol 1984; 64(2): 151–154.

15. Jenkins S, Olive DL, Haney AF. Endometriosis: pathogenetic implications of the anatomic distribution. Obstet Gynecol 1986; 67(3): 335–338.

16. Te Linde RW, Scott RB. Experimental endometriosis. Am J Obstet Gynecol 1950; 60: 1147–1173.

17. Olive DL, Henderson DY. Endometriosis and müllerian anomalies. Obstet Gynecol 1987; 69(3 Pt 1): 412–415.

18. Regidor PA, Vogel C, Regidor M, et al. Expression pattern of integrin adhesion molecules in endometriosis and human endometrium. Hum Reprod Update 1998; 4(5): 710–718.

19. van der Linden PJ, de Goeij AF, Dunselman GA, et al. Expression of integrins and E-cadherin in cells from menstrual effluent, endometrium, peritoneal fluid, peritoneum, and endometriosis. Fertil Steril 1994; 61(1): 85–90.

20. Rai V, Hopkisson J, Kennedy S, et al. Integrins alpha 3 and alpha 6 are differentially expressed in endometrium and endometriosis. J Pathol 1996; 180(2): 181–187.

21 Starzinski-Powitz A, Handrow-Metzmacher H, Kotzian S. The putative role of cell adhesion molecules in endometriosis: can we learn from tumour metastasis? Mol Med Today 1999; 5: 304–309.

22. Scotti S, Regidor PA, Schindler AE, et al. Reduced proliferation and cell adhesion in endometriosis. Mol Hum Reprod 2000; 6(7): 610–617.

23. Gaetje R, Kotzian S, Herrmann G, et al. Nonmalignant epithelial cells, potentially invasive in human endometriosis, lack the tumor suppressor molecule E-cadherin. Am J Pathol 1997; 150(2): 461–467.

24. Starzinski-Powitz A, Gaetje R, Zeitvogel A, et al. Tracing cellular and molecular mechanisms involved in endometriosis. Hum Reprod Update 1998; 4(5): 724–729.

25. Kupker W, Schultze MA, Diedrich K. Paracrine changes in the peritoneal environment of women with endometriosis. Hum Reprod Update 1998; 4(5): 719–723.

26. Fukaya T, Sugawara J, Yoshida H, et al. Intercellular adhesion molecule-1 and hepatocyte growth factor in human endometriosis: original investigation and a review of literature. Gynecol Obstet Invest 1999; 47 (Suppl 1): 11–16.

27. Vigano P, Infantino M, Lattuada D, et al. Intercellular adhesion molecule-1 (ICAM-1) gene polymorphisms in endometriosis. Mol Hum Reprod 2003; 9(1): 47–52.

28. Osteen KG, Keller NR, Feltus FA, et al. Paracrine regulation of matrix metalloproteinase expression in the normal human endometrium. Gynecol Obstet Invest 1999; 48 (Suppl 1): 2–13.

29. Kokorine I, Nisolle M, Donnez J, et al. Expression of interstitial collagenase (matrix metalloproteinase-1) is related to the activity of human endometriotic lesions. Fertil Steril 1997; 68(2): 246–251.

30. Bruner KL, Matrisian LM, Rodgers WH, et al. Suppression of matrix metalloproteinases inhibits establishment of ectopic lesions by human endometrium in nude mice. J Clin Invest 1997; 99(12): 2851–2857.

31. Lebovic DI, Mueller MD, Taylor RN. Immunobiology of endometriosis. Fertil Steril 2001; 75(1): 1–10.

32. Oosterlynck DJ, Cornillie FJ, Waer M, et al. Women with endometriosis show a defect in natural killer activity resulting in a decreased cytotoxicity to autologous endometrium. Fertil Steril 1991; 56(1): 45–51.

33. Hill JA, Faris HM, Schiff I, et al. Characterization of leukocyte subpopulations in the peritoneal fluid of women with endometriosis. Fertil Steril 1988; 50(2): 216–222.

34. Oral E, Arici A. Pathogenesis of endometriosis. Obstet Gynecol Clin North Am 1997; 24(2): 219–233.

35. McLaren J. Vascular endothelial growth factor and endometriotic angiogenesis. Hum Reprod Update 2000; 6(1): 45–55.

36. Vigano P, Gaffuri B, Somigliana E, et al. Expression of intercellular adhesion molecule (ICAM)-1 mRNA and protein is enhanced in endometriosis versus endometrial stromal cells in culture. Mol Hum Reprod 1998; 4(12): 1150–1156.

37. Garcia-Velasco JA, Arici A, Zreik T, et al. Macrophage derived growth factors modulate Fas ligand expression in cultured endometrial stromal cells: a role in endometriosis. Mol Hum Reprod 1999; 5(7): 642–650.

38. Gazvani R, Templeton A. New considerations for the pathogenesis of endometriosis. Int J Gynaecol Obstet 2002; 76(2): 117–126.

39. Sinaii N, Cleary SD, Ballweg ML, et al. High rates of autoimmune and endocrine disorders, fibromyalgia, chronic fatigue syndrome and atopic diseases among women with endometriosis: a survey analysis. Hum Reprod 2002; 17(10): 2715–2724.

40. Hughesdon PE. The structure of endometrial cysts of the ovary. J Obstet Gynaecol Br Emp 1957; 64: 481–487.

41. Brosens IA, Puttemans PJ, Deprest J. The endoscopic localization of endometrial implants in the ovarian chocolate cyst. Fertil Steril 1994; 61(6): 1034–1038.

42. Vercellini P, Aimi G, De GO, et al. Is cystic ovarian endometriosis an asymmetric disease? Br J Obstet Gynaecol 1998; 105(9): 1018–1021.

43. Vercellini P, Pisacreta A, Vicentini S, et al. Lateral distribution of nonendometriotic benign ovarian cysts. BJOG 2000; 107(4): 556–558.

44. Rosenfeld DL, Lecher BD. Endometriosis in a patient with Rokitansky–Küster–Hauser syndrome. Am J Obstet Gynecol 1981; 139(1): 105.

45. Sampson JA. Perforating haemorrhagic (chocolate) cysts of the ovary. Arch Surg 1921; 3: 245–323.

46. Jain S, Dalton ME. Chocolate cysts from ovarian follicles. Fertil Steril 1999; 72(5): 852–856.

47. Nisolle M. Ovarian endometriosis and peritoneal endometriosis: are they different entities from a fertility perspective? Curr Opin Obstet Gynecol 2002; 14(3): 283–288.

48. Meyer R. Uber den staude der frage der adenomyosites adenomyoma in allgemeinen und adenomyometritis sarcomastosa. Zentralbl Gynakol 1919; 36: 745–750.

49. Motta PM, Van Blerkom J, Mekabe S. Changes in the surface morphology of ovarian germinal epithelium during the reproductive life and in some pathological conditions. Submicroscopy Cytol 1992; 99: 664–667.

50. Donnez J, Nisolle M, Gillet N, et al. Large ovarian endometriomas. Hum Reprod 1996; 11(3): 641–646.

51. Mayr D, Amann G, Siefert C, et al. Does endometriosis really have premalignant potential? A clonal analysis of laser-microdissected tissue. FASEB J 2003; 17(6): 693–695.

52. Wu Y, Basir Z, Kajdacsy-Balla A, et al. Resolution of clonal origins for endometriotic lesions using laser capture microdissection and the human androgen receptor (HUMARA) assay. Fertil Steril 2003; 79: 3–7.

53. Tamura M, Fukaya T, Murakami T, et al. Analysis of clonality in human endometriotic cysts based on evaluation of X chromosome inactivation in archival formalin-fixed, paraffin-embedded tissue. Lab Invest 1998; 78(2): 213–218.

54. Jimbo H, Hitomi Y, Yoshikawa H, et al. Evidence for monoclonal expansion of epithelial cells in ovarian endometrial cysts. Am J Pathol 1997; 150: 1173–1178.

55. Swiersz LM. Role of endometriosis in cancer and tumor development. Ann N Y Acad Sci 2002; 955: 281–292.

56. Goumenou AG, Arvanitis DA, Matalliotakis IM, et al. Loss of heterozygosity in adenomyosis on hMSH2, hMLH1, p16Ink4 and GALT loci. Int J Mol Med 2000; 6(6): 667–671.

57. Jiang X, Hitchcock A, Bryan EJ, et al. Microsatellite analysis of endometriosis reveals loss of heterozygosity at candidate ovarian tumor suppressor gene loci. Cancer Res 1996; 56(15): 3534–3539.

58. Obata K, Hoshiai H. Common genetic changes between endometriosis and ovarian cancer. Gynecol Obstet Invest 2000; 50 (Suppl 1): 39–43.

59. Thomas EJ, Campbell IG. Molecular genetic defects in endometriosis. Gynecol Obstet Invest 2000; 50 (Suppl 1) 44–50.

60. Bischoff FZ, Heard M, Simpson JL. Somatic DNA alterations in endometriosis: high frequency of chromosome 17 and p53 loss in late-stage endometriosis. J Reprod Immunol 2002; 55(1–2): 49–64.

61. Kosugi Y, Elias S, Malinak LR, et al. Increased heterogeneity of chromosome 17 aneuploidy in endometriosis. Am J Obstet Gynecol 1999; 180(4): 792–797.

62. Shin JC, Ross HL, Elias S, et al. Detection of chromosomal aneuploidy in endometriosis by multi-color fluorescence in situ hybridization (FISH). Hum Genet 1997; 100(3–4): 401–406.

63. Prowse AH, Fakis G, Manek S, et al. Allelic loss studies do not provide evidence for the "endometriosis-as-tumor" theory. Fertil Steril 2005; 83: 1134–1143.

64. Sampson JA. Intestinal adenomas of endometrial type. Arch Surg 1922; 5: 21–27.

65. Cullen TS. The distribution of adenomyomata containing uterine mucosa. Arch Surg 1920; 1: 215–283.

66. Brosens I. Endometriosis rediscovered? Hum Reprod 2004; 19(7): 1679–1680.

67. Vercellini P, Aimi G, Panazza S, et al. Deep endometriosis conundrum: evidence in favor of a peritoneal origin. Fertil Steril 2000; 73(5): 1043–1046.

68. Donnez J, Nisolle M, Smoes P, et al. Peritoneal endometriosis and 'endometriotic' nodules of the rectovaginal septum are two different entities. Fertil Steril 1996; 66(3): 362–368.

69. Koninckx PR, Martin DC. Deep endometriosis: a consequence of infiltration or retraction or possibly adenomyosis externa? Fertil Steril 1992; 58(5): 924–928.

70. Zondervan KT, Cardon LR, Kennedy SH. The genetic basis of endometriosis. Curr Opin Obstet Gynecol 2001; 13: 309–314.

71. Moen MH, Magnus P. The familial risk of endometriosis. Acta Obstet Gynecol Scand 1993; 72(7): 560–564.

72. Simpson JL, Elias S, Malinak LR, Buttram-VC J. Heritable aspects of endometriosis. I. Genetic studies. Am J Obstet Gynecol 1980; 137(3): 327–331.

73. Coxhead D, Thomas EJ. Familial inheritance of endometriosis in a British population: a case control study. J Obstet Gynaecol 1993; 13: 42–44.

74. Kennedy S, Hadfield R, Westbrook C, et al. Magnetic resonance imaging to assess familial risk in relatives of women with endometriosis. Lancet 1998; 352(9138): 1440–1441.

75. Treloar SA, O'Connor DT, O'Connor VM, et al. Genetic influences on endometriosis in an Australian twin sample. Fertil Steril 1999; 71(4): 701–710.

76. Zondervan KT, Weeks DE, Colman R, et al. Familial aggregation of endometriosis in a large pedigree of rhesus macaques. Hum Reprod 2004; 19(2): 448–455.

77. Rier SE, Martin DC, Bowman RE, et al. Endometriosis in rhesus monkeys (Macaca mulatta) following chronic exposure to 2,3,7,8-tetrachlorodibenzo-p-dioxin. Fundam Appl Toxicol 1993; 21(4): 433–441.

78. Guo SW. The link between exposure to dioxin and endometriosis: a critical reappraisal of primate data. Gynecol Obstet Invest 2004; 57: 157–173.

79. Zondervan KT, Cardon LR, Kennedy SH. What makes a good case-control study? Design issues for complex genetic traits such as endometriosis. Hum Reprod 2002; 17: 1415–1423.

80. Zondervan KT, Cardon LR, Kennedy SH. Development of a web site for the genetic epidemiology of endometriosis. Fertil Steril 2002; 78(777): 781.

81. Kennedy S, Mardon H, Barlow D. Familial endometriosis. J Assist Reprod Genet 1995; 12(1): 32–34.

82. Treloar SA, Do KA, O'Connor VM, et al. Predictors of hysterectomy: an Australian study. Am J Obstet Gynecol 1999; 180(4): 945–954.

83. Kennedy S, Bennett S, Weeks DE. Affected sib-pair analysis in endometriosis. Hum Reprod Update 2001; 7(4): 411–418.

84. Treloar S, Hadfield R, Montgomery G, et al. The International Endogene Study: a collection of families for genetic research in endometriosis. Fertil Steril 2002; 78(4): 679–685.

3 Pathogenesis of peritoneal endometriosis

Michelle Nisolle and Jean-Michel Foidart

Introduction

Transplantation theory

The transplantation theory, proposed by Sampson in 1927, involves the dissemination of viable epithelial and stromal endometrial cells via the fallopian tubes into the abdominal cavity and the implantation of these cells into the peritoneum, leading eventually to endometriotic lesions.[1] According to this theory, retrograde menstruation, peritoneal adhesion of shed endometrial tissue, and cells outgrowth are the three essential steps resulting in endometriosis.

Halme et al showed that retrograde menstruation is a common and physiologic occurrence in menstruating women with patent tubes (90% of cases) (Figure 3.1).[2] Anatomic alterations of the pelvis that promote tubal reflux of menstrual endometrium increase the incidence of endometriosis, as observed in adolescents with genital tract obstructions.[3,4] Human peritoneal fluid endometrial cells were found to be viable in culture.[5]

Retrograde menstruation is not sufficient to induce peritoneal endometriosis since it occurs in over 90% women, whereas the rate of peritoneal endometriosis is much lower (2–10% in women of reproductive age, 30% in infertile patients, and 10–70% in women with chronic pelvic pain).[6]

One explanation is that endometriosis could be dependent not only upon the quantity of endometrial tissue reaching the peritoneal cavity but also of the decrease in apoptotic regurgitated cells and also on the decreased capacity of the immune system to eradicate the refluxed menstrual debris.

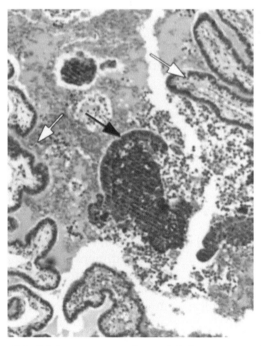

Figure 3.1 Salpingectomy performed during menstruation for a tubal myoma. Endometrial tissue (black arrow) is observed in the tubal ampulla (white arrows).

Other theories

Although the transplantation theory is the most widely accepted one, other theories are not mutually exclusive and have been proposed to explain the pathogenesis of endometriosis since its first detailed description by von Rokitansky.[7]

The celomic metaplasia theory, proposed by Meyer in 1919, suggests that the coelomic cavity contains cells able to differentiate into endometrial tissue under the influence of unknown factors.[8] This theory is supported by the description of cases of endometriosis in which retrograde menstruation does not occur (Rokitansky–Küster–Hauser syndrome) and cannot be explained by Sampson's theory.[9]

The induction theory proposes that menstrual endometrium produces substances that induce peritoneal tissues to form endometriotic lesions.[10]

The embryonic remnants theory suggests that endometriosis results from pluripotent embryonic stem cells, which could differentiate into functioning endometrium. This theory could explain the development of endometriosis located in the rectovaginal septum.[11]

The lymphatic and vascular metastasis theories propose a dissemination of endometrial cells through lymphatics and blood vessels and explain the development of endometriosis outside the pelvis as in pulmonary parenchyma, bone, biceps muscle, peripheral nerves, and the brain.[12,13]

Histopathology

A classification of peritoneal endometriotic lesions as red, black and white lesions has been described according to the difference in the stromal vascularization[14] (Figures 3.2 and 3.3).

Two-dimensional evaluation of the stromal vascularization and the three-dimensional reconstruction of tissue architecture from serial sections demonstrate an obvious similarity between eutopic endometrium and red peritoneal lesions.[15] The red lesions are considered as arising from recently implanted regurgitated endometrial cells.[11] A hypothesis of evolution of peritoneal endometriosis, based on the difference in activity observed in the three types of lesions has been described.[11] Red flame-like lesions and glandular excrescences represent the first stage of the disease. The peritoneal infiltration by the lesion is

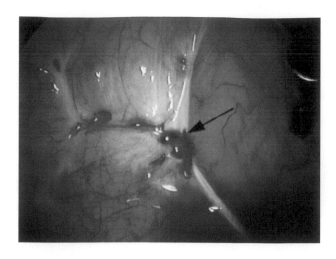

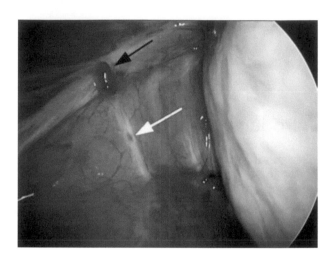

Figure 3.2 Macroscopic aspects of red peritoneal endometriotic lesions (black arrow) and white peritoneal lesions (white arrow).

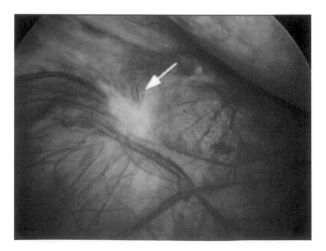

Figure 3.3 Macroscopic aspects of white peritoneal endometriotic lesions (white arrow).

responsible for the presence of intraluminal debris and its black appearance. Subsequent fibrosis explains its white aspect.

Differences in the vessel maturation index, represented by the presence of vascular smooth cells surrounding the endothelial cells, were noted between red and black peritoneal lesions. These data suggest that they could represent different stages of the spontaneous evolution of endometriotic implants, with red lesions being the first stage with dilated and isolated endothelial cells while mature vessels were observed in black lesions.[16]

Analogy with the neoplastic process: the seed and soil theory

Stephen Paget's 1989 proposal that metastasis depends on cross-talk between selected cancer cells ('the seeds') and specific organ microenvironments ('the soil') still holds forth today. It is known that the potential of a tumor cell to metastasize depends on its interactions with host cells that promote tumor cell growth, survival, angiogenesis, and invasion.[17,18] Similarly the ectopic implantation of endometrial cells onto peritoneum, ovary, bladder, and the rectovaginal septum and successful formation of an endometriotic nodule require complex interactions between competent living endometrial epithelial cells and perhaps also stromal cells (seed) and adequate microenvironmental host cells.

As in metastasis formation, mechanical arrest of endometrial cells or tumor cells at distant sites from the tissue of origin may occur without specificity. However, the subsequent proliferation and growth into secondary lesions is influenced by specific organ host cells.

The process of cancer metastasis consists of a long series of sequential and interrelated steps that also occur during endometriosis.[19] Each of these steps can be rate limiting, as a failure or an insufficiency at any of the steps can stay the entire process. As in a primary tumor, endometrial cells in their eutopic localization undergo progressive growth, become vascularized, and then detach to migrate at distant sites. As for the success of metastasis formation, endometrial cells must survive outside the endometrium; they must arrest, implant, evade the host defence, induce angiogenesis, and undergo proliferative growth.

Endometrial cells therefore require various properties that are also shared by metastatic cells, such as adhesive characteristics, invasive capacity, and immune resistance to natural killer cells.[20,21]

Host cells include epithelial cells of the mesothelium, fibroblasts, vascular endothelial cells, and infiltrating leukocytes. The microenvironment of the 'soil' must be favorable for endometrial cells to adhere and invade the host tissue. In other words, the outcome of endometriosis depends on multiple interactions ('cross-talks') of endometriotic cells with homeostatic mechanisms, which they can usurp. Therapy of endometriosis, therefore, should be targeted not only against the endometriotic cells themselves but also against the homeostatic factors that promote endometrial cell adhesion, survival, angiogenesis invasion, and immune tolerance.

The seed: endometrial cells

Adhesion

In-vivo models
In the baboon (*Papio anubis*, *Papio cynocephalus*), spontaneous endometriosis has been described as well as induced endometriosis by intrapelvic seeding of menstrual endometrium, which supports Sampson's theory.[22–24]

Nude mice represent a well-known model of experimental endometriosis, and several investigators have described the transplantation of proliferative or secretory human endometrium with an implantation rate varying from 33% to 87%.[25,26]

Attachment of endometrial tissue and cell viability have been detected as early as 1 day after subcutaneous transplantation of proliferative or secretory human endometrium. Degenerative changes were observed in the central part of the transplant, probably caused by ischemia.[27]

Transplantation of human menstrual endometrium also resulted in the development of endometriosis within 24 hours.[28] The high vascular endothelial growth factor (VEGF) score observed in stromal cells suggests that an active vascular network is a necessary condition for the survival of the graft. In freshly implanted endometriotic lesions, an extensive proliferation rate was observed in glandular cells (Figure 3.4). Two distinct roles were attributed to glandular and stromal cells: glandular cells showing high rates of proliferative activity should be involved in the growth of the lesion; however,

(a)

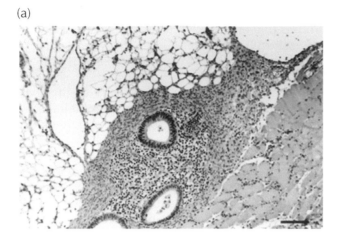

(b)

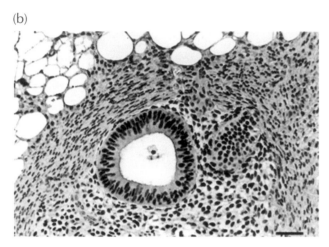

Figure 3.4 (a,b) Immunohistochemical staining for Ki-67 in transplanted endometrial explants. Ki-67 is expressed in both glandular epithelium and stroma. (Reproduced from Nisolle et al[26] with permission of European Society of Human Reproduction and Embryology and Oxford Press/Human Reproduction.)

stromal cells should be responsible for the first step of attachment of endometrial fragments.[28]

The role of both endometrial cell types for ectopic implantation was recently confirmed by Beliard et al, who investigated the role of different cellular types: transplantation of mixed cultures of stromal and epithelial cells resulted in the development of endometriotic-like nodules in nude mice; on the contrary, transplantation of isolated stromal and/or isolated epithelial cells was found to be unsuccessful.[29]

The success of implantation was dependent not only on the cooperativeness between stromal and epithelial endometrial cells but also on the endocrine environment of endometrial cells (pretreatment of cells with estrogen alone or with estrogen and progestin increasing the implantation rate). Such cooperation between epithelial cells and stromal cells probably involves a cross-talk between both cell types through the secretion of growth factors, cytokines and/or chemokines.[30]

Alternatively, the contribution of stromal cells to epithelial cell adhesion could be the secretion of extracellular matrix (ECM) components, or the release of proteases leading to ECM remodeling and formation of an appropriate microenvironment for epithelial cell implantation, proliferation, and organization into endometrial glands. Such epithelial–stromal cooperation has been demonstrated for the implantation of tumor cells in an ectopic site.[31]

In-vitro models

Some authors evaluated the attachment of endometrial fragments to an amniotic membrane.[32,33] The endometrium was found to adhere to surfaces not coated with amniocytes and to areas where the amniotic epithelium was damaged. They concluded that an intact epithelial layer of amniocytes prevented endometrial attachment. They also measured the adhesion of proliferative phase endometrium of women without endometriosis to peritoneal explants.[34] They hypothesized that trauma to the mesothelial lining was a prerequisite for endometrial cell adhesion, as endometrial fragments attached only at locations where the mesothelium was absent.

In contrast to these findings, Witz et al demonstrated that endometrial epithelial cells and endometrial stromal cells were capable of adhering to the intact mesothelium within 1 hour.[35,36] In their study, by using confocal laser scanning microscopy and electron microscopy of peritoneal explants, they demonstrated an intact layer of viable mesothelial cells beneath sites of endometrial attachment and a transmesothelial invasion occurring within 18 hours.

Recently, Beliard et al have set up an in-vitro model suitable for evaluating the adhesion of human endometrial cells to peritoneum and the effect of various cytokines on the adhesion process.[37] Endometrial cells were labeled with [111]indium, a radionuclide widely used to trace leukocytes and platelets. Cultured endometrial cells were confronted in vitro with mouse peritoneum pre-exposed in vivo for 24 hours to the following proinflammatory cytokines: interleukins IL-1β and IL-6, tumor necrosis factor alpha (TNF-α), and transforming growth factor (TGF)-β$_1$.

A moderate increase of endometrial cell adhesion to the peritoneum in response to the addition of TGF-β, IL-1β, IL-6, and TNF-α was observed, suggesting that proinflammatory cytokines may play a role in the development of endometriosis.

Molecular mechanisms

A large number of adhesive proteins and proteoglycans have been determined biochemically during the last decade. Among these macromolecules, laminin and fibronectin are two major adhesion glycoproteins that play a key role in epithelial cell attachment to basement membranes and stromal cell adhesion to the interstitial matrix, respectively. Laminin and fibronectin exercise their functions through cell surface molecules of the integrin family.[38] The distribution of both laminin and fibronectin and their receptors was found to be identical in endometriosis and endometrium, except for fibronectin receptors.[38] The expression of $\alpha4\beta1$ and $\alpha5\beta1$ persisted around endometriotic glands, whereas it was absent from endometrial glands. These data suggested that fibronectin receptors could play a role in the persistence of endometriotic lesions.

No difference in the pattern of localization for the adhesive glycoproteins and for the integrins was observed between the eutopic endometrium from fertile women and from women with endometriosis.

Non-integrin proteins (the 67 kDa laminin receptor (LR), galectin-3, and galectin-1) are also capable of binding to laminin, displaying a multidomain complex structure. They are involved in cancer progression through their capacity to modulate tumor cells' extracellular matrix interactions.[39,40]

Changes in the pattern of cell surface laminin-binding proteins have already been documented in diverse malignant human tumors: 67 LR expression increases with the acquisition of the metastatic phenotype, while galectin-3 expression is down-regulated.[39,40]

Endometriotic tissue (superficial lesions and rectovaginal nodules) and eutopic endometrium expressed galectin-3 but not 67 LR, suggesting that galectin-3 could contribute to the attachment of both endometrial and endometriotic cells to the extracellular matrix. The similar expression of these laminin-binding proteins between superficial and rectovaginal endometriosis may suggest that invasive behavior of endometriotic cells does not require a repertoire of laminin-binding proteins similar to that of cancer cells (Beliard, pers comm).

Naturally, shed endometrium expresses at least six integrins involved in adhesion to ECM components.[41] By performing blocking studies, it was demonstrated that $\alpha6\beta1$ integrin may play a key role in the adhesion of menstrual tissue to laminin and may be of pivotal importance in the very early phases of the development of endometriosis.

The presence of integrins ($\alpha2\beta1$, collagen–laminin receptor, and $\alpha3\beta1$, collagen–laminin–fibronectin receptor) on the cell surface of mesothelial cells has been demonstrated in vivo and in vitro, suggesting a role for these molecules in adhesion to the basement membrane.[42]

Invasion

E-cadherins

In order to penetrate deeply in the host tissues, endometrial epithelial cells must detach from their neighboring partners to which they are connected via E-cadherins.

Cadherins are calcium-dependent transmembrane cell–cell adhesion molecules. E-cadherin mediates cell–cell interaction by homophilic interactions and is expressed in the epithelial cell-to-cell boundaries of the endometrium.[38]

Differences in invasiveness properties between endometrial cells of women with or without endometriosis have been suggested by using an in-vitro collagen invasion assay.[43] A higher proportion of potentially invasive E-cadherin-negative epithelial cells from human endometriotic biopsies have been observed when compared to human endometrial biopsies. In epithelial cancer, loss of E-cadherin expression is known to be involved in the acquisition of an invasive phenotype. It is postulated to constitute a crucial mechanism in the pathogenesis of endometriosis. However, by immunohistochemistry of constituted lesions, E-cadherin was found to display a similar pattern of expression in epithelial glandular cells of endometriosis and endometrium.[38]

Polymorphism in the promoter region of the E-cadherin gene is responsible for interindividual variation in the production of E-cadherin and in turn leads to individual susceptibility to epithelial dysfunctions. It has been demonstrated that a single nucleotide polymorphism in the E-cadherin gene promoter alters transcriptional activities.[44]

Such mutation of the E-cadherin gene has not yet been evaluated in endometriotic tissue.

Expression of matrix metalloproteinases

Matrix metalloproteinases (MMPs) are a family of endopeptidases that play a role in the degradation and turnover of ECM proteins. Their action is regulated by specific tissue inhibitors of metalloproteinases (TIMPs).

In the endometrium, MMPs are involved in matrix remodeling associated with perimenstrual phases.[45] They can be divided into several distinct subgroups based on substrate specificity or structural similarities: collagenases (MMP1, 8, and 13); gelatinases (MMP2 and 9); stromelysins (MMP3, 7, 10, and 11); and membrane-type MMPs (MT-MMP1–6). An additional miscellaneous group of MMPs includes MMP12, MMP18, and MMP19–26.

Three distinct patterns of MMP and two patterns of TIMPs expression have been described in cycling endometrium:[46]

1. MMPs restricted to the menstrual period (MMPs1, 3, 8, 9, and 12)
2. MMP and TIMPs expressed throughout the cycle (MMP2, MT1-MMP, MT2-MMP, MMP19, TIMP1 and TIMP2)
3. MMPs predominantly expressed during the proliferative phase (MMP7, MMP11, MMP26, and MT3-MMP)
4. TIMP3, which showed significant modulations, with maximum expression during the late secretory and menstrual phase.

The cyclic expression of MMP by human endometrium has also been suggested to play a role in the invasive process necessary to establish endometriosis. Although endometrial expression of the MMP family is normally regulated during the menstrual cycle, altered patterns of MMP and TIMP expression have been reported in eutopic and ectopic endometrial tissues from patients with endometriosis.

The levels of MMP2 and MMP9 which have the highest enzymatic activities against type IV collagen were found to be elevated in ectopic endometrium.[47]

A correlation of MMP1 expression with activity of endometriotic tissue has been demonstrated by the MMP1 mRNA expression in red peritoneal and ovarian endometriosis, whereas it was not detectable in black peritoneal and rectovaginal lesions.[48] MMP1 and MMP2 protein were found to be highly expressed in endometriotic tissues when compared with entopic endometrium, whereas expression of TIMP1 and TIMP2 proteins were significantly reduced.[49,50]

Very recently, Chung et al described higher MMP9 and lower TIMP3 mRNA expression in ectopic and eutopic endometrium from endometriosis patients compared with that observed in patients without endometriosis, suggesting that increased proteolytic activity of the endometrium could result in the development of endometriosis.[51] Expression of MMP11 mRNA has been identified in the eutopic endometrium from women with endometriosis, whereas it is not expressed in women without endometriosis.[52]

Treatment of endometrium with TIMP1 in vitro followed by intraperitoneal injections of TIMP1 was shown to reduce the development of endometriosis in nude nice after intraperitoneal transplantation of human endometrial tissue.[53] Eutopic endometrium and ectopic tissue from women with endometriosis were found to exhibit patterns of altered MMP (MMP3 and MMP7) regulation in vivo.[54] A lack of responsiveness to progesterone was demonstrated in vitro, associated with a failure to suppress MMP expression and enhanced ability of the tissue to establish experimental endometriosis.

Finally, beyond their clinical connective tissue-degrading functions, MMPs regulate the activities of bioactive molecules by proteolytic processing. For example, MMPs mediate cell surface-receptor cleavage and release, cytokine and chemokine activation and inactivation, and the release of apoptotic ligands (see 'Apoptosis of Cytotoxic T Lymphocytes' section).

Angiogenesis

Once implantation has occurred, the further growth of the lesions will depend on the formation of new capillaries. Indeed, the establishment of a new blood supply is essential for the survival of the implant and the development of endometriosis. Angiogenesis is a complex process involving a number of different functions: proliferation, migration and extension of endothelial cells; adherence of these cells to the ECM; remodeling of this matrix; and formation of a lumen.[55]

Soluble substances involved in angiogenesis have been detected in the peritoneal fluid of women with endometriosis.[56,57] These angiogenic factors could be produced by peritoneal macrophages, retrogradely menstruated endometrial cells, and/or the ectopic endometriotic lesions themselves.[58]

Several angiogenic factors have been identified, including acid and basic fibroblast growth factors (FGF-α, FGF-β), platelet-derived endothelial cell growth factor (PD-ECGF), TGF-α, TGF-β, TNF-α, and VEGF.[55] VEGF is a multifunctional family of cytokines that is expressed in both epithelial and mesenchymal cells in a wide variety of tissues and in many tumors. The angiogenic actions of VEGF are thought to be mediated primarily by two cell surface receptors termed VEGF-R1 and VEGF-R2.[59] After receptor activation in endothelial cells, a number of cellular responses occur, playing a role in angiogenesis and tissue remodeling (induction of urokinase and urokinase receptors, tissue plasminogen activators (PA), PA inhibitors, metalloproteinase activity, vascular cell adhesion molecule 1 (VCAM-1), and intercellular adhesion molecule 1 (ICAM-1) expression).[60]

VEGF immunostaining has been observed in the epithelium of endometriotic implants, particularly in red peritoneal lesions.[61]

Moreover, VEGF, in addition to being angiogenic, causes increased permeability of the capillary bed, leading to a leakage of fibrin products into the extracellular space, which will increase the recruitment of macrophages and their secretion of TNF-α.[55] This, in addition to its angiogenic activity, promotes adhesion of human endometrial stromal cells to peritoneal mesothelial cells in vitro in a dose-dependent fashion.[62]

Growth

Effect of estrogen
Estrogens regulate the growth, differentiation, and function of eutopic endometrium. Both estrogen receptors ER-α and ER-β play a key role in eutopic endometrium growth regulation. Although both ER-α and ER-β are expressed in the endometrium, ER-α is the predominant isoform.[63] Matzuzaki et al compared mRNA levels of ER-α and ER-β and noted that both eutopic endometrium and endometriotic lesions show predominantly higher levels of ER-α than ER-β.[64] The relative ratio of ER-α to ER-β mRNA was significantly higher in red peritoneal lesions than in black lesions and ovarian endometriotic cysts. A similar ER-α/ER-β mRNA ratio was observed in proliferative eutopic endometrium and red peritoneal lesions. These data suggested that ER-α may play an essential role in the development and growth of endometriosis.

Variations in the levels of enzymes involved locally in steroidogenesis function have also been proposed as an explanation for a production of estradiol in the endometriotic implant responsible for its growth independently of the plasma levels of estrogen. The conversion of androstendione and testosterone to estrone and estradiol is catalyzed by aromatase, which is expressed in human tissues and cells (ovarian granulosa cells, placental syncytiotrophoblast, adipocytes, skin fibroblasts, and brain).[65]

Aromatase activity is absent in normal endometrium but aberrant aromatase expression in stromal cells has been described in endometriotic lesions, resulting in higher local production of estradiol.[66,67]

New evidence suggests also that prostaglandin E_2 (PGE_2) might up-regulate the expression of aromatase in endometriotic stromal cells, leading to endogenous steroid synthesis.[68] Moreover, cytokines (TNF-α and IL-1β) also stimulate the expression of prostaglandin synthase 2, which in turn increases the production of PGE_2.[69]

Another intrinsic molecular aberration has been observed in endometriotic implants: endometriotic glandular cells are deficient in 17β-hydroxysteroid dehydrogenase type 2, which converts E_2 (estradiol) to estrone in the eutopic endometrium in response to progesterone. This enzymatic deficiency results therefore in an increased local production of estradiol and contributes to the development of endometriosis.[67]

Effect of progesterone
Studies comparing eutopic and ectopic endometrium showed that hormonally induced changes in endometriosis did not correlate with the corresponding endometrium. During the luteal phase, ectopic endometrium did not reveal morphologic secretory changes, mitoses were still present and it was suggested that this hormonal independence was associated to the persistence of progesterone receptor (PR) and possibly to its biologic inactivity.[70,71]

Two PR isoforms have subsequently been identified, PR-A and PR-B. They are functionally different: PR-B is a stronger activator of progesterone target genes, whereas PR-A acts as a dominant repressor of PR-B. The alteration in the ratio of PR-A to PR-B in endometriotic tissue (presence of the inhibitory PR isoform PR-A and the absence of the stimulatory isoform PR-B) may be a possible explanation for tissular progesterone resistance.[72] This progesterone resistance has been suspected by the observation of the persistence of PR in endometriotic tissue during the late secretory phase, whereas there was a down-regulation of PR in eutopic endometrium.[70]

Deficiency of 17β-hydroxysteroid dehydrogenase type 2 in endometriosis impairs the inactivation of estradiol to estrone and may be a consequence of insensitivity to progesterone.[73]

Apoptosis

Normal cells require mitogenic growth signals to proliferate. These signals are transmitted into the cell by transmembrane or nuclear-cytosolic receptors that bind distinct classes of signaling molecules: diffusible growth factors, ECM components, steroids, and cell-to-cell adhesion/interaction molecules.[20] Multiple antiproliferative signals operate also to maintain cellular quiescence and tissue homeostasis. The signals include both soluble growth inhibitors and immobilized inhibitors embedded in the ECM and on the surface on nearby cells. These growth-inhibitory signals, like their positively acting counterparts, are received by transmembrane cell surface receptors coupled to intracellular signaling circuits.

The ability of endometriotic cell proliferations to expand in number is determined not only by the rate of cell proliferation but also by the rate of cell attrition. Programmed cell death, i.e. apoptosis, represents a major source of attrition.

Apoptosis is a programmed cell death that results in cell disparition without inflammatory reaction. Several proteins, including bcl-2 and p53, regulate this complex process. The p53 and bcl-2 proteins can be regarded as positive and negative regulators of cell death, respectively.[74]

A decrease in apoptosis might lead to ectopic survival and implantation of endometriotic cells and development of endometriosis.

Different studies comparing apoptosis in endometrium from patients with or without endometriosis led to controversial results. Dmowski et al. found that spontaneous apoptosis is decreased in the endometrial glands of women with endometriosis, indicating that increased viability of endometrial cells shed during menses facilitates their survival and implantation.[75] Recently, Braun et al demonstrated that apoptotic cells and macrophages numbers were positively correlated in the eutopic endometrium of women with and without endometriosis.[76] The number of apoptotic cells and the macrophage content in the endometrium of women with endometriosis was found to be significantly reduced compared to that of healthy women, predominantly during the early proliferative phase. Therefore, it was hypothesized that the reduction in apoptosis in the endometrium of women with endometriosis may be related to reduced macrophage trafficking.

On the other hand, Jones et al did not report significant differences in apoptotic cell rate in both types of endometrium.[77] Beliard et al evaluated apoptotic markers (tunel, bcl-2) concomitantly with steroid hormone receptors and cellular proliferation in endometrium from patients with or without endometriosis and did not find any significant difference in the rate of apoptosis.[78] These data indicate that ectopic implantation of endometrium could not be the consequence of a decrease in apoptosis in endometrium. This is also in agreement with in-vitro and in-vivo previous studies that showed that perimenstrual endometrium from women without endometriosis is able to adhere to the peritoneum.[26–34]

Markers of apoptosis were also assessed in peritoneal endometriosis and in the corresponding endometrium throughout the menstrual cycle. A reduction of apoptosis in endometriotic lesions was observed when compared to the eutopic endometrium suggesting the dissemination and implantation of these cells to ectopic sites.[78] These results are consistent with previous reports.[77]

Genetic alterations

Kao et al investigated differentially regulated genes in endometrium from women with or without endometriosis by applying paralleled gene expression profiling using high-density oligonucleotide microarrays.[79] Their data support dysregulation of select genes, leading to an inhospitable environment for implantation, as well as genes contributing to the pathogenesis of endometriosis, including aromatase, progesterone receptor, and angiogenic factors.[79] Identification and validation of selected genes and their functions will contribute to uncovering mechanisms underlying the pathogenesis of endometriosis and providing potential new targets for diagnosis and intervention.

The soil: host cells

The peritoneal response to the invasion of regurgitated menstrual debris is directed towards incapacitation, destruction, and removal of these cells.

The defective immunosurveillance may lead to decreased clearance of menstrual debris from the peritoneal cavity and may allow for attachment of ectopic endometrium to peritoneal surfaces. An inadequate response of this defense mechanism has been suggested as a facilitating factor for the development of endometriosis.[80,81] It also could promote the persistence and growth of ectopic endometrial tissue.[82]

Macrophages, which constitute the dominant cell type in the peritoneal fluid cell population, are involved in phagocytosis and in the initiation of the inflammatory response.[80]

Peritoneal fluid from patients with endometriosis was shown to contain high levels of peritoneal macrophages and inflammatory cytokines probably produced by these cells.[80,83] These activated peritoneal macrophages as well as endometriotic cells are hypothesized to secrete various cytokines with pleiotropic biologic activities. Among these cytokines, IL-1, TNF-α, and IL-8 seem to play pivotal roles in the development and persistence of the endometriotic lesions.

Tumor necrosis factor-alpha

The elevated TNF-α concentrations in peritoneal fluid of patients with endometriosis when compared with controls suggest that this cytokine contributes to a peritoneal microenvironment favoring the implantation of endometrial cells.[84]

TNF-α, a proinflammatory cytokine, activates inflammatory leukocytes and stimulates macrophages to produce other cytokines such as IL-1, IL-6, and more TNF-α. IL-1 also acts on mononuclear cells to increase further production of IL-1 and IL-6. Moreover, IL-1α and TNF-α are known to regulate MMP and TIMP production, suggesting their role in the establishment of endometriosis.[85]

Interleukin-8

In-vitro production of other macrophage secretory products such as IL-6 and IL-8 have also been described in patients with endometriosis.[84,86–88] A significant correlation between peritoneal fluid (PF) IL-8 concentration and the stage of endometriosis has been found, suggesting that IL-8 is an important angiogenic factor that promotes the neovascularization and proliferation of ectopic endometrial implants.[84] IL-8 is a chemoattractor and activator of neutrophils and is a potent angiogenic agent. The potential cellular sources of IL-8 that may contribute to its high level in the PF of women with endometriosis are endometrial cells, mesothelial cells and peritoneal macrophages.[86,87]

It has recently been demonstrated that IL-8 increased MMP2 and 9 activities and the invasive capability of endometrial stromal cells in culture,

suggesting a pivotal role for IL-8 in the pathogenesis of endometriosis.[89]

Monocyte chemotactic protein 1

The macrophage products IL-1β and TNF-α stimulate endometrial epithelial and mesothelial cells as well as endometriotic cells to produce monocyte chemotactic protein 1 (MCP-1), a proinflammatory and angiogenic cytokine.[90]

Increased concentrations of MCP-1 in PF have been reported in patients with endometriosis when compared with healthy women.[87]

Peritoneal macrophages of women with endometriosis showed an increased capacity to secrete MCP-1 and a tendency for an increased secretion of macrophage migration inhibition factor (MIF) when compared with healthy women.[90]

Macrophage migration inhibitory factor

MIF may play a role in activating and retaining peritoneal macrophages and in activating T lymphocytes.

Moreover, MIF may also contribute to the development and the growth of ectopic endometrial tissue as it is able to stimulate endothelial cell proliferation in vitro and to induce angiogenesis in vivo. MIF is expressed in glandular epithelial cells, endothelial cells, macrophages, and T lymphocytes of the stroma. MIF expression was found to be significantly higher in red lesions than in black or white lesions.[91] This could reflect the role of MIF in promoting and maintaining a higher degree of vascular development and suggests that MIF may play a role in active angiogenesis and inflammatory process as observed in endometriosis.[91]

RANTES

Leukocytes and macrophages accumulate in ectopic endometrium and secrete cytokines (IL-1, IL-6, IL-8, TNF-α, and RANTES).[92]

RANTES (regulated upon activation, normal T-cell expressed and secreted) is a T-lymphocyte product involved in macrophage recruitment and activation. Increased PF concentrations of RANTES have been found in patients with endometriosis. Stromal cells from both endometriotic lesions and eutopic endometrium have also been shown to produce RANTES, and this production is increased by TNF-α and interferon-γ in culture.[93]

Apoptosis of cytotoxic T lymphocytes

Fas (CD95 or APO-1) is a type I membrane receptor protein, 45 kDa in size, expressed in various tissues and cells such as thymus, liver, heart, and kidney.[94] It is structurally related to the TNF receptor and is also expressed by leukocytes, macrophages, and immune effector cytolytic T cells.[95] Fas-bearing cells undergo apoptotic cell death when they interact with its ligand, called Fas ligand (FasL).[96]

FasL is a type II membrane protein that belongs to the TNF family.[97] It is predominantly expressed in activated T cells, activated macrophages, and lymphocytes. The system Fas–FasL makes use of membrane-bound molecules related to the immune cytotoxicity. The immune effector cell expresses both the T-cell receptor and a FasL. Upon activation, it would recognize the target cells which express the major histocompatibility complex (MHC) antigens and Fas. The Fas-bearing cells would then undergo apoptosis (Figure 3.5).[98]

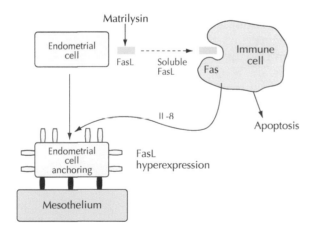

Figure 3.5 FasL complex and resistance to immune surveillance. Endometrial cells express small amount of Fas ligand and matrilysin. This MMP cleaves the Fas ligand. The soluble Fas ligand forms a complex with Fas at the surface of immune cells, which either undergo apoptosis or overproduce IL-8. This proinflammatory cytokine stimulates adhesion of the endometrial cells to the mesothelium. This, in turn, stimulates the expression of Fas-ligand, further promoting the resistance to immune surveillance. FasL = Fas ligand; IL = interleukin; MMP = matrix metalloproteinase

In the context of endometriosis, epithelial and stromal cells express high levels of membrane-bound FasL that is proteolytically cleaved by matrilysin (MMP7) and released into the PF and plasma.[99,100]

Activated PF macrophages and lymphocytes may also contribute to the elevated levels of soluble FasL.[97,101] This soluble FasL may bind to the immune cells that express Fas at their surface and provokes increased apoptosis of these cells, thereby preventing the immune rejection of regurgitated endometrial cells.

The formation of a complex Fas–FasL at the surface of immune cells may paradoxically result in secretion of IL-8 instead of causing programmed cell death.[102] These cytokines may then stimulate the adhesion of endometrial cells onto the mesothelium. The attachment of the endometrial stromal cells to the peritoneum during retrograde menstruation could lead to an increase in the expression of FasL.[103] This induction of FasL expression by adhesion of endometrial stromal cells to the ECM may thus lead to a positive feedback, allowing the development of endometriosis (see Figure 3.5). Garcia-Velasco et al noted elevated soluble FasL in serum and peritoneal fluid of women with moderate to severe endometriosis when compared to that observed in women in early-stage disease or disease-free women, confirming a dysregulation of apoptosis in the development of endometriosis.[104]

Collectively, these data indicate that secretion of various cytokines by endometriotic cells and inflammatory cells into the peritoneal cavity lead to proliferation of implants, angiogenesis, and chemoattraction of leukocytes to these foci of peritoneal inflammation.[82] Therefore, a positive feedback loop could explain the maintenance and progressive growth of the lesions. But it is still unclear whether the alterations of peritoneal macrophages' activation, recruitment, and cytokine synthesis observed in women with endometriosis is due to endometriosis or is the cause of the disease.

Therapeutic perspectives

Until now the medical treatment of endometriosis has been based on the hormonal responsiveness of the endometriotic tissue (hypoestrogenic environment or progestin-dominant environment). But hormonal therapy only suppresses symptoms; it is not able to eradicate the ectopic implant. Therapy of endometriosis, therefore, should be targeted not only against the endometriotic cells themselves but also against the homeostatic factors that growth promote cell adhesion, survival, angiogenesis, invasion, and immune tolerance.

Aromatase inhibitors

Aromatase inhibitors could theoretically be candidate drugs in the treatment of endometriosis in cases of resistance to standard regimens in postmenopausal women.

The suppression of extraovarian aromatase activity in the endometriotic lesion could explain the successful treatment observed in postmenopausal women.[105]

Further studies are required to determine the precise role of aromatase inhibitors in premenopausal women. A pilot study performed in 10 premenopausal women previously treated both medically and surgically for endometriosis seems to be efficacious in reducing symptoms and laparoscopically visible endometriotic lesions.[106]

Selective progesterone receptor modulators (SPRMs)

Progesterone receptor modulators (PRMs) are progesterone receptor ligands that can produce different effects:[107,108]

1. Pure antagonists of progesterone action, by prevention of PR binding to the progesterone response element (PRE) or by prevention of transcription, even PR binding to the progesterone element has occurred.
2. Agonists, partial agonists, or antagonists, by variable alteration of gene expression. Improvement in symptoms has been obtained in women with endometriosis who received mifepristone (5 or 50 mg/day for 6 months or 100 mg/day for 3 months).[109,110] The success of mifepristone can be related to its antiproliferative effect and to its promoting apoptotic effect by *bax* overexpression, the apoptosis-promoting gene and by down-regulating *bcl*-2. Mifepristone mediates this effect by increasing nuclear factor-kappa B (NF-κB) binding activity.[111]

MMPS Inhibitors (MMPIs)

Theoritically, inhibition of MMPs might be effective in the development of endometriosis.[53] Such drugs decrease the tumoral cell invasion and migration, neoangiogenesis, chemotaxis of inflammatory and immune cells, release and activation of cytokines, growth factors and FasLs. However, first-generation (broad-spectrum) MMPIs were associated with side effects such as muscular pain and articular stiffness. Trials with second-generation (selective MMPIs) are in progress in various cancer treatments.[112]

Tumor necrosis factor alpha inhibitors

Recombinant human TNF binding protein-1 has been evaluated in the treatment of endometriosis.

TNF-α has two membrane-bound receptors (type I and type II). The soluble form of both receptors, deriving from the shed extracellular portion of TNF receptors, binds with high affinity to TNF, thereby hampering the binding of the cytokine to the cell-associated receptor.[113]

In-vitro studies on proliferation of endometrial tissue demonstrated that the soluble TNF receptor reduced the proliferation-enhanced activity of PF from women with endometriosis.[114]

Specific anti-TNF-α therapy has been evaluated in animal models. In rat models of endometriosis, recombinant human TNF binding protein-1 (soluble form of TNF receptor type I) was shown to reduce the size of endometriotic-like foci 9 days after autologous transplantation of uterine tissue.[115] In baboons, recombinant protein (r-hTBP-1) reduced the stage, the volume of endometriotic lesions, and the adhesions 25 days after the transplantation.[116] The efficacy of 8 weeks of treatment with Etanercept (soluble form of the TNF-α receptor) in reducing the amount of spontaneously occurring active endometriosis in the baboon was recently demonstrated after 8 weeks of treatment.[117]

In humans, these drugs are used only in rheumatoid arthritis (Remicade (infliximab), Etanercept), but limiting factors such as the cost and secondary effects are encountered.[118]

Immunomodulators

Several compounds (cytokines and synthetic immunomodulators) that have immune-enhancing properties have been investigated in the treatment of endometriosis: the cytokines IL-12 and interferon-α2b, and two synthetic immunomodulators, the guanosine analogue loxoribine and the acetylcholine nicotinic receptor agonist levamisole.[113] In murine model of induced endometriosis, it has been demonstrated that IL-12 could prevent the establishment of endometriosis.[119]

In a murine model, intraperitoneal or subcutaneous administration of recombinant human interferon–α2b showed a reduction of the growth of endometrial fragments intraperitoneally transplanted.[120]

Synthetic immunomodulators have also been investigated in animal models of endometriosis. Regression of both stromal and epithelial components of endometrial explants was observed in a rat model of endometriosis treated with loxoribine, a synthetic immunomodulator.[121] On the other hand, the administration of levamisole was found to be ineffective.

Antiangiogenic agents

Angiostatic therapy has been recently described to be effective in a nude mouse model.[122] A significant decrease in the number of endometriotic lesions has been observed, under the effect of the angiostatic compounds antihuman vascular endothelial growth factor, TNP-470, Endostatin, and Anginex. The angiostatic compounds also significantly decreased microvessel densities and the number of immature vessels (negative for the α-smooth muscle actin). These data confirm that inhibitors of angiogenesis effectively interfere with the maintenance and growth of endometriosis.[123]

Conclusion

Extensive pathogenic studies in recent years have largely contributed to more precisely delineating the key features of ectopic endometrial implantation and growth. In particular, the roles of cytokines and the escape from immune rejection are being elucidated. The molecular mechanisms of implantation, migration–invasion angiogenesis, and growth apoptosis are being characterized with the aim of designing new more specific targets.

Despite a better understanding of the pathophysiology of endometriosis, it becomes evident that several positive feedback loops are responsible for the maintenance and growth of the constituted lesions. It appears, therefore, that the rationale of treatment should be based upon surgical eradication of the lesions, with additional medical therapy aimed at preventing recurrence.

Acknowledgments

This work was supported by grants from the Fond National de la Recherche Scientifique (FNRS, Belgium): Fonds de la Recherche Scientifique Médicale (Grants Nos 3.4595.98, 3.4608.01, and 3.4531.02), Conventions Télévie (Grant No. 7.4535.98), Crédits aux Chercheurs (Grants Nos 1.5115.02 and 1.5068.05).

REFERENCES

1. Sampson JA. Peritoneal endometriosis due to menstrual dissemination of endometrial tissue into the peritoneal cavity. Am J Obstet Gynecol 1927; 14: 422–469.
2. Halme J, Hammond MG, Hulka JF, et al. Retrograde menstruation in healthy women and in patients with endometriosis. Obstet Gynecol 1984; 64: 151–154.
3. Sanfilippo JS, Wakim NG, Schikler KN, et al. Endometriosis in association with uterine anomaly. Am J Obstet Gynecol 1986; 154: 39–43.
4. Olive DL, Henderson DY. Endometriosis and müllerian anomalies. Obstet Gynecol 1987; 69: 412.
5. Kruitwagen RF, Poels LG, Willemsen WN, et al. Endometrial epithelial cells in peritoneal fluid during the early follicular phase. Fertil Steril 1991; 55: 297–303.
6. Lapp T. ACOG issues recommendations for the management of endometriosis. American College of Obstetricians and Gynecologists. Am Fam Physician 2000; 62: 1431–1434.
7. Von Rokitansky C. Ueber Uteusdrusen-Neubildung in Uterus and Ovarialsarcomen [Uterine gland proliferation in uterine and ovarian sarcomas]. Zeitschrift Gesellschaft fur Aerzte zu Wien 1860; 37: 577.
8. Meyer R. Ueber den Stand der Frage der Adenomyositis und Adenomyome in Algemeinen und Insbesondere ueber Adenomyositis seroepitheliasis und Adenomyometritis sacromatosa. Zbl Gynaekol 1919; 43: 745–750.
9. Rosenfeld DL, Lecher BD. Endometriosis in a patient with Rokitansky–Küster–Hauser syndrome. Am J Obstet Gynecol 1981; 139: 105.
10. Merrill JA. Endometrial induction of endometriosis across Millipore filters. Am J Obstet Gynecol1966; 94: 780–789.
11. Nisolle M, Donnez J. Peritoneal endometriosis, ovarian endometriosis, and adenomyotic nodules of the rectovaginal septum are three different entities. Fertil Steril 1997; 68: 585–596.

12. Halban J. Hysteroadenosis metastatica, Die lymphogene Genese der sog. Adenofibromatosis heterotopica. Arch Gynecol 1925; 124: 457–482.

13. Javert CT. Observations on the pathology and spread of endometriosis based on the theory of benign metastasis. Am J Obstet Gynecol 1951; 62: 477–487.

14. Nisolle M, Casanas-Roux F, Anaf V, et al. Morphometric study of the stromal vascularization in peritoneal endometriosis. Fertil Steril 1993; 59: 681–684.

15. Nisolle M, Casanas-Roux F, Donnez J. Peritoneal endometriosis: new aspects in two-dimensional and three-dimensional evaluation. In: Sutton C, Diamond M, eds. Endoscopic surgery for gynaecologists. Philadelphia: WB Saunders; 1993: 207–214.

16. Matsuzaki S, Canis M, Murakami T, et al. Immunohistochemical analysis of the role of angiogenic status in the vasculature of peritoneal endometriosis. Fertil Steril 2001; 76: 712–716.

17. Fidler IJ. Seed and soil revisited: contribution of the organ microenvironment to cancer metastasis. Surg Oncol Clin N Am 2001; 10(2): 257–269.

18. Fidler IJ. The pathogenesis of cancer metastasis: the seed and soil hypothesis revisited. Nature Reviews 2003; 3: 1–6.

19. Reddi AH, Roodman D, Freeman C, et al. Mechanisms of tumor metastasis to the bone: challenges and opportunities. J Bone Miner Res 2003; 18(2): 190–194.

20. Hanahan D, Weinberg RA. The hallmarks of cancer. Cell 2000; 100: 57–70.

21. Varma R, Rollason T, Gupta KJ, et al. Endometriosis and the neoplastic process. Reproduction 2004; 127: 293–304.

22. D'Hooghe TM, Bambra CS, Cornillie FJ, et al. Prevalence and laparoscopic appearance of spontaneous endometriosis in the baboon (Papio anubis, Papio cynocephalus). Biol Reprod 1991; 45: 411–416.

23. D'Hooghe TM, Bambra CS, Suleman MA, et al. Development of a model of retrograde menstruation in baboons. Fertil Steril 1994; 62: 635–638.

24. D'Hooghe TM, Bambra CS, Raeymaekers BM, et al. Intrapelvic injection of menstrual endometrium causes endometriosis in baboons (Papio cynocephalus and Papio anubis). Am J Obstet Gynecol 1995; 173: 125–134.

25. Bergqvist A, Jeppsson S, Kullander S, et al. Human endometrium transplanted into nude mice. Histologic effects of various steroid hormones. Am J Pathol 1985; 119: 336–344.

26. Nisolle M, Casanas-Roux F, Marbaix E, et al. Transplantation of cultured explants of human endometrium into nude mice. Hum Reprod 2000; 15: 572–577.

27. Aoki D, Katsuki Y, Shimizu A, et al. Successful heterotransplantation of human endometrium in SCID mice. Obstet Gynecol 1994; 83: 220–228.

28. Nisolle M, Casanas-Roux F, Donnez J. Early-stage endometriosis: adhesion and growth of human menstrual endometrium in nude mice. Fertil Steril 2000; 74: 306–312.

29. Beliard A, Noel A, Goffin, F et al. Role of endocrine status and cell type in adhesion of human endometrial cells to the peritoneum in nude mice. Fertil Steril 2002; 78: 973–978.

30. Singer CF, Marbaix E, Kokorine I, et al. Paracrine stimulation of interstitial collagenase (MMP-1) in the human endometrium by interleukin 1 alpha and its dual block by ovarian steroids. Proc Natl Acad USA 1997; 94(19): 10341–10345.

31. Noel A, Kebers F, Maquoi E, et al. Cell-cell and cell-matrix interactions during breast cancer progression. Curr Top Pathol 1999; 93: 183–193.

32. Groothuis PG, Koks CA, de Goeij AF, et al. Adhesion of human endometrium to the epithelial lining and extracellular matrix of amnion in vitro: an electron microscopic study. Hum Reprod 1998; 13: 2275–2281.

33. Koks CA, Groothuis PG, Dunselman GA, et al. Adhesion of shed menstrual tissue in an in-vitro model using amnion and peritoneum: a light and electron microscopic study. Hum Reprod 1999; 14: 816–822.

34. Groothuis PG, Koks CA, de Goefje AF et al. Adhesion of human endometrial fragments to peritoneum in vitro. Fertil Steril 1999; 71: 1119–1124.

35. Witz CA, Montoya-Rodriguez IA, Schenken RS. Whole explants of peritoneum and endometrium: a novel model of the early endometriosis lesion. Fertil Steril 1999; 71: 56–60.

36. Witz C, Thomas MR, Montoya-Rodriguez IA, et al. Short-term culture of peritoneum explants confirms attachment of endometrium to intact peritoneal mesothelium. Fertil Steril 2001; 75: 385–390.

37. Beliard A, Noel A, Goffin F, et al. Adhesion of endometrial cells labelled with [111]indium-tropolonate to peritoneum: a novel in vitro model to study endometriosis. Fertil Steril 2003; 79: 724–729.

38. Beliard A, Donnez J, Nisolle M, et al. Localization of laminin, fibronectin, E-cadherin and integrins in endometrium and endometriosis. Fertil Steril 1997; 67(2): 266–272.

39. Van den Brule FA, Berchuck A, Bast RC, et al. Differential expression of the 67-kD laminin receptor and 31-kD human laminin-binding protein in human ovarian carcinomas. Eur J Cancer 1994; 30A(8): 1096–1099.

40. Van den Brule FA, Waltregn D, Castronovo V. Increased expression of galectin-1 in carcinoma-associated stroma predicts poor outcome in prostate carcinoma patients. Pathol 2001; 193(1): 80–87.

41. Koks CA, Groothuis PG, Dunselman GA, et al. Adhesion of menstrual endometrium to extracellular matrix: the possible role of integrin alpha6beta1 and laminin interaction. Mol Hum Reprod 2000; 6: 170–177.

42. Witz CA, Takahashi A, Montoya-Rodriguez IA, et al. Expression of the alpha2beta1 and alpha3beta1 integrins at the surface of mesothelial cells: a potential attachment site of endometrial cells. Fertil Steril 2000; 74: 579–584.

43. Gaetje R, Kotzian S, Herrmann G, et al. Non malignant epithelial cells, potentially invasive in human endometriosis, lack the tumor suppressor molecule E-cadherin. Am J Pathol 1997; 150: 461–467.

44. Li LC, Chui RM, Sasaki M, et al. A simple nucleotide polymorphism in the E-cadherin gene promoter alters transcriptional activities. Cancer Res 2000; 60: 873–876.

45. Marbaix E, Kokorine I, Moulin P, et al. Menstrual breakdown of human endometrium can be mimicked in vitro and is selectively and reversibly blocked by inhibitors of matrix metalloproteinases. Proc Natl Acad Sci USA 1996; 93: 9120–9125.

46. Goffin F, Munaut C, Frankenne F, et al. Expression pattern of metalloproteinases and tissue inhibitors of matrix-metalloproteinases in cycling human endometrium. Biol Reprod 2003; 69: 976–984.

47. Chung HW, Lee JY, Moon H-S, et al. Matrix metalloproteinase-2, membranous type I matrix metalloproteinase, and tissue inhibitor of metalloproteinase-2 expression in ectopic and eutopic endometrium. Fertil Steril 2002; 78: 787–795.

48. Kokorine I, Nisolle M, Donnez J, et al. Expression of interstitial collagenase (matrix metalloproteinase-1) is related to the activity of human endometriotic lesions. Fertil Steril 1997; 68: 246–251.

49. Wenzl RJ, Heinzl H. Localization of matrix metalloproteinase-2 in uterine endometrium and ectopic implants. Gynecol Obstet Invest 1998; 45: 253–257.

50. Gottschalk C, Malberg K, Arndt M, et al. Matrix metalloproteinases and TACE play a role in the pathogenesis of endometriosis. Adv Exp Med Biol 2000; 477: 483–486.

51. Chung HW, Wen Y, Chun SH, et al. Matrix metalloproteinase-9 and tissue inhibitor of metalloproteinase-3 mRNA expression in ectopic and eutopic endometrium in women with endometriosis: a rationale for endometrioric invasiveness. Fertil Steril 2001; 75: 152–159.

52. Bruner-Tran K, Webster-Clair D, Osteen KJ. Experimental endometriosis: the nude mouse as a xenograft host. Ann N Y Acad Sci 2002; 955: 328–339.

53. Bruner KL, Matrisian LM, Rodgers WH, et al. Suppression of matrix metalloproteinases inhibits establishment of ectopic lesions by human endometrium in nude mice. Clin Invest 1997; 99: 2851–2857.

54. Bruner-Tran KL, Eisenberg E, Yeaman GR, et al. Steroid and cytokine regulation of matrix metalloproteinase expression in endometriosis and the establishment of experimental endometriosis in nude mice. J Clin Endocrinol Metab 2002; 87: 4782–4791.

55. Folkman J, Shing Y. Angiogenesis. J Biol Chem 1992; 267: 10931–10934.

56. Oosterlynck DJ, Meuleman C, Sobis H, et al. Angiogenic activity of peritoneal fluid from women with endometriosis. Fertil Steril 1993; 59: 778–782.

57. McLaren J, Prentice A, Charnock-Jones DS, et al. Vascular endothelial growth factor (VEGF) concentrations are elevated in peritoneal fluid of women with endometriosis. Hum Reprod 1996; 11: 220–223.

58. Oosterlynck DJ, Cornillie FJ, Waer M, et al. Immunohistochemical characterization of leucocyte subpopulations in endometriotic lesions. Arch Gynecol Obstet 1993; 253: 197–206.

59. Smith SK. Angiogenesis, vascular endothelial growth factor and the endometrium. Hum Reprod Update 1998; 4: 509–519.

60. Hyder SM and Stancel GM. Regulation of angiogenic growth factors in the female reproductive tract by estrogens and progestins. Mol Endocrinol 1999; 13: 806–811.

61. Donnez J, Smoes P, Gillerot S, et al. Vascular endothelial growth factor (VEGF) in endometriosis. Hum Reprod 1998; 13: 1686–1690.

62. Zhang R, Wild R, Ojago JA. Effect of tumor necrosis factor-α on adhesion of human endometrial stromal cells to peritoneal mesothelial cells: an in vitro system. Fertil Steril 1993; 59: 1196–1201.

63. Enmark E, Pelto-Huikko M, Grandien K. Human estrogen receptor β-gene structure, chromosomal localization, and expression pattern. J Clin Endocrinol Metab 1997; 82: 4258–4265.

64. Matsuzaki S, Murakami T, Uehara S, et al. Expression of estrogen receptor alpha and beta in peritoneal and ovarian endometriosis. Fertil Steril 2001; 75: 1198–1205.

65. Bulun SE, Zeitoun KM, Takayama K, et al. Estrogen biosynthesis in endometriosis: molecular basis and clinical relevance. J Mol Endocrinol 2000; 25: 35–42.

66. Noble LS, Simpson ER, John A, et al. Aromatase expression in endometriosis. J Clin Endocrinol Metab 1996; 81: 174–179.

67. Bulun SE, Gurates B, Fang Z, et al. Mechanisms of excessive estrogen formation in endometriosis. J Reprod Immunol 2002; 55: 21–33.

68. Noble LS, Takayama K, Zeitoun KM, et al. Prostaglandin E2 stimulates aromatase expression in endometriosis-derived stromal cells. J Clin Endocrinol Metab 1997; 82: 600–606.

69. Chen DB, Yang ZM, Hilsenroth R, et al. Stimulation of prostaglandin (PG) F2 alpha and PGE2 release by tumour necrosis factor-alpha and interleukin-1 alpha in cultured human luteal phase endometrial cells. Hum Reprod 1995; 10: 2773–2780.

70. Nisolle M, Casanas-Roux F, Wyns C, et al. Immunohistochemical analysis of estrogen and progesterone receptors in endometrium and peritoneal endometriosis: a new quantitative method. Fertil Steril 1994; 4: 751–759.

71. Nisolle M, Casanas-Roux F, Donnez J. Immunhistochemical analysis of proliferative activity and steroid receptor expression in peritoneal and ovarian endometriosis. Fertil Steril 1997; 68: 912–917.

72. Attia GR, Zeitoun K, Edwards D, et al. Progesterone receptor isoform A but not B is expressed in endometriosis. J Clin Endocrinol Metab 2000; 85: 2897–2902.

73. Zeitoum K, Bulun S. Aromatase: a key molecule in the pathophysiology of endometriosis and a therapeutic target. Fertil Steril 1999; 72: 961–969.

74. Stewart BW. Mechanisms of apoptosis: integration of genetic, biochemical, and cellular indicators. J Natl Cancer Inst 1994; 86: 1286–1296.

75. Dmowski WP, Ding J, Shen J. Apoptosis in endometrial glandular and stromal cells in women with and without endometriosis. Hum Reprod 2001; 16: 1802–1808.

76. Braun DP, Ding J, Shen J, et al. Relationship between apoptosis and the number of marcophages in eutopic endometrium from women with and without endometriosis. Fertil Steril 2002; 78: 830–835.

77. Jones RK, Searle RF, Stewart JA, et al. Apoptosis, bcl-2 expression and proliferative activity in human endometrial stroma and endometrial granulated lymphocytes. Biol Reprod 1998; 58: 995–1002.

78. Beliard A, Noel A, Foidart JM. Reduction of apoptosis and proliferation in endometriosis. Fertil Steril 2004; 82: 80–85.

79. Kao LC, Germeyer A, Tulac S, et al. Expression profiling of endometrium from women with endometriosis reveals candidate genes for disease based implantation failure and infertility. Endocrinology 2003; 144 (7): 2870–2881.

80. Haney AF, Muscato JJ, Weinberg JB. Peritoneal fluid cell populations in infertility patients. Fertil Steril 1981; 35: 696–698.

81. Dmowski WP, Gebel HM, Braun DP. The role of cell-mediated immunity in pathogenesis of endometriosis. Acta Obstet Gynecol Scand 1994; 159: 7–14.

82. Lebovic DI, Mueller MD, Taylor RN. Immunobiology of endometriosis. Fertil Steril 2001; 75: 1–10.

83. Hill JA, Faris HM, Schiff I, et al. Characterization of leukocyte subpopulations in the peritoneal fluid of women with endometriosis. Fertil Steril 1988; 50: 216–222.

84. Ryan IP, Tseng JF, Schriock ED, et al. Interleukin-8 concentrations are elevated in peritoneal fluid of women with endometriosis. Fertil Steril 1995; 63: 929–932.

85. Bullimore DW. Endometriosis is sustained by tumour necrosis factor-alpha. Med Hypotheses 2003; 60(1): 84–88.

86. Arici A, Tazuke SI, Attar E, et al. Interleukin-8 concentrations are elevated in peritoneal fluid of women with endometriosis and modulation of interleukin-8 expression in human mesothelial cells. Mol Hum Reprod 1996; 2: 40–45.

87. Arici A. Local cytokines in endometrial tissue: the role of interleukin-8 in the pathogenesis of endometriosis. Ann N Y Acad Sci 2002; 955: 101–109.

88. Iwabe T, Harada T, Tsudo T, et al. Pathogenetic significance of increased levels of interleukin-8 in the peritoneal fluid of patients with endometriosis. Fertil Steril 1998; 69: 924–930.

89. Mulayim N, Savlu A, Guzeloglu-Kayisli O, et al. Regulation of endometrial stromal cell matrix metalloproteinase activity and invasiveness by interleukin-8. Fertil Steril 2004; 81(Suppl): 904–911.

90. Akoum A, Kong J, Metz C, et al. Spontaneous and stimulated secretion of monocyte chemotectic protein-1 and macrophage migration inhibitory factor by peritoneal macrophages in women with and without endometriosis. Fertil Steril 2002; 77: 989–994.

91. Kats R, Metz C, Akoum A. Macrophage migration inhibitory factor is markedly expressed in active and early-stage endometriotic lesions. J Clin Endocrinol Metab 2002; 87: 883–889.

92. Witz CA, Montoya IA, Dey TD, et al. Characterization of lymphocyte subpopulations and T cell activation in endometriosis. Am J Reprod Immunol 1994; 32: 173–179.

93. Hornung D, Ryan IP, Chao VA, et al. Immunolocalization and regulation of the chemokine RANTES in human endometrial and endometriosis tissues and cells. J Clin Endocrinol Metab 1997; 82: 1621–1628.

94. Watanabe-Fukanaga R, Brannan CI, Itoh N, et al. The cDNA structure, expression, and chromosomal assignment of the mouse Fas antigen. J Immunol 1992; 148: 1274–1279.

95. Itoh N, Yonehara S, Ishii A, et al. The polypeptide encoded by the cDNA for human cell surface antigen Fas can mediate apoptosis. Cell 1991; 66: 233.

96. Nagata S. Fas and Fas-ligand: a death factor and its receptor. Adv Immunol 1994; 57: 129–135.

97. Suda T, Okasaki T, Naito Y, et al. Expression of the Fas-ligand in T cell linage. J Immunol 1995; 154: 3806–3813.

98. Rouvier E, Luciani MF, Goldstein P. Fas involvement in Ca2-independent T cell-mediated cytotoxicity. J Exp Med 1993; 1: 195–200.

99. Powell WC, Fingleton B, Wilson CL, et al. The metalloproteinase matrilysin proteolytically generates active soluble Fas-ligand and potentiates epithelial cell apoptosis. Curr Biol 1999; 9: 1441–1447.

100. Kayagaki N, Kawasaki A, Ebata T, et al. Metalloproteinase mediated release of human Fas-ligand. J Exp Med 1995; 182: 1777–1783.

101. Nagata S, Goldstein P. The Fas death factor. Science 1995; 267: 1449–1456.

102. Abreu M, Vidrich A, Lynch D, et al. Divergent induction of apoptosis and interleukin-8 secretion in HT-29 cells in response to TNF-alpha and ligation of Fas antigen. J Immunol 1995; 155: 4147–4154.

103. Selam B, Kayisli UA, Garcia-Velasco JA, et al. Extracellular matrix-dependent regulation of Fas ligand expression in human endometrial stromal cells. Biol Reprod 2002; 66: 1–5.

104. Garcia-Velasco JA, Mulayim N, Kayisli UA, et al. Elevated soluble Fas ligand levels may suggest a role for apoptosis in women with endometriosis. Fertil Steril 2002; 78: 855–859.

105. Takayama K, Zeitoum K, Gunby RT, et al. Treatment of severe postmenopausal endometriosis with an aromatase inhibitor. Fertil Steril 1998; 69: 709–713.

106. Ailawadi RK, Jobanputra S, Kataria M, et al. Treatment of endometriosis and chronic pelvic with letrozole and norethindrone acetate: a pilot study. Fertil Steril 2004; 81: 290–296.

107. Spitz IM. Progesterone antagonists and progesterone receptor modulators: an overview. Steroids 2003; 68: 981–993.

108. Olive DL, Lindheim SR, Pritts EA. New medical treatments for endometriosis. Best Pract Res Clin Obstet Gynaecol 2004; 18(2): 319–328.

109. Kettel LM, Murphy AA, Morales AJ, et al. Treatment of endometriosis with the antiprogesterone mifepristone (RU486). Fertil Steril 1996; 65: 23–28.

110. Kettel LM, Murphy AA, Morales AJ, et al. Preliminary report on the treatment of endometriosis with low-dose mifepristone (RU486). Am J Obstet Gynecol 1998; 178: 1151–1156.

111. Han S, Sidell N. RU486-induced growth inhibition of human endometrial cells involves the nuclear factor-kappa B signaling pathway. J Clin Endocrinol Metab 2003; 88: 713–719.

112. Noel A, Maillard C, Rocks SN, et al. Membrane asssociated proteases and their inhibitors in tumour angiogenesis. J Clin Pathol 2004; 57: 577–584.

113. Vignali M, Infantino M, Matrone R, et al. Endometriosis: novel etiopathogenetic concepts and clinical perspectives. Fertil Steril 2002; 78: 665–678.

114. Braun DP, Ding J, Dmowski WP. Peritoneal fluid-mediated enhancement of eutopic and ectopic endometrial cell proliferation is dependent on tumor necrosis factor-alpha in women with endometriosis. Fertil Steril 2002; 78(4): 727–732.

115. D'Antonio M, Martelli F, Peano S, et al. Ability of recombinant human TNF binding protein-1 (r-hTBP-1) to inhibit the development of experimentally-induced endometriosis in rats. J Reprod Immunol 2000; 48: 81–98.

116. D'Hooghe TM, Cuneo S, Nugent N, et al. Recombinant human TNF binding protein-1 (r-hTBP-1) inhibits the development of endometriosis in baboons: a prospective, randomized, placebo- and drug-controlled study. Fertil Steril 2001; 76: S1.

117. Barrier BF, Bates CW, Leland MM, et al. Efficacy of anti-tumor necrosis factor therapy in the treatment of spontaneous endometriosis in baboons. Fertil Steril 2004; 81(S1): 775–779.

118. Kaiser MJ, Malaise MG. [How I treat rheumatoid arthritis. The arrival of a new therapeutic era: anti-tumor necrosis factor alpha antibodies]. Rev Med Liège 2002; 57(8): 486–492. [in French]

119. Somigliana E, Vigano P, Rossi G, et al. Endometrial ability to implant in ectopic sites can be prevented by interleukin-12 in a murine model of endometriosis. Hum Reprod 1999; 14: 2944–2950.

120. Ingelmo JM, Quereda F, Acièn P, et al. Intraperitoneal and subcutaneous treatment of experimental endometriosis with recombinant human interferon-α2b in a murine model. Fertil Steril 1999; 71: 907–911.

121. Keenan JA, Williams-Boyce PK, Massey PJ, et al. Regression of endometrial explants in a rat model of endometriosis treated with the immune modulators loxoribine and levamisole. Fertil Steril 1999; 72: 135–141.

122. Nap AW, Griffioen AW, Dunselman GA, et al. Antiangiogenesis therapy for endometriosis. J Clin Endocrinol Metab 2004; 89: 1089–1095.

123. Hull ML, Charnock-Jones DS, Chan CL, et al. Antiangiogenic agents are effective inhibitors of endometriosis. J Clin Endocrinol Metab 2003; 88: 2889–2899.

4 Animal studies

Cleophas M Kyama, Jason M Mwenda, and Thomas M D'Hooghe

Introduction

Endometriosis can be defined as the presence of endometrial glandular and stromal cells outside the uterine cavity. The prevalence of the disease in the general population is unknown, but among women with infertility the prevalence has been shown to range from 13–33%.[1] Endometriosis is a progressive disease in 40–50% of women of reproductive age.[2] The most frequent sites of implantation are the pelvic area and the peritoneum. The disease varies in appearance from a few minimal lesions on pelvic linings to massive ovarian endometriotic cysts that distort tubo-ovarian architecture and characteristic extensive adhesions often involving bowel, bladder, and ureter.[3] Efforts geared towards early diagnosis and treatments of endometriosis have been hampered by lack of proper methods to study and manage the disease in humans.

The approach to management of the disease demands consideration of factors such as symptoms, stage of the disease, age, and reproductive desires of patient. Surgical treatment of endometriosis may be effective in reducing dysmenorrhea, dyspareunia, non-menstrual pelvic pain, and dyschezia.[4,5] Appropriate animal models provide important in vivo systems to investigate and develop better techniques for proper surgical management of endometriosis. This chapter highlights the role of animal models in addressing the unresolved issues related to pathogenesis and management of human endometriosis.

Animal models in the management of endometriosis

Endometriosis remains an enigma in regard to etiology, characteristics, and prognosis. Some risk factors identified in women with endometriosis, such as long duration of uninterrupted menstruation, have also been identified in non-human primates with spontaneous endometriosis, including rhesus macaques[6] and baboons.[7,8] Animal models are important in biomedical research because disease presentation in these models may mimic the pathophysiologic features observed in humans. Experience over the years has shown animal models provide an excellent in-vivo model system to investigate and develop better surgical procedures in management of human endometriosis.

Role of animal models in endometriosis research

Chronic pelvic pain (CPP), emotional distress, and associated infertility are hallmarks of endometriosis among women of reproductive age. Although endometriosis has been well described and known since 1896,[9] the current knowledge on the relationship between endometriosis and infertility as well as between endometriosis and pain are still poorly understood.

Adequate knowledge regarding management of pathophysiology-associated infertility and/or pain and spontaneous evolution of the disease has been hampered by the following factors. First, there is a lack of positive correlation between stages of disease and the severity of pain. The staging of disease is based on the criteria of the revised American Fertility Society (r-AFS) classification system I.[10] This classification may be useful to document the extent and severity of the disease, but has remained somewhat unsatisfactory, due to lack of reproducibility. Furthermore, a negative correlation between the stage of endometriosis and infertility has been described[1] but the correlation between the stage of endometriosis and pain is more controversial. Secondly, the gold standard for diagnosis is laparoscopy, a technique that is not only invasive but also is not commonly available in most health facilities in developing countries. In women, it is difficult to carry out controlled experimental studies and it is not possible to monitor the true prevalence or progression of endometriosis without performing repeated laparoscopies that are unacceptable due to ethical reasons. Since spontaneous endometriosis occurs in humans and non-human primates only, non-human primate models may help our understanding of etiology, spontaneous evolution, and physiopathology of endometriosis.

Rodent models

The most extensively used rodent models in the experimental study of endometriosis include the rat, rabbit, the hamster,[11–13] the nude mouse, and the severe combined immunodeficient (SCID) mouse.[14,15] Rodent models offer some advantages because they are cheap and easy to manipulate. However, rodent models have numerous drawbacks for endometriosis studies: they exhibit a wider phylogenetic gap with humans, lack a menstrual cycle, do not develop spontaneous endometriosis, and are a small animal and thus do not allow repeated surgical interventions. The rat ovulates spontaneously but its luteal phase is shorter than that of humans, whereas the rabbit lacks a luteal phase. Endometriosis is induced surgically through autotransplantation of endometrial fragments in both rodents,[11] which is not physiologic, consequentially leading to severed uterus and additional complications associated with adhesions, which may interfere with fertility. The endometriotic lesions consist of cysts containing clear serous fluid in the rat, whereas vascularized hemorrhagic solid masses observed in the rabbit are quite different from the variety of pigmented and nonpigmented lesions exhibited in human endometriosis.[3,16]

Therefore, the surgical induction of endometriosis in these rodent models does not result in the true features of human endometriosis disease. As an alternative, the use of immunocompromised animals, such as the athymic (nude) mouse and the SCID mouse as models for endometriosis[14,15] has gained much interest. The advantage of these models is that they do not reject xenographic human endometrial tissue,[17] which can be introduced subcutaneously or into the peritoneal cavity. The nude mouse model has been utilized as a human endometrial tissue recipient to examine the role of steroid-regulated endometrial matrix metalloproteinases (MMPs) in the establishment of experimental endometriosis.[18] In the nude mouse model, ectopic adhesion of endometrial cells to the peritoneum and the formation of endometriotic-like lesions involve cooperation of epithelial and stromal cells through secretion of growth factors, cytokines and/or chemokines.[17,19] It is still controversial whether the data generated from this rodent model can be extrapolated to the human disease situation given the wide species difference between mice and humans.

Nonhuman primate models for endometriosis

Nonhuman primates are valuable models for biomedical research because they exhibit similar anatomic, immunologic, reproductive, and physiologic characteristics to humans and also because of the phylogenetic relationship.[20] The use of nonhuman primates is limited due to high cost of primate experimentation and maintenance in captivity. Hence, primate studies have been tailored to unravel critical questions that cannot be answered using the other experimental animals. Endometriosis occurs exclusively in menstruating species, including nonhuman primates and humans. Nonhuman primates, although expensive to maintain in captivity, offer unique advantages in endometriosis research when compared to rodents:

1. They have a close phylogenetic relatedness to human and a comparable menstrual cycle.
2. They develop spontaneous endometriosis.[21]
3. Induced endometriosis mimics human disease.[12,22,23]
4. The similar immunologic parameters and cross-reactivity of most antihuman antibodies to nonhuman primate cell surface antigens may lead to a better understanding of some immunologic aspects of endometriosis.[24,25]

Studies on rhesus monkeys and cynomolgus monkeys

Until 12 years ago, most endometriosis research had been done on rhesus and cynomolgus monkeys.[26,27] Limited studies on endometriosis had also been done using the De Brazza monkey,[28] an endangered species.

Rhesus monkeys

The occurrence of spontaneous endometriosis in rhesus monkeys has enabled scientists to investigate the genetic epidemiology of this disease[29] and the endometrial implants are morphologically identical to human endometriosis.[6] The exposure of rhesus monkeys to 0, 5, or 25 ppt TCDD (parts per trillion 2,3,7,8-tetrachlorodibenzo-p-dioxin) via their food for approximately 4 years demonstrated a dose-dependent increase in incidence and severity of endometriosis when they were assessed for spontaneous endometriosis 10 years after withdrawal of treatment.[30] Spontaneous endometriosis in the rhesus monkey has been associated with irradiation, but only after at least 6 years of exposure.[31] Rhesus monkeys share many similarities with humans, especially reproductive physiology. Menarche in rhesus monkey occurs at about 3 years of age, the length of the menstrual cycle is about 28 days, and menstrual bleeding lasts for about 4 days.[6]

Cynomolgus monkeys

Natural progression of experimental endometriosis in cynomolgus monkeys has been reported, but complete regression of macroscopic disease after pregnancy occurred in monkeys with minimal and mild disease,[32] suggesting that pregnancy exerts a beneficial effect on endometriosis.

Is the baboon the best nonhuman primate model to study endometriosis?

The baboon is one of the Old World primate species and is widely used in biomedical and behavioral research. Baboons are abundant in the African savannah land and breed fairly well in captivity[33] as opposed to the rhesus monkey, whose seasonal breeding may be disrupted when housed indoors and maintained under constant light/dark and temperature/humidity environment.[29] Baboons adapt well in captivity and they have a complex behavioral and social life.[34]

Extensive studies carried out at the Institute of Primate Research (IPR), Nairobi, Kenya have demonstrated that the baboon is a better model for studies on human endometriosis than the rhesus and cynomolgus monkeys,[35] as reviewed in the following sections of this chapter:

- Baboons have 42 chromosomes, a very close phylogenetic homology to the 46 chromosomes in humans, and share many genetic characteristics to humans.[36]
- The reproductive anatomy and physiology of baboons is well documented and include similar menstrual cycle characteristics to that of women.[20] Baboons have a menstrual cycle of 33 days, which is the similar to humans. Perineal skin inflation and deflation in the baboon, with relative precision, correspond to the follicular and luteal phases, respectively, enabling noninvasive follow-up of menstruation and follicular and luteal phases.
- The baboon has been demonstrated as a model for studies in cardiovascular and endoscopic surgery, endocrinology, teratology, and toxicology.[37]
- The baboon menstrual cycle continues throughout the year, even in captivity, as opposed to the rhesus monkey, whose breeding season can be interrupted in captivity.
- Baboons are large primates and versatile, allowing repeated sampling and performance of even complicated surgical procedures.[38]
- Accessibility of the baboon uterine cavity, through the cervix, permits sampling of endometrium without hysterotomy.[39]
- Endometriosis in the baboon is associated with lesions which undergo active remodeling, with some disappearing while other new lesions are formed.[40] Some lesions develop more aggressively and progress to the typical or colored lesions found in women.[16]
- Baboons experience a high prevalence of spontaneous endometriosis.[41]
- Laparoscopic appearances, pathologic aspects, and pelvic localization of the implants (Figure 4.1) are similar to those of the human disease.[42]

(a)

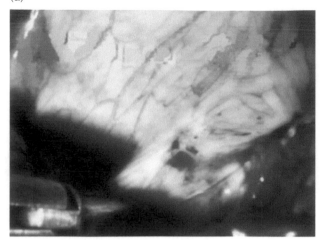

(b)

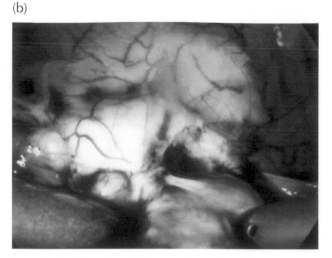

Figure 4.1 (a and b) Endometriotic lesions surrounded by fibrosis and adhesions from baboons with induced endometriosis after intrapelvic injection of menstrual endometrium.

Prevalence of spontaneous endometriosis in rhesus monkeys and baboons

Most studies on the prevalence of endometriosis among nonhuman primates have mainly focused on baboons and rhesus monkeys.

Rhesus monkeys

The prevalence of spontaneous endometriosis in rhesus macaques at necropsy has been reported for macaques ≥10 years in colony to be 31.4%,[6] whereas the prevalence among animals that had reached at least 10 years was 29%.[43] In another study, clinical endometriosis was diagnosed by laparoscopy in 16/37 (43%) macaques from the breeding colony and was confirmed by histologic examination biopsies collected from these animals. The disease was classified as minimal (40%), mild (25%), moderate (10%), or severe (25%). The most common sites of endometriosis were the serosal surface of the uterus (75%) and the posterior cul-de-sac (75%).[44]

Baboons

In our previous studies, we have shown that baboons of proven fertility have a prevalence of 25% spontaneous endometriosis with laparoscopic appearance (see Figure 4.1) and pelvic localization similar to that found in human disease.[41] The prevalence of endometriosis in baboons without previous hysterotomy (8%) was comparable to the reported 7.5% prevalence of endometriosis in asymptomatic women undergoing sterilization.[45]

Effect of age, duration of captivity, and pregnancy on the prevalence of endometriosis in non-human primates

An increased prevalence of endometriosis (27%) has been observed in baboons that had been maintained in captivity for more than 2 years.[39] Among rhesus monkey, prevalence of endometriosis increased with age from about 10% among those aged 10–12 years to about 40% among those aged 15 years or older at death.[6] This could be caused by the high number of menstrual cycles in captivity without interruption by pregnancy, which does not occur in the wild where they are mostly pregnant or breast-feeding. It is also possible that the increased prevalence may be due to captivity-associated stress. Due to limited social interactions and constrained physical exercise, baboons in captivity may lead a stressful lifestyle,[7] which may be an exposing risk factor for development of endometriosis. Recent studies suggest that immune dysfunction may be associated with a stressful lifestyle, and thus suboptimal immune functions may be associated with the pathogenesis of endometriosis.[46]

Endometriosis is thought to undergo regression during pregnancy in women and in cynomolgus monkeys with experimental endometriosis.[32] Conversely, other investigators reported enlargement of endometriotic lesions during the first trimester and regression during the remaining part of pregnancy.[47] However, studies done in 1997 in the baboon have shown that pregnancy may not have a significant effect on endometriosis during the first and second trimester.[48]

Spontaneous evolution of endometriosis in nonhuman primates

According to the current knowledge about endometriosis in women, the natural history of endometriosis seems to have been poorly studied. Endometriosis appears to be a dynamic disease that is progressive in some women,[49] static in some, and resolves in others.[50]

In baboons, spontaneous endometriosis has been reported to be a progressive disease.[51] Serial laparoscopic observations were performed over a 30-month period in 13 baboons with spontaneous endometriosis. During each laparoscopy, the pelvis was examined for the presence of endometriosis; the number, size, and type of endometriotic implants were noted on a pelvic map; the endometriosis score and stage was calculated according to the r-AFS.[10] An increase in the number of endometriotic lesions was observed in baboons after 10 months with spontaneous endometriosis compared to the number of lesions scored during the first laparoscopy.[5] The remodeling, defined by transition of lesions between typical, subtle, and suspicious implants, was observed in 23% of lesions. A study of 24 baboons, with an initially normal pelvis, demonstrated a cumulative endometriosis incidence of 29% and 64% within 12 and 32 months, respectively.[52] This study suggests that endometriosis is a dynamic and moderately progressive disease, with periods of development and regression and with active remodeling between different types of lesions,[51] as seen in women with endometriosis.[53]

Pathogenesis of endometriosis

Major investigations are now focused on trying to understand the pathogenesis of endometriosis. The theory that has gained most supportive evidence for the pathogenesis of peritoneal endometriosis is Sampson's theory[54] of retrograde menstruation. This theory is supported by several factors: first, retrograde menstruation occurs in 70–90% of women[55] and 83% of female baboons.[39] Secondly, women with early menarche, short

cycle, and long duration of menstrual flow are perceived to be at higher risk of disease development.[56] Obstructed menstrual outflow, probably associated with increased retrograde menstruation, has been associated with endometriosis in 77% of patients with functional endometrium and patent tubes, and in up to 89% of those with hematocolpos/hematometra.[57]

Retrograde menstruation is a widely accepted and proposed mechanism that may explain the presence of endometrial cells in the extrauterine site.[54] An experiment to support the Sampson hypothesis was done by intrapelvic injection of menstrual endometrium in baboons, which caused extensive peritoneal endometriosis with adhesions.[1,23,35] However, this theory does not account for the fact that these misplaced cells survive in women with endometriosis and not in healthy women. Based on studies done in both humans and baboons, an immunologic etiology has been proposed, as demonstrated by increased inflammatory parameters in subjects with endometriosis when compared with controls.[58,59]

Endometriosis-associated infertility

Endometriosis occurs in 30–40% of women with infertility. The severe form of this condition has been associated with scarring and adhesions in the pelvis, leading to mechanical blockage, prevention of the fusion of sperm and egg, and disruption of normal pelvic anatomy. Other studies have shown that women with endometriosis are much more likely to be infertile, even when they ovulate and have anatomically patent fallopian tubes.[60]

Indeed, endometriosis has been associated with infertility even in the absence of adhesions or anatomic distortion of pelvis. Infertility of women with minimal endometriosis has been suggested to be caused by ovulatory dysfunction.[61] Koninckx et al[62] suggested minimal endometriosis-associated infertility might be due to luteinized unruptured follicle (LUF) syndrome. A study done on cynomolgus monkeys with endometriosis showed that impaired fertility appeared to be mediated primarily by failure of follicular rupture and/or pelvic adhesion.[63] In this study, an LUF was noted in 5 of 10 cycles in monkeys with endometriosis and in 3 of the 6 cycles in animals with severe cases, whereas no LUF was reported in controls or animals with microscopic and mild endometriosis.[63] In baboons, serial laparoscopies were carried out to investigate the re-epithelialization of the ovulation stigma during the luteal phase in baboons.[64] If a fresh ovulation, stigma was observed in baboons within 5 days after ovulation; it diminished in size but remained visible up to 8, 12, and 16 days after ovulation in 91%, 75%, and 50% of animals, respectively.[64]

If the data obtained in baboons can be extrapolated to the clinical investigation of the infertile woman, it would appear that laparoscopies performed for the documentation of a fresh ovulation stigma should be done as early after ovulation as possible, preferably immediately.[64] D'Hooghe et al[39,65] reported a higher incidence and recurrence of corpus luteum without fresh ovulation stigma in baboons with mild endometriosis than in controls, and this was associated with a reduced egg recovery. This study suggested that the existence of the LUF syndrome could be a contributing factor to mild endometriosis-associated subfertility.

However, in baboons minimal endometriosis appears not to be associated with infertility. Baboons with minimal endometriosis had a cycle fecundity rate of 18%, whereas baboons with a normal pelvis had a cycle fecundity rate of 24%,[66] which relatively corresponds to the normal monthly fecundity rate (MFR) of 20% observed in fertile women and in patients with minimal endometriosis.[67] However, mild, moderate, or severe endometriosis in baboons is associated with infertility, even in the absence of ovarian endometriotic cysts.[66,68]

Endometriosis-associated pelvic pain

CPP is a major health problem. It is the reason for 10% of all outpatient visits to a gynecologist, as well as being responsible for approximately 40% of laparoscopies and 10–15% of hysterectomies.[69]

Endometriosis has been associated with CPP in women of reproductive age. Other clinical symptoms of endometriosis are dysmenorrhea, dyspareunia, and chronic nonmenstrual pain.[70] Endometriosis may invoke several mechanisms that may provoke pain, including peritoneal inflammation, infiltration and tissue damage, delivery of tissue mediators of pain, adhesion, and scar formation.[70] Among nonhuman primates, endometriosis-associated pain may be a cause of discomfort. Reports from rhesus macaques with

spontaneous endometriosis has suggested altered behavior likely to be related to discomfort, abdominal distention due to pelvic mass, and, occasionally, cachexia due to full thickness of bowel involvement.[72]

In a randomized, double-blind trial of laparoscopic treatment with the carbon dioxide laser, Sutton and colleagues[4] reported a 72.5% reduction or resolution of symptoms among patients with endometriosis and pelvic pain when compared with 22.6% among controls after 6 months. Pain scores may be used to compare treatments for pelvic pain and provide useful information for preoperative counseling.[73] The management of endometriosis in women with CPP is dependent on the patient's age, her desire for childbearing, the severity of pain, and the response to previous treatment.[71]

Baboon model to evaluate the safety and efficacy of new methods in the treatment of endometriosis and associated infertility and pelvic pain

Although endometriosis-related infertility is poorly understood, surgery appears to be the primary choice of treatment. Endometriosis is also characterized by painful periods (dysmenorrhea), pain during sexual intercourse (dyspareunia), and CPP. Current treatment is limited because the causes of the disease are not well understood. These treatment regimens include hormonal drugs to suppress the menstrual cycle, surgical ablation of the endometriotic lesions, or, finally, as definitive treatment with hysterectomy and removal of ovaries.

Future potential targets in the management of endometriosis may include nonsurgical and nonhormonal methods to eliminate pain and improve fertility. These have been reviewed extensively recently.[58,74,75] In the future, the baboon model for endometriosis should be used to test new drugs in the prevention or treatment of endometriosis and of endometriosis-associated subfertility.[58] Since intrapelvic injection of menstrual endometrium causes moderate to severe endometriosis in most baboons, it is possible to either do prevention studies (prevent attachment of menstrual endometrium on the uterine peritoneum) or treatment studies (reduce extent of induced endometriosis after medical or surgical therapy).[58] Furthermore, placebo-controlled randomized trials can be done to evaluate the effect of new antiendometriosis drugs on endometriosis-associated subfertility with the possibility of complete standardization for the degree of endometriosis (after intrapelvic injection of menstrual endometrium). For the presence of ovulation – this can be interpreted based on the perineal cycle; perineal skin inflation and deflation, in the female baboons, with relative precision, correspond to the follicular and luteal phases, respectively, enabling noninvasive follow up menstruation, and ovulation is know to occur about 3 days before perineal deflation, with a margin of error of 2 days[76] – and for male factors (timed intercourse with male baboon of proven fertility, controlled by behavioral observation and postcoital test, as described before).[58]

Intrapelvic injection of menstrual endometrium also allows the possibility of studying early endometrial–peritoneal interaction at short-term intervals during in-vivo culture and could give a very important insight into the early development of endometriotic lesions[58] and offer better understanding of the role of endometrium, peritoneum, and peritoneal fluid in the onset of endometriosis. This would be very important in assessing the validity of the Sampson hypothesis.

Conclusion

Endometriosis is a debilitating condition among women of reproductive age and a major disease burden on healthcare systems worldwide. Several animal models have been used to study the pathophysiology of endometriosis. Extensive experimental studies, using baboons and other nonhuman primate models support the superiority of the baboon model for better understanding of human endometriosis. Indeed, spontaneous or induced endometriosis in baboons shares important morphologic and clinical features with the disease in women, as has been reviewed extensively. Currently, baboons appear to be the best models for the evaluation of endometriosis-associated subfertility and for the preclinical evaluation of new medical methods to prevent the onset of endometriosis or to cure established endometriosis.

Acknowledgments

Thomas M D'Hooghe has been supported by grants from the Leuven Research Council (1999–2008) and from the Flemish Fund for Scientific Research (1999–2003). He is a part-time (50%) senior clinical investigator on the pathogenesis of endometriosis funded by the Flemish Fund for Scientific Research (1998–2007).

REFERENCES

1. D'Hooghe TM, Debrock S, Hill JA, et al. Endometriosis and subfertility: is the relationship resolved? Semin Reprod Med 2003; 21: 243–254.

2. D'Hooghe TM, Hill JA. Endometriosis. In: Berek JS, Adashi EY, Hillard PA, eds. Novak's gynecology, 13th edn. Philadelphia: Lippincott, Williams, and Wilkins; 2002:931–972.

3. Jansen RPS. Russell P. Nonpigmented endometriosis: clinical, laparoscopic and pathologic definition. Am J Obstet Gynecol 1986; 155: 1160–1163.

4. Sutton CJ, Ewen SP, Whitelaw N, et al. Prospective, randomized, double-blind, controlled trial of laser laparoscopy in the treatment of pelvic pain associated with minimal, mild, and moderate endometriosis. Fertil Steril 1994; 62: 696–700.

5. Garry R, Clayton R, Hawe J. The effect of endometriosis and its radical laparoscopic excision on quality of life indicators. Br J Obstet Gynaecol 2000; 107: 44–54.

6. Zondervan KT, Weeks DE, Colman R, et al. Familial aggregation of endometriosis in a large pedigree of rhesus macaques. Hum Reprod 2004; 19: 448–455.

7. D'Hooghe TM, Bambra CS, De Jonge I, et al. The prevalence of spontaneous endometriosis in the baboon increases with the time spent in captivity. Acta Obstet Gynecol Scand 1995; 75: 98–101.

8. Dick EJ, Hubbard GB, Martin LJ, et al. Record review of baboons with histologically confirmed endometriosis in a large established colony. J Med Primatol 2003; 32: 39–47.

9. Cullen TS. Adeno-myoma uteri diffusum benignum. Johns Hopkins Hosp Rep 1896; 6: 133–157.

10. American Fertility Society. Revised American Fertility Society classification of endometriosis. Fertil Steril 1985; 43: 351–352.

11. Vernon MW, Wilson EA. Studies on the surgical induction of endometriosis in the rat. Fertil Steril 1985; 44: 684–694.

12. Mann DR, Collins DC, Smith MM, et al. Treatment of endometriosis in Rhesus monkeys: effectiveness of a gonadotropin-releasing hormone agonist compared to

treatment with a progestational steroid. J Clin Endocrinol Metab 1986; 63: 1277–1283.

13. Werlin LB, Hodgen GD. Gonadotropin-releasing hormone agonist suppresses ovulation, menses, and endometriosis in monkeys: an individualized, intermittent regimen. J Clin Endocrinol Metab 1983; 56: 844–848.

14. Zamah NM, Dodson MG, Stephens LC, et al. Transplantation of normal and ectopic human endometrial tissue into athymic nude mice. Am J Obstet Gynecol 1984; 149: 591–597.

15. Bergqvist A, Jeppson S, Kullander S, et al. Human uterine endometrium and endometriotic tissue transplanted into nude mice: morphologic effects of various steroid hormones. Am J Pathol 1985; 121: 337–341.

16. Martin DC, Hubert GD, Vander Zwaag R, et al. Laparoscopic appearances of peritoneal endometriosis. Fertil Steril 1989; 51: 63–67.

17. Bruner-Tran KL, Webster-Clair D, Osteen KG. Experimental endometriosis: the nude mouse as a xenographic host. Ann N Y Acad Sci 2002; 955: 328–339.

18. Bruner KL, Matrisian LM, Rodgers WH, et al. Suppression of matrix metalloproteinases inhibits establishment of ectopic lesions by human endometrium in nude mice. J Clin Invest 1997; 99: 2851–2857.

19. Beliard A, Noel A, Goffin F, et al. Adhesion of endometrial cells labeled with 111Indium-tropolonate to peritoneum: a novel in vitro model to study endometriosis. Fertil Steril 2003; 79: 724–729.

20. Stevens VC. Some reproductive studies in the baboon. Hum Reprod Update 1997; 3: 533–540.

21. Merrill JA. Spontaneous endometriosis in the Kenya baboon (Papio doguera). Am J Obstet Gynecol 1968; 101: 569–570.

22. Jacobson VC. The intraperitoneal transplantation of endometrial tissue in the rabbit. Arch Pathol Lab Med 1926; 1: 169–174.

23. D'Hooghe TM, Bambra CS, Raeymaekers BM, et al. Intrapelvic injection of menstrual endometrium causes endometriosis in baboons (Papio cynocephalus, Papio anubis). Am J Obstet Gynecol 1995; 173: 125–134.

24. D'Hooghe TM, Hill JA, Ousterlynck DJ, et al. Effect of endometriosis on white blood cell subpopulations in the peripheral blood and peritoneal fluid of baboons. Hum Reprod 1996; 11: 1736–1740.

25. D'Hooghe TM, Bambra CS, Ling Xiao, et al. The effect of menstruation and intrapelvic injection of endometrium on peritoneal fluid parameters in the baboon. Am J Obstet Gynecol 2001; 184: 917–925.

26. Lindberg BS, Busch C. Endometriosis in rhesus monkey. Ups J Med Sci 1984; 89: 129–134.

27. Fanton JW, Hubbard GB. Spontaneous endometriosis in cynomolgus monkey. Lab Anim Sci 1983; 33: 597–601.

28. Binhazim AA, Tarara RP, Suleman MA. Spontaneous external endometriosis in a De Brazza's monkey. J Comp Pathol 1989; 101: 471–474.

29. Zondervan K, Cardon L, Desrosiers R, et al. The genetic epidemiology of spontaneous endometriosis in the rhesus monkey. Ann N Y Acad Sci 2002; 955: 233–238.

30. Rier SE. The potential role of exposure to environmental toxicants in the pathophysiology of endometriosis. Ann NY Acad Sci 2002; 955: 201–212.

31. Wood DH. Long-term mortality and cancer-risk in irradiated rhesus monkeys. Radiat Res 1991; 126: 132–140.

32. Schenken RS, Williams RF, Hodgen G. Effect of pregnancy on surgically induced endometriosis in cynomolgus monkey. Am J Obstet Gynecol 1987; 157: 1392–1396.

33. Birrell AM, Hennessy A, Gillin A, et al. Reproductive and neonatal outcomes in captive bred baboons (Papio hamadryas). J Med Primatol 1996; 25: 287–293.

34. Smith K, Alberts SC, Altmann J. Wild female baboon bias their social behaviour towards paternal half sister. Proc R Soc Lond B Biol Sci 2003; 270: 503–510.

35. D'Hooghe TM. Clinical relevance of the baboon as a model for the study of endometriosis. Fertil Steril 1997; 68: 613–625.

36. Marks J. Evolutionary tempo and phylogenetic inference based on primate karyotes. Cytogenet Cell Genet 1982; 34: 261–264.

37. D'Hooghe TM, Bambra CS, Farah IO, et al. High intraabdominal pressure: effects on clinical parameters and lung pathology in baboons (Papio cynocephalus and Papio anubis) Am J Obstet Gynecol 1993; 169: 1352–1356.

38. Isahakia MA, Bambra CS. Primate models for research in reproduction. In: Alexander NJ, Speiler JM, Waites GMH, eds. Gamete interaction: prospects for immunocontraception. New York: Wiley-Liss; 1990: 487–500.

39. D'Hooghe TM, Bambra CS, Raeymaekers BM, et al. Increased incidence and recurrence of retrograde menstruation in baboons with spontaneous endometriosis. Hum Reprod 1996; 11: 2022–2025.

40. D'Hooghe TM, Bambra CS, Isahakia M, et al. Evolution of minimal endometriosis in the baboon (Papio anubis, Papio cynocephalus) over a 12-month period. Fertil Steril 1992; 58: 409–412.

41. D'Hooghe TM, Bambra CS, Cornillie FJ, et al. Prevalence and laparoscopic appearance of spontaneous endometriosis in the baboon (Papio anubis, Papio cynocephalus). Biol Reprod 1991; 45: 411–416.

42. Cornillie FJ, D'Hooghe TM, Bambra CS, et al. Morphological characteristics of spontaneous endometriosis in the baboon (Papio anubis and Papio cynocephalus). Gynecol Obstet Invest 1992; 34: 225–228.

43. Hadfield RM, Yudkin PL, Coe CL, et al. Risk factors for endometriosis in the rhesus monkey (Macaca mulatta): a case-control study. Hum Reprod Update 1997; 3: 109–115.

44. Rippy MK, Lee DR, Pearson SL, et al. Identification of rhesus macaques with spontaneous endometriosis. J Med Primatol 1996; 25: 346–355.

45. Kirshon B, Poindexter AN 3rd, Fast J. Endometriosis in multiparous women. J Reprod Med 1989; 34: 215–217.

46. D'Hooghe TM, Bambra CS, Raeymaekers BM, et al. The

effects of immunosuppresion on development and progression of endometriosis in baboons (*Papio anubis*). Fertil Steril 1995; 64: 172–178.

47. McArthur JW, Ulfeelder H. The effect of pregnancy upon endometriosis. Obstet Gynecol Surv 1965; 20: 709–733.

48. D'Hooghe TM, Bambra CS, De Jonge I, et al. Pregnancy does not affect endometriosis in baboons (*Papio anubis*, *Papio cynocephalus*). Arch Gynecol Obstet 1997; 261: 15–19.

49. Chatman DL, Ward AB. Endometriosis in adolescents. J Reprod Med 1982; 27: 156–160.

50. Sutton CJG, Pooley AS, Ewen SP, et al. Follow-up report on randomised, controlled trial of laser laparoscopy in the treatment of pelvic pain associated with minimal to moderate endometriosis. Fertil Steril 1997; 68: 1070–1074).

51. D'Hooghe TM, Bambra CS, Raeymaekers BM, et al. Serial laparoscopies over 30 months show that endometriosis in captive baboons (*Papio anubis*, *Papio cynocephalus*) is a progressive disease. Fertil Steril 1996; 65: 645–649.

52. D'Hooghe TM, Bambra CS, Raeymaekers BM, et al. The cumulative incidence rate of endometriosis in baboons (*Papio anubis*, *Papio cynocephalus*) with an initially normal pelvis is 70% after 30 months. Obstet Gynecol 1996; 88: 462–466.

53. Wiegerinck MA, Van Dop PA, Brosens IA. The staging of peritoneal endometriosis by the type of active lesion in addition to the revised American Fertility Society classification. Fertil Steril 1993; 60: 461–464.

54. Sampson JA. Peritoneal endometriosis due to menstrual dissemination of endometrial tissue into the pelvic cavity. Am J Obstet Gynecol 1927; 14: 422–469.

55. Blumenkrantz MJ, Gallagher N, Bashore RA, et al. Retrograde menstruation in women undergoing chronic peritoneal dialysis. Obstet Gynecol 1981; 142: 890–895.

56. Cramer DW, Missmer SA. The epidemiology of endometriosis. Ann N Y Acad Sci 2002; 955: 11–22.

57. Olive DL, Henderson DY. Endometriosis and müllerian anomalies. Obstet Gynecol 1987; 69: 412–415.

58. D'Hooghe TM. The future of endometriosis research. Proceedings of the Vth Conference The Uterus and Human Reproduction. Session 'Anatomy and Physiology', San Giovanni in Marignano, Italy, June 5, 2004. Ann N Y Acad Sci 2004; 1034: 316–325.

59. Kyama CM, Debrock S, Mwenda JM, et al. Potential involvement of the immune system in the development of endometriosis. Reprod Biol Endocrinol 2003; 1: 123.

60. Harada T, Iwabe T, Tarakawa N. Role of cytokines in endometriosis. Fertil Steril 2001; 76: 1–10.

61. Tummon IS, Maclin VM, Radwanksa E, et al. Ovulatory dysfunction in women with minimal endometriosis or unexplained infertility. Fertil Steril 1988; 50: 716–720.

62. Koninckx PR, De Moor P, Brosens IA. Diagnosis of the luteinized unruptured follicle syndrome by steroid hormone assays on peritoneal fluid. Br J Obstet Gynaecol 1980; 87: 929–934.

63. Schenken RS, Asch RH, Williams RF, et al. Etiology of infertility in monkeys with endometriosis: luteinized unruptured follicles, luteal phase defects, pelvic adhesions, and spontaneous abortions. Fertil Steril 1984; 41: 122–130.

64. D'Hooghe TM, Bambra CS, Raeymaekers BM, et al. Disappearance of the ovulation stigma in baboons (*Papio anubis*, *Papio cynocephalus*) as determined by serial laparoscopies during the luteal phase. Fertil Steril 1996; 65: 1219–1223.

65. D'Hooghe TM, Bambra CS, Raeymaekers BM, et al. Incrased incidence and recurrence of recent corpus luteum without ovulation stigma (luteinized unruptured follicle syndrome?) in baboons with endometriosis. J Soc Gynecol Investig 1995; 3: 140–144.

66. D'Hooghe TM, Bambra CS, Koninckx PR. Cycle fecundity in baboons of proven fertility with minimal endometriosis. Gynecol Obstet Invest 1994; 37: 63–65.

67. Rodriguez-Escudero FJ, Neyro JL, Corcostegui B, et al. Does minimal endometriosis reduce fecundity? Fertil Steril 1988; 50: 522–524.

68. D'Hooghe TM, Bambra CS, Raeymaekers BM, et al. A prospective controlled study over 2 years shows a normal monthly fertility rate (MFR) in baboons with stage I endometriosis and a decreased MFR in primates with stage II and stage III–IV disease. Fertil Steril 1996; 66: 809–813.

69. Gelbaya TA, El-Halwagy HE. Focus on primary care: chronic pelvic pain in women. Obstet Gynecol Surv 2001; 56: 757–764.

70. Milingos S, Protopapas A, Drakakis P, et al. Laparoscopic management of patients with endometriosis and chronic pelvic pain. Ann N Y Acad Sci 2003; 997: 269–273.

71. Porpora MG, Gomel V. The role of laparoscopy in the management of pelvic pain in women of reproductive age. Fertil Steril 1997; 68: 765–779.

72. MacKenzie WF, Casey HW. Animal model of human disease. Endometriosis. Animal model: endometriosis in rhesus monkeys. Am J Pathol 1975; 80: 341–344.

73. Abbott J, Hawe J, Shaltoot N, et al. Pelvic pain scores in women without pelvic pathology. J Am Assoc Gynecol Laparosc 2002; 9: 414–417.

74. D'Hooghe TM, Debrock S, Kyama CM, et al. Baboon model for fundamental and preclinical research in endometriosis. Gynecol Obstet Invest 2004; 57: 43–45.

75. D'Hooghe TM, Mwenda JM, Hill JA, et al. A critical review of the use and application of the baboon as a model for research in women's reproductive health. Gynecol Obstet Invest 2004; 57: 1–60.

76. Hendrickx AG, ed. Reproduction methods. In: Embryology of the baboon. Chicago: University of Chicago Press; 1971: 1–44.

5 Outcome measures

Ray Garry and Roger Hart

Introduction

Endometriosis may produce a variety of different symptoms of varying severity and lesions of variable distribution and extent. With such protean manifestations, there is confusion about how to classify the disease and how to measure the effectiveness of individual treatments. This chapter seeks to describe a workable clinical classification and to review various outcome measures that might be employed to determine the optimum therapeutic approach for this most confusing of conditions.

Background

The disorder we call endometriosis can be a condition that presents as an incidental finding in asymptomatic women or as a disorder of such severity that the sufferer's quality of life (QoL) is destroyed. Diagnosis of the extent and location may be simple and self-evident or complex in the extreme. Treatments may be cheap or extraordinarily expensive. Mild analgesic agents and/or simple hormone therapy may be appropriate in many cases, whereas for others nothing less than major extirpative surgery will suffice. Therapeutic operations may take a few minutes or many hours. In this confused situation the wrong therapeutic option is often chosen.

Clinical classification: two types of endometriosis

The majority of patients with endometriosis have only minor degrees of the disease associated with mild or moderately severe symptomatology. The absolute prevalence is unknown and is dependent on the clinical source of the patients. The presence of superficial endometriosis in asymptomatic infertile patients varies between 20 and 50%[1] and even among women unexposed to spermatozoa, deposits were found in 32% of cases.[2] Similar lesions were found in 2–5% of patients having sterilization procedures.[3] Multiple superficial deposits scattered widely across the pelvis, broad ligaments, ovaries, and abdominal cavity are features of this type of lesions.[4]

Sampson first used the term endometriosis to describe the finding of endometrial glands and stroma outside the uterus (Figure 5.1). The classic illustrations of Sampson show small blood-filled lesions on the peritoneum, the ovary (Figure 5.2), and the surface of the bowel. Subsequently, laparoscopic studies have revealed several variations in the gross morphology of such peritoneal endometriosis.[5–9] The characteristic histology is of deposits of endometrial-like glands and stroma (Figure 5.3), sometimes with evidence of menstrual shedding.[10] Even these peritoneal lesions have recently been shown to also contain smooth muscle cells, but in this situation this element is

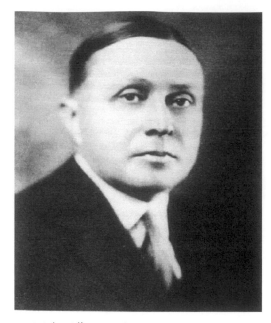

Figure 5.1 John Albertson Sampson.

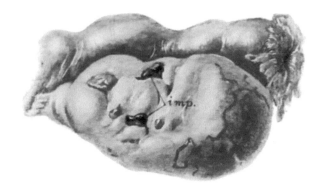

Figure 5.2 Sampson's illustration of superficial endometriotic implants.

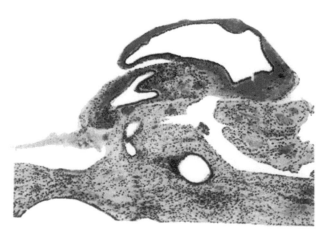

Figure 5.3 Sampson's illustration of a typical superficial endometriotic implant.

usually not clinically apparent.[11] These superficial lesions may be symptomatic and associated with both infertility and pain.

Various medical treatments, including progestogens,[12] danazol,[13] oral contraceptives,[14] and gonadotropin-releasing hormone (GnRH) agonists[15] have been shown to be effective, with none being more efficacious than the others. CO_2 laser ablation is effective in relieving pain associated with minimal, mild, and moderate endometriosis.[16] Laparoscopic surgery[17] but not medical therapy[18] has also been shown to be of benefit in treating infertility associated with superficial disease. However, a proportion of superficial lesions are asymptomatic and the clinical importance of this group has been questioned. A study from Norway demonstrated that there appears to be little risk that asymptomatic minimal endometriotic lesions will become symptomatic[19] and a study from the UK showed that minimal endometriosis was not significantly associated with pelvic pain.[20]

The second clinical manifestation of endometriosis is that associated with more severe symptoms and signs. Thomas Cullen (Figure 5.4) described a condition that he called adenomyoma of the rectovaginal septum.[21] He characterized these lesions as tumors of nonstriped muscle, with islands of

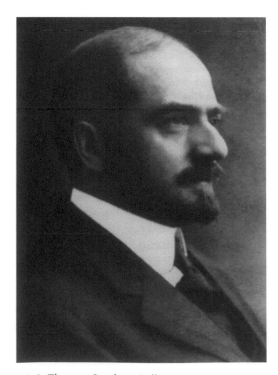

Figure 5.4 Thomas Stephen Cullen.

uterine mucosa scattered throughout them, that arise from behind the cervix and spread laterally to blend with the anterior wall of the rectum and the uterosacral ligaments. He noted that the disease might also invade the broad ligaments, encircle the ureter, and break through into the vagina (Figure 5.5). He commented that:

> Many will have undoubtedly seen these lesions, but may not have recognized them. They are of unusual importance, and if overlooked will, in time, cause the patient to become a chronic invalid.

He ventured the view that

> In less than 10 years, I feel sure that the surgeon will recognize and operate on these 'adenomyomas of the rectovaginal septum' long before the wall of the rectum or the broad ligament have been involved.

Sadly 83 years later, these views seem rather optimistic, for this type of lesion is frequently missed and/or subjected to multiple ineffective therapies. These adenomyomas require surgical removal that has been shown to be effective in a number of large series[22–25] and most recent in a placebo-controlled randomized controlled trial (RCT).[26]

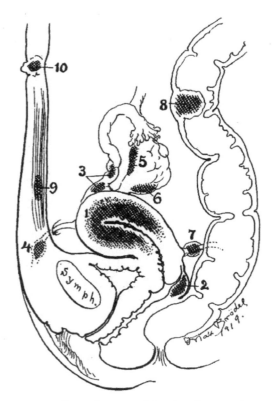

Figure 5.5 Cullen's diagram of the distribution of adenomyomas (1–10).

Cullen's term of adenomyoma is purely descriptive and gives no hint as to the possible source or cause of the lesion. These lesions show marked fibrosis in almost every case and are associated with smooth muscle metaplasia in 88% of cases in addition to the classical combination of endometrial glands and stroma.[27] These tumors have a substantial mass that can usually be palpated on careful vaginal examination. Such deeply located endometriosis is found only in the cul-de-sac (55%), the uterosacral ligaments (34%), and the uterovesical fold (11%).[28] This group found no deep lesions of endometriosis in the ovarian fossa or scattered across the peritoneum. The intensity of the patient's pain is strongly correlated with the depth of the lesion.[28–30] This type of lesion produces not only intense dysmenorrhea but also severe nonmenstrual pain, dyspareunia, and dyschesia.[24,31] The location of the lesion is correlated with the nature of the symptoms, e.g. dyspareunia is associated with uterosacral involvement and noncyclical pelvic pain and dyschesia with bowel involvement.[32] In addition to various types of pain, patients with deep endometriosis have profound disturbance in quality of life and sexual activity, as assessed by a number of validated instruments.[25,31,33] In a series of patients with this type of deeply infiltrating endometriosis, 58% of patients had disease principally in the uterosacral ligaments, 18% in the cul-de-sac, 16% involving the bowel, and 8% in the bladder.[34] The histology of this type of lesion has been described repeatedly over the years.[21,23,27,29,35–37] The nodules have three histologic components characterized by endometrial-like glands and stroma surrounded by much fibrosis and smooth muscle hyperplasia.[11] This type of histologic lesion can be best described as an adenomyoma.

It is well recognized that endometriosis is associated with infertility. Reduced chances of conception appear to be associated with both superficial and deep phenotypes of endometriosis. Despite the clinical importance of this symptom, its presence or absence does not seem to help in the clinical classification of endometriosis and so a more detailed review of this major area has not been performed in this study.

Although deep cul-de-sac endometriosis or adenomyoma can cause severe pain and distress, such lesions alone seldom threaten survival. However, some aggressive forms of adenomyoma may be potentially life-threatening conditions, e.g. when the bowel, ureter, and bladder are involved or when the lesions undergo malignant transformation.[38]

The intestines are involved in between 5 and 15% of patients with symptomatic endometriosis[39] but usually it is only the serosal surface of the bowel that is involved and, for example, only 5.4% of 3037 cases of endometriosis were of sufficient severity to require a laparotomy in one series.[40] Such lesions produce anatomical distortion and associated bowel dysfunction that may be improved by correction of the anatomy without the need for excisional bowel surgery.[23,36] Deeper colorectal endometriosis may, however, produce an obstructive syndrome and/or cyclical rectal bleeding. Formal bowel resection is then required.[40–42] This is required in about 0.2 and 16% of those with adenomyoma.[33,34,43] It was noted in Donnez's series[23] that no case of bowel involvement was found without associated adenomyoma. The histology of this type of lesion was clearly described by both Cullen[21] and Sampson.[35] Cullen described a case:

> . . . who had a recto-vaginal growth of typical adenomyatous tissue and a separate tumour that projected into the sigmoid that consisted of normal rectal mucosa but with greatly thickened muscular tissue. Scattered throughout the muscular tissue were uterine glands surrounded by the characteristic stroma.

The rectovaginal lesion and the lesion within the bowel had identical histologic features predominated by muscular hyperplasia that both authorities termed adenomyoma. It is clear that bowel endometriosis is usually multifocal, and effective therapy will need to remove all deposits.[34,42] Malignant change in colonic endometriosis has been documented. The rate of progression is unknown but is uncommon. In a recent series, 17 cases were reviewed, of whom 9 developed in patients taking unopposed estrogens.[43] A similar lesion has been described after using long-term tamoxifen therapy[44] and a clear cell carcinoma of the rectum has also been described in a 40-year-old woman with severe endometriosis treated on a long-term basis with medroxyprogesterone acetate.[45]

The need for syndromes

What then can we conveniently and accurately call these two types of endometriosis? In the absence of an agreed etiologic mechanism or unambiguous symptomatology or even a concise agreed anatomic description, it is perhaps pragmatic at this stage to classify the disease according to the sum of the anatomic location, clinical findings, and associated histologic appearances. Such a collection of symptoms, signs, and findings is a syndrome. Endometriosis appears to be two different syndromes, currently collected under the single 'endometriosis' terminology.[46]

The first syndrome may be defined as the combination of symptoms suggestive of endometriosis together with tender palpable nodular or indurative lesions in the deep pelvis. Such nodules are associated with the histologic finding of marked fibromuscular hyperplasia containing islands of endometrium-like glands. This collection of findings is precisely that described by Cullen in 1920. We would therefore suggest this collection of signs and symptoms be called Cullen's syndrome. The incidence of this syndrome is not known, but probably represents a fairly small proportion of all cases of endometriosis, with estimates of between 1/170 and 1/3800 women.[47] Cullen's syndrome, although relatively infrequent, will include many of those with the more severe symptoms, almost all those at risk of developing malignancy, and all those at risk of lower bowel and urinary tract involvement.

The other syndrome also consists of the symptoms of infertility and/or chronic pelvic pain with dysmenorrhea and dyspareunia. This syndrome is, however, associated with the absence of deep pelvic local tenderness, induration, or nodule formation. This condition is usually associated with the laparoscopic appearances of multiple classical superficial clear, red, black, or white lesions. The histology of such lesions is characterized by the findings of superficial deposits containing endometrial-like glands and stroma. These lesions have little or no associated myohyperplasia and are the same as those described by Sampson. This syndrome of pelvic pain without focal nodular lesions could therefore be known as Sampson's syndrome, and is associated with more minor symptoms, less structural changes in the pelvis, and substantially less risk of major complications.

These suggestions are made in an attempt to familiarize doctors without a special interest in endometriosis with the important realities of differing clinical degrees of endometriosis. Of course from an expert's view this clinical classification is inherently inaccurate and will only produce a fairly crude subdivision. Severe cases may be missed and there will be inaccuracies in assignment and some overlap, with both 'syndromes' occasionally coexisting. Many cases will have evidence of both superficial and deep disease, and it is quite probable that some lesions will evolve from one syndrome to the other over the course of time. In such circumstances the presence of the clinically most severe group (Cullen's syndrome) would take precedent. This classification makes no attempt to determine the origin of the lesions. They may represent different aspects of a single disease continuum or two (or three) completely different disease processes.

Despite these weaknesses and problems, we believe it is important to classify endometriosis into one of these two clinical syndromes in order that those with minor disease are not over-investigated and/or treated, while ensuring that those with major and potentially serious lesions are rapidly recognized and treated appropriately by those equipped to do so as early as possible in the course of the disease.

Outcome measures

How can we best assess the magnitude of the impact of these forms of endometriosis on a patient and how can we determine the relative effectiveness of various interventions?

Essentially we can look at:

1. change in symptoms
2. complications and adverse outcomes associated with treatments
3. changes in health-related QoL instruments
4. cost-effectiveness analysis.

Change in symptoms

Endometriosis is associated with pain and reduction in fertility potential. The most simple, and to some the most important, method of assessment of treatment effectiveness is whether it improves the chances of the patient becoming pregnant. Using this measure, hysterectomy is obviously completely inappropriate and all forms of drug therapy are also completely ineffective during the treatment course and have been shown to produce no improvement in conception rates following completion of the therapy. In contrast, laparoscopic ablation has been shown to improve fertility prospects in women with mild and moderate endometriosis[17] and more extensive laparoscopic excision improves fertility chances in women.[25]

Redwine has demonstrated that endometriosis is associated with a number of different types of pain.[22] Dysmenorrhea and painful menstruation is often the most severe and important pain element, although many women with endometriosis also suffer from nonmenstrual pelvic pain, deep dyspareunia, and various forms of menstrual-related bowel pain and dyschesia. To fully assess the impact of any treatment for endometriosis, each of these elements of pain must be individually assessed. This is usually done using some form of pain score.[22,25] Several drugs, including oral contraceptives, progestogens, danazol, and various GnRH agonists, have been shown to be equally effective in relieving elements of endometriotic pain,[15] but recurrence of pain within a few months of discontinuing the treatment is usual. Hysterectomy completely and permanently relieves the symptom of dysmenorrhea but often leaves other elements of the pain complex unaffected. There are numerous examples in the literature of aggressive disease persisting and progressing after hysterectomy and so hysterectomy alone cannot be considered a complete therapy for all cases of endometriosis and it is obviously contraindicated in the many patients wishing to preserve their fertility potential.

Laparoscopic ablation and excision have been shown to be effective in relieving many elements of the endometriosis pain symptom complex. For example, the effectiveness of laparoscopic excision in a 2–5-year study from our own unit[25] showed highly significant reductions in all elements of pain. The visual analogue pain scores of 135 women who had laparoscopic excision of endometriosis demonstrated a fall from 9 to 3.3 for dysmenorrhea, 8 to 3 for nonmenstrual pelvic pain, 7 to 0 for dyspareunia, and 7 to 2 for dyschesia. All these differences from pre-treatment to long-term post-treatment values were significant at the $p < 0.0001$ level. However, the chance of requiring further surgery 5 years after the initial surgical intervention was 36%, and so this method of intervention can also not be considered a completely effective intervention in all cases.

Complications and adverse events

Although both medications and surgery are widely advocated as alternative therapies for the management of endometriosis, there has never been an RCT comparing the relative efficacy of each.

Intuitively, extensive laparoscopic excision must be associated with significant risk of surgical complications, but this has not been formally tested. The two small placebo-controlled trials[16,26] that have been published reported no major complications but were grossly underpowered to detect small but important rates of major complications. In our larger prospective study of 135 cases, one patient suffered an unintended injury to her rectum that was repaired laparoscopically at the time of the original surgery as was a single injury to the bladder. In addition, 4% of women required a blood transfusion and the only other complication encountered was of a perforation by the Valtchev manipulator of the uterine fundus. We can conclude that there is a risk of major surgical complications associated with laparoscopic excision but the risk is fairly low and can in most cases be managed without long-term consequence to the patient. The surgical complications associated with hysterectomy by every method are now well documented.[48] These relatively rare surgically induced complications associated with laparoscopic excision and hysterectomies, however performed, are potentially serious and could be fatal.

In contrast, although the various medical therapies employed are seldom if ever associated with very serious complications, the incidence of troublesome long-term side effects is much greater. Unhappiness with side effects such as weight gain, menstrual disturbances, mood changes, or hot flashes is responsible for a high rate of failure to complete the prescribed course of medication.

When using complications as an outcome measure in comparing the effectiveness of different treatment approaches for endometriosis, it would appear that the informed consumer must choose between the fairly rare risk of the major complications associated with surgery that can usually be remedied without long-term sequelae and the much more common and troublesome but non-life-threatening complications associated with medication.

Changes in health-related quality of life

The ultimate reason why most women seek treatment for their endometriosis is that the symptoms of pain, infertility, dyspareunia, and/or bowel problems materially affect their day-to-day QoL. It is therefore logical to determine the effectiveness of differing treatments in influencing validated QoL instruments.

Using EQ-5Dindex and EQ-5Dvas, along with SF12-PCS and SF-12 MCS, quality of life instruments we have recently demonstrated that all stages of endometriosis produce marked impairment in many aspects of health-related QoL.[25] Surgical excision of all possible lesions dramatically improves every component investigated and in most circumstances restores the QoL measures to the values reported by a healthy normal population, Surgical excision produced improvements in QoL for every AFS (American Fertility Society)

stage, but was particularly effective in stage 4 disease. Such excisional surgery has also been shown to improve a woman's sexual experience and has lightheartedly been described as surgical 'Viagra' as in both our prospective and randomized control trials we demonstrated that surgical excision increased the pleasure, reduced the discomfort, and increased the frequency of sexual intercourse when compared to both placebo control and preoperative findings.

The norgestrel intrauterine system has also been shown in a single RCT to produce improvements in QoL instruments (but not pain scores) of a similar magnitude and may therefore in some circumstances be considered an appropriate alternative to surgical excision.[49] Our study clearly demonstrates that endometriosis is a most severe disease that seriously reduces a sufferer's quality of life and that laparoscopic excision substantially improves all aspects of this.[25]

Cost-effectiveness analysis

Most clinicians have over the years striven to demonstrate the evidence for the clinical effectiveness of procedures and, until recently, such evidence of clinical efficacy was all that was required to justify the introduction of a new technique into clinical practice. In the evolving delivery of health care, most healthcare providers, and particularly the UK National Health Service, now demand that evidence of the relative cost-effectiveness is also provided in addition to data on clinical effectiveness in order to drive the introduction of new techniques. Many papers include a passing reference to the costs of particular procedures and, on the basis of a superficial comparison, go on to assert that a particular treatment or approach has been shown to be cost-effective.

A formal cost-effectiveness analysis (CEA) evaluates both costs and healthcare outcomes to compare alternative healthcare programs. Costs will always include all direct costs but in the NHS and many private healthcare systems loss of productivity costs are not included in the analysis. This is a contentious issue for the overall cost of an illness and its treatment clearly includes the loss to society and the individual of their labor and the consequent income generated. However, organizations such as the UK Department of Health and many large health insurance bodies, who frequently commission CEAs, are parochially only interested in the cost to their particular budget and are not concerned by the global costs to society of an illness and its treatment. This neglect of total costs will frequently unfairly discriminate against certain treatments such as laparoscopic interventions compared with open abdominal procedures. For example in a recent CEA of different methods of hysterectomy that the senior author contributed to[50] we concluded that the cost-effectiveness of laparoscopic hysterectomy (LH) was finely balanced when compared to a total abdominal hysterectomy (TAH) when using a health service perspective to analyze the data. However, we also observed that women who had an LH took fewer days off work than women who underwent an abdominal procedure [77.8 days (CI 39.5) vs 94.87 days (CI 60.0)]. Clearly, if a monetary value was assigned to this lost productivity, the CEA for LH would be significantly strengthened.

When a new healthcare intervention is compared with the 'gold standard' therapy in a formal cost-effectiveness analysis, there are four possible outcomes:

1. The new therapy may be both more effective and cheaper. In this circumstance, the new technique is said to dominate the existing standard.
2. The new technique may be more clinically effective but also more costly than the standard therapy.
3. The new technique may be less effective but also cheaper than the existing standard.
4. The new technique may be less effective and also more expensive than the standard therapy. In this circumstance, the new treatment is dominated by the gold standard.

When the new therapy dominates the existing therapy, the novel treatment will always be preferred and, conversely, when it is dominated it should never be used. In some circumstances a new treatment that is less effective but significantly cheaper than its precursor may be selected: for example, when widespread or national use of vast quantities of a therapy is needed. In the most usual circumstance, a new technique is introduced that is more effective clinically but also more expensive than its comparator. In these last two circumstances, those who fund health care must make a balanced decision between costs and clinical efficacy.

We have discussed the technicalities of performing a valid CEA in some detail because of the frequency with which such terms are used inappropriately, often resulting in misleading conclusions. This is particularly true when considering the treatment of pain associated with endometriosis. To illustrate the problem I quote in its entirety the summary of a paper entitled, 'The

cost-effective approach to the management of endometriosis' by CA Winkel:[51]

Recent studies have demonstrated that surgical therapy offers no better results in terms of pain relief than medical therapy with gonadotrophin releasing hormone agonists. Surgical therapy requires considerable experience and expertise on the part of the surgeon and the results are likely to be operator dependent. The results of the very best surgeons, as published in the medical literature, cannot be replicated by the average gynaecologist. Medical treatment on the other hand is not operator dependent. The efficacy of clinical diagnosis given a thorough examination has been proved and the outcomes of empiric medical therapy with gonadotrophin releasing hormone agonists are substantial. Given the similar results obtained with GnRH agonists and surgical intervention and the fact that medical treatment is less expensive, primary therapy with GnRH agonists appears to be the most cost-effective approach to the management of endometriosis and pelvic pain.!! [authors punctuation]

This paper is one of the very few that attempts to evaluate the cost-effectiveness of medical and surgical treatments for endometriosis. Unfortunately, it illustrates many of the problems associated with an inadequate CEA and, in our opinion, the conclusions made in it cannot be justified from the data available.

No randomized trial comparing medical and surgical interventions in the management of endometriosis has yet been undertaken. Most of the drug-related trials that have been reported lasted for only 3–6 months of therapy and the longest trial so far reported has been 12 months. The results were reported during or immediately after the end of the therapeutic course and no trial has looked at symptom control long after discontinuing therapy. Yet the data that are available suggest that symptoms almost invariably return within 6 months of discontinuing medical therapy.

To make a meaningful determination of the most effective and cost-effective therapy for endometriosis requires prolonged follow-up of at least 5 and preferably 10 or more years. To calculate the health-related costs it is essential to know the respective symptom recurrence rates of the two approaches. We would also need to determine the rates of subsequent surgery after initial medical therapy and the need for medical therapy and repeat surgery after primary surgery. It is clearly absurd to suggest that medical therapy is more cost-effective at the end of a 6-month course of GnRH therapy if within a year of discontinuing the treatment 80% of the patients required surgical management. These data are not available and, without it, it is impossible to make a meaningful cost-effectiveness comparison.

Some of those who favor a primary surgical approach for established endometriosis have at least attempted to determine the incidence of requiring further intervention after surgery. Redwine reported that 19% of his patients required further surgery within 7 years of the primary operation.[2] We obtained rather worse results in our group, where we found that almost one-third of our patients required some further intervention within 5 years of the first operation.[25] Neither of these groups, however, presented data on how many patients required postoperative medical therapy and, without such fundamental data, it is again not possible to begin to calculate the cost-effectiveness of either type of intervention. This is of course even more apparent when attempting to calculate the cost-effectiveness of medical therapies. It is possible that most, if not all, patients with established endometriosis will require surgery shortly after completing one or more courses of medication. If this speculation is indeed true, then the cost-effectiveness of the medical approach would be very low indeed. In fact, in such circumstances medical therapy would appear to be just an expensive surgical pre-medication. Without the necessary data, such conclusions are highly speculative but are at least as likely to be correct as those contrary opinions that were speculated in the paper cited above.

The data currently available are more helpful in regard to the relative cost-effectiveness of the various treatments for infertility associated with endometriosis. Medical therapy in these circumstances has been shown to be of no value and is not indicated, but there is real doubt about whether an infertile patient with endometriosis should proceed directly to in vitro fertilization (IVF) or would benefit more by primary surgery aimed at removing the cause of the problem in its entirety. When the infertility coexists with significant pain and other major symptoms of endometriosis, the authors believe that treating the cause is more rational than managing one symptom and leaving the disease to progress. This hypothesis is as yet completely untested in an RCT. The principal clinical dilemma today remains the best management when infertility associated with endometriosis is the predominant symptom.

In a formal but simulated model, a CEA of endometriosis excision against IVF by Philips et al,[52] the group subdivided endometriosis into three levels of mild, moderate, and severe. In the case of mild and moderate endometriosis, the authors calculated that surgery would be more effective than IVF. In mild endometriosis, they calculated that IVF at less than 2 cycles would be dominated by surgery. Expected outcomes are lower and the costs are higher with IVF. At two cycles and more, expected outcomes are higher with IVF but the additional costs are such that the average cost per pregnancy will always be higher. The average cost per pregnancy calculated in 2000 is £2393 (surgery) and £8377–£9400 (IVF 1–4 cycle). The same result occurs in the case of moderate endometriosis. IVF at less than 2 cycles is dominated by surgery. The average costs per pregnancy are higher than for mild disease: £8673 (surgery), £10 416–£11 750 (IVF 1–4 cycles). In the case of severe endometriosis, the author assumes poor outcomes and the cost per pregnancy is high for both treatments' pregnancy. With their assumptions, the expected cost per pregnancy is £34 692 (surgery) and £19 488 (IVF). However, they point out that in fact surgery will be more cost-effective option if:

- the success rate of surgery exceeds 11.4%
- the success rate of IVF is less than 6.5% per cycle
- the cost of surgery is less than £364
- the cost of full IVF treatment is more than £4859.

It must be emphasized that this study is a mathematical calculation based on a series of decision-analytical models that have been developed to reflect current diagnostic and treatment pathways for couples with infertility. These are not actual calculations and are based on many assumptions, some of which are tenuous. The analysis, however, indicates the scope of a full CEA and the type of results that may be expected.

It is clear that in most modern healthcare systems the personal preferences and beliefs of individual specialists will be subjected to restrictions based on the cost-effectiveness of alternative therapeutic options. It is therefore essential that influential clinicians become familiar with the techniques of CEA and ensure that the therapeutic approaches they recommend are cost-effective. There is a great sparsity of such information available at the present time and much work needs to be done in almost every area. Nowhere is the need for this greater than in the management of endometriosis, where currently various authors are suggesting that a strong case has been made for the primary and empirical use of medical therapies in preference to surgical excision. In fact, there is as yet no such evidence and the probability is that with reasonable surgical approach the opposite is in fact true.

Conclusions

The optimum method of treatment will depend in part on the outcome measure selected. Preference for the relief of presenting symptoms, improvement in quality of life, nature and extent of associated complications, or the cost-effectiveness of each modality may determine the treatment approach selected. The surgical approach to treatment of endometriosis has been shown to be better than placebo for the management of both pelvic pain and infertility. Its superiority to medical therapy and IVF in the management of endometriosis-associated infertility is also clear, but the respective role of these two interventions in the management of pelvic pain remains uncertain. The necessary evidence is missing, and suitable RCT and CEA have not yet been performed. Enthusiasts tend to adopt any approach that suits our personal biases in the absence of authoritative data. The need is therefore to undertake further careful RCT and CEA trials of these important and conflicting therapeutic options.

REFERENCES

1. ACOG practice Bulletin. Medical management of endometriosis. Int J Gynaecol Obstet 2000; 71: 183–196.

2. Matorras R, Rodriguez F, Pijoan JI, et al. Women who are not exposed to spermatozoa and infertile women have similar rates of stage 1 endometriosis. Fertil Steril 2001; 76: 923–928.

3. Strathy JH, Molgaard CA, Coulman CB. Endometriosis and infertility: a laparoscopic study of endometriosis among fertile and infertile women. Fertil Steril 1982; 39: 667–672.

4. Sampson JA. Peritoneal endometriosis due to the menstrual dissemination of endometrial tissue into the peritoneal cavity. Am J Obstet Gynecol 1927; 14: 422–469.

5. Jansen RP, Russell P. Nonpigmented endometriosis: clinical, laparoscopic and pathologic definition. Am J Obstet Gynecol 1986; 15: 1154–1159.

6. Redwine DB. The distribution of endometriosis in the pelvis by age group and fertility. Fertil Steril 1987; 47: 173–175.

7. Stripling MC, Martin DC, Chatman DL. Subtle appearances of pelvic endometriosis. Fertil Steril 1988; 49: 427–438.

8. Martin DC, Hubert GD, Van der Zwaay R. Laparoscopic appearances of peritoneal endometriosis. Fertili Steril 1989; 51: 984–988.

9. Nisolle M, Paindaveine B, Bourdon A, et al. Histologic study of peritoneal endometriosis in infertile women. Fertil Steril 1990; 53: 984–988.

10. Sampson JA. Benign and malignant implants in the peritoneal cavity and their relationship to certain ovarian tumors. Surg Gynecol Obstet 1924; 38: 287–311.

11. Anaf V, Simon P, El Nakadi I, et al. Relationship between endometriotic foci and nerves in rectovaginal endometriotic nodules. Hum Reprod 2000; 15: 1744–1750.

12. Prentice A, Deary AJ, Bland E. Progestagens and antiprogestagens for pain associated with endometriosis. Cochrane Database System Rev 2000; CD 002122.

13. Selak V, Farquhar C, Prentice A, et al. Danazol for pelvic pain associated with endometriosis. Cochrane Database System Rev 2001; CD 000068.

14. Moore J, Kennedy S, Prentice A. Modern combined oral contraceptives for pain associated with endometriosis (Cochrane review). Cochrane Library Issue 2. Oxford: Update Software, 2003.

15. Prentice A, Deary AJ, Goldbeck-Wood S, et al. Gonadotrophin-releasing hormone analogues for pain associated with endometriosis (Cochrane review). Cochrane Library, Issue 2. Oxford: Update Software; 2003.

16. Sutton CJ, Ewen SP, Whitelaw N, et al. Prospective randomized, double-blind controlled trial of laser laparoscopy in the treatment of pelvic pain associated with minimal, mild, and moderate endometriosis. Fertil Steril 1994; 62: 696–700.

17. Marcoux S, Maheux R, Berabe S. Laparoscopic surgery in infertile women with minimal or mild endometriosis. Canadian Collaborative Group on Endometriosis. N Engl J Med 1997; 337: 217–222.

18. Hughes E, Fedorkow D, Collins J, et al. Ovulation suppression for endometriosis. Cochrane Database System Rev 2000; 2: CD000155.

19. Moen MH, Stokstad S. A long term follow-up study of asymptomatic endometriosis diagnosed incidentally at sterilisation. Fertil Steril 2002; 78: 773–776.

20. Thorton JG, Morley S, Lilleyman J, et al The relationship between laparoscopic disease, pelvic pain and infertility: an unbiased assessment. Eur J Obstet Gynecol Reprod Biol 1997; 74: 57–62.

21. Cullen TS. The distribution of adenomyomas containing uterine mucosa. Arch Surg 1920; 1: 215–283.

22. Redwine DB. Conservative laparoscopic excision of

endometriosis by sharp dissection: life table analysis of re-operation and persistent or recurrent disease. Fertil Steril 1991; 56: 628–634.

23. Donnez J, Nisolle M, Gillerot S, et al. Rectovaginal septum adenomyotic nodules: a series of 500 cases. Br J Obstet Gynaecol 1997; 104: 1014–1018.

24. Redwine DB. Conservative laparoscopic excision of endometriosis by sharp dissection: life table analysis of re-operation and persistent or recurrent disease. Fertil Steril 1991; 56: 628–634.

25. Abbott JA, Hawe J, Clayton RD, et al. The effects and effectiveness of laparoscopic excision of endometriosis: a prospective study with 2–5 year follow-up. Hum Reprod 2003; 18: 1922–1927.

26. Abbott J, Hawe J, Hunter D, et al. Laparoscopic excision of endometriosis: a randomised, placebo-controlled trial. Fertil Steril 2004; 82: 878–884.

27. Itoga T, Matsumoto T, Takeuki H, et al. Fibrosis and smooth muscle metaplasia in rectovaginal endometriosis. Pathol Int 2003: 53: 371–375.

28. Cornillie FJ, Oosterlynck D, Lauweryns JM, et al. Deeply infiltrating pelvic endometriosis: histological and clinical significance. Fertil Steril 1990; 53: 978–983.

29. Koninckx PR, Martin DC. Deep endometriosis: a consequence of infiltration or retraction or possibly adenomyosis externa? Fertil Steril 1992; 58: 924–928.

30. Chapron C, Fauconnier A, Dubuisson JB, et al. Deep infiltrating endometriosis; relation between severity of dysmenorrhoea and extent of disease. Hum Reprod 2003; 18: 760–766.

31. Garry R, Clayton R, Hawe J. The effect of endometriosis and its radical laparoscopic excision on quality of life indicators. BJOG 2000; 107: 44–54.

32. Fauconnier A, Chapron C, Dubuisson JB, et al. Relationship between pain symptoms and the anatomic location of deep infiltrating endometriosis. Fertil Steril 2002; 78: 719–726.

33. Redwine DB, Wright JT. Laparoscopic treatment of complete obliteration of the cul-de-sac associated with endometriosis: long-term follow-up of en bloc resection. Fertil Steril 2001; 76: 359–365.

34. Chapron C, Fauconnier A, Vieira M, et al. Anatomical distribution of deeply infiltrating endometriosis: surgical implications and proposition for a classification. Hum Reprod 2003; 18: 157–161.

35. Sampson JA. Perforating hemorrhagic (chocolate) cysts of the ovary. Their importance and especially their relation to pelvic adenomas of endometriotic type (adenomyoma of the uterus, rectovaginal septum, sigmoid etc.). Arch Surg 1921; 3: 245–322.

36. Reich H, McGlynn F, Salvat J. Laparoscopic treatment of cul-de-sac obliteration secondary to retrocervical deep fibrotic endometriosis. J Reprod Med 1991; 36: 516–522.

37. Brosens IA, Brosens JJ. Redefining endometriosis: Is deep endometriosis a progressive disease? Hum Reprod 2000; 15: 1–7.

38. Garry R. Endometriosis: an invasive disease. Gynecol Endoscopy 2001; 10: 79–82.

39. Jubanyik KJ, Comite F. Extrapelvic endometriosis. Obstet Gynecol Clin North Am 1997; 24: 411–440.

40. Weed J, Ray JE. Endometriosis of the bowel. Obstet Gynecol 1987; 69: 727–730.

41. Possover M, Diebolder H, Plaul K, et al. Laparoscopically assisted vaginal resection of rectovaginal endometriosis. Obstet Gynecol 2000; 96: 304–307.

42. Kavallaris A, Kohler C, Kune-Heid R, et al. Histopathological extent of rectal invasion by rectovaginal endometriosis. Hum Reprod 2003; 18: 1323–1327.

43. Jones KD, Owen E, Berresford A, et al. Endometrial adenocarcinoma arising from endometriosis of the rectosigmoid colon. Gynecol Oncol 2002; 86: 220–222.

44. Bese T, Simsek Y, Bese N, et al. Extensive pelvic endometriosis with malignant change in tamoxifen-treated postmenopausal women. Int J Gynecol Cancer 2003; 13: 376–380.

45. Pokieser W, Schmerker R, Kisser M, et al. Clear cell carcinoma arising in endometriosis of the rectum following progestin therapy. Pathol Res Pract 2002; 198: 121–124.

46. Garry R. The endometriosis syndromes: a clinical classification in the presence of aetiological confusion and therapeutic anarchy. Hum Reprod 2004; 19: 760–768.

47. Martin DC, Batt RE. Rectocervical, retrovaginal pouch and rectovaginal septum endometriosis. J Am Assoc Gynecol Laposc 2001; 8: 12–17.

48. Garry R, Fountain J, Mason S, et al. The eVALuate study: two parallel randomised trials, one comparing laparoscopic with abdominal hysterectomy, the other comparing laparoscopic with vaginal hysterectomy. BMJ 2004; 328: 129–133.

49. Vercellini P, Frontino G, De Giorgi O, et al Comparison of a levenonorgestrel-releasing intra-uterine device versus expectant management after conservative surgery for symptomatic endometriosis: a pilot study. Fertil Steril 2003; 80: 305–309.

50. Sculpher M, Manca A, Abbott J, et al. Cost effectiveness analysis of laparoscopic hysterectomy compared with standard hysterectomy: results from a randomised trial. BMJ 2004; 328: 134–137.

51. Winkel CA. A cost-effective approach to the management of endometriosis. Curr Opin Obstet Gynecol 2000; 12: 317–320.

52. Philips Z, Barraza-Llorens M, Posnett J. Evaluation of the relative cost-effectiveness of treatments for infertility in the UK. Hum Reprod 2000; 15: 95–106.

6 Data collection in surgical studies and evidence-based medicine

David L Olive, Steven R Lindheim, and Elizabeth A Pritts

Surgery is often practiced by the clinicians as an art: a skill that is learned, perfected by innovation and repetition, and finally taught in an apprenticeship-like process. However, physicians have now come to recognize that surgery can in fact be practiced in a scientific manner. Critical evaluation of indications, techniques, and complications by established methods of investigations has led to an improvement in the quality of surgical care delivery.

To truly understand the science of surgery requires a solid grasp of hypothesis formulation, study design, and study analysis. The principles of evidence-based medicine should be implemented to evaluate the available literature. Finally, a thorough knowledge of the unique assets and complexities of surgical trials must be considered. These factors, when brought to bear upon the value of available evidence, will help the discerning reader determine the applicability of a study to individual practice or patient.

This chapter will endeavor to provide the rationale, structure, and tools for analyzing surgical research. It will also provide guidelines for those wishing to conduct such research in the future.

What is evidence-based medicine?

Evidence-based medicine is defined as:

the conscientious, explicit, and judicious use of the current best evidence in making decisions about the care of individual patients and populations.[1]

Proficiency and judgment acquired through clinical experience, or internal clinical expertise, must be integrated with external clinical evidence drawn from relevant research, especially from patient-centered studies.

This description helps define what evidence-based medicine is not. It is not a replacement for individual expertise. Without experience and diagnostic skill, even the best evidence can be mishandled or used inappropriately. Evidence-based medicine is also not costly; rather, it reduces costs by improving outcomes. It is not burdensome; in fact, audits of evidence-based practice in general medicine,[2] general practice,[3] and psychiatry[4] show that it can be practiced easily in a busy clinical setting. In such situations, 80% of patients received interventions that could be supported by medical literature.[5] Finally, evidence-based medicine is not restricted to randomized clinical trials (RCTs) and meta-analyses; it involves using the best external evidence, whatever that might be.

This approach differs from the traditional approach to medical care. In the past, our education and hence our practice patterns rested on four assumptions:

- individual clinical experience provides the foundation for diagnosis, treatment, and prognosis
- pathophysiology provides the scientific foundation for practice

- clinical experience and personal or collective judgment equip practitioners to evaluate new tests and procedures
- experience and thorough mastery of subject areas supply the foundation for practice guidelines.

In this paradigm, a clinician unsure about a decision would consult an authority figure, such as a book chapter, an experienced colleague, or a respected elder clinician. However, such advice may or may not be based on comprehensive knowledge and it may or may not be based on current information. Thus, the value of this authoritative consult may be suspect.

Evidence-based medicine rests on a different set of assumptions. First, experience and the development of clinical instincts are crucial to becoming a competent physician, as many aspects of practice cannot or will not be adequately tested. At the same time, systematic attempts to record observations in a reproducible and unbiased fashion markedly increase the confidence one can have about those observations. In the absence of systematic study, one must be cautious about interpreting information derived from clinical experience and intuition, as it may be misleading. Secondly, knowledge and understanding of pathophysiology are necessary but are insufficient to guide clinical practice. Finally, formal rules of evidence are prerequisites to understanding the literature on diagnosis, treatment, and prognosis.

It follows that clinicians should regularly consult the literature in attempting to provide optimal patient care. It also follows that they must be prepared to live with uncertainty and to acknowledge that management decisions are often made in the face of relative ignorance. The new paradigm puts a lower value on authority, but does not reject what can be learned from experienced teachers and colleagues. A final assumption of the paradigm is that physicians whose practice is based on understanding the underlying evidence will provide superior patient care.

Research design

Formulating an hypothesis

The first question to be asked of any investigative endeavor is, 'What is the hypothesis?' The hypothesis to be tested ultimately will influence subsequent design and analysis, and a clear determination of the outset of the study will often prevent the investigator from becoming bogged down

with tangential issues. When reviewing studies already conducted, the discerning reader must likewise ask what hypothesis is being tested; lack of clarity regarding this point is often indicative of a 'shotgun' approach by the authors, who are looking for anything significant to help justify use of a procedure.

Once an hypothesis is raised, the next decision involves selection of the appropriate outcome measure. Examples of such measures in surgery may include pregnancy rates (for treatment of fertility problems), pain relief (for treatment of pain syndrome), or even operating time or blood loss (when comparing endoscopy to laparotomy). Whatever outcome measure is selected, it must address the original hypothesis. For instance, if it is hypothesized that the endoscopic myomectomy will increase subsequent fertility when compared to laparotomy, it is inappropriate to use intraoperative blood loss as a primary outcome measure for this effect.

Types of clinical trials

Research design may be divided into two categories: descriptive, such as delineation of prognostic factors or the clinical course of a disease; and analytic, in which an interventional cause–effect relationship is investigated. The latter category encompasses those studies evaluating the role of surgery in the treatment of gynecologic disease. Within the category of analytic research, there are two basic structures: the experimental trial and the observational survey.[6] A study design qualifies as an experimental trial when more than one study group is involved and when study subjects are allocated to each of the study groups in a random fashion. If, on the other hand, only a single study group is evaluated or if treatment options are assigned not randomly but for a reason, the research is an observational survey.

Observational surveys can be classified further by when the data were collected in relation to the present time (real-time relationship). Studies with data accumulated in the past, prior to hypothesis development, can be called retrospective, whereas those performed after the study was conceived and designed are termed prospective.[7,8]

Another way to classify observational surveys is by their research pursuit direction, i.e. from what point in the diagnosis–treatment–outcome continuum was the patient selected for inclusion in the study.[8,9] If the subject was selected based on a diagnosis or treatment modality and was subsequently followed for outcome evaluation, the direction is termed antecedent-to-outcome, or *cohort*. Conversely, if a study enrolls patients because of a given outcome and then follows their records back to see what treatment was administered, the research pursuit direction is outcome-to-antecedent, or *trohoc*.

The primary advantage of a study performed in present time (the randomized trial and the prospective cohort study) is the ability to collect data in a complete and dependable fashion. Thus, the presence or absence of a factor of importance in the study can be determined uniformly and without bias among study participants. Furthermore, since the means of evaluation are determined before initiation of data collection, uniformity of outcome assessment is more likely in this situation. Despite these advantages, there are problems with prospective trials. Experimental studies are expensive, time-consuming, and often of insufficient size to address adequately the hypothesis being tested. They may also be so rigid in their inclusion criteria that the results only apply to a very narrow subset of the patient population. Prospective cohort studies suffer from the lack of random assignment of patients, with the resulting bias sure to affect study results. Both study types must make allowances for the failure of some subjects to complete the designated study protocol.

In the retrospective study, data are gleaned from medical records or patient recall; both can be significantly unreliable to the point of severely prejudicing the conclusions. In addition, these studies are limited to those methods of evaluation recorded in the chart, prompting questions about any preexisting conditions that may or may not have been recorded, the degree and intensity of observation, and whether or not there was uniformity of outcome assessment. Although such studies are rapid and inexpensive to perform, the results are often highly suspect due to these shortcomings in design.

Control groups

To determine the value of a therapeutic maneuver, it must be clear as to what would have happened had the therapy not been administered. This concept, the determination of baseline values as a source of comparison, is termed *control*.[8] A study may be controlled in a variety of ways or it may remain uncontrolled; the decision as to whether and how to control a trial can impact greatly on the value of a clinical investigation.

In endoscopic treatment trials, the appropriate choice of a control group depends on the hypoth-

esis being tested. If the study is an attempt to study the efficacy of endoscopic treatment, one must consider what is known to occur in the absence of treatment or with alternative treatment. If it is well known that the absence of treatment never leads to a favorable outcome, demonstration of an improvement via endoscopy would require only evidence that successful outcome follows endoscopic intervention, without the need for a comparable control group of untreated patients. For example, if the hypothesis is that women with bilateral distal tubal obstruction will have increased pregnancy rates following laparoscopic cuff salpingostomy, any pregnancies resulting after the procedure can be deemed to have resulted from the procedure itself, as no woman would achieve pregnancy without surgery.

Conversely, if the study hypothesis is that women with unilateral distal tubal obstruction will have increased pregnancy rates following laparoscopic cuff salpingostomy, the issue is quite different. In this situation, untreated women will achieve pregnancy; the question is whether or not they will do it more often after surgery. To test this hypothesis, a control group of untreated women is essential so that the baseline success rate can be identified, and it can be seen if the treated group performs better.

If, however, a standard treatment exists that is of known efficacy, the hypothesis to be tested may not be whether the intervention is efficacious but rather how it compares to standard therapy. For the above example of bilateral distal tubal obstruction, control group selection might include women undergoing microsurgical cuff salpingostomy or even in vitro fertilization. Pregnancy rate would certainly be one outcome measure; but others might include cost, recovery time, and complication rates. Again, the outcome measure(s) selected depend on the precise hypothesis under consideration.

Aside from the composition of the control group, the method of accumulating controls is an important issue. In a randomized therapeutic trial, patients are arbitrarily allocated to either the experimental or the control group. This method is optimal in that it minimizes effects of confounding variables on the outcome measure.[10] However, many reports are not of this design but rather exist as observational surveys. For such trials, patients may be assigned at the same time to either the experimental or the control group, but the assignment is based upon clinical discretion rather than random assignment. This type of control group is referred to as *concurrent* and *nonrandomized*. This method of control has the obvious limitation of the introduction of bias due to the method of allocation.[11,12] Clearly, the factors that influence a clinician to place the patient in one group or the other might also affect the rate of successful outcome in the two groups.

Another type of control group is the *historical control*. With this technique, patients treated with the experimental procedure are compared to subjects previously treated with the control approach. Thus, the two groups are not treated during the same time span but rather sequentially. Historical control creates many difficulties, including the fact that the historical data are usually gathered retrospectively, with all the inherent problems of a retrospective study. Furthermore, other substantive factors may have changed over time besides the therapeutic change under study; these factors may contribute to significant alterations in the outcome of the study.

Confounding variables

Patient characteristics known to effect the outcome measure in a surgical treatment trial may have a substantial impact on study results. For example, if the outcome measure is pregnancy, variables such as age, duration of infertility, gravidity, and additional infertility factors might have a considerable effect. The best way to minimize the effect of confounders on a study outcome is the randomized experimental design discussed earlier. Random allocation of subjects should virtually equalize the effects of such confounding variables – whether known to the investigator or not! However, even with randomization, there is the possibility that some critical factor may unduly influence one group over another. To protect against this, the prevalence of all known confounding variables should be assessed for each study group. If the research involves a nonrandomized but comparative trial, specific regression techniques can be utilized to help determine the value of treatment independent of such confounders. A thorough understanding of biases present in the study population will always aid in determining the applicability of results to specific clinical circumstances.

Analyzing a study

In research involving surgery, there are two types of outcome measures. The first type involves measures related to the surgical procedure or the immediate postoperative period. In this situation, there is a one-to-one relationship between the procedure and the outcome measure, and standard statistical techniques are applicable. Examples include such outcomes as time of surgery, amount of blood loss, number of lymph nodes recovered, agreement of surgical and tissue diagnosis, and length of hospital stay.

A second type of outcome measure is much more complex: the time-dependent outcome. With this measure, the result may vary given the length of follow-up after surgery. Thus, the outcome at 1-month postoperatively may differ from that of 6–12 months following surgery. Most outcomes related to symptom relief fall into this category. Examples include pregnancy, pain relief, restoration of continence, and reduction/elimination of abnormal uterine bleeding. Statistical methodology applied to these types of trials differs markedly in that follow-up time must be considered; methods that fail to take this factor into consideration prove grossly inadequate in analyzing such data.

Significance and power

In the comparison of the results of two treatments (or one treatment vs no therapy), absolutely conclusive results are not attainable. Instead, one must play the odds when trying to decide if success rates differ. The key to determining this is *statistical significance*, a concept which states that, given the available data, the odds overwhelmingly favor there being a real difference between two groups. Generally, statistical significance requires that, given an observed difference between two treatments, it will in fact be a *real* difference (rather than just a statistical fluke) at least 95% of the time.

Occasionally, a study suggests a difference in success between treatments, yet in reality there is not one. This is called a type I statistical error. The rate for a type I error in a given experiment is termed the α value and is generally set at no more than 5%.

Some studies suggest no difference in success between treatments. However, occasionally a real difference will exist despite a failure to demonstrate this in a treatment trial. The chances of this occurring is called a type II statistical error. The rate for a type II error in a given experiment is termed the β value and a maximum chance is generally set at not more than 20%. In such a situation, the statistical power to avoid a type II error is $1-\beta$ (at least 80% in most settings).[13]

Significance and power are two critical concepts that must be clearly delineated in a treatment trial. If a study presumes to show a difference between treatments, it is imperative to know whether statistical significance was achieved and, if so, what was the preset α value. If the authors claim no difference, one must ask if the study achieved reasonable power in avoiding a type II error given the sample size and significance threshold. It is all too often the case that a poorly conceived study fails to demonstrate a significant difference between treatments, yet is not of sufficient power to exclude with reasonable certainty that such a difference exists. These investigations are of little value to anyone and generally serve only to muddle the literature. This highlights the importance of thoroughly planning an investigation prior to its initiation, emphasizing the inherent value of the prospective approach.

The surgical randomized clinical trial

Gathering evidence to evaluate surgical procedures provides clinicians with perhaps their greatest challenge. As with other aspects of medicine, surgical care is subject to great variations. Comparative assessment of competing operative methods of medical vs surgical intervention involves studying the effect on a highly variable process. Such a task can be both difficult and frustrating.

Surgeons initially believed that results of operations could be evaluated and compared by retrospective analysis of large series of patients. Unfortunately, large collections of clinical observations meticulously analyzed repeatedly failed to supply conclusive answers.[14]

During the last quarter century, surgeons toyed with concepts of randomized trials involving surgical procedures. The tool proved powerful in other arenas, and its inherent logical appeal provides a strong incentive to budding surgical investigators.

A surgical RCT is defined as an experiment to evaluate a surgical procedure. It may compare two or more operative procedures or it may compare a surgical procedure with other types of interven-

tions. The outcome usually measures which intervention is more effective. Unfortunately, the surgical RCT has a number of difficulties which must be considered.

Bias in patient selection

Patient selection may be subject to the biases of both participating surgeons and referring physicians. When referring physicians realize a study is under way, referral patterns may be altered to reflect their preconceived ideas. A particularly common pattern is diversion of high-risk patients away from the study center, leaving a population of low-risk patients to enroll. Such bias increases the chance of type II statistical error. Participating physicians, too, can contribute to selection bias. This is particularly true when inclusion or exclusion criteria are not sufficiently specific to remove subjective assessment. Even systematic exclusion of a type of patient may lead to problems; although all groups' postrandomization may be comparable, they may not be generalizable.

Bias in allocation to treatment groups

Proper assignment of patients to treatment groups may eliminate physician bias, but it cannot eliminate patient bias. Patients may, after randomization, refuse to participate due to a desire to receive one of the tested therapies. This rarely occurs when two medical therapies are evaluated, but is much more common when dissimilar treatments (surgery vs medical) are compared.

Nonadherence to the assigned therapy is another type of bias. The effect is termed crossing over and it can be a major problem when comparing surgery with medical intervention, because it generally arises when medical therapy fails to control disease progressions and the subject crosses over to surgery. When this occurs, the medical therapy group is composed predominantly of those for whom the treatment was successful, and a false impression of the value is developed.

Problems of statistical analysis

Two problems frequently arise in this arena: type II errors due to inadequate study design and failure to use intention-to-treat analysis. Type II (false-negative) errors can occur in trials when the study population is low risk compared with the general population (infrequent terminal event), when the sample is too small, and when follow-up is too short. Such errors should be held to a minimum with proper planning and trial design.

A difficulty in the analysis phase is caused by exclusion of patients after randomization but before treatment. This is a particular problem with surgical trials, in that a lag period often exists between randomization and surgery. Note that a general rule is that subgroups cannot be defined by events after randomization; inclusion of all subjects in the analysis of the group to which they were randomized is called intention-to-treat and is an important concept in study analysis.

Difficulties in blinding

In medical trials, unbiased assessment of results such as pain relief or symptomatic improvements is often greatly facilitated by blinding patients and physicians to the intention. In surgical trials, this is often difficult and may be impossible. It is not possible to avoid having the surgeon know which procedure was performed, and it is often difficult to find an objective, blinded assessor. Patients, too, often cannot be blinded if different surgical approaches are required for two compared procedures. It follows that in many surgical RCTs the outcome measure must be restricted to objectively measurable results, which is clearly a down side given today's penchant for quality of life assessment.

Influence of skill and experience

With surgical procedures, in contrast to medical trials, skill affects the treatment itself, not the way in which it is perceived by the patient. Obviously, it cannot be neutralized by blinding. For this reason, correctly performed surgical RCTs by different physicians may yield drastically different results.[15]

Randomization of the first patient may be impossible

This issue is particularly important for innovative surgical techniques. Whenever a new procedure requires training to perfect it, randomized evaluation must be delayed until after the evolutionary phase. Initially, patients may be carefully chosen and the procedure varied as necessary. If a surgical RCT is performed before the surgery is standardized, the results will probably be invalidated even before the conclusion of the study due to changes in technique and results. Thus, pilot studies and innovative periods are a must with many surgical developments.

Systematic bias in random-order operations design

In this design, an envelope is opened as an operation reaches a certain stage, thus determining how a surgeon should proceed.[15] Although popular with statisticians, this design has several drawbacks. First, there is systematic bias in favor of the procedure most participating surgeons performed before the trial; familiarity with a procedure construes a definite advantage in outcome. Secondly, there is a systematic bias in favor of the technically easier procedure as the learning curve will be steeper and this will be reflected in results. If information is to be gleaned about the value of the surgery rather than its learning characteristics, this issue is problematic.

Need for large numbers

Because surgical skill affects results of a surgical RCT, it is imperative to minimize this effect. If only a few surgeons participate in a trial, one or two with special talents may unduly influence the overall results.

Whereas many of these problems of surgical RCTs seem overwhelming, they are in fact possible to deal with. The most important aspect is to be aware of the issues. When potential biases are recognized, steps can be taken to overcome them. For example, to guard against outlier surgical skill, multicenter trials with many participating surgeons are clearly beneficial.[16] To protect against premature RCTs in the evolutionary phase of a procedure, a prerandomization period for training should be allowed and the trial begun only when all surgeons agree the procedure has reached steady state.

Problems with random-order operations design are moot if the innovative or more complex procedure performs better, but if this is not the case, it may be advisable to consider alternative designs. One such option is the nonrandomized surgeon's design.[15] Here, surgeons who generally perform procedure A would perform only this procedure, and those used to performing procedure B would perform only that one. Patients are randomly allocated to either group. In this way, all surgeons perform procedures they are familiar with, and no ethical concerns are raised about substandard experience or confidence. The drawback of this design is that it must be shown that the two groups of surgeons are very similar in level of training.

Thus, every effort should be made to balance the experts.

Despite the difficulty of the surgical RCT, it is clearly of benefit to perform such studies. Comparisons of results from RCTs with those of nonrandomized studies repeatedly confirmed that the treatment effect is exaggerated by nonrandomized designs.[17] In fact, the difference in proportion of treatment successes may be doubled by nonrandomized controlled trials or externally controlled trials compared with RCTs. For this reason, results of the surgical RCT should be highly sought after as evidence.

Overviews of surgical interventions are hampered by the shortage of surgical RCTs and the unpredictable effects of other designs. Furthermore, the quality of surgical RCTs is far below that of trials involving medical therapy. Few surgical RCTs were multicenter, initial establishment of sample size was performed in only 11%, and double-blinding was present in only one-third of trials where blinding was feasible.[14] In addition, sample size calculations are frequently not provided, resulting in type II errors being highly likely.[18]

Surgical investigation carries with it a number of inherent difficulties, and to forget this fact is to criticize the surgical literature in a cavalier and unfair manner. Surgery has an immediate risk, whereas drugs often do not. Surgery entails craftsmanship to a much larger extent than does drug administration. Finally, surgery requires training. For these reasons, it is important to adapt methods of RCTs to surgical procedures, for the value of this design is without question. With continued interest in these design concepts, increases in the number and quality of surgical RCTs should be forthcoming.

In recognition of the frequent problems associated with poor design and analysis of RCTs (particularly surgical RCTs), the Consolidated Standards of Reporting Trials (CONSORT) Statement has been developed by researchers and editors to improve RCT report quality.[19] These guidelines comprise a 22-item checklist and study flow diagrams to help authors include information essential to assess the design, conduct, analysis, and interpretation of the trial.

Quality of evidence

Given the large number of issues inherent in study design to evaluate treatments, how does the discerning reader rank the importance of the various studies while attempting to formulate an overall recommendation from the literature? One simple method would be to rank papers according to the simple hierarchy presented earlier: first, RCTs; secondly, observational studies; and thirdly, survey (descriptive studies). A recent publication expanded this categorization to five levels of importance:[20] RCTs with low α and β errors (e.g., $p < 0.01$ and power $> 90\%$); RCTs with a higher α and β errors; nonrandomized concurrent prospective cohort studies; nonrandomized historically controlled cohort studies; and uncontrolled studies and surveys.

Finally, the US Preventive Services Task Force provided a means by which to assess the strength of accumulated literature on a given topic.[21] It is centered on the quality of the best study on a particular subject, and results in the following classification scheme:

I. Evidence obtained from one properly designed, randomized, controlled trial.
II-1. Evidence obtained from a well-designed controlled trial without randomization.
II-2. Evidence obtained from well-designed cohort or case control studies, preferably from more than one center or research group.
II-3. Evidence obtained from several timed series with or without the intervention. Dramatic results in uncontrolled experiments, such as results of introduction of penicillin treatment in the 1940s could also be regarded as this type of evidence.
III. Opinions of respected authorities based on clinical experience, descriptive studies, or reports of expert committees.

The role of evidence-based medicine in surgery

While the medical literature is growing in its capacity to address the many aspects of surgical care, the question arises as to how these principles should be applied to practice. The solution to this query is not an easy one. Research studies are often exercises in the execution of an experiment in a small, tidy, narrow universe; the real world rarely intrudes. However, our clinical practices are littered with exclusions and exceptions: those patients that do not exactly fit the studies but nevertheless seem to be overly plentiful in your community.

The successful surgeon combines a number of factors into the equation that, when solved, points toward the proper path. These factors must include the surgical literature, but also unique or unusual patient characteristics. In addition, surgeons must factor in their own skill and comfort levels with a technique or procedure, the surgical environment of the facility in which they operate, and the available equipment. Only when all of these variables are taken into account, can the surgeon truly make the clinical decision considered optimal for an individual patient.

REFERENCES

1. Evidence-Based Medicine Working Group. Evidence based medicine: a new approach to teaching the practice of medicine. JAMA 1992; 268: 2420–2425.

2. Ellis J, Mulligan I, Rowe J, et al. Inpatient general medicine is evidence based. Lancet 1995; 346: 407–470.

3. Gill P, Dowell AC, Neil RD, et al. Evidence-based general practice: a retrospective study of interventions in one training practice. BMJ 1996; 312: 819–821.

4. Geddes JR, Game D, Jenkins NE. In-patient psychiatric care is evidence-based. Proceedings of the Royal College of Psychiatrists Winter Meeting, Stratford, UK, January 23–25, 1996.

5. Cooke IE, Sackett DL. Evidence-based obstetrics and gynaecology. Baillière's Clin Obstet Gynaecol 1996; 10: 535–549.

6. Feinstein AR. Clinical biostatistics. XLIV. A survey of the research architecture used for publications in general medical journals. Clin Pharmacol Ther 1978; 24: 117–125.

7. Feinstein AR. Clinical biostatistics. XLVIII. Efficacy of different research structures in preventing bias in the analysis of causation. Clin Pharmacol Ther 1979; 26: 129–141.

8. Feinstein AR. Clinical biostatistics. LVII. A glossary of neologisms in quantitative clinical science. Clin Pharmacol 1981; 30: 564–577.

9. Olive D. Analysis of clinical fertility trials: a methodologic review. Fertil Steril 1987; 45: 157.

10. Feinstein AR. Clinical biostatistics. XXIV. The role of randomization in sampling, testing, allocation, and credulous idolatry (conclusion). Clin Pharmacol Ther 1973; 14: 1035–1051.

11. Student. The Lanarkshire milk experiment. Biometrika 1931; 23: 398–404.

12. Smithells RW, Sheppard S, Schorah CJ, et al. Possible prevention of neural-tube defects by periconceptional vitamin supplementation. Lancet 1980; 1: 339–340.

13. Cohen J. Statistical power analysis for the behavioral sciences. Hillsdale, NJ: Lawrence Erlbaum Associates; 1998.

14. Solomon MJ, Laxamana A, Devore L, et al. Randomized controlled trials in surgery. Surgery 1994; 115: 707–712.

15. Van der Linden W. Pitfalls in randomized surgical trials. Surgery 1980;87:258–262.

16. Koops HS. Surgical quality control in an international randomized clinical trial. Eur J Surg Oncol 1992; 18: 525–529.

17. Miller JN, Colditz GA, Mosteller F. How study design affects outcomes in comparisons of therapy. II. Surgical Stat Med 1989; 8: 455–466.

18. Maggard MA, O'Connell JB, Liu JH, et al. Sample size calculations in surgery: Are they done correctly? Surgery 2003; 134: 275–279.

19. Moher D, Schulz KF, Altman DG for the CONSORT group. The CONSORT Statement: revised recommendations for improving the quality of reports of parallel-group randomized trials. Lancet 2001; 357: 1191–1194.

20. Cook DJH, Guyatt GH, Laupacis A, et al. Rulers of evidence and clinical recommendations on the use of antithrombolic agents. Chest 1992; 102: 305S–311S.

21. Grimes DA. Introducing evidence-based medicine into a department of obstetrics and gynecology. Obstet Gynecol 1995; 86: 451–457.

SECTION II
Surgical Treatment

7 Preoperative investigations

Karen Kinkel, Jan Brosens, and Ivo Brosens

Introduction

The gold standard for the diagnosis of endometriosis is laparoscopy. As laparoscopy is an invasive procedure, the diagnosis is often combined with surgical treatment. Although this combined approach may be justifiable, it does not conform with the standard stratification for a surgical procedure that proceeds from diagnosis, to assessment of therapeutic options, and, finally, to operative intervention with informed patient consent.

Endometriosis is a complex pathology that affects reproductive function and often involves other pelvic structures. It is therefore important, especially in the case of severe endometriosis, to provide adequate information on the type and extent of the proposed surgery and to give the patient an opportunity to seek a second opinion or referral to a center of surgical excellence. A detailed history and gynecologic examination may point towards the presence of endometriosis but will yield little or no information on the type or extent of the lesions.

This chapter describes preoperative investigations that may be helpful to determine the presence of endometriosis as well as the type and severity of disease. Although new developments in the field of diagnostic serum and endometrial markers for endometriosis are briefly described, we will focus on the role of preoperative imaging.

Markers of endometriosis

Serum markers

Ideal serum markers for endometriosis should exhibit high sensitivity and specificity, have excellent prognostic value, and provide a good correlation between the levels and severity of disease. Such markers could be used not only for the diagnosis of endometriosis but also for monitoring disease progression and response to medical or surgical treatment.

Peripheral blood levels of cancer antigen 125 (CA-125) have been extensively investigated for the diagnosis of endometriosis. CA-125 is a high molecular weight membrane glycoprotein and is expressed in all tissues derived from embryonic coelomic epithelium, including endometrium, endocervix, fallopian tubes, peritoneum, pleura, and pericardium. In patients with advanced endometriosis, CA-125 levels are elevated predominantly during the first few days of the menstrual cycle. However, elevated serum concentrations of CA-125 are not specific for endometriosis and are also associated with many epithelial cancers as well as with benign gynecologic and non-gynecologic disorders such as adnexitis, pancreatitis, pregnancy, and ovarian hyperstimulation syndrome. After meta-analysis, Mol et al[1] concluded that, despite its limited diagnostic performance, the routine use of serum CA-125 measurement is justified in patients with suspected endometriosis. It may be particularly useful to identify patients with grade III/IV endometriosis who are likely to benefit from early surgical intervention. In patients with severe endometriosis, the monitoring of CA-125 after surgery can be useful for the detection of recurrences during their follow-up.

Harada et al[2] recently compared the clinical value of measuring CA-19.9 vs CA-125 serum levels and suggested that CA-19.9 is potentially a more useful marker for determining the severity of the disease. Bedaiwy et al[3] found that by measuring serum interleukin (IL)-6 and peritoneal fluid tumor necrosis factor alpha (TNF-α) levels, it was possible to discriminate between patients with endometriosis and those without. However, Somigliana et al[4] found that combining CA-125, CA-19.9, and IL-6 measurements did not increase the diagnosis accuracy of either early or advanced endometriosis when compared to CA-125 alone.

Anti-endometrial and anti-carbonic anhydrase antibodies have also been investigated for their diagnostic potential in women with endometriosis, but the technical difficulty is too high for general application. Increased leptin levels in serum and peritoneal fluid have also been reported in patients with endometriosis, but follow-up studies failed to confirm an association between pelvic endometriosis and elevated leptin levels.[5]

Endometrial markers of endometriosis

Many recent studies have shown that there are profound biochemical abnormalities in the eutopic endometrium of women with endometriosis.[6] Comparative analysis between endometrial samples from endometriosis and disease-free patients have revealed differences in the expression of many cellular factors, including cytokines and growth factors, adhesion molecules, proteolytic enzymes and their inhibitors, enzymes involved in oxidative stress responses, and transcription factors. However, attempts to exploit these molecular differences for diagnostic purposes have been largely unsuccessful for several reasons. First, the level of expression of a given gene may vary considerably between individuals and between biopsy samples. Secondly, an abnormal expression pattern is often confined to a certain phase of the cycle. Thirdly, the altered expression pattern may be too subtle to be used as a discriminatory marker. Finally, the expression profiles of many endometrial factors have only been determined by immunostaining. This approach is not only time-consuming but the assessment of immunoreactivity is, to a certain degree, subjective

and observer-dependent. Hence, the lack of easy, reliable, and quantitative techniques to assess expression levels in biopsy material restricts the use of endometrial markers.

Recent studies have reported that aromatase P450, the enzyme that catalyzes the conversion of C19 steroids (androstenedione and testosterone) to estrone (E1), is expressed in the eutopic endometrium of women with endometriosis but not in endometria of disease-free controls. Furthermore, aromatase P450 mRNA expression appears to be independent of the phase of the cycle, rendering it a potential 'ideal' marker that does not require quantitation or timed biopsy samples. In a retrospective study, Kitawaki and coworkers reported that detection of P450arom protein in endometrial biopsy samples could be used as an outpatient screening test for endometriosis, with a sensitivity and specificity of 91% and 100%, respectively.[7] However, a prospective study reported that endometrial P450arom mRNA expression, detected by reverse transcriptase-polymerase chain reaction (RT-PCR) and Southern blot analysis, is not confined to women with endometriosis but is also associated with most hormone-dependent proliferative disorders of the uterus, including leiomyomata, adenomyosis, and proximal tubal disease.[8] As a diagnostic marker for endometriosis, P450arom mRNA expression yielded a sensitivity of 82%, a specificity of 59%, a positive predictive value of 76%, and a negative predictive value of 67%. If additional uterine pathology was taken into account, the sensitivity increased to 84%, the specificity to 72%, the positive predictive value to 87%, but the negative predictive value remained unchanged (67%). The authors concluded that although endometrial P450arom gene expression is predictive of the presence of pelvic disease, the relative high incidence of false negatives and lack of specificity is likely to impair clinical application.

Functional genomics and proteomics

Microarray technology allows simultaneous analysis of the expression of large numbers of genes. This technology has been used to characterize the expression of genes, gene families, and signal tranduction pathways in the endometrium of women with endometriosis. In a parallel high-density oligonucleotide microarray study, Kao et al[9] found that 91 genes, out of 12 686 genes analyzed, were significantly higher expressed in eutopic endometrium from endometriosis patients, whereas the expression of 115 genes was decreased more than two-fold. The data support the hypothesis that endometriosis is associated with dysregulation of specific gene sets, leading to an inhospitable environment for implantation. Some of the genes that were found to be aberrantly expressed have been implicated in embryo attachment, embryo toxicity, immune dysfunction, and apoptotic responses, whereas others are likely to contribute to the pathogenesis of endometriosis, including aromatase P450, progesterone receptor, and angiogenic factors.

There is increasing evidence to suggest that endometriosis is a polygenic and multifactorial disease, indicating that multiple distinct pathways could be involved in its pathogenesis. At present, functional genomics and proteomics are being applied in all areas of medicine, including in the search for novel diagnostic modalities of endometriosis.

Imaging techniques

Endometriosis has various phenotypes. However, the current terminology used to describe different types of endometriosis is confusing and includes superficial, deep, pseudo-deep, free, enclosed, invasive, metaplastic, and progressive lesions. From a functional viewpoint, an endometriotic lesion can be classified as predominantly hemorrhagic and pseudocystic or predominantly fibromuscular and nodular.[10] Imaging techniques are increasingly accurate in identifying the dominant phenotype of the lesions by the presence of hemorrhagic and the fibromuscular components, which allow for a more rational classification of the endometriotic lesion.

Superficial peritoneal and ovarian endometriosis

Superficial peritoneal and ovarian endometriosis and endometriotic adhesions are not detectable by transvaginal ultrasound (TVU). Magnetic resonance (MR) imaging also fails to detect subtle endometriotic lesions, although fat-saturated MR imaging, when compared to conventional MR imaging, greatly improves the detection rate of small hemorrhagic lesions (± 4 mm) from 4% to 50%.[11] The poor accuracy of MR imaging to diagnose superficial endometriosis is explained by the small size of the implants and the fact that cross-sectional images are routinely obtained at 5 mm intervals. Moreover, red, black, and white lesions have variable degrees of endometriotic components, including endometrial-like tissue, blood, myofibroblasts, and fibrosis. Furthermore, superficial endometriotic implants can easily be confused with other pelvic structures such as blood vessels, and adhesions, especially after pelvic surgery.

The endometrial cyst of the ovary

Pathologic appearances
The endometrial cyst of the ovary represents a complex hemorrhagic and adhesive type of endometriosis. The macroscopic and microscopic features of ovarian endometriomas have been described in detail by histologic examination of extirpated in-situ specimens[12,13] and in vivo by ovarioscopy combined with targeted biopsies.[14] There is strong evidence to suggest that more than 90% of ovarian endometriomas are pseudocysts, characterized by invagination of the ovarian cortex. These pseudocysts are sealed off at the site of invagination (so-called 'site of perforation') by adhesions and are lined by a mucosa that resembles the superficial endometrium of the uterus. There is no evidence that the endometriotic tissue lining the cavity of the pseudocyst actually invades the ovarian stroma.[13]

The structure of the ovarian endometrioma can vary greatly. In older symptomatic women the wall of the pseudocyst is often characterized by thick fibrosis and scanty endometriotic tissue. The implants at the site of invagination often consist of normal endometrial tissue with evidence of menstrual shedding. These endometriomas are typically adherent to the pelvic side wall and, in most cases, adenomyotic lesions are present in the adherent tissue.[12] It is very likely that pain associated with these advanced endometriomas originates from the adenomyotic lesion rather than the cystic endometrioma.

Asymptomatic endometriomas are increasingly diagnosed in young women with infertility at TVU. At ovarioscopy, the wall of the endometriomas often has the same marble-white color as the outer ovarian cortex and is lined by a reddish, highly vascularized mucosa. Targeted biopsies of these lesions have confirmed that the wall is ovarian cortex and that most of the wall is lined by a thin rim of mucosa containing a surface epithelium and stroma. In younger women, adenomyotic lesions are usually absent in the adherent tissue.

Large multilocular cysts often consist of endometriomas combined with a hemorrhagic corpus luteum or lutein cyst. A recent corpus luteum can open into an endometrioma and show colonization by endometriotic epithelium that originates from the endometrioma. Such colonization of a corpus luteum could result into a deep intraovarian endometrioma. A major challenge is to correlate the ultrasound characteristics with specific histologic pathology found in targeted biopsies or in ovarian specimens with in-situ endometriomas.

Ultrasound diagnosis

The characteristic features of endometriomas are the presence of diffuse, low-level internal echoes and hyperechoic foci in the wall (Figure 7.1). The pathologic significance of increased wall thickness, nodularity, and hyperechoic foci remains speculative and the diagnostic potential of other possible discriminatory factors, such as location, lesion shape, and position, have yet to be determined.

Using a standardized checklist, Patel et al[15] found that an adnexal mass with low-level internal echoes and absence of particular neoplastic features is highly likely to be an endometrioma, especially if the cyst is multilocular or if hyperechoic foci are present in the cyst wall. A variety of ovarian cysts can mimic the appearance of an endometrioma, including corpus luteum and lutein cysts, teratomas, cystadenomas, ovarian fibroids, tubo-ovarian abscesses, and carcinomas (Figures 7.2 and 7.3). A repeat ultrasound is highly recommended for unilocular cysts with low-level internal echoes but without wall nodularity or hyperechoic foci. If papillary structures protruding from the internal cyst wall are visualized, ovarian malignancy, such as endometrioid carcinoma, needs to be excluded.

(a)

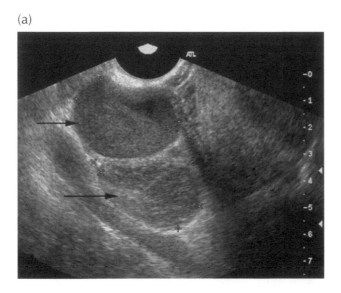

(b)

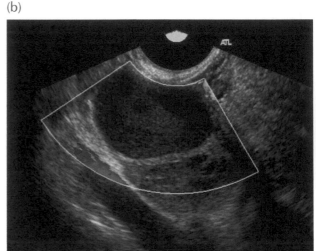

(c)

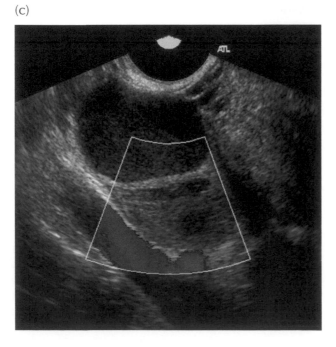

Figure 7.1 A 37-year-old woman with dysmenorrhea. (a) Axial TVU image of the right ovary demonstrating two cystic structures (arrows) with layers of different echogenicity, corresponding to blood of various ages in two contiguous endometriomas. (b and c) The corresponding color Doppler image, demonstrating absent flow in each cyst, confirming, in the absence of intracystic solid tissue, the benign nature of the cyst.

(a)

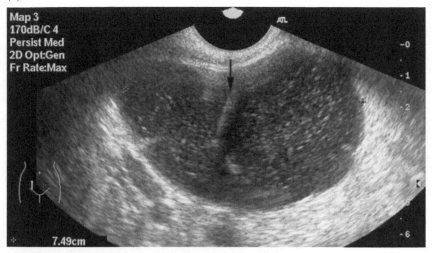

(b)

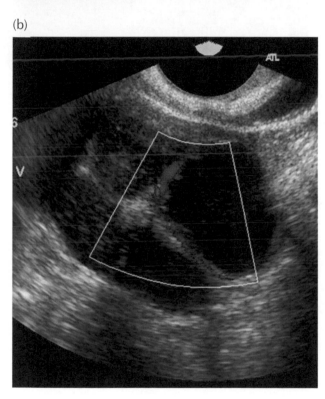

Figure 7.2 A 36-year-old asymptomatic woman with a complex ovarian cyst on ultrasound. (a) Axial TVU image of the right ovary, demonstrating a multilocular cyst with punctuated hypoechoic content and thin septations (arrow). Differential diagnoses include mucinous cyst, endometrioma, dermoid cyst, or cancer. (b) Hypervascularity within two septations, which increases the suspicion for malignancy. Pathologic examination of this right ovary demonstrated a benign multilocular mucinous tumor which can mimic the ultrasound appearance of ovarian cancer.

TVU has important limitations in the detection of ovarian endometriomas. Moore et al[16] identified 38 papers related to the diagnosis of endometriosis by ultrasound scan, but considered only seven studies sufficiently sound for further analysis. The authors concluded that TVU appears to be a useful test both to make and to exclude the diagnosis of an ovarian endometrioma. However, the mean size of the endometriomas included in the seven studies reviewed varied between 4 and 6 cm. Therefore, TVU may accurately identify endometriomas but only if sufficiently large (Table 7.1). Recently, we confirmed that 77% of the endometriomas smaller than 2 cm were not detected preoperatively by TVU (unpublished data). The specificity of TVU is also likely to be reduced in postoperative patients with recurrent hemorrhagic cysts. It has been reported that up to 73% of the recurrent hemorrhagic ovarian cysts after ovarian surgery for endometriomas are actually lutein cysts that may persist for several months. TVU combined with transvaginal aspiration of such persisting postoperative hemorrhagic cysts can be used for measurement of CA-125 levels in the aspirate, which may help to differentiate a recurrent endometrioma from a lutein cyst.

Whether color Doppler study adds to the diagnostic efficiency of TVU remains uncertain. Guerriero et al[20] reported that endometriomas are associated with 'poor' blood supply, whereas other ovarian cysts, and particularly malignant tumors, are

(a)

(b)

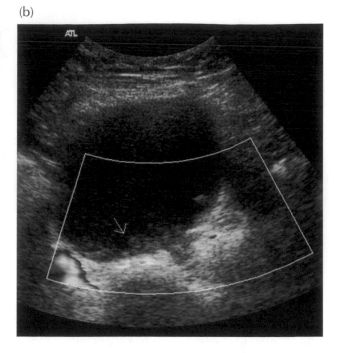

Figure 7.3 A 43-year-old woman with chronic pelvic pain. (a) Sagittal TVU image of the right ovary, demonstrates a large complex cyst with a heterogeneous content, resembling a hair ball associated with a cystic teratoma. (b) Axial color Doppler image of the same cyst shows an irregular inner wall simulating cancer (white arrow); however, the absence of color Doppler flow within the mural projections decreases the suspicion of malignancy. Surgery and pathologic examination of the right ovary identified a large endometrioma with an irregular inner wall.

Table 7.1 Accuracy of ultrasound for the diagnosis of ovarian endometriomas

Study	Number	Size (mm)		Sensitivity (%)	Specificity (%)
		Mean	Range		
Kurjak and Kupesic[17]	103	55	18–160	84	97
Guerriero et al[18]	29	40	SD: 10	84	95
Alcazar et al[19]	27	unknown		89	91
Guerriero et al[20]	58	40	SD: 16	81	96

Table 7.2 Accuracy of magnetic resonance imaging for the diagnosis of hemorrhagic endometriosis

Study	Location	Size	Sensitivity %	Specificity %
Zawin et al[22]			71	82
Arrivé et al[23]			64	60
Takahashi et al[11]		<5 mm	49	Fat-saturated
		5–10 mm	100	Fat-saturated
Stratton et al[24]			69	75
Togashi et al[25]	Ovary	Unknown	90	98
Stratton et al[24]	Ovary	1–9 cm		77

characterized by a 'rich' vascularization pattern, often with detectable arterial flow in the papillary structures or echogenic areas of the cyst. The characteristic vascular pattern of an endometrioma has been described as 'pericystic flow at the level of the ovarian hilus'.

Several scoring systems have been proposed to improve the diagnosis and differentiate between malignant and benign adnexal masses, although complex scoring systems are unlikely to be clinically useful. From a meta-analysis, Kinkel et al[21] concluded that a combination of ultrasound techniques and a diagnostic algorithm performs significantly better than morphologic assessment, color Doppler flow imaging, or Doppler ultrasound indexes alone in characterizing ovarian masses.

Magnetic resonance imaging

Several investigators have evaluated the accuracy of MR imaging for the diagnosis of hemorrhagic endometriosis (Table 7.2). In a preoperative study of 16 endometriomas, ranging in size from 1 to 9 cm in diameter, MR imaging detected 77% of lesions.[24] Despite the limited size of these studies, it appears likely that MR imaging is a useful technique to detect endometriomas of 1 cm diameter or more.

Endometriomas can present either as a homogeneously high signal intensity mass on T1-weighted MR images, a low signal intensity mass with focal high signal intensity areas on T2-weighed images, or as a mass with a mixed signal intensity pattern (Figure 7.4). Endometriomas may

(a)

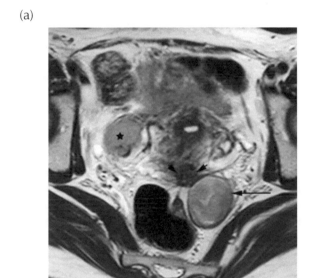

(b)

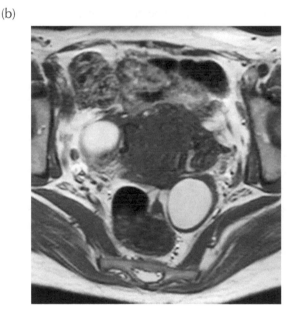

(c)

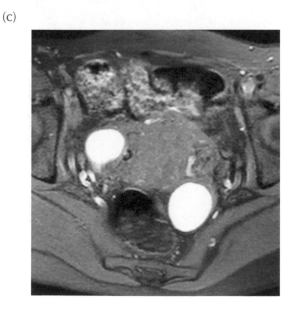

Figure 7.4 A 37-year-old woman with bilateral endometrioma. (a) A T2-weighted axial MR image demonstrates two endometriomas with heterogeneous (left endometrioma, black arrow) and homogenous cyst content (right endometrioma, star), respectively. A T2-hypointense nodule (arrowheads) between the posterior wall of the uterus and the left ovary corresponded to a large adenomyotic nodule of the posterior pelvis at surgery. (b) The corresponding native T1-weighted axial image, taken at the same level as image in (a), demonstrating hyper-signal intensity of the cystic content of both endometriomas. (c) The hyper-signal intensity appearance persists on axial fat-suppressed T1-weighted images. The hyperintense tubulous structures lateral to both ovaries reflect blood flow in pelvic vessels.

also manifest as multiple, homogeneously high signal intensive cysts on T1-weighted images (Figure 7.5). Some authors have described a thickened hypointense cyst wall on T2-weighted images with a retracted part producing the typical appearance of a 'grain de cafè' (coffee bean). This area of retraction is likely to represent the site of invagination.

The features of endometriomas on MR imaging are largely based on the detection of chronic and recurrent bleeding in the lesion. If a bleeding occurred recently, the cyst content will have a high-signal intensity in both types of sequences. Frequently, the cavity is filled with blood of different ages.

Endometriosis of the posterior pelvis

Physical examination is often inadequate to evaluate the extent of infiltrating endometriosis in the posterior pelvis. Imaging techniques are increasingly accurate in diagnosing the extent of endometriosis in the posterior pelvis.

Histopathology

Posterior pelvis endometriosis consists predominantly of myoproliferative lesions interspersed with a sparse amount of glandular and stromal tissue and microendometriomas. Thomas Cullen coined the term 'adenomyoma' for lesions of this type.[26] Hence, the terms 'adenomyoma' or 'adenomyosis' not only describes uterine lesions but also myoproliferative endometriotic lesions in other pelvic structures or organs. Like uterine adeno-

myosis, these lesions have no capsule and are in continuity with the surrounding fibromuscular or muscular structures.

Itoga et al[27] recently described in detail the fibrosis and smooth muscle metaplasia that characterizes rectovaginal endometriosis. Immunostains were used to study 90 rectovaginal tissue specimens obtained from 37 affected women. Fibrosis was present in 89 specimens. The intensity of fibrosis differed greatly in specimens from area to area. In mild cases, collagen fibers were present around the endometriotic tissue, but in severe cases they extended into the surrounding fat and connective tissue. Increasing amount of endometriotic tissue correlated with increasing degree of fibrosis. Smooth muscle metaplasia, defined as aggregated smooth muscle not associated with blood vessels, was always detectable within the fibrotic areas. The degree of smooth muscle metaplasia correlated significantly with the degree of fibrosis.

'Rectovaginal septum' endometriosis is often a misnomer as the endometriotic lesions do not infiltrate the rectovaginal septum. However, adenomyotic lesions may be found in close proximity to the upper part of the septum.[28] Consequently, the rectovaginal septum appears distinct and regular on MR imaging. Involvement of the rectovaginal septum by endometriosis can be identified as an extension of the larger lesions located at the uterosacral ligaments, the pouch of Douglas, or the anterior rectal wall. Infiltrating posterior pelvis endometriosis can also extend into the cervix, rectal wall, and laterally into the parametrium, and even involve the ureters.

(a)

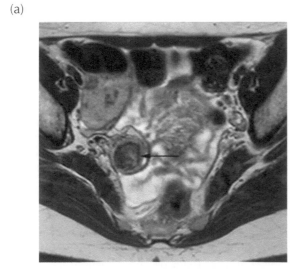

(b)

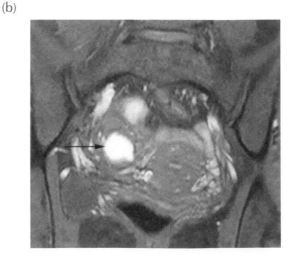

Figure 7.5 A 32-year-old woman with chronic pelvic pain and dyspareunia. (a) An axial T2-weighted MR image of a 3 cm right endometrioma with a thick capsule apparent as a hypointense peripheral ring (arrow). (b) The hyper-signal intensity of the cyst on coronal fat-suppressed T1-weighted images (arrow) confirms that it is filled with blood.

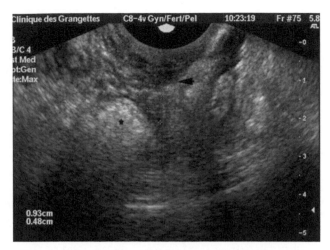

Figure 7.6 Axial image of rectal endometriosis on TVU. The hypoechoic structure between calipers corresponds to the thickened rectal wall. The rectum is easily identified due to air within the rectal lumen (black star). The adenomyotic nodule is located posterior to the cervix (black arrowhead).

However, it is important to remember that endometriotic infiltration of the posterior pelvis is not destructive and that fat tissue is not invaded. The inability of endometriotic lesions to infiltrate fat tissue may explain why women with a low body mass index (BMI) are more at risk of developing posterior pelvis endometriosis than those with a higher BMI.

Transvaginal ultrasound

Recent ultrasound studies have focused on determining the extent of posterior pelvis involvement in the presence of endometriosis. On TVU, adenomyotic nodules can appear as solid hypoechoic lesions ranging from 0.5 to 4 cm (Figure 7.6). The larger nodules may be adherent to the anterior rectal wall. Characteristically, these lesions are more painful when TVU examination is performed during menstruation. In a controlled prospective study of 142 women with symptomatic endometriosis Bazot et al[29] found that TVU accurately diagnosed intestinal and bladder endometriosis, but is less accurate for uterosacral, vaginal lesions and those in close proximity to the rectovaginal septum involvement.

Magnetic resonance imaging

MR imaging is increasingly used to determine preoperatively the presence and extent of posterior pelvis endometriosis. The technique is superior over TVU, as it is less operator-dependent and can provide more objective documentation.

Endometriosis of the uterosacral ligaments appears on MR imaging as a retrocervical nodularity with a signal intensity similar to that of normal uterosacral ligaments (Figure 7.7a). Chapron et al[28] have detailed the MR appearances of rectovaginal endometriotic nodules, varying between 2.0 and 2.5 cm, in 8 affected patients. On a T1-weighted image the signal intensity of the lesion is iso-intense to that of the myometrium with possible hyperintensive spots which remain visible in the fat-suppressed sequences, indicating the presence of microendometriomas. On the T2-weighed images the signal intensity of the nodules is iso- or hypointense, when compared to the myometrium, with hyperintensive spots (Figure 7.7b). The nodules have an irregular contour and are indistinguishable from the uterovaginal structures. In some cases a hyper-signal intensity transition zone

(a)

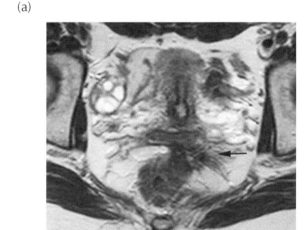

(b)

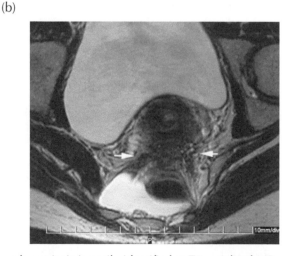

Figure 7.7 Thickening of uterosacral ligaments due to posterior endometriosis is easily identified at T2-weighted MR images. (a) An axial T2-weighted image shows unilateral hypointense thickening of the left uterosacral ligament (arrow), which extends to the adjacent rectal wall. (b) Bilateral thickening of the initial portion of both uterosacral ligaments (white arrows) at axial T2-weighted images extends into the pouch of Douglas.

can be identified between the rectum and the nodule which has been termed the 'safety margin'. In other cases, this 'safety margin' is not seen and thickening of the rectum wall is noticed. The 'safety margin' is likely to represent interposing fat tissue. The retraction between the torus uterinum, the endometriotic nodule, and the rectum results in obliteration of the pouch of Douglas. This can give a false impression that the lesion is located below the pouch and infiltrates the perirectal space with thickening and rigidity of the rectum wall. False-negative and false-positive results can occur in patients with a retroverted uterus or in the presence of an endometrioma that masks the insertion or proximal part of the uterosacral ligaments.[30] Bazot et al[31] found recently that imaging demonstrates high accuracy in prediction of deep pelvic endometriosis in specific locations (Table 7.3).

Protocol for magnetic resonance imaging of pelvic endometriosis

The routine technical imaging protocol for suspicion of posterior endometriosis in the pelvic cavity includes the use of a pelvic phase array coil and T2-weighted spin echo sequences – reception time (TR) 4000 ms and echo time (TE) 90 ms – in three imaging planes with at least one parallel and one perpendicular slice orientation to the endometrial lining of the uterine cavity. Standard section thickness of 5 mm may need to be decreased to 3 mm if a small nodule of posterior endometriosis is suspected. The imaging plane that demonstrates best the pathologic structure is repeated three times: a native T1-weighted sequence, a fat-suppressed T1-weighted sequence, and a fat-suppressed T1-weighted sequence with injection of gadolinium, particularly if extension to the bladder or rectal wall is suspected. Prior fasting and intramuscular injection of 1 mg of glucagon or an inhibitor of peristalsis reduces bowel movement artifacts that decrease imaging quality. Imaging during menstruation is not recommended, as fresh blood up to 8 days old has low-signal intensity at T1-weighted MR imaging instead of the classical hyper-signal intensity indicative of older blood.

Rectosigmoid endometriosis

Posterior pelvis endometriosis can also affect the rectosigmoid colon, appendix, and ileum. At those locations it can cause marked overgrowth and retraction of the external muscular wall of the bowel. These lesions may be constricting or may produce an intraluminal filling defect, resembling colon carcinoma. However, unlike colon carcinoma, endometriosis does not breach the bowel mucosa or cause mucosal ulcerations.

Endorectal ultrasound

Rectal endoscopic ultrasound has been found useful in the preoperative evaluation of rectal wall involvement in endometriosis.[32,33] In a small study, Koga et al[34] detected infiltrating rectosigmoid endometriosis through a combination of TVU and transrectal ultrasonography. A hypoechoic irregularly shaped area corresponded to a layer of hypertrophic muscular propria, whereas a hyperechoic rim represented the layer consisting of mucosa, submucosa, and serosa. Bazot et al[35] compared the accuracy of TVU and rectal endoscopic sonography for the diagnosis of endometriosis involving the bowel. In a study of 30 patients, TVU was as efficient as rectal endoscopic sonography. However, the main limitation of TVU is the inability to determine the exact distance of the rectal lesions from the anal margin or to evaluate the depth of rectal wall involvement.

As TVU is as efficient as rectal endoscopic sonography for detecting bowel involvement, it should be used as the first-line procedure. Rectal endoscopic sonography can be recommended for cases

Table 7.3 Accuracy of magnetic resonance imaging for the diagnosis of adenomyotic endometriosis according to localization[31]

Localization	Sensitivity %	Specificity %	Accuracy %
Uterosacral ligaments	76	83	80
Rectovaginal	80	98	97
Rectosigmoid	88	98	95
Bladder	88	99	98
Vagina	76	95	93

in which colorectal involvement is suspected or prior to surgery.

Magnetic resonance imaging

Bowel wall thickening and possible T2- or T1-hyperintensive cysts within the bowel wall are characteristic MR imaging signs (Figure 7.8). In most cases the rectum is retracted towards the uterus, yielding a triangular aspect with the tip of the triangle pointing forward. Intravenous contrast injection and rectal opacification with water enema has been suggested to improve confirmation of bowel involvement and avoid false-positive findings. In a preliminary comparative study, Chapron et al[36] found that the sensitivity and negative predictive value of rectal endoscopic ultrasonography were higher than those of MR imaging, suggesting that rectal endoscopic ultrasonography performs better than MR imaging in the diagnosis

of rectal involvement for patients presenting with severe posterior pelvic endometriosis.

Bladder endometriosis

Nodular bladder endometriosis is not easily palpable on vaginal examination. Patients typically present with dysmenorrhea combined with urinary symptoms such as micturation frequency. TVU may reveal a solid nodule within the posterior bladder wall if the bladder is slightly filled. Color Doppler studies may detect low-to-moderate vascularization of the lesion and the mild pressure of the vaginal probe often elicits focal pain.

In a series of 12 patients with nodular bladder endometriosis, varying between 10 and 31 mm in diameter, TVU examination was found to be normal in four patients, whereas MR imaging, using a

(a)

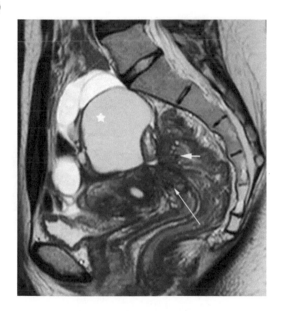

(b)

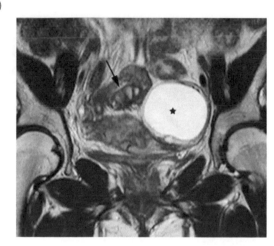

(c)

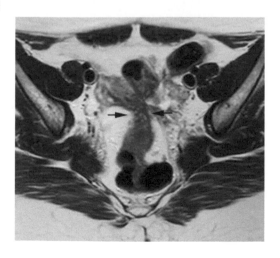

Figure 7.8 Endometriosis of the rectosigmoid in three different patients. (a) Sagittal T2-weighted MR image demonstrating a multilocular endometrioma (white star) and severe posterior endometriosis affecting the sigmoid (short white arrow) and cervix (long white arrow). (b) Coronal T2-weighted image shows a large left endometrioma (asterisk) with adjacent thickening of the sigmoid wall (arrow), which also contains hyperintense cystic structures due to invading endometriosis. (c) Axial T2-weighted image shows a stricture of the sigmoid bowel (between black arrows) in a patient with severe peritoneal endometriosis and adhesions. The bowel wall contains very small hyperintense cysts due to chronic bleeding.

body coil, enabled visualization of all lesions[37] (Figure 7.9). Furthermore, the use of an endocavitary coil was found to be superior to a body coil in determining the extent of infiltration of the bladder wall. MR imaging characteristics of bladder endometriosis included irregular posterior wall thickening and T1 hyperintensive spots within the thickened bladder wall. Coils are the part of the MRI imaging that receive the magnetic field changes inside the body and transmit them to the computer reconstructing them into an image. A body coil is nothing else than the part of the MR tunnel that captures overall MR field changes inside the tunnel. More recent coils are designed to one part of the body only, such as the head, wrist or pelvic coils. Endocavitary coils are coils that are covered by a condom and introduced by the radiologist into the rectum or the vagina to increase information close to this region. Comparative studies on the combination of the body coil plus endovaginal coil vs a pelvic coil alone have not been done.

Obstructive uropathy secondary to endometriosis

Ureteral obstruction is an infrequent, but serious complication of posterior pelvis endometriosis. Involvement of posterior pelvis or ovarian endometriosis may result in extrinsic compression of the ureteric wall.[38] Less commonly, the endometriosis is intrinsic, resulting in a thickened ureteric wall with fibrosis and proliferation of the ureteric muscularis (Figure 7.10). The risk of obstructive uropathy increases in the presence of nodular posterior pelvis endometriosis larger than 3 cm.[39]

Extrinsic ureteral endometriosis is more frequent than intrinsic lesions and is commonly caused by endometrioma formation. Ureter-obstructing endometriomas have been described many years after hysterectomy and bilateral salpingo-oophorectomy during long-term unopposed estrogen or combined estrogen-progestin replacement

(a)

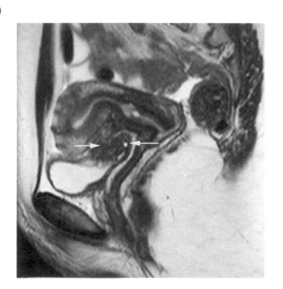

(b)

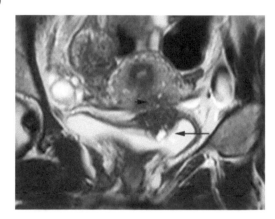

(c)

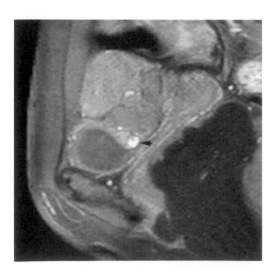

Figure 7.9 Bladder endometriosis in a 29-year-old woman with dysuria during menstruation. (a) This sagittal T2-weighted image shows a thickening of the upper posterior bladder wall (arrows) with a hyperintense spot within the detrusor. (b) The coronal T2-weighted image demonstrates hypointensity with a hyperintense locus within the submucosal portion of the lesion (long arrow). The anterior myometrium demonstrates associated external adenomyosis (short arrow). (c) The sagittal fat-suppressed T1-weighted image confirms the presence of blood within this submucosal portion of the bladder wall (arrow).

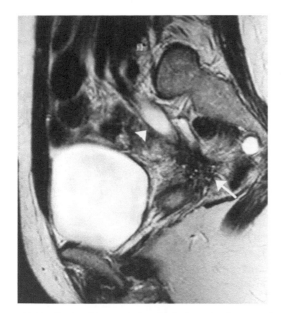

Figure 7.10 Sagittal T2-weighted MR image of ureteral endometriosis (white arrow), identified as a solid tubular hypointense structure with irregular borders containing small hyperintense cysts. Ureteral dilatation is seen above the suspicious nodule (white arrowhead).

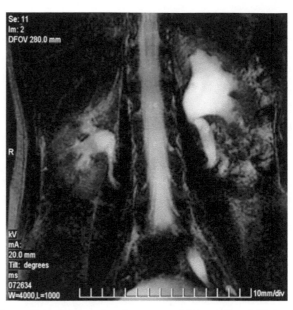

Figure 7.11. MR urography (coronal T2-weighted thick sections) demonstrating unilateral left hydronephrosis due to external ureteral obstruction by endometriomas.

therapy.[40] Small endometriomas obstructing the ureter can be detected by MR imaging.[41] MR imaging is therefore useful for both the diagnosis and monitoring the response to medical therapy of an obstructing periureteric endometrioma. MR urography can also be used to visualize associated hydronephrosis (Figure 7.11).

Conclusion

TVU is a useful technique for the detection of endometriomas of the ovaries and endometriotic lesions of the bladder and pouch of Douglas. However, the ability of ultrasound to visualize adenomyotic lesions located in the posterior pelvis is limited. MR imaging of the pelvis detects small endometriomas and will yield accurate information on the presence and extent of adenomyotic pelvic endometriosis. Other associated lesions such as adenomyosis of the uterus can be diagnosed with greater specificity and reproducibility by MR imaging when compared to TVU.[42,43]

It is important to inform the radiologist adequately of the presenting symptoms and clinical findings as this will determine the most appropriate imaging protocol. For instance, if endometriosis is sus-

pected to involve the bowel then preparation with rectal water enema and intravenous contrast injection are indicated. Although image acquisition can be easily standardized at any MRI unit, prior experience in gynecologic imaging will greatly determine the diagnostic accuracy.[44]

Preoperative knowledge of the endometriotic lesions will help in determining the best surgical approach, thereby reducing the incidence of inadequate or partial surgical treatment of patients with more severe disease. Needless to say, this approach will also reduce the cost and suffering associated with inadequate treatment.

With the introduction of new medical treatments for severe endometriosis, such as aromatase inhibitors,[45] the real challenge today is tailoring treatment, whether surgical, medical, or combined, to individual patient needs and wishes. Too often, patients are not informed of the extent of surgery required or offered a referral to a surgical center of excellence. Preoperative diagnosis of severe endometriosis, including hemorrhagic as well as adenomyotic lesions, is increasingly feasible. It is likely that gynecologists in the future will make much more use of specialized women's imaging centers to diagnose and stage pelvic endometriosis.

REFERENCES

1. Mol BW, Bayram N, Lijmer JG, et al. The performance of CA-125 measurement in the detection of endometriosis: a meta-analysis. Fertil Steril 1998; 70: 1101–1108.

2. Harada T, Kubota T, Asi T. Usefulness of CA19-9 versus CA125 for the diagnosis of endometriosis. Fertil Steril 2002; 77: 733–739.

3. Bedaiwy MA, Falcone T, Sharma RK, et al. Prediction of endometriosis with serum and peritoneal fluid markers: a prospective controlled trial. Hum Reprod 2002; 17: 426–431.

4. Somigliana E, Viganò P, Tirelli AS, et al. Use of the concomitant serum dosage of CA 125, CA 19-9 and interleukin-6 to detect the presence of endometriosis. Results from a series of reproductive age women undergoing laparoscopic surgery for benign gynecologic conditions. Hum Reprod 2004; 19: 1871–1876.

5. Vigano P, Somigliana E, Matrone R, et al. Serum leptin concentrations in endometriosis. J Clin Endocrinol Metab 2002; 87: 1085–1087.

6. Brosens IA, Brosens JJ. Redefining endometriosis: is deep endometriosis a progressive disease? Hum Reprod 2000; 15: 1–3.

7. Kitawaki J, Kusuki I, Koshiba H, et al. Detection of aromatase cytochrome P-450 in endometrial biopsy specimens as a diagnostic test for endometriosis. Fertil Steril 1999; 72: 6.

8. Dheenadayalu K, Mak I, Gordts S, et al. Aromatase P450 messenger RNA expression in eutopic endometrium is not a specific marker for pelvic endometriosis. Fertil Steril 2002; 78: 825–829.

9. Kao LC, Germeyer A, Tulac S, et al. Expression profiling of endometrium from women with endometriosis reveals candidate genes for disease-based implantation failure and infertility. Endocrinology 2003; 144: 2870–2881.

10. Brosens I. The classification of endometriosis revisited. Lancet 1993; 341: 630.

11. Takahashi K, Okada M, Okada S, et al. Studies on the detection of small endometrial implants by magnetic resonance imaging using a fat saturation technique. Gynecol Obstet Invest 1996; 41: 203–206.

12. Sampson JA. Perforating hemorrhagic (chocolate) cysts of the ovary. Arch Surg 1921; 3: 245–323.

13. Hughesdon PE. The structure of endometrial cysts of the ovary. J Obstet Gynaecol Br Emp 1957; 44: 481–487.

14. Brosens IA, Puttemans PJ, Deprest J. The endoscopic localization of endometrial implants in the ovarian chocolate cyst. Fertil Steril 1994; 61: 1034–1038.

15. Patel MD, Feldstein VA, Chen DC, et al. Endometriomas: diagnostic performance of US. Radiology 1999; 210: 739–745.

16. Moore J, Copley S, Morris J, et al. A systematic review of the accuracy of ultrasound in the diagnosis of endometriosis. Ultrasound Obstet Gynecol 2003; 20: 630–634.

17. Kurjak A, Kupesic S. Scoring system for prediction of ovarian endometriosis based on transvaginal color and pulsed Doppler sonography. Fertil Steril 1994; 62: 81–88.

18. Guerriero S, Mais V, Ajossa S, et al. Transvaginal ultrasonography combined with CA-125 plasma levels in the diagnosis of endometrioma. Fertil Steril 1996; 65: 293–298.

19. Alcazar J L, Laparte C, Jurado M, et al. The role of transvaginal ultrasonography combined with colour velocity imaging and pulsed Doppler in the diagnosis of endometrioma. Fertil Steril 1997; 67: 487–491.

20. Guerriero S, Ajossa S, Mais V, et al. The diagnosis of endometriomas using colour Doppler energy imaging. Hum Reprod 1998; 13: 1691–1695.

21. Kinkel K, Hricak H, Lu Y, et al. US characterization of ovarian masses: a meta-analysis. Radiology 2000; 217: 803–811.

22. Zawin M, McCarthy S, Scoutt L, et al. Endometriosis: appearance and detection at MR imaging. Radiology 1989; 171: 693–696.

23. Arrivé L, Hricak H, Martin M. Pelvic endometriosis: MR imaging. Radiology 1989; 171: 687–692.

24. Stratton P, Winkel C, Premkumar A, et al. Diagnostic accuracy of laparoscopy, magnetic resonance imaging, and histopathologic examination for the detection of endometriosis. Fertil Steril 2003; 79: 1078–1085.

25. Togashi K, Nishimura K, Kimura I, et al. Endometrial cysts: diagnosis with MR imaging. Radiology 1991; 180: 73–78.

26. Cullen TS. The distribution of adenomyoma containing uterine mucosa. Arch Surg 1920; 1: 215–283.

27. Itoga T, Matsumoto T, Takeuchi H, et al. Fibrosis and smooth muscle metaplasia in rectovaginal endometriosis. Pathol Int 2003; 53: 371–375.

28. Chapron C, Liaras E, Fayet P, et al. Magnetic resonance imaging and endometriosis: deeply infiltrating endometriosis does not originate from the rectovaginal septum. Gynecol Obstet Invest 2002; 53: 204–208.

29. Bazot M, Thomassin I, Hourani R, et al. Diagnostic accuracy of transvaginal sonography for deep pelvic endometriosis. Ultrasound Obstet Gynecol 2004; 24: 180–185.

30. Kinkel K, Chapron C, Balleyguier C, et al. Magnetic resonance imaging characteristics of deep endometriosis. Hum Reprod 1999; 14: 1080–1086.

31. Bazot M, Darai E, Hourani R, et al. Deep pelvic endometriosis: MR imaging for diagnosis and prediction of extension of disease. Radiology 2004; 232: 379–389.

32. Abrao MS, Neme RM, Averbach M, et al. Rectal endoscopic ultrasound with a radial probe in the assessment of rectovaginal endometriosis. J Am Assoc Gynecol Laparosc 2004; 11: 50–54.

33. Doniec JM, Kahlke V, Peetz F, et al. Rectal endometriosis: high sonsitivity and specificity of endorectal ultrasound with an impact for the operative management. Dis Colon Rectum 2003; 46: 1667–1673.

34. Koga K, Osuga Y, Momoeda M, et al. Characteristic images of deeply infiltrating rectosigmoid endometriosis on transvaginal and transrectal ultrasonography. Hum Reprod 2003; 18: 1328–1333.

35. Bazot M, Detchev R, Cortez A, et al. Transvaginal sonography and rectal endoscopic sonography for the assessment of pelvic endometriosis: a preliminary comparison. Hum Reprod 2003; 18: 1686–1692.

36. Chapron C, Vieira M, Chopin N, et al. Accuracy of rectal endoscopic ultrasonography and magnetic resonance imaging in the diagnosis of rectal involvement for patients presenting with deeply infiltrating endometriosis. Ultrasound Obstet Gynecol 2004; 24: 175–179.

37. Balleyguier C, Chapron C, Dubuisson JB, et al. Comparison of magnetic resonance imaging and transvaginal ultrasonography in diagnosing bladder endometriosis. J Am Assoc Gynecol Laparosc 2002; 9: 15–23.

38. Donnez J, Brosens I. Definition of ureteral endometriosis? Fertil Steril 1997; 68: 178–179.

39. Donnez J, Nisolle M, Squifflet J. Ureteral endometriosis: a complication of rectovaginal endometriotic (adenomyotic) nodules. Fertil Steril 2002; 77: 32–37.

40. Brosens I. Endometriosis – a disease because it is characterized by bleeding. Am J Obstet Gynecol 1997; 176: 263–267.

41. Deprest J, Marchal G, Brosens I. Obstructive uropathy secondary to endometriosis. N Engl J Med 1997; 337: 1174–1175.

42. Dueholm M, Lundorf E, Sorensen JS, et al. Reproducibility of evaluation of the uterus by transvaginal sonography, hysterosonographic examination, hysteroscopy and magnetic resonance imaging. Hum Reprod 2002; 17: 195–200.

43. Dueholm M, Lundorf E, Hansen ES, et al. Magnetic resonance imaging and transvaginal ultrasonography for the diagnosis of adenomyosis. Fertil Steril 2001; 76: 588–594.

44. Bazot M, Darai E, Clement de Givry S, et al. Fast breath-hold T2-weighted MR imaging reduces interobserver variability in the diagnosis of adenomyosis. Am J Roentgenol 2003; 180: 1291–1296.

45. Soysal S, Soysal ME, Ozer S, et al. The effects of post-surgical administration of goserelin plus anastrozole compared to goserelin alone in patients with severe endometriosis: a prospective randomized trial. Hum Reprod 2004; 19: 160–167.

8 Open pelvic surgery for endometriosis

David H Oram and Barnaby D Rufford

Introduction

Endometriosis in a significant number of women is a chronic progressive disease with the overwhelming symptom being intractable pain. Hormonal therapy and conservative surgery, either local excision or ablation, offer temporary relief but this is often short-lived and relapse rates are high. When symptomatic relief becomes more important than fertility preservation, surgery, in the form of pelvic clearance followed by hormone replacement therapy (HRT), must be contemplated. The nature of the disease process itself, and the effects of previous surgery – extensive adhesions and fibrotic tissues are the rule – make this definitive surgery extremely challenging. It is therefore axiomatic that experienced surgeons should perform such procedures, and it is for this reason that many of these cases of end-stage disease gravitate to gynecologic oncologists for this form of surgical management.

Prevalence

Endometriosis has been variously estimated to affect between 1–2%[1,2] and 7–10%[3] of women of reproductive years, and up to 45%[4,5] if laparoscopic visualization of lesions regardless of symptoms is the parameter assessed. Studies have estimated that at least 9% of all gynecologic surgery is performed for this disease.[3] Estimates vary considerably regarding the percentage of women with diagnosed endometriosis who will ultimately require surgery in the form of hysterectomy and

bilateral salpingo-oophorectomy, with reported figures ranging between 12 and 55%.[6–8] The numbers obviously increase with advancing age, with one study reporting 83% of women with endometriosis over 39 years undergoing a pelvic clearance.[9]

Endometriosis is the fifth commonest reason for the performance of hysterectomy in the UK (5.4%), following fibroids (38.5%), menstrual problems (35.3%), prolapse (6.5%), and cancer (5.6%).[10] The same epidemiologic study reported that the peak age for hysterectomy for endometriosis was 40–44 years. In this study population, 92.1% of women underwent a total abdominal hysterectomy, 6.9% underwent a vaginal hysterectomy, 1.0% had a subtotal hysterectomy, and bilateral salpingo-oophorectomy accompanied the procedure in 33.7% of cases.[10]

Preoperative assessment

By the time the point is reached when hysterectomy and bilateral salpingo-oophorectomy is being considered, virtually all patients will have endured years of pain. They will have undergone initial diagnostic investigations, repeated courses of hormonal therapies, and very often several laparoscopies. They may have endured the anguish of subfertility and perhaps submitted themselves to numerous attempts at assisted conception. At this stage they are also a very well-informed group. Although detailed counseling regarding all aspects of pelvic clearance and possible long-term HRT is of course essential, the decision to proceed to definitive surgery is usually patient-led, and once made is associated with feelings of relief rather than despair.

The extent of the disease process can and should be assessed as much as possible preoperatively, and potential surgical difficulties anticipated, so that the nature and extent of the surgery can be discussed with the patient in advance, and informed consent obtained. In this context, clinical assessment is often unhelpful. It can of course indicate the size and fixity of the uterus and associated pelvic masses, and perhaps help to determine the most appropriate abdominal incision, but it does not give an accurate assessment of the true extent of the disease process, including adhesion formation and the problems that are likely to be encountered at laparotomy. The most helpful factor in this regard is the pictorial or video record that is now so frequently obtained at a preceding laparoscopy. Such information will alert the operating surgeon in advance of the need perhaps to involve colleagues from other disciplines, such as colorectal and urological surgery, if techniques such as bowel resection and reanastomosis, stoma formation, and urinary diversion do not fall within their compass.

Preoperative investigations should include a complete blood count, serum urea and electrolytes, and blood should be cross-matched. Serum cancer antigen CA-125 levels, although not good at making, or indeed confirming, a diagnosis of endometriosis, are often elevated, sometimes markedly in active and extensive disease. Levels above 6000 IU/ml[11] have been reported, but even moderately elevated levels in the presence of bilateral complex ovarian masses identified on ultrasound can be somewhat alarming. CA-125 levels have, however, been shown to correlate with the American Society of Reproductive Medicine defined stages of disease, and levels of >65 IU/ml have been used as a preoperative predictor of women who should undergo bowel preparation.[12] It is also argued that CA-125 is an inexpensive, relatively noninvasive test that might be used to rationalize the practice of laparoscopy by identifying patients who would most benefit from the procedure. Serum CA-19-9 levels have also been reported as correlating significantly with the stage of disease and, as such, may be used as an adjunct to predict the anticipated severity of the disease in the preoperative work-up.[13]

Some time might have elapsed since the last surgical assessment, and imaging techniques such as transvaginal ultrasound, computed tomography (CT), or magnetic resonance imaging (MRI) scanning may be employed to help plan surgical management. Although CT imaging is not particularly good at characterizing pelvic masses, both ultrasound and MRI are of value in this regard. MRI has limitations in the identification of small peritoneal foci of disease and adhesions, but nevertheless there is a 95% concordance with subsequent surgical findings.[14] Endovaginal ultrasound and MRI can be utilized to detect, stage, and follow up disease in the rectovaginal septum,[15] and MRI has a high accuracy in predicting deep pelvic endometriosis in specific locations such as the uterosacral ligaments, the rectosigmoid, and the bladder.[16]

As well as cross-sectional imaging, the renal tract should be specifically imaged to identify the course of the ureters, and an intravenous urogram should be requested. A chest X-ray is advisable. Further investigations such as endoscopic assessment of the bladder or bowel are dictated by the clinical situation. Some surgeons favor the insertion of ureteric stents, but in the majority of cases this should not be necessary.

The bowel should be prepared prior to surgery, and a regimen such as sodium picosulfate and magnesium citrate (Picolax) can be given on the day before surgery together with a phosphate enema that evening.

The incision

The choice lies between a vertical lower midline incision and a transverse suprapubic approach that includes a muscle-splitting option. The transverse incision with division of the rectus abdominus muscle provides a perfectly good view of the pelvic organs with acceptable access but if it is anticipated that extensive or defunctioning bowel surgery will be required then the vertical incision provides far more flexibility. The choice of incision is not only influenced by the anticipated extent of disease but also by factors such as the size of the patient, the size and mobility of the pelvic organs, and the presence of existing scars. If doubt exists over the adequacy of the access, the vertical incision should be selected.

The surgical procedure

The paramount aim of the surgical procedure is to achieve total eradication of all disease. That having been said, definitive surgery in the form of pelvic clearance for advanced stage endometriosis can be extremely challenging, requiring a difficult combination of patience and perseverance, and courage and caution on the part of the operating surgeon. A balance needs to be struck between an awareness of the ease with which bowel or ureteric damage can occur, and the knowledge that successful removal of the uterus, and in particular the ovaries, is the only way in which the patient's intractable pain can be cured.

The concept of removing ovaries in relatively young women has always been, and still is, controversial. On the one hand, there are those who would urge the preservation of some ovarian tissue on the basis that this will avoid the early introduction of HRT, and suggest the need for reoperation, due to problems arising in residual ovaries is as low as 1–3%.[17] They would also argue that persistence or reactivation of patients' endometriosis and associated symptoms is no different if stimulated by either exogenous or endogenous estrogens. On the other hand, there is a counter argument, and other data exist to suggest that reoperation rates for persistent symptoms related to conserved ovaries is of the order of 7.6%;[18] in one study, 45% of women required repeat laparotomy for pain associated with adhesions and the residual ovary syndrome.[19] In a further study of 109 women,[20] 85 of whom had no ovarian tissue at the end of laparotomy and 24 women had some residual tissue, only 1 patient required further laparotomy following commencement of HRT in the no residual tissue group, whereas 6 women (25%) required further surgery for recurrence of endometriosis and pelvic pain in the group where ovarian tissue was left behind. All the women in the group who had had all of their ovarian tissue removed reported excellent symptomatic relief.

In the decision-making equation, there is also the now well-described concept of potential malignant transformation of endometriosis. This was first described in 1925 by Sampson,[21] who acknowledged that ovarian adenocarcinoma could arise in areas of endometriosis. However, it was not until 1961 that the term endometrioid adenocarcinoma of the ovary was agreed.[22] Overall, the malignant potential of endometriosis is low. However, endometrioid tumors are variously reported to account for between 16 and 30% of all ovarian carcinomas.[23–26] Two modes of histogenesis are possible: either from the epithelium of antecedent endometriosis or from the surface of the epithelium of the ovary. Some form of pelvic endometriosis is identified in 28% of cases of endometrioid ovarian cancer[26] but an origin from an endometriotic cyst itself is demonstrable in only 5–10% of cases.[27]

Many women, by the time they get to the point of undergoing definitive pelvic surgery for intractable symptoms, have undergone several surgical procedures in the past, and view the prospect of pelvic clearance as a surgical finale after many miserable years and do not want to run the risk of the need for further surgery in the future. However, on questioning retrospectively, it has been shown that over 60% of women regret having their ovaries removed, and this figure is unrelated to parity or the number of previous surgical procedures, but was significantly related to the age at which hysterectomy was performed.[20] Not surprisingly, the younger women expressed greater regret.

The decision to perform oophorectomy at the time of hysterectomy should therefore be taken on an individual basis following a detailed discussion with the patient about all of these issues. In practice, it is the authors' experience that this decision-making process is not as difficult as it might seem. Patients are usually motivated towards definitive surgery, and at that surgery the usual finding is of diseased ovaries buried in dense adhesions and chronically inflamed tissues. Symptomatic relief will not be obtained until they are painstakingly released and removed.

On opening the abdomen, the usual finding is one of dense and widespread adhesions, usually matting loops of small bowel together, which frequently obscure the pelvic organs. The adhesions themselves are not of the flimsy, easily separated, type but are most commonly fibrotic, and reflect years of chronic inflammatory response. Consequently the surgical procedure usually commences by meticulous sharp dissection of 'woody' adhesions in an attempt to separate loops of bowel in order to gain access to the pelvis. Tissue planes are obscured and the problem of 'serosal stripping' of the bowel is frequently encountered. In many instances the problem is so bad that considerable time is spent performing adhesiolysis before the fundus of the uterus becomes visible. The ovaries themselves are frequently not visible, but can occasionally be palpated buried in a mass of adhesions and stuck bowel, or are frequently densely adherent to the posterior leaf of the broad ligament and pelvic side wall. They may also be retroperitoneal in position, and on one occasion in the authors' experience were eventually located in the inguinal canal.

The immediate challenge is therefore to identify some semblance of normal anatomy, and in this regard the successful identification of round ligaments on either side is both helpful and uplifting. Once found, the round ligaments can be transected and the retroperitoneal space can be entered. This is an area that frequently has been unaffected by the disease process and once entered often assists further surgical progression. In some circumstances, however, the chronic inflammatory process has also affected the tissues in the retroperitoneal area, and these are fibrotic and difficult to dissect, and in many ways are similar tissues to those encountered in patients who have previously undergone pelvic radiotherapy. The importance of entering the retroperitoneal space in the area of the pelvic side walls, however, is that it allows identification of the ureters on both sides. This is essential before the ovaries can be mobilized. It is not sufficient to identify the ureters in the region of the bifurcation of the iliac arteries because they can be kinked, distorted, and pulled out of normal position by the fibrotic process and as a result can easily be inadvertently caught in a surgical clamp at any point in the pelvis. It is therefore very important to expose the ureter throughout its length in the pelvis on both sides before transecting any pedicles.

The next challenge is to identify and mobilize the ovaries on both sides. This often requires painstaking and courageous dissection because of the nature of the tissue the surgeon is dealing with, the absence of surgical planes, and the proximity of the bowel. Once achieved, however, the infundibulopelvic ligaments can usually be easily identified, transected, and ligated, with the ureters under direct vision. The remainder of the surgery should be directed towards restoring as much normal anatomy as possible before proceeding to hysterectomy. This often requires releasing loops of bowel which may be adherent to the fundus and posterior wall of the uterus, to the cervix and the pouch of Douglas, and to the bladder anteriorly. Once this is achieved, the hysterectomy is usually accomplished uneventfully.

Occasionally, if anatomic landmarks are still uncertain or somewhat obscured, the easier option, having deflected the bladder, is to identify the longitudinal fibers of the vagina anteriorly. This allows the surgeon to open the vagina safely and confidently, and thereafter a retrograde hysterectomy can be performed. A subtotal hysterectomy is rarely necessary and, in the authors' opinion, should be avoided if at all possible. On the whole it is a bad operation, and should problems with the cervical stump occur at a later date, effective treatment in the form of both surgery and radiotherapy is extremely complicated. As a rule, therefore, it is usually best to persevere with the definitive surgery that was originally planned. Leaving the cervix behind can only be justified if its removal would result in a significant risk of

organ damage, or bleeding that will be difficult to access to control.

Bowel resection, reanastomosis, and a protective defunctioning stoma is infrequently required, but is indicated if there has been surgical trauma to a segment or segments of bowel on mobilization. It may also be required if there is an area of marked stenosis secondary to fibrosis, or if active endometriosis involves specific sites such as the colon and rectum. There is data from several studies that confirm the efficacy of bowel resection, in order to eradicate all visible endometriosis, in producing symptomatic relief, and in improving the quality of life.[28–30]

Adhesion formation as a consequence of endometriosis, and indeed all surgical procedures associated with its treatment, is a real and widespread problem. The SCAR[31] study which reported in 1999, defined the extent of the problem by demonstrating that over one-third (34.7%) of 29 790 patients who underwent open surgery were readmitted a mean of 2.1 times for complications related to adhesions over a 10-year follow-up period. By the time most patients with end-stage endometriosis undergo pelvic clearance, adhesion formation is usually well established and widespread in the abdomen and pelvis. Nevertheless, following this definitive surgery, it is sensible to do everything possible to prevent further adhesion formation and the associated complications that may ensue. In this regard, at the end of the surgical procedure, as well as ensuring meticulous hemostasis, the use of antiadhesion or adjuvant adhesion-reducing preparations should be considered. These generally fall into two categories: physical barriers and solutions. Physical barriers such as Seprafilm (hyaluronic acid carboxymethylcellulose film), although difficult to handle, may be used to try to prevent adhesions in a specific site. Otherwise, for more widespread adhesion prevention, intra-abdominal solutions such as Adept (icodextrin 4% solution) can be instilled into the peritoneal cavity and left in situ at the time of peritoneal closure.

Postoperative hormone replacement therapy

There is still considerable debate regarding the use of HRT following total abdominal hysterectomy and bilateral salpingo-oophorectomy for endometriosis. Many authorities advocate the use of low-dose estrogen replacement only, being fearful of the risk of stimulation of recurrence of the disease process, and the associated symptoms. Others suggest the concomitant administration of progestogens in the hope that these will have a suppressant affect. Furthermore, it is frequently recommended that HRT should not be commenced for a period of time, usually 6 months, postoperatively. However, this practice is purely arbitrary and no data exist which definitively supports this recommendation. There is, however, evidence to suggest that estrogen therapy does not stimulate progression or recurrence of disease, providing all ovarian tissue has been removed.[20] Consensus of a number of reports is that the use of combined testosterone/estradiol implants in the immediate postoperative period is safe practice.

REFERENCES

1. Simpson JL, Elias S, Malinak LR, et al. Heritable aspects of endometriosis. I. Genetic studies. Am J Obstet Gynecol 1980; 137(3): 327–331.

2. Strathy JH, Molgaard CA, Coulam CB, et al. Endometriosis and infertility: a laparoscopic study of endometriosis among fertile and infertile women. Fertil Steril 1982; 38(6): 667–672.

3. Darbois Y. Etiological factors of endometriosis. Contrib Gynecol Obstet 1987; 16: 1–6.

4. Sangi-Haghpeykar H, Poindexter AN 3rd. Epidemiology of endometriosis among parous women. Obstet Gynecol 1995; 85(6): 983–992.

5. Balasch J, Creus M, Fabregues F, et al. Visible and non-visible endometriosis at laparoscopy in fertile and infertile women and in patients with chronic pelvic pain: a prospective study. Hum Reprod 1996; 11(2): 387–391.

6. Schenken RS, Malinak LR. Reoperation after initial treatment of endometriosis with conservative surgery. Am J Obstet Gynecol 1978; 131(4): 416–424.

7. Spangler DB, Jones GS, Jones HW Jr. Infertility due to endometriosis. Conservative surgical therapy. Am J Obstet Gynecol 1971; 109(6): 850–857.

8. Pratt JH, Williams TJ. Indications for complete pelvic operations and more radical procedures in the treatment of severe or extensive endometriosis. Clin Obstet Gynecol 1980; 23(3): 937–950.

9. Puolakka J, Kauppila A, Ronnberg, L. Results in the operative treatment of pelvic endometriosis. Acta Obstet Gynecol Scand 1980; 59(5): 429–431.

10. Vessey MP, Villard-Mackintosh L, McPherson K, et al. The epidemiology of hysterectomy: findings in a large cohort study. Br J Obstet Gynaecol 1992; 99(5): 402–407.

11. Kashyap RJ. Extremely elevated serum CA125 due to endometriosis. Aust N Z J Obstet Gynaecol 1999; 39(2): 269–270.

12. Cheng YM, Wang ST, Chou CY. Serum CA-125 in preoperative patients at high risk for endometriosis. Obstet Gynecol 2002; 99(3): 375–380.

13. Harada T, Kubota T, Aso T. Usefulness of CA19-9 versus CA125 for the diagnosis of endometriosis. Fertil Steril 2002; 78(4): 733–739.

14. Zanardi R, Del Frate C, Zuiani C, et al. Staging of pelvic endometriosis based on MRI findings versus laparoscopic classification according to the American Fertility Society. Abdom Imaging 2003; 28(5): 733–742.

15. Hoogeveen M, Dorr PJ, Puylaert JB. Endometriosis of the rectovaginal septum: endovaginal US and MRI findings in two cases. Abdom Imaging 2003; 28(6): 897–901.

16. Bazot M, Darai E, Hourani R, et al. Deep pelvic endometriosis: MR imaging for diagnosis and prediction of extension of disease. Radiology 2004; 232(2): 379–389.

17. Wheeler JM, Malinak LR. Recurrent endometriosis: incidence, management, and prognosis. Am J Obstet Gynecol 1983; 146(3): 247–253.

18. Brosens IA, Boeckx W, Page G. Microsurgery of ovarian endometriosis. Hum Reprod 1988; 3(3): 365–366.

19. Montgomery JC, Studd JW. Oestradiol and testosterone implants after hysterectomy for endometriosis. Contrib Gynecol Obstet 1987; 16: 241–246.

20. Henderson AF, Studd JWW, Watson N. A retrospective study of oestrogen replacement therapy following hysterectomy for endometriosis. Proceedings of the ICI Conference on Endometriosis, September 1989, 1990: 133–142.

21. Sampson JA. Endometrial carcinoma of the ovary arising in endometrial tissue in that organ. Arch Surg 1925; 10: 1–72.

22. Scully RE, Richardson GS, Barlow JF. The development of malignancy in endometriosis. Clin Obstet Gynecol 1966; 9(2): 384–411.

23. Czernobilsky B, Silverman BB, Mikuta JJ. Endometrioid carcinoma of the ovary. A clinicopathologic study of 75 cases. Cancer 1970; 26(5): 1141–1152.

24. Kurman RJ, Craig JM. Endometrioid and clear cell carcinoma of the ovary. Cancer 1972; 29(6): 1653–1664.

25. Long ME, Taylor HC, Jr. Endometrioid carcinoma of the ovary. Am J Obstet Gynecol 1964; 90: 936–950.

26. Russell P. The pathological assessment of ovarian neoplasms. I: Introduction to the common 'epithelial' tumours and analysis of benign 'epithelial' tumours. Pathology 1979; 11(1): 5–26.

27. Scully RE. Ovarian tumors. A review. Am J Pathol 1977; 87(3): 686–720.

28. Bailey HR, Ott MT, Hartendorp P. Aggressive surgical management for advanced colorectal endometriosis. Dis Colon Rectum 1994; 37: 747–753.

29. Urbach DR, Reedijk M, Richard CS, et al. Bowel resection for intestinal endometriosis. Dis Colon Rectum 1998; 41: 1158–1164.

30. Redwine DB, Wright JT. Laparoscopic treatment of complete obliteration of the cul-de-sac associated with endometriosis: long-term follow-up of en bloc resection. Fertil Steril 2001; 76: 358–365.

31. Ellis H, Moran BJ, Thompson JN, et al. Adhesion-related hospital readmissions after abdominal and pelvic surgery: a retrospective cohort study. Lancet 1999; 353(9163): 1476–1480.

9 Adhesions: an update

Vikas Sachar, Michael P Diamond, and Christopher Sutton

Pelvic adhesions can be the result of pelvic inflammation, endometriosis, or surgical trauma. Even when surgery is performed with strict adherence to microsurgical principles, postoperative adhesions occur in 51–100% of cases.[1] Adhesions resulting from surgical procedures may cause considerable pain and impair fertility. Subsequent surgical procedures become more difficult and occasionally emergency exploratory laparotomy for bowel obstruction is necessary. Complications such as these can present at any time, and are a lifetime concern for patients having even one laparotomy.[2,3] In fact, adhesions causing postoperative bowel obstruction more than 10 years after the initial surgery have been reported.[2,3] Clinically, adhesions may affect the practicing obstetrician during a repeat cesarean section by preventing emergency delivery, thereby placing the fetus at risk, increasing operative time, and increasing risk to the mother with higher risk of injury to the bladder, bowel, and uterus upon re-entry. Similarly, the practicing gynecologist may be affected by adhesions causing pelvic and abdominal pain and even intestinal obstruction decades after the initial surgery. The cost of caring for these complications has been estimated at $1.3 billion annually.[4] The significant socioeconomic cost of adhesions has prompted over a century of published literature documenting the search for operative strategies which may lead to a safe reduction or prevention of adhesions. These strategies have focused on minimizing surgical trauma, the use of barriers to prevent adhesions, and the use of medications both locally and systemically. In this article we will present the different modalities available to the obstetrician/gynecologist to prevent and treat adhesions, and discuss the evidence in the literature supporting or refuting them.

Pathophysiology

Adhesion formation can be considered to be the result of a normal physiologic response to a peritoneal insult gone unchecked. The most common cause of adhesions is previous surgery; other etiologies include infection, chemical irritation, trauma, endometriosis, and foreign body reactions. Cutting, surgical denudation, ischemia, dessication, or abrasion can cause peritoneal trauma during surgery. Injury to intact peritoneum creates two raw edges, and intiates a complex cascade of events which involves a subsequent increase in vessel permeability, release of inflammatory cells, an increase in leukotrienes and prostaglandins, and a decrease in plasminogen activity.[5] The peritoneal defect is initially sealed by a proteinaceous exudate consisting of fibrin deposits, leukocytes, and macrophages. Normal peritoneum contains high levels of plasmin and other fibrinolytic agents, but it may be absent or reduced at injured sites. With normal healing, the fibrin is completely degraded by plasmin, the principal agent in the fibrinolytic process; however, any abnormality of this process will result in fibrin deposition onto adjoining damaged surfaces. Recombinant tissue plasminogen activator has been used as an agent in reducing postoperative pelvic adhesions in the rabbit, and confirmed by second-look laparoscopy.[6,7] However, clinical trials demonstrating efficacy have yet to be reported. Poor oxygenation of the tissue, tissue trauma, and foreign bodies such as sutures can cause an imbalance in the healing pathway, which leads to a decrease in the amount of plasminogen, thereby leading to the organization of the unlysed fibrin with an invasion of fibroblasts, deposition of collagen, and formation of blood vessels. It is the presence and organization of fibrin that is thought to initiate this activation of the adhesion cascade, with the resultant adhesion formation completed within a week.[8] The pathogenesis of adhesion formation following surgery therefore appears to require the presence of a deperitonealized area due to trauma, peritoneal inflammation, a reduction in peritoneal fibrinolytic activity, and the formation of fibrin bands.

Current adhesion prevention modalities are aimed at targeting particular key steps in the fibrin formation cascade, and also at the physical separation of the two raw peritoneal surfaces.

Adhesion prevention modalities

The objective of the use of antiadhesion adjuvants is to eliminate or reduce the incidence and severity of postoperative adhesions while retaining normal healing and avoiding infection. Pelvic adhesions can cause infertility and pain. Accordingly, by eliminating or reducing the incidence of adhesions, there should be a benefit noted in fertility rates as well as a reduction in pain. Microsurgical technique tenets include minimizing serosal trauma, using atraumatic instruments, inert suture material, careful tissue handling, prevention of tissue desiccation and ensuring meticulous hemostasis are thought to reduce but not completely prevent the occurrence of adhesions.[9] Considerable experimental evidence indicates that peritoneal suturing increases adhesion formation.[10] Accordingly, this practice is slowly falling out of favor for the purposes of reducing adhesion development. Other approaches used to decrease the formation of adhesions in addition to microsurgical techniques are hydroflotation, use of gels, and the use of sheets or films as physical barriers.[11]

Surgical adjuvants

Hydroflotation
With this technique, the viscera are 'floated' and separated by a large volume of liquid drawn into the abdomen. Dextran is a polysaccharide solution that in a more concentrated (32%) solution with

10% dextrose is known as Hyskon (32% dextran 70, Pharmacia, Piscataway, NJ). This substance is used with the hysteroscope as an aid in distending the uterine cavity for hysteroscopic procedures. Gynecologic surgeons have also used Hyskon intraperitoneally as adjuvant therapy for the prevention of adhesions in a non-FDA (Food and Drug Administration)-approved manner. When placed within the peritoneal cavity, dextran 70 can last up to 4 days and causes an osmotically induced transudation of several hundred milliliters of water into the cavity, causing the abdominal contents to 'float' apart from each other or from peritoneal surfaces. This theoretically reduces the likelihood of adhesion formation.[12,13] A review of animal studies revealed a reduction in adhesion formation with the use of dextran 70, but the human studies are less consistent.[14] Two of the largest randomized controlled trials in patients to evaluate dextran 70-induced hydroflotation failed to show any significant difference in the reduction of adhesions at second-look laparoscopy when compared to their respective controls of saline and lactated Ringer's solution.[15] The Adhesion Study Group, however, found a reduction in adhesion formation in patients who received dextran 70 before abdominal closure, as compared to saline.[16] However, dextran 70 use has been limited by its association with a number of complications, including pleural effusion, pulmonary edema, elevated liver enzymes, ascites, labial edema, and rarely anaphylactic shock.[17–19] This product is not approved for use with an indication of adhesion reduction or prevention.

In the United States crystalloid solutions are the most commonly used surgical adjuvant to reduce adhesion development. These substances are mistakenly believed by some to be effective by creating a state of hydroflotation. Physiologically, they must be present for 3–5 days, as this is the time required for remesothelialization of the peritoneal defect to occur in uncomplicated circumstances.[11,20] However, studies suggest that fluid absorption by the peritoneal cavity occurs at a rate of 30–35 ml/h.[22] If one were to hope to support the crystalloid solution hydroflotation theory during remesothelialization, then there would have to be approximately 3000 ml of fluid left within the patient at the time of the initial injury to the peritoneum to have sufficient hydroflotation present up to about 3 days later. Some surgeons have done this at the end of the primary procedure prior to closing the abdomen. However, instilling this amount of fluid usually requires full paralysis of the abdominal musculature, which may prolong the operative and recovery times.[21] This is not a practical option. In a rat model, however, Ringer's lactate instillation has been shown to decrease adhesion formation and reformation.[24] This may be due to the intrinsic difficulty in comparing animal model systems to human systems, as well as differences in fluid reabsorption by the peritoneum in the animal. A compilation of four clinical studies demonstrated adhesion reformation in up to 80% of the patients treated with crystalloid adjuvants.[23] It has also been reported that instillation of normal saline (300–500 ml) after laparoscopic ovarian drilling for polycystic ovaries reduced adhesion formation; however the findings from this study could not be reproduced.[25] However, a meta-analysis of 13 randomized clinical studies conclusively showed no reduction in adhesion formation with instillation of lactated Ringer's solution or saline.[16] The use of intraperitoneal crystalloid solution is not approved by the FDA for adhesion prevention and these data do not support their use for postoperative adhesion prevention.

Laparoscopy

Laparoscopy reduced postoperative adhesion formation in a randomized trial by Lundorff and colleagues[26] comparing 73 patients diagnosed with ectopic pregnancy, who were assigned to treatment with laparoscopy or laparotomy with a second-look procedure 12 weeks later. Patients treated in the laparoscopic arm developed significantly fewer adhesions than the patients treated by laparotomy. Furthermore, the patients that did develop adhesions in the laparoscopic arm had reduced adhesion scores.[26] However, although it may be associated with significant reduction in adhesion scores, it does not appear that laparoscopic adhesiolysis results in a greater reduction of postoperative adhesion reformation than is able to be achieved by laparotomy.[27,28] De-novo adhesions are observed at the time of early second-look procedures at sites within the pelvis that did not have adhesions at the time of initial laparotomy. De-novo adhesion formation after operative laparoscopy has been reported to occur in only 12% of patients vs 50% of patients after laparotomy, but after laparoscopic adhesiolysis 97% of patients developed postoperative adhesions within 3 months at the same sites for which they underwent the initial procedure.[27] The overall reformation rate suggests laparoscopy is not effective by itself in eliminating all adhesions. Furthermore, the benefits of laparoscopic surgery, such as reduced postoperative pain, reduced morbidity, and decreased length of stay, have solidified the role of laparoscopy as an option in clinical surgery.[29]

Adhesion barriers

Barriers and adhesion prevention

Upon examination of the physiologic basis of adhesion formation, different aspects in the adhesion formation cascade have been targeted in order to inhibit their development. It has been demonstrated by electron microscopy that adhesion formation does not progress after a mesothelial cell layer covers a foreign mesh at approximately 1 week.[31] Theoretically, the independent healing of each of the traumatized peritoneal surfaces separated by a physical barrier prevents fibrin bridges from forming. In the United States there are two synthetic barriers currently approved with an indication to reduce postoperative adhesions: modified hyaluronic acid (HA) with carboxymethylcellulose (CMC) and oxidized regenerated cellulose (ORC). We also examine expanded polytetrafluorethylene (PTFE), which although not FDA-approved for use in adhesion prevention, has been utilized in certain instances. Finally, we will also discuss a prototypical broad peritoneal barrier, which is in the form of ferric hyaluronate gel, which was approved by the FDA, but was subsequently withdrawn and is not currently available.

ORC is commercially available as Interceed (TC7) (Ethicon, Somerville, NJ). It can be cut as necessary, requires no suturing, is absorbable, and may be applied via the laparoscope, although it is not approved for that use as such application may impair its efficacy.[30,32] It is applied over raw surfaces at the conclusion of surgery once hemostasis has been achieved and all irrigation fluid and instillates have been removed from the peritoneal cavity with the patient in reverse Trendelenburg position. Cut pieces of Interceed are applied to completely cover the area at risk, and moistened with irrigating solution to further ensure adherence to the application site. The most important step to maximize the efficacy of Interceed is hemostasis, as the presence of bleeding renders it ineffective.[33] Interceed is a procoagulant and causes fibrin deposition at sites of incomplete hemostasis. Accordingly, Interceed saturated with blood loses its ability to reduce subsequent adhesion formation. Fibroblasts then grow along the strands of fibrin, triggering the adhesion cascade with subsequent collagen deposition and vascular proliferation.[32,34,35] Interceed that turns dark brown or black within 1–2 minutes following application to the raw surface indicates incomplete hemostasis. If this occurs, the Interceed should be removed, hemostasis achieved, and then a new piece of Interceed should be placed.

Numerous studies have shown the benefit of Interceed in decreasing the appearance and severity of postoperative adhesions. The Interceed Adhesion Barrier Study Group randomly assigned 74 infertility patients from 9 investigational centers to receive Interceed on either the left or right pelvic side wall at treatment laparotomy, with the contralateral untreated side serving as a control.[36] These patients had bilateral pelvic side wall adhesions. At second-look laparoscopy, up to 14 weeks after the initial surgery, it was found that Interceed reduced adhesion formation by 90% compared with the control side and, furthermore, was associated with significant reduction in the extent and the severity of postsurgical pelvic adhesions.

Heparin is one of the most frequently used adjuncts in combined regimens with Interceed, and in animal studies has been demonstrated to have synergistic effects in reducing adhesion formation.[37–39] Human studies have been mixed, however, with one study showing a significant reduction, and another only showing a reduction in adhesions that was not significant as compared to Interceed alone.[40] There are many mechanisms by which heparin may exert a beneficial effect. Heparin in combination with antithrombin III inhibits clotting by enhancing serine esterase activity, thereby reducing the deposition of fibrin strands which serve as triggers for the adhesion cascade.[41] Secondly, heparin directly stimulates plasminogen activator activity and increases the action of plasminogen, which enhances fibrinolysis and, accordingly, decreases adhesion formation.[42] Thirdly, heparin may possibly stimulate macrophages to secrete plasminogen activator.[43] Finally, heparin may prevent adhesions by binding to fibroblast growth factor, which stimulates wound healing.[44] Although this combination therapy is not FDA-approved, clearly this adjunct deserves further clinical research.

Wiseman et al conducted a meta-analysis testing the hypothesis that Interceed is safe and effective for the prevention of postsurgical adhesions.[44] Data from seven studies ($n = 389$) were used and the anatomic sites examined for adhesion reduction at second-look laparoscopy included the ovaries, pelvic side walls, fallopian tubes, fimbriae, and uterus. They found a statistically significant reduction of 24% ($p < 0.001$) in adhesion incidence in the Interceed-treated group compared to the untreated control group. Furthermore, only four adverse events – atelectasis, postoperative ileus, fever, and abdominal pain – and hemoglobin reduction were reported in a meta-analysis of 10 studies ($n = 560$).[44] These adverse events were consistent with events typically seen after surgery and thought not to be secondary to the use

of Interceed by the investigators.[44] Overall, Interceed more than doubled the chance that a site will be adhesion-free.

Farquhar and colleagues[9] assessed the effect of mechanical barriers on postoperative adhesion reformation in women undergoing pelvic surgery. They examined randomized controlled trials of women of reproductive age undergoing pelvic surgery with adhesion barriers vs no treatment. Fifteen randomized controlled trials were included. There were six trials that compared Interceed vs no treatment at laparoscopy. Analysis of these trials showed the Interceed-treated group with a reduced incidence of adhesions vs the control group. The Interceed-treated group had decreases in both de-novo adhesions, OR (95% CI) = 0.31 (0.12, 0.79), and the reformation of adhesions, OR (95% CI) = 0.19 (0.09, 0.42), compared with the control group. Six trials reported on Interceed vs no treatment following laparotomy for adhesiolysis and ovarian surgery. The use of Interceed resulted in a reduction in the incidence of adhesions compared with no treatment: OR (95% CI) = 0.39 (0.28, 0.55).

Adhesions are thought to adversely affect fertility by interfering with ovum pickup by the fimbriae. The most common site of adhesion formation in the pelvis is the ovary.[37] However, there are few adhesion prevention studies with pregnancy as the primary outcome. Giannacodimos et al performed laser drilling in 40 patients with polycystic ovarian disease, after which Interceed was applied around the entire ovarian surface in each patient.[45] Within 2 years, 24 patients (60%) became pregnant and, of these, 20 were delivered by cesarean section. Postoperative adhesions were observed in 3 of 20 patients (15%), and the remaining 17 (85%) had no adhesions present. The limitation of this study, however, is the lack of a control group; accordingly, limited conclusions can be made from the results.[45,46]

In a study by Sawada et al, 38 women were followed for 2 years after undergoing reproductive surgery.[47] The procedures were all laparotomies and comprised myomectomy (19), cystectomy (5), tuboplasty (10), and uteroplasty (4). The patients were divided into two randomized groups: 23 cases had the surgical site completely covered with Interceed and 15 control cases had no intervention. Pregnancy and postoperative adhesions were the measured outcomes. Within the 2-year follow-up period, 18 (78%) of the Interceed-treated patients achieved pregnancy compared with 7 (47%) of the control group. Second-look laparoscopy in 23 patients revealed postoperative adhesions in 6 of the 16 patients treated with

Interceed, a significant improvement (p <0.04) when compared with the control group, in which 6 of the 7 control patients had postoperative adhesions.[47] The authors concluded that the significantly higher rate of pregnancy may be explained by the use of Interceed in reducing postoperative adhesions. Clearly, Interceed appears to decrease adhesion reformation in the studies mentioned above. Incomplete hemostasis and barrier migration may explain why adhesion development is only reduced and not eliminated.

Preclude

Expanded PTFE is marketed as Preclude (Gore-Tex Surgical Membrane, WL Gore and Associates, Inc., Flagstaff, AZ). It must be sutured in place, is inert, and permanent (unless subsequently surgically removed). Preclude is approved for use for peritoneal repair, but not for adhesion reduction per se. Its initial approved use was for cardiovascular surgery as a graft for reconstruction of the pericardium or vessels. However it has also been utilized as an adjuvant during abdominal and pelvic surgery. When placed over traumatized tissue it has been shown to reduce adhesion formation and reformation, regardless of whether hemostasis has been achieved.[48,49] However, a 'membrane' which is in essence an adhesion usually forms over the Preclude. A multicenter clinical study found Preclude decreased both postmyomectomy adhesions and pelvic side-wall adhesions at second-look laparoscopy in 18 patients.[50]

A randomized clinical trial (n = 32) directly compared Preclude and Interceed in patients undergoing pelvic adhesiolysis.[51] Each patient had both Preclude placed on one side wall, and Interceed on the other. At second-look laparoscopy (n = 29), both Interceed and Preclude were associated with improved adhesion scores, and reduced area of adhesions, but Preclude was associated with a greater benefit. More side walls covered with Preclude had no adhesions (21 vs 7) as compared to Interceed. However, whether adhesions would develop following removal of Preclude in this study is unknown. The authors attributed some of the benefit of Preclude over Interceed to the fact that Preclude is effective in an environment in which complete hemostasis has not been obtained, whereas Interceed is not.

The Myomectomy Adhesion Multicenter Study group performed myomectomies on 28 patients who were randomized to have Preclude sutured over the uterine incision, or no barrier.[52] At second-look laparoscopy, the patients who had Preclude-covered suture sites had 55% more adhesion-free sites (p <0.01) as compared to the control with only 7% adhesion-free sites.[52] As Preclude is a permanent material, it has generally been removed at second-look laparoscopy. Concern over this is twofold: first, the very act of removal may create new surgical trauma sufficient to result in the formation of adhesions; secondly, the morbidities associated with a second surgery and its associated costs. Haney evaluated this concern in two women who had initial laparotomies with Preclude, subsequent laparoscopy for Preclude removal, and then had a third-look laparoscopy for unrelated medical conditions.[53] His findings were consistent with animal studies, in that no postoperative adhesions were associated with the removal of Preclude by laparoscopy.[53,54] Until the long-term effects of a nonabsorbable barrier in the pelvis are known, the removal of Preclude may be a significant barrier to its widespread use.

Seprafilm

Seprafilm (HAL-F, Genzyme Corp, Cambridge, MA) is composed of HA and CMC. It is a nontoxic, nonimmunogenic, biocompatible, and biodegradable material, which has been modified to prolong its intraperitoneal residence time. Support for the prevention of postoperative adhesions by Seprafilm has been found in clinical studies in both general surgery and gynecology.[55,56] It turns into a gel within 24 hours after placement and provides protection for the traumatized tissue it covers for up to 7 days.[31] Similar to Interceed, Seprafilm is completely cleared from the body in 28 days[33] and, similar to Preclude, it can be used in the presence of blood.[55] Diamond conducted a multicenter trial in which 127 patients undergoing myomectomy were randomized to Seprafilm covering the uterine incision vs no barrier.[55] At second-look laparoscopy, significantly more uteri of patients in the Seprafilm group were adhesion-free than the control group. Furthermore, adhesion area and severity were also reduced in the Seprafilm-treated patients; however, the differences reached statistical significance only for the anterior uterus.[55]

Becker and colleagues randomly assigned Seprafilm to 175 patients with ulcerative colitis or familial polyposis who were scheduled for colectomy and ileal pouch–anal anastomosis with diverting-loop ileostomy.[56] Before abdominal closure, patients were randomly assigned to receive or not receive Seprafilm. At ileostomy closure 8–12 weeks later, laparoscopy was used to evaluate the incidence, extent, and severity of adhesion formation to the midline incision. The incidence of patients with one or more adhesions to the midline incision was significantly reduced from 94% in the control group to 49% in the Seprafilm group (p <0.00000000001). No adhesions were found in 43 of the 85 patients who received Seprafilm, as compared to only 5 of the 90 control patients. Furthermore, the extent and severity of postoperative adhesions were significantly less in the Seprafilm group. Between the study groups, no statistically significant difference was found in the incidence of any adverse reaction (p <0.05).[56] Abscess development was 4.9% overall, with 7 of the 91 patients in the Seprafilm developing abscesses and 2 of the 92 patients in the control group. Most of these patients recovered with conservative management. This rate was marginally higher than the rates reported in a different study of patients undergoing colectomy and ileal pouch–anal anastomosis.[57] Overall, the number of adverse events did not differ significantly between the Seprafilm group and the control group.

Other studies have raised concerns of the effectiveness of Seprafilm in abdominal bowel surgery,[58] and its safety there. Khaitan et al examined 17 female and 2 male patients with a diagnosis of intractable pain typical of adhesions, which had made them narcotic-dependent.[59] These patients had a history of numerous previous abdominal surgeries, with an average of 6.4 procedures (range 1–14).[59] All patients underwent laparoscopic adhesiolysis with placement of Seprafilm laparoscopically. Three patients had their procedure converted to laparotomy, secondary to complications ranging from severe dense adhesive disease to inadvertent enterotomy. Two patients' postoperative course was complicated by the formation of an enterocutaneous fistula that healed with nonoperative management, and one patient who had an intra-abdominal hematoma. About a year after their procedure, patients were asked subjective questions relating to pain, diet, symptoms, narcotic use, and satisfaction with the procedure; all but five of the patients were significantly improved, and 14 (74%) patients were very pleased with their procedure. Three patients continue to require narcotics regularly, whereas two other patients were explored laparoscopically and found to have no intra-abdominal adhesions. It was the authors' recommendation that Seprafilm placement may increase the likelihood of a leak from repaired enterotomies when placed directly over the enterotomy repair. Furthermore, they did not recommend Seprafilm next to or on an enterotomy repair.[59]

Animal studies examining this adverse reaction have been mixed. A study by Bowers et al compared irradiated rats that had undergone a distal ileal resection with an end-to-end ileoileostomy and had their anastomosis wrapped in Seprafilm with rats that did not have Seprafilm.[60] The results showed 13 of 14 (93%) rats treated with Seprafilm had perianastomotic abscesses, which was significantly more (p <0.0001) than the control group (n = 50), which had 11 perianastomotic abscesses (24%).[60] Irradiation of this study population, however, may have been an independent risk factor for abscess formation. Moreira et al evaluated the safety of Seprafilm after myotomy and enterotomy in rabbits and did not find any increase in abscess formation.[61] They did find Seprafilm significantly reduced postsurgical adhesion formation in the myotomy group; however, their study failed to find any significant difference in postsurgical adhesion formation in the Seprafilm-treated enterotomy group as compared to the control group.[61]

Recently, however, Beck et al addressed the safety of Seprafilm in abdominopelvic surgery of the intestine.[62] In this controlled trial of 1791 patients undergoing abominopelvic surgery were blindly randomized to Seprafilm or to a no treatment control group before abdominal closure. The incidence of abscess was not significantly different between the Seprafilm-treated group (4% vs 3%) and the control group. However in a subpopulation of patients in whom Seprafilm was wrapped around a fresh bowel anastomosis, leak related events, which included anastomotic leak, fistula, peritonitis, abscess and sepsis occurred more frequently (p ≤0.05).[62]

Gels

A liquid formation of modified HA (Sepracoat, Genzyme Corp, Cambridge, MA) showed promising preclinical and clinical results in the reduction of postoperative adhesions,[63] but was withdrawn a few years ago after the FDA rejected it for lack of efficacy data.

Another gel, Intergel (ferrous sulphate hyaluronic acid) (Gynecare, Johnson & Johnson, Somerville, NJ), has recently been withdrawn because of problems with increased postoperative pain and rare reports of sclerosing peritonitis. Another gel to enter the marketplace is SprayGel adhesion barrier (Confluent Surgical, Inc., Waltham, MA), which consists of two aqueous solutions containing modified polyethylene glycol molecules that react rapidly and form an absorbable hydrogel polymer when sprayed together. These liquids are sprayed onto tissue using an applicator which can be passed through a 5 mm trocar. When sprayed onto the tissue with an air pump, the two liquids polymerize to form a gel that effectively coats and adheres to the surfaces where the surgical trauma has taken place. One of the liquids contains methylene blue to ensure that the entire surface is adequately covered and, after about 5 days, the hydrogel layer is absorbed and subsequently undergoes complete renal clearance. For polymerization to take place, the CO_2 pneumoperitoneum has to be evacuated and replaced by oxygen via an air pump, which takes about 2 minutes. SprayGel has been evaluated in the porcine model and has been shown to be efficacious insofar as 90% of the untreated sites had adhesions compared with 30% of the treated sites.[64] Clinical studies in Kiel and Bordeaux have demonstrated the ease of use of this material and second-look laparoscopies support the claim of complete hydrogel absorption with evidence of normal healing. Efficacy studies, although impressive, have only been presented as a congress poster[65] and, as yet, there have been no published randomized controlled studies to demonstrate efficacy.

The most recent gel to enter into this potentially lucrative market is Hyalobarrier Gel (Baxter, Pisa, Italy), which is a biodegradable gel of autocross-linked HA. The gel is highly viscous and easy to apply via a 5 mm cannula; it effectively coats the operated area and is therefore site-specific. It appears to me (C.S.) safe and the only adverse reactions have been a few cases of mild postpartum pyrexia, which resolved spontaneously.

One randomized prospective controlled trial from Italy[66] on 36 patients undergoing laparoscopic myomectomy were divided randomly – one-half treated with this HA gel and the others had no antiadhesion agent. At second-look laparoscopy, 60–90 days later, the treated group had significantly less postoperative adhesions (27.8% vs 77.8%). This study also found that adhesion formation was significantly higher in patients treated with interrupted figure-of-eight sutures than with subserous sutures. An exciting new application for this agent is in the prevention of intrauterine adhesions that occur following hysteroscopic adhesiolysis. Of all the possible adhesion barriers, this is the only one that is suitable for this particular application and one randomized controlled trial has testified to its use following hysteroscopic adhesiolysis.[67]

Iso-osmotic solutions

For many years laparoscopic surgeons have used Hartmann's solution (Ringer's lactate) as an irrigant fluid and many add 5 IU of heparin per liter,

which appears to help in limiting the formation of large blood clots that can be difficult to remove. Reich introduced a concept of hydroflotation at the end of his advanced laparoscopic procedures and often left 1–2 L of Ringer's lactate solution in the abdominal cavity for hydroflotation, to try and prevent subsequent adhesion formation.[6] Ultrasonic studies of fluid absorption have shown that most of this fluid is absorbed within 72 hours, which is too soon to adequately prevent the formation of fibrinous adhesions. A new glucose polymer solution, Adept (4% icodextrin, Shire Pharmaceuticals, Basingstoke, Hants, UK) has been used extensively on patients for peritoneal dialysis and, since observers have commented on the lack of adhesion formation in patients undergoing repeated passage of catheters for renal dialysis, it was suggested that this may well be an ideal solution for the prevention of adhesions. Icodextrin is an α 1–4-linked glucose polymer produced by the hydrolysis of corn starch and fractionated by membrane separation technology to produce material with the desired molecular weight distribution. Icodextrin is a substrate for amylase, which is widely distributed throughout the body but is not present in the human peritoneal cavity.[69] Therefore, when icodextrin is instilled intraperitoneally, it is largely retained within the peritoneal cavity, absorption of the polymer occurring gradually via the lymphatic system into the systemic circulation. Icodextrin is then readily metabolized by amylase to oligosaccharides, which are cleared by further metabolism to glucose. Studies of fluid dynamics show that a 1 L volume of icodextrin placed into the peritoneal cavity at the end of surgery would stay in situ during the time of maximum adhesion formation, up to 3–5 days postsurgery.[70–73] Early preclinical studies using controlled studies on animal models have demonstrated significant reduction in adhesion formation and particularly a very large reduction in nonsurgical site adhesions. The advantage of Icodextrin is that it probably stays in the peritoneal cavity for about 7 days and not only prevents apposition of traumatized surgical surfaces but also, by producing a prolonged hydroflotation effect, possibly also decreases de-novo adhesion formation at distant sites. Since Adept was introduced into the UK in late summer 2000, it has been our (C.S.) primary method for adhesion prevention, together with careful laparoscopic surgical technique. We (C.S.) have been impressed with its ease of use and have also noticed that the irrigant solution appears to stop capillary oozing, which may be one of the mechanisms in its favor. It is certainly more uncomfortable for the patient than heparinized Ringer's lactate, since it takes 7 days to be absorbed, and the patient is aware of fluid moving around inside her peritoneal cavity. It can also cause diaphragmatic irritation and referred pain to the shoulders, and patients should be advised to try to sleep upright for the first week following surgery. The solution will also leak from the small laparoscopic incisions and patients must be warned of this and advised to change the dressings regularly until the wound has healed. In spite of these postoperative problems, we (C.S.) have found that it has been very well tolerated by patients, particularly if it can be explained to them that these minor problems are of little significance if adhesion reformation can be prevented. We have not yet had the opportunity to have any second-look procedures but have video recorded all the procedures where icodextrin has been used and it will be possible to carefully analyze the patients who require clinically indicated second-look surgery at sometime in the future.

Preclinical efficacy studies on animal models (rabbit uterine horn and rabbit side-wall formation and reformation model) have been shown to reduce the incidence and extent of adhesions.[74] Thus far, only one clinical efficacy study has been performed and that was a comparative, randomized study comparing 4% icodextrin solution with Ringer's lactate solution during adnexal surgery performed by laparoscopy.[75] A reduction in the number, extent, and severity of adhesions and the adhesion scores were demonstrated between first surgery and second-look surgery in 12 of the 27 (44%) of the women in the icodextrin group compared with 6 of 26 (23%) in the controlled group. Preliminary data from the large double-blind randomized US multi-centre study in gynaecologic laparoscopy was presented at the International Society for Gynecologic Endoscopy meeting in London (Figure 9.1)[76,77] in April 2005. The data from this study indicate a significant reduction in the incidence of adhesions throughout the peritoneal cavity and we await the full publication of this study as well as a similar European study which should report in 2006.

Icodextrin appears to be safe and easy to use. I (C.S.) was one of the lead coordinators of a large prospective study involving 376 hospitals throughout Europe to investigate the safety and acceptance of icodextrin by gynecologic and general surgeons and the side effects and tolerability by patient questionnaire. This study involved 4000 patients and there were no serious adverse reactions. The general consensus was that it was safe and easy to use and the side-effect profile was no more than one would expect with Ringer's lactate solution and the incidence of vulval edema was possibly even lower. A recent paper by a group of colorectal surgeons[78] has presented the cost-effectiveness data for icodextrin and, since it has a good safety profile, we await the efficacy studies with great interest.

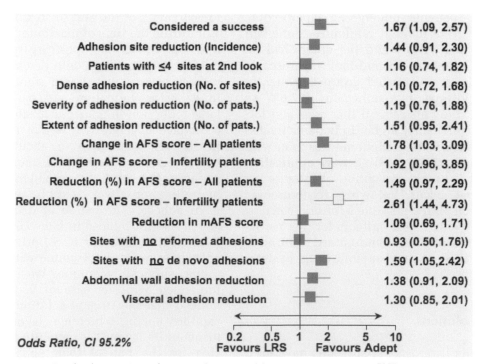

Figure 9.1 Clinical benefit of Adept (4% icodextrin solution): odds ration (CI = 95.2%) [76,77] (reproduced with permission from ML Laboratories plc, Blaby, Leicestershire UK).

Conclusion

A number of human interventional trials and animal studies have evaluated techniques and technologies designed to prevent and reduce postsurgical adhesions. Although many options are available for adhesion prevention, each option has limitations. None of the barriers or adjuvant therapies is completely effective. The fabric nature of Interceed can make passage through a laparoscopic port cumbersome;[79] furthermore, its ineffectiveness in the absence of complete hemostasis has been well documented in the literature and may explain its reduction but not complete elimination of postsurgical adhesions. Interceed absorbs water and sticks to any surface, but in the presence of excess irrigation fluid, barrier migration can occur and may also contribute to Interceed's failure. The time taken to place Interceed is reported to be less than 9 minutes.[80] This is a much shorter time span than it takes to perform a second laparoscopy, as with Preclude. Preclude, however, has an advantage in that it is unaffected by the presence of blood and, secondly, it is sutured in place, therefore eliminating the chance of barrier migration. However, it is permanent unless surgically removed, and is often engulfed by an adhesion-like membrane. Seprafilm has been proven to prevent adhesion formation after abdominopelvic surgery, is effective in the presence of blood, is biodegradable, and does not need to be sutured in place. Its use in gynecologic surgery does not appear to have the same safety concerns as compared to colorectal surgery: additional studies are needed to confirm this. There is no role for crystalloid solutions or dextran in preventing adhesion development. Studies of heparin and other agents as a combination adjuvant therapy with barriers warrant further evaluation. The impact of the voluntary withdrawal of Intergel[81] secondary to adverse outcomes raises issues in the off-label use of barrier adjuvants before FDA approval. Financially, the cost of Interceed is approximately $170 per sheet, and the costs of Preclude are even higher, compounded by the need for a second laparoscopy if it is to be removed. However, if these barriers accomplish what they are designed to do, the avoidance of future adhesiolytic surgery and morbidity outweighs these fiscal issues.

Ultimately, the best adhesion prevention agent may be a site- and patient-specific combination of barriers with drugs or biologic agents. Importantly, an antiadhesion adjuvant used for the purpose of prevention of postsurgical adhesions must be considered secondary to the use of microsurgical technique. Meticulous hemostasis and gentle tissue handling to the extent possible for the procedure to be performed are critical for limiting initial peritoneal injury. Thus, preventing postsurgical adhesions remains an art, rather than a science.

REFERENCES

1. Diamond M, Daniel JF, Feste J, et al. Adhesion reformation and de novo adhesion formation prevention after reproductive pelvic surgery. Fertil Steril 1987; 47: 864–866.

2. Ellis H, Moran BJ, Thompson JN, et al. Adhesion-related hospital readmissions after abdominal and pelvic surgery: a retrospective cohort study. Lancet 1999; 353: 1476–1480.

3. Lower AM, Hawthorn RJS, Ellis H. The impact of adhesions on hospital readmissions over ten years after 8849 open gynecologic operations: an assessment from the Surgical and Clinical Adhesions Research Study. Br J Obstet Gynaecol 2000; 107: 855–862.

4. Ray NF, Denton WG, Thamer M, et al. Abdominal adhesiolysis: inpatient care and expenditures in the United States in 1994. Am Coll Surg 1998; 186: 1–9.

5. Thompson JN, Paterson-Brown S, Harbourne T, et al. Reduced human peritoneal plasminogen activating activity: possible mechanism of adhesion formation. Br J Surg 1989; 76: 382–384.

6. Doody KJ, Dunn RC, Buttram VC Jr. Recombinant tissue plasminogen activator reduces adhesion formation in a rabbit uterine horn model. Fertil Steril 1989; 51: 509–512.

7. Menzies, D, Ellis H. Intra-abdominal adhesions and their prevention by topical tissue plasminogen activator. J R Soc Med 1989; 82: 534–535.

8. Dijkstra FR, Nieuwenhuijzen M, Reijnen MM. Recent clinical developments in pathophysiology, epidemiology, diagnosis and treatment of intra-abdominal adhesions. Scand J Gastroenterol Suppl 2000; 35(Suppl 232): 52–59.

9. Farquhar C, Vanderkerckhove P, Watson A, et al. Barrier agents for preventing adhesions after surgery for subfertility. Cochrane Database Syst Rev 2003; 3: 1–49.

10. Duffy DM, diZerega GS. Is peritoneal closure necessary? Obstet Gynecol Surv 1994; 49: 817–822.

11. Menzies D, Ellis H. Intestinal obstruction from adhesions – how big is the problem? Ann R Coll Surg Engl 1990; 72: 60–63.

12. DeCherney A, Hurd W, Pagidas K, et al. Techniques and tools to prevent pelvic adhesions. An Expert Panel. OBG Manage 2003; 15: 20–40.

13. Wiseman D. Polymers for the prevention of surgical adhesions. In: Domb AJ, ed. Polymeric site-specific pharmacotherapy. New York: John Wiley and Sons; 1994: 370–421.

14. Krinsky A, Haseltine F, DeCherney A. Peritonal fluid accumulation with dextran 70 instilled at time of laparoscopy. Fertil Steril 1984; 41: 647–649.

15. Pfeffer W. Adjuvants in tubal surgery. Fertil Steril 1980; 33: 245–256.

16. Watson A, Vanderkerckhove P, Lilford R. Liquid and fluid agents for preventing adhesions after surgery for subfertility. Cochrane Database Syst Rev 2003; 3: 1–49

17. Adhesion Study Group. Reduction of postoperative pelvic adhesions with intraperitoneal 32% dextran 70: a prospective, randomized clinical trial. Fertil Steril 1983; 40: 612–619.

18. Adoni A, Addatto-Levy R, Mogle P, et al. Postoperative pleural effusion caused by dextran. Int J Gynecol Obstet 1980; 18: 243–247.

19. Magyar D, Hayes M, Spiritos N, et al. Is intraperitoneal dextran 70 safe for routine gynecologic use? Am J Obstet Gynecol 1985; 152: 198–201.

20. Borten M, Seibert C, Taymor M. Recurrent anaphylactic reaction to intraperitoneal dextran 70 used for prevention of postsurgical adhesions. Obstet Gynecol 1983; 61: 755–757.

21. Duffy DM, diZerega GS. Adhesion controversies: pelvic pain as a cause of adhesions, crystalloids in preventing them. J Reprod Med 1996; 5: 19–26.

22. Shear L, Swartz C, Shinaberger JA, et al. Kinetics of peritoneal fluid absorption in adult man. N Engl J Med 1965; 272: 123–127.

23. Wiseman D, Trout JR, Diamond M. The rates of adhesion development and the effects of crystalloid solutions on adhesion development in pelvic surgery. Fertil Steril 1998; 70: 702–711.

24. diZerega GS, Campeau JD. Use of instillates to prevent intraperitoneal adhesions. Infertil Reprod Med Clin N Am 1994; 5: 463–478.

25. Naether OGL. Significant reduction of adnexal adhesions following laparoscopic electrocautery of the ovarian surface (LEOS) by lavage and artificial ascites. Gynaecol Endosc 1995; 4; 17–19.

26. Lundorff P, Hahlin M, Kallfelt B, et al. Adhesion formation after laparoscopic surgery in tubal pregnancy: a randomized trial versus laparotomy. Fertil Steril 1991; 55: 911–915.

27. Operative Laparoscopy Study Group. Postoperative adhesion development after operative laparoscopy: evaluation at early second-look procedures. Fertil Steril 1991; 55: 700–704.

28. Luciano AA, Maier DB, Kock EI, et al. A comparative study of postoperative adhesions following laser surgery by laparoscopy versus laparotomy in the rabbit model. Obstet Gynecol 1989; 74: 220–224.

29. Hidlebaugh DA, Vulgaropulos S, Orr RK. Treating adnexal masses. Operative laparoscopy versus laparotomy. J Reprod Med 1997; 47: 551–558.

30. Baptista ML, Bonsack MW, Felemoviscius I, et al. Abdominal adhesions to prosthetic mesh evaluated by laparoscopy and electron microscopy. J Am Coll Surg 2000; 190: 271–280.

31. Liakakos T, Thomakos N, Fine PM, et al. Peritoneal adhesions: etiology, pathophysiology, and clinical significance. Recent advances in prevention and management. Dig Surg 2001; 18: 260–273.

32. Wiseman DM, Gottlick LE, Diamond MP. Effect of thrombin-induced hemostasis on the efficacy of an absorbable adhesion barrier. J Reprod Med 1992; 37: 766–770.

33. De Cherney AH, di Zerega GS. Clinical problem of intraperitoneal postsurgical adhesion formation following general surgery and the use of adhesion prevention barriers. Surg Clin North Am 1997; 77: 671–688.

34. Wiseman D. Polymers for the prevention of surgical adhesions. In: Domb AJ, ed: Polymeric site-specific pharmacotherapy. New York: John Wiley and Sons; 1994: 370–421.

35. Prevention of postsurgical adhesions by INTERCEED(TC7), an absorbable adhesion barrier: a prospective randomized multicenter clinical study. INTERCEED(TC7) Adhesion Barrier Study Group. Fertil Steril 1989; 51: 933–938.

36. Diamond MP, Linsky CB, Cunningham T, et al. Synergistic effects of Interceed (TC7) and heparin in reducing adhesion formation in the rabbit uterine horn model. Fertil Steril 1991; 55: 389–394.

37. Diamond MP, Linsky CB, Cunningham T, et al. Adhesion reformation: reduction by the use of Interceed (TC7) plus heparin. J Gynecol Surg 1991; 7: 1–6.

38. Sahin Y, Saglam A. Synergistic effects of carboxymethylcellulose and low molecular weight heparin in reducing adhesion formation in the rat uterine horn model. Acta Obstet Gynecol Scand 1994; 73: 70–73.

39. Reid RL, Lie K, Spence JE, et al. Clinical evaluation of the efficacy of heparin-saturated Interceed for prevention of adhesion reformation in the pelvic sidewall of the human. In: Diamond MP, diZerega GS, Linsky CB, et al, eds. Gynecologic surgery and adhesion prevention. New York: Wiley-Liss; 1993: 261–264.

40. Reid RL, Hahn PM, Spence JE, et al. A randomized clinical trial of oxidized regenerated cellulose adhesion barrier (Interceed, TC7) alone or in combination with heparin. Fertil Steril 1997; 67: 23–29.

41. Andrade-Gordon P, Strickland S. Interaction of heparin with plasminogen activators and plasminogen. Biochemistry 1986; 25: 4033–4040.

42. Orita H, Campeau JD, Gale J, et al. Differential secretion of plasminogen activator activity by postsurgical activated macrophages. J Surg Res 1986; 41: 569–573.

43. Markwardt F, Klocking HP. Heparin-induced release of plasminogen activator. Haemostasis 1977; 6: 370–374.

44. Wiseman DM, Trout JR, Franklin R, et al. Metaanalysis of the safety and efficacy of an adhesion barrier (Interceed TC7) in laparotomy. J Reprod Med 1999; 44: 325–331.

45. Giannacodimos G, Douligeris N, Lappas K. Prevention of

postsurgical adhesions by Interceed (TC7) in polycystic ovary syndrome treated by CO_2 laser vaporization laparoscopy. In Proceedings of the Eighth Annual Meeting of the European Society of Human Reproduction and Embryology, 1992: 61. [Abstract]

46. diZerega GS. Use of adhesion prevention barriers in ovarian surgery, tubalplasty, ectopic pregnancy, endometriosis, adhesiolysis, and myomectomy. Curr Opin Obstet Gynecol 1996; 8(3): 230–237.

47. Sawada T, Nishizawa H, Nishio E, et al. Postoperative adhesion prevention with an oxidized regenerated cellulose adhesion barrier in infertile women. J Reprod Med 2000; 45: 387–389.

48. Haney AF, Doty ED. Murine peritoneal injury and de novo adhesion formation caused by oxidized-regenerated cellulose (Interceed TC7) but not expanded polytetrafluoroethylene (Gore-Tex surgical membrane). Fertil Steril 1992; 57: 202–208.

49. Boyers SP, Diamond MP, DeCherney AH. Reduction of postoperative adhesions in the rabbit with Gore-Tex surgical membrane. Fertil Steril 1988; 49: 1066–1070.

50. Prophylaxis of pelvic sidewall adhesions with Gore-Tex surgical membrane: a multicenter clinical investigation. The Surgical Membrane Study Group. Fertil Steril 1992; 57: 921–923.

51. Haney AF, Hesla J, Hurst BS, et al. Expanded polytetrafluoroethylene (Gore-Tex) Surgical Membrane is superior to oxidized regenerated cellulose (Interceed TC7) in preventing adhesions. Fertil Steril 1995; 63: 1021–1026.

52. An expanded polytetrafluoroethylene barrier (Gore-Tex Surgical Membrane) reduced post-myomectomy adhesion formation. Myomectomy Adhesion Multicenter Study Group. Fertil Steril 1995; 63: 491–493.

53. Haney AF. Removal of surgical barriers of expanded polytetrafluoroethylene at second-look laparoscopy was not associated with adhesion formation. Fertil Steril 1997; 68: 721–723.

54. Grow DR, Seltman HJ, Coddington CC, et al. The reduction of postoperative adhesions by two different barrier methods versus control in cynomolgus monkeys: a prospective randomized, crossover study. Fertil Steril 1994; 61: 1141–1146.

55. Diamond MP. Reduction of adhesions after uterine myomectomy by Seprafilm membrane (HAL-F): a blinded, prospective, randomized multicenter clinical study. Fertil Steril 1996; 66: 904–910.

56. Becker JM, Dayton MT, Fazio VW, et al. Prevention of postoperative abdominal adhesions by a sodium hyaluronate based bioresorbable membrane: a prospective, randomized, double-blind multicenter trial. J Am Coll Surg 1996; 183: 297–306.

57. Kelly KA, Pemberton JH, Wolff BG, et al. Ileal pouch–anal anastomosis. Curr Probl Surg 1992; 64: 64–131.

58. Wietske WV, Tseng LNL, Eijkman HJM, et al. Fewer intraperitoneal adhesions with use of hyaluronic acid-carboxymethylcellulose membrane; a randomized clinical trial. Ann Surg 2002; 235: 193–199.

59. Khaitan L, Scholz S, Houston H, et al. Results after laparoscopic lysis of adhesions and placement of Seprafilm for intractable abdominal pain. Surg Endosc 2003; 17: 247–253.

60. Bowers D, Raybon RB, Wheeless CR Jr. Hyaluronic acid-carboxymethylcellulose film and perianastomotic adhesions in previously irradiated rats. Am J Obstet Gynecol 1999; 181: 1335–1338.

61. Moreira H Jr, Wexner SD, Yamaguchi T, et al. Use of bioresorbable membrane (sodium hyaluronate + carboxymethylcellulose) after controlled bowel injuries in a rabbit model. Dis Colon Rectum 2000; 43: 182–187.

62. Beck DE, Cohen Z, Fleshman JW, et al for the Adhesion Study Group Steering Committee. A prospective, randomized, multicenter, controlled study of the safety of Seprafilm adhesion barrier in abdominopelvic surgery of the intestine. Dis Colon Rectum 2003; 46: 1310–1319.

63. Burns JW, Skinner K, Colt MJ, et al. A hyaluronate based gel for the prevention of postsurgical adhesions: evaluation in two animal species. Fertil Steril 1996; 66: 814–821.

64. Ferland R, Mulani D, Campbell PK. Evaluation of a sprayable polyethylene glycol adhesion barrier in a porcine efficacy model. Hum Reprod 2001; 16(12): 2718–2723.

65. Mettler L, Audebert A, Lehmann-Willenbrock E, et al. A prospective clinical trial of SprayGel as a barrier to adhesion formation: interim analysis. Poster and presentation at the 10th Congress of the European Society for Gynecologic Endoscopy, Lisbon, Portugal. Bologna: Monduzzi Editore; 2001.

66. Pellicano M, Bramante S, Cirillo D, et al. Effectiveness of autocrosslinked hyaluronic acid gel after laparoscopic myomectomy in infertile patients: a prospective, randomised, controlled study. Fertil Steril 2003; 80(2): 441–444.

67. Acunzo G, Guida M, Pellicano M, et al. Effectiveness of auto-cross-linked hyaluronic acid gel in the prevention of intrauterine adhesions after hysteroscopic adhesiolysis: a prospective randomised study. Hum Reprod 2003; 18(9): 1918–1921.

68. Reich H. New techniques in advanced operative laparoscopy. In: Sutton CJG, ed. Baillière's Clin Obstet Gynaecol 1989; 3: 655–681.

69. Davies DS. Kinetics of icodextrins. Perit Dial Int 1994; 14: S45–S50.

70. Rosen DMB, Sutton CJG. Outcome measures and adhesion formation: pain and postsurgical adhesion. In: diZerega GS, ed. Peritoneal surgery. New York: Springer-Verlag; 1999: 321–327.

71. deZerega GS. Biochemical events in peritoneal tissue repair. Eur J Surg 1997; S577: 10–16.

72. Harris ES, Morgan RF, Rodeheaver GT. Analysis of the kinetics of peritoneal adhesion formation in the rat and evaluation of potential antiadhesive agents. Surgery 1995; 117: 663–669.

73. Gilbert JA, Peers EM, Brown CB, et al. Intraperitoneal

fluid dynamics of 4% icodextrin in non-ESRC patients. Perit Dial Int 1999; 19: S79.

74. Verco SJS, Peers EM, Brown CB, et al. Development of a novel glucose polymer solution (icodextrin) for adhesion prevention: pre-clinical studies. Hum Reprod 2000; 15(8): 1764–1772.

75. diZerega G, Verco SJS, Young P, et al. A randomized controlled pilot study of the safety and efficacy of 4% icodextrin solution (Adept) in the reduction of adhesions following laparoscopic gynecologic surgery. Hum Reprod 2002; 17: 1031–1038.

76. Peers E, Brown CB. Adept Adhesion Study Group. Adept (4% icodextrin): change in American Fertility Society score in a large, multicentre, randomised, double-blind clinical trial. Abstract F11.02 presented at the 14th Annual Congress of the International Society for Gynecologic Endoscopy; 3–6 April 2005, London.

77. Peers E, Brown CB. Adept Adhesion Study Group. Adept (4% icodextrin): significantly reduces post-surgical adhesion incidence in a large randomized, double-blind clinical trial. Abstract F13.05 presented at the 14th Annual Congress of the International Society for Gynecologic Endoscopy; 3–6 April 2005, London.

78. Wilson MS, Menzies D, Knight AD, et al. Demonstrating the clinical use and cost effectiveness of adhesion reduction strategies. Colorectal Dis 2002; 4: 355–360.

79. Tulandi T, Collins J, Burrows E, et al. Treatment-dependent and treatment-independent pregnancy among women with periadnexal adhesions. Am J Obstet Gynecol 1990; 162: 354–357.

80. Pados G, Camus M, De Munck L, et al. Laparscopic application of Interceed (TC7). Hum Reprod 1992; 7: 1141–1143.

81. Ethicon Communication. Urgent voluntary market withdrawal of Gynecare Intergel Adhesion Prevention Solution. March 28, 2003.

10 The role of perioperative medical therapy

Cindy Farquhar

Introduction

The commonly adopted approaches to endometriosis have been either medical therapy or surgery, which is usually laparoscopic. Medical therapy induces atrophy within the hormonally dependent ectopic endometrium. Surgery usually involves either destroying the endometriotic implant by ablation or excising the lesion. Surgery is also used to alleviate symptoms by dividing adhesions and interrupting neural pathways. Unfortunately, neither management approaches are a guarantee against recurrence of endometriosis and the condition is rarely considered cured.

The failure rates with medical therapy following cessation of the treatment may be as high as 50% in the 12–24 months following treatment.[1–3] This recurrence of symptoms may in part be because large lesions respond poorly to medical therapy. Furthermore, hormonal suppression does not influence the extent of adhesions, which are often associated with large lesions. These high rates of recurrence following medical therapy have led to a greater role for surgery. The surgery may be performed laparoscopically or as an open procedure. The methods of treatment are varied, including excision and laser or diathermy ablation with or without adhesiolysis.[4] Recurrence of endometriosis following laparoscopic surgery is common – even in the hands of the very experienced laparoscopic surgeon the cumulative recurrence rate after 5 years is nearly 20%.[5,6] A recent small study has shown a return of dysmenorrhea in 45% of women within 1 year of laparoscopic surgery who received no other treatment.[7] Disappointment

with these results has led gynecologists to consider if a combination of medical and surgical therapy may have advantages, and in recent years there has been interest in combining medical and surgical therapy in an attempt to reduce recurrence of endometriosis.

This chapter aims to evaluate the use of medical therapy before or after, or before and after, surgery for endometriosis. In order to evaluate perioperative medical therapy where possible, evidence from randomized controlled trials (RCTs) will be used.

Options for perioperative medical therapy

The aim of medical treatment is to suppress menstruation and induce atrophy of the endometriotic implants. Medical therapy for endometriosis without surgery will be covered in a separate chapter and it is not planned to repeat information on medical therapy from that chapter. Treatment options for perioperative medical therapy include the oral contraceptive pill, progestogens, androgenic agents, and gonadotropin-releasing hormone (GnRH) agonists. All these options suppress ovarian activity, although the extent to which they achieve this varies between treatments. Side-effect profiles are also variable; progestogens are associated with irregular menstrual bleeding, weight gain, mood swings, and decreased libido. The side effects associated with danazol, the most commonly used androgenic agent, include skin changes, weight gain, and occasionally deepening of the voice. GnRH analogues dramatically lower estrogen levels by suppression of the hypothalamic–pituitary–ovarian axis. Side effects include the development of menopausal symptoms and the loss of bone mineral density with long-term use (both reversible), which may be managed by using estrogen therapy in an add-back regimen. GnRH analogues are given by injections or nasal spray.

GnRH analogues are often considered the 'gold standard' treatment in endometriosis because, when compared to progestogens and danazol, the suppression of ovarian function as measured by estradiol levels is greatest with the GnRH analogue. However, in comparative clinical studies all the medical therapies are effective in relieving pain and inducing atrophy, although few studies report the laparoscopic scores following treatment.[8–10] There is also no evidence that one GnRH analogue is superior to another.

Two approaches to perioperative medical therapy have been considered. One is the preoperative use of medical therapy (usually for 3 months), which may decrease the severity of the endometriosis and the size of endometriomas, making complete removal of endometriosis during laparoscopic surgery easier.[11,12] However, possible disadvantages of preoperative medical therapy, especially with danazol or GnRHs, are the adverse effects associated with these medications, which may influence women's willingness to continue to use the therapy. Furthermore, preoperative therapy means a delay of surgery. The second approach is to provide postoperative medical therapy for 3–6 months. This approach has the potential advantage of treating microscopic endometriosis, which may not have been visible at the time of surgery. In addition, it may induce the suppression of lesions that cannot be surgically removed and should reduce the risk of recurrence of endometriosis.[13,14]

Preoperative medical therapy

Should women with known endometriosis have medical therapy for 3 months prior to scheduled surgery? The aim of such therapy is to reduce the extent of endometriosis and, in particular, the size of endometriomas, making complete removal of the endometriosis during laparoscopic surgery feasible. If this approach is successful, a reduction in recurrence rates and an improvement in pregnancy rates should occur.

The ideal study design to answer this question would be an RCT of women with known endometriosis who were planning to have surgery and who were randomly assigned to medical therapy or a placebo for 3 months. Concealment of allocation and blinding of the surgeons would be important in the study design. The primary outcome measures should include laparoscopic scores, ease of surgery, recurrence of the endometriosis at least 12 months later, and the pregnancy rate.

There is only one RCT of preoperative medical therapy.[15] This RCT comprised 80 women with infertility, who were less than 35 years of age, with laparoscopically confirmed ovarian endometriotic cysts that were initially drained and flushed out. The patients were then randomized to receive a subcutaneous GnRH analogue (goserelin) implant 4-weekly for 12 weeks or no treatment. Twelve weeks after the first-look laparoscopy, another laparoscopy was performed, during which a biopsy was done, endometriosis vaporized, and the cyst wall vaporized using a laser. It is not clear if the surgeons were aware of which women received the GnRH analogue or not. The outcome measure was the laparoscopic scoring (American Fertility Society; AFS), which was performed by the same two observers. A statistically significant reduction in total AFS scores was reported, with a weighted mean difference (WMD) of -9.60 in the score (95% CI, -11.42 to -7.78). There was also a statistically significant reduction in implant AFS scores (WMD, -8.70; 95% confidence interval (CI), -10.67 to -6.73), but no difference between the groups with regard to adhesion AFS scores (WMD, -0.90; 95% CI, -3.42 to 1.62). No pregnancy or recurrence outcomes were reported.

Postoperative medical therapy

Eight RCTs of postoperative medical therapy have been undertaken: three compared different medical therapies with placebo[16–18] and five trials compared with no treatment.[19–23] These studies have been summarized in a systematic review[24] and are listed in Table 10.1. The treatment periods varied from 3 to 6 months. Two studies compared intranasal nafarelin (400 µg/day) with placebo, over a period of 6 months[16] or 3 months.[17] The other placebo-controlled trial of postsurgical medical therapy had two treatment arms (medroxyprogesterone acetate 100 mg/day and danazol 600 mg/day for 6 months) and a placebo arm.[18] The remaining studies compared postoperative medical therapy with no treatment and therefore were unblinded studies. In one

Table 10.1 Characteristics of included studies

Study	Methods	Participants	Interventions	Outcomes
Preoperative therapy Donnez 1994[15]	RCT Unclear if blinded occurred Single center Belgium	Eighty infertile women (<35 years old) with endometriomata at the time of laparoscopy	Medical therapy prior to surgery, with subcutaneous goserelin 4 weekly × 4 ($n = 40$) vs no therapy ($n = 40$)	AFS scores and ovarian cysts diameter
Postoperative therapy Bianchi 1999[19]	RCT Unclear if blinded Single center in Italy	Seventy-seven women with endometriosis	Postsurgical medical therapy comparing danazol oral 600 mg daily for 3/12 ($n = 36$) with no treatment ($n = 41$)	Pain recurrence AFS scores Pregnancy rates Adverse events of medication
Busacca 2001[20]	RCT Unclear if blinded Single center in Italy	Eighty-nine women with laparoscopic diagnosis of endometriosis stage III–IV Exclusion criteria: previous medical or surgical treatment for endometriosis	Postsurgical medical therapy comparing leuprolide acetate SC 3.5 mg 4 weekly × 3 doses ($n = 44$) with no treatment ($n = 45$)	Pelvic pain recurrence at 18/12 ASRM scores: objective disease recurrence Cumulative pregnancy rates at 18/12
Hornstein 1997[16]	RCT Multicentered study in the USA	One hundred and nine women with endometriosis	Postsurgery medical therapy comparing nafarelin nasal 400 µg daily for 6/12 ($n = 49$) with placebo ($n = 44$)	Pain Physician scores for tenderness and induration on physical examination at end of treatment and 6/12 after treatment
Loverro 2001[21]	RCT Unclear if blinded Single center in Italy	Sixty-two women with moderate–severe endometriosis	Postsurgery medical therapy with triptorelin SC 3.75 mg every 4 weeks for 3 months ($n = 33$) vs no treatment	Pain Pregnancy rates

Table 10.1 Characteristics of included studies (cont.)

Study	Methods	Participants	Interventions	Outcomes
Muzii 2000[22]	RCT Unclear if blinded Two centers in Italy	Seventy women with moderate to severe dysmenorrhea and/or chronic pelvic pain, not desiring fertility	Postsurgical medical therapy with cyclic monophasic oral contraceptive pill (ethinyl estradiol 0.03 mg, gestodene 0.075 mg) for 21 days with 7 pill-free days for 6/12 ($n = 35$) vs no treatment ($n = 35$)	Recurrence of pain and time to recurrence Recurrence of cysts
Parazzini 1994[17]	Double-blind RCT Multicentered trial in Italy	Seventy-five women with unexplained infertility for at least 1 year, with/without chronic pelvic pain, moderate to severe endometriosis	Postsurgical medical therapy with nafarelin nasal 400 μg daily for 3/12 ($n = 36$) vs placebo ($n = 39$)	Pain (multidimensional and 10-point linear scale) score Pregnancy rates Adverse drug outcome
Telimaa 1987[18]	Double-blind RCT Single center in Finland	Sixty women with advanced endometriosis	Postsurgical medical therapy with danazol oral 600 mg daily for 180 days ($n = 20$). MPA 100 mg daily for 180 days ($n = 20$) or placebo ($n = 20$)	Pain scores AFS scores Pregnancy rates Patient satisfaction Adverse drug outcomes
Vercellini 1999[23]	Double-blind RCT Multicentered trial in Italy	Two hundred and sixty-nine women with endometriosis and chronic pelvic pain	Postsurgical medical therapy with goserelin SC 3.6 mg every 4 weeks for 6 months ($n = 133$) vs no treatment ($n = 134$)	Pain recurrence Pregnancy rates
Pre-versus postoperative medical therapy				
Audebert 1998[25]	Double-blind RCT	Fifty-five women with stage III–IV endometriosis, pelvic pain, dysmenorrhea or dyspareunia	Preoperative medical treatment with nafarelin nasal 400 μg daily for 6/12 vs postoperative medical treatment with nafarelin nasal 400 μg daily for 6/12	Pain (dysmenorrhea, dyspareunia), tenderness, pelvic induration AFS scores: global, adhesions, endometriosis Ease of surgery

AFS = American Fertility Society; MPA = medroxyprogesterone acetate; RCT = randomized controlled trial; SC = subcutaneous.
ASRM = American Society Reproductive Medicine

study, postoperative danazol, 600 mg/day for 3 months was compared with surgery alone.[19] In three studies, postoperative GnRHs (leuprolide, triptorelin, and goserelin, respectively) administered subcutaneously every 4 weeks for a period of 3 months, were compared with surgery alone.[20,21,23] One study compared surgery plus 6 months of therapy with low-dose cyclical oral contraceptives with surgery alone.[22]

In the five unblinded trials comparing postoperative medical therapy with surgery alone (no medical therapy), there was no evidence of a statistically significant reduction in pain recurrence at 12 months (risk ratio (RR), 0.76; 95% CI, 0.52 to 1.10) although the difference at 24 months approached statistical significance (RR, 0.70; 95% CI, 0.47 to 1.03).[24] There was no evidence of a statistically significant difference between the use of these medical therapies after surgery compared to surgery alone, with regard to disease recurrence (RR, 1.02; 95% CI, 0.27 to 3.84) or pregnancy rates (RR, 0.78; 95% CI, 0.50 to 1.22).

In the three blinded studies, postoperative medical therapy was compared to surgery plus placebo.[16–18] There was no evidence of a statistically significant difference between medical therapy and placebo with regard to the measures for pain: multidimensional pain score WMD −0.40 (95% CI, −2.15 to 1.35); linear scale score 0.10 (95% CI, −2.24 to 2.44); change in pain −0.40 (95% CI, −1.48 to 0.68). There was no evidence of a statistically significant difference between medical therapy and placebo for pregnancy rates (RR, 1.05; 95% CI, 0.44 to 2.51) or total AFS scores (WMD, −2.10; 95% CI, −4.56 to 0.36).[24]

In summary, there is insufficient evidence to support the case of medical therapy postoperatively. Further well-designed studies are needed to establish the role of postoperative medical therapy in preventing recurrence of endometrosis or improving pregnancy rate.

Preoperative medical therapy compared with postoperative medical therapy

One study of 55 women with endometrosis that compared medical therapy with intranasal nafarelin administered for 6 months before surgery with intranasal nafarelin administered for 6 months after surgery did not show evidence of a difference between the groups with regard to pain.[25] There was no dysmenorrhea reported after treatment in either group and no difference between presurgical therapy and postsurgical therapy with regard to pelvic pain or pelvic tenderness.

Levonorgestrel intrauterine system following surgery for endometriosis

Although the intrauterine device was originally designed as a method of contraception, with the addition of progesterone to the device it can now be used for managing menstrual disorders, particularly menorrhagia.[26] The levonorgestrel intrauterine system (LNG-IUS) is a device which releases 20 µg of levonorgestrel per day and has been shown to result in a profound reduction in menstrual blood loss in women with menorrhagia:[27,28] 25% of the women using the LNG-IUS were amenorrheic after 1 year's use[28] while still continuing to ovulate. The LNG-IUS, which has to be replaced every 5 years, has also been reported to improve dysmenorrhea.[28] A major disadvantage of the device is frequent and variable intermenstrual bleeding and spotting during the first few months of use. Its use in women with endometriosis has been less well documented, but one recent RCT has suggested benefit in women with endometriosis.[7] Forty women were randomized to either LNG-IUS or not following surgery for endometriosis. Moderate or severe dysmenorrhea recurred in 2 of 20 (10%) subjects in the postoperative LNG-IUS group and 9/20 (45%) in the surgery-only group.[7] It has also been used in women with rectovaginal endometriosis with good effect, although the study was small and not randomized.[29]

Adverse events

A balance sheet of harms and benefits of pre- and postoperative medical therapy for women with endometrosis is presented in Table 10.2.

Conclusions

Overall, there is a paucity of well-designed research in the area of perioperative medical therapy in women with endometriosis. In the only study comparing preoperative medical therapy with surgery alone, laparoscopic scores were the only outcomes reported and it is not known if the improvements in score in the medical therapy

Table 10.2 Balance sheet of harms and benefits for pre- and postoperative medical therapy for women with endometriosis

Therapy	Benefits	Harms
Preoperative therapy (GnRHa CIRCT)	Improved laparoscopic scores No other benefits yet proven	Adverse events (hot flushes) Inconvenience of regular medications Delay in surgery Cost
Postoperative therapy GnRH (6 RCTs)	None proven	Adverse events (hot flushes, vaginal dryness) Inconvenience of regular medications Delayed fertility Cost
MPA (1 RCT)	None proven	Adverse events (weight gain, bloating) Inconvenience of regular medications Delayed fertility Cost
Danazol (2 RCTs)	None proven	Adverse events (hyperandrogenism) Inconvenience of regular medications Delayed fertility Cost
OC pill (1 RCT)	None proven	Adverse events Inconvenience of regular medications Delayed fertility Cost
Levonorgestrel intrauterine system (1 RCT)	Significant reduction in dysmenorrhea	Irregular bleeding Amenorrhea Delayed fertility Cost

GnRHa = gonadotropin-releasing hormone agonists; MPA = medroxyprogesterone acetate; OC pill = oral contraceptive; RCT = randomized controlled trial.

group were associated with better outcomes for the patients. Although there were eight RCTs comparing postoperative hormonal suppression of endometriosis with surgery alone (either no medical therapy or placebo), five of them were unblinded and therefore limited in value. Furthermore, the included studies were small and of variable quality. Overall, these studies did not demonstrate benefit for the outcomes of pain, pregnancy rates, and disease recurrence.

In summary, there is no evidence of benefit with the use of medical treatment after surgery in women with endometriosis. When used prior to surgery, medical therapy was shown to improve AFS scores. However, there is no evidence that medical therapy pre- or postsurgery influences disease recurrence or improves pregnancy rates. No conclusions can be drawn with respect to the outcomes of facilitating surgery, duration of surgery, postoperative complications, or levels of satisfaction of women participants from the trials included in this review. The role of the LNG-IUS for postoperative management in those women who do not desire pregnancy, although promising, requires further investigation with more RCTs and longer follow-up.

There is a need for further research to be conducted in this area. However, there are significant challenges. For example, while the outcome desired by surgeons may be a reduction in the extent of endometriosis, it is unlikely that many women will consent to undergo second-look laparoscopy. Maintaining blinding is also difficult due to the adverse effects associated with hormonal suppression which may be obvious to both the patient and investigator. Women with subfertility due to endometriosis may also not accept treatment that may improve pain and other symptoms but reduces or delays their chance of conceiving.

In spite of these difficulties, it would be valuable to have well-designed and adequately powered trials to determine if there is a significant benefit in medical therapy before or after surgery for endometriosis. Consistency in the methods of assessing outcomes, with respect to pain and the extent of endometriosis from AFS scores, would also help in being able to combine and to compare the results of studies.

REFERENCES

1. Barbieri RL. Endometriosis. Current treatment approaches. Drugs 1990; 39(4): 502–510.
2. Dlugi AM, Miller JD, Knittle J. Lupron depot (leuprolide acetate for depot suspension) in the treatment of endometriosis: a randomized, placebo-controlled, double-blind study. Lupron Study Group. Fertil Steril 1990; 54: 419–427.
3. Fedele L, Bianchi S, Bocciolone L, et al. Buserelin acetate in the treatment of pelvic pain associated with minimal and mild endometriosis: a controlled study. Fertil Steril 1993; 59: 516–521.
4. Sutton CJG, Pooley AS, Ewen SP, et al. Follow-up report on a randomized controlled trial of laser laparoscopy in the treatment of pelvic pain associated with minimal to moderate endometriosis. Fertil Steril 1997; 68: 1070–1074.
5. Redwine DB. Conservative laparoscopic excision of endometriosis by sharp dissection: life table analysis of reoperation and persistent or recurrent disease. Fertil Steril 1991; 56(4): 628–634.
6. Redwine DB, Wright JT. Laparoscopic treatment of complete obliteration of the cul-de-sac associated with endometriosis: long-term follow-up of en bloc resection. Fertil Steril 2001; 76(2): 358–365.
7. Vercellini P, Frontino G, De Giorgi O, et al. Comparison of a levonorgestrel-releasing intrauterine device versus expectant management after conservative surgery for symptomatic endometriosis: a pilot study. Fertil Steril 2003; 80(2): 305–309.
8. Prentice A, Deary AJ, Goldbeck-Wood S, et al. Gonadotrophin-releasing hormone analogues for pain associated with endometriosis. Cochrane Database Syst Rev 2000; 2: CD000346.
9. Prentice A, Deary AJ, Bland E. Progestagens and anti-progestagens for pain associated with endometriosis. Cochrane Database Syst Rev 2000; 2: CD002122.
10. Selak V, Farquhar C, Prentice A, et al. Danazol for pelvic pain associated with endometriosis. Cochrane Database Syst Rev 2001; 4: CD000068.
11. Hemmings R. Combined treatment of endometriosis, GnRH agonists and laparoscopic surgery. J Reprod Med 1998; 43(2 Suppl): 316–320.
12. Donnez J, Lemaire-Rubbers M, Karaman Y, et al. Combined (hormonal and microsurgical) therapy in infertile women with endometriosis. Fertil Steril 1987; 48(2): 239–242.
13. Kettel LM, Murphy AA. Combination medical and surgical therapy for infertile patients with endometriosis. Obstet Gynecol Clin North Am 1989; 16: 167–177.
14. Thomas EJ. Combining medical and surgical treatment for endometriosis: the best of both worlds? Br J Obstet Gynaecol 1992; 99(Suppl 7): 5–8.

15. Donnez J, Anaf V, Nisolle M, et al. Ovarian endometrial cysts: the role of gonadotropin-releasing hormone agonist and/or drainage. Fertil Steril 1994; 62(1): 63–66.

16. Hornstein MD, Hemmings R, Yuzpe AA, et al. Use of nafarelin versus placebo after reductive laparoscopic surgery for endometriosis. Fertil Steril 1997; 68(5): 860–864.

17. Parazzini F, Fedele L, Busacca M, et al. Postsurgical medical treatment of advanced endometriosis: results of a randomized clinical trial. Am J Obstet Gynecol 1994; 171: 1205–1207.

18. Telimaa S, Ronnberg L, Kauppila A. Placebo-controlled comparison of danazol and high-dose medroxyprogesterone acetate in the treatment of endometriosis after conservative surgery. Gynecol Endocrinol 1987; 1(4): 363–371.

19. Bianchi S, Busacca M, Agnoli B, et al. Effects of 3 month therapy with danazol after laparoscopic surgery for stage III/IV endometriosis: a randomized study. Hum Reprod 1999; 14(5): 1335–1337.

20. Busacca M, Somigliana E, Bianchi S, et al. Post-operative GnRH analogue treatment after conservative surgery for symptomatic endometriosis stage III–IV: a randomized controlled trial. Hum Reprod 2001; 16(11): 2399–2402.

21. Loverro G, Santillo V, Pansini MV, et al. Are GnRH agonists helpful in the therapy of endometriosis after surgical treatment? Hum Reprod 2001; 16(1 Suppl): 96.

22. Muzii L, Marana R, Caruana P, et al. Postoperative administration of monophasic combined oral contraceptives after laparoscopic treatment of ovarian endometriomas: a prospective, randomized trial. Am J Obstet Gynecol 1999; 183(3): 588–592.

23. Vercellini P, Crosignani PG, Fadini R, et al. A gonadotrophin-releasing hormone agonist compared with expectant management after conservative surgery for symptomatic endometriosis. Br J Obstet Gynaecol 1999; 106: 672–677.

24. Yap C, Furness S, Farquhar C. Pre and postoperative medical therapy for endometriosis surgery. Cochrane Database Syst Rev 2004; 3: CD003678.

25. Audebert A, Descamps P, Marret H, et al. Pre or post-operative medical treatment with nafarelin in stage III–IV endometriosis: a French multicenter study. Obstet Gynecol 1998; 79: 145–148.

26. Lethaby AE, Cook I, Rees M. Progesterone/progestogen releasing intrauterine systems for heavy menstrual bleeding. Cochrane Database Syst Rev 1999; 4: CD002126.

27. Bergquist C. Effects of nafarelin versus danazol on lipids and calcium metabolism. Am J Obstet Gynecol 1990; 162: 589–591.

28. Andersson K, Odlind V, Rybo G. Levonorgestrel-releasing and copper-releasing (Nova T) IUDs during five years of use: a randomized comparative trial. Contraception 1994; 49: 56–72.

29. Fedele L, Bianchi S, Zanconato G, et al. Use of a levonorgestrel releasing intrauterine device in the treatment of rectovaginal endometriosis. Fertil Steril 2001; 75: 485–488.

SECTION III
Surgical Treatment by Laparoscopy

11 Overview of laparoscopic techniques for endometriosis surgery

Mauro Busacca and Michele Vignali

Introduction

Endometriosis is today one of the most frequent indications for gynecologic surgery worldwide. Endometriosis is a benign disease that must be treated when at least two signs are present:

- infertility
- pain

The aim of this chapter is to overview the surgical techniques and modalities employed in the treatment of advanced endometriosis, particularly ovarian endometriosis, deep endometriosis, and recurrent endometriosis.

There is still a great debate on the best way to treat surgically minimal and mild endometriosis and on the results in terms of infertility and pelvic pain.

During the past 15 years, the potential for treating endometriosis at the same time as diagnostic laparoscopy has increased dramatically. Complication rates due to laparoscopy appear to be equivalent to, or less frequent, than those associated with laparotomy, although strict comparative data are unavailable. We must stress that the results in achieving pregnancy or in pain reduction are comparable when performed either by laparoscopy or laparotomy, but the advantages to the patient when the disease is treated by minimally invasive techniques are considerable.

It has been demonstrated that all the surgical procedures employed for advanced endometriosis can be performed via laparoscopy. Nevertheless, these procedures are extremely difficult and must be performed only by well-trained and expert laparoscopic surgeons and these techniques are not available in all hospitals but only in special centers.

Deep endometriosis

Deep endometriosis is a peculiar form of endometriosis: it is very active, penetrating below the surface of the peritoneum for more than 5 mm.[1] These lesions are more commonly located

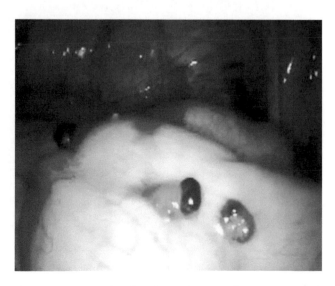

Figure 11.1 Superficial endometriotic implants on sigmoid serosa.

at the level of uterosacral ligaments and the pouch of Douglas,[2] but often may extend along the rectovaginal septum and may infiltrate and extend posteriorly into the rectum and sigmoid, leading to cul-de-sac obliteration (Figure 11.1).[3,4] Deep infiltrating endometriosis strongly correlates with pelvic pain and severe dyspareunia.[5] The exact mechanism by which deep endometriotic lesions cause pelvic pain is not well defined[6] and, because the specific depth of infiltration is not addressed in the revised American Fertility Society (r-AFS),[7] several studies have reached conflicting results when correlating the severity of pain with stage.[8-12]

Recently, it has been suggested that the fibrosis surrounding rectovaginal endometriotic nodules could entrap nerve structures, exerting a certain pressure on nerve ganglia, which could explain the pain symptoms associated with this type of disease.[13] Although chronic pelvic pain, dysmenorrhea, and dyspareunia are the most frequent symptoms, dyschezia and rectal bleeding can occur when the rectum is infiltrated.[14]

Pelvic tenderness and nodularities at pelvic examination have been directly correlated with the frequency and severity of deep dyspareunia,[15] (Figure 11.2) and recently Chapron et al demonstrated a straight association between severity of dyspareunia and the severity of adnexal adhesion and obliteration of the pouch of Douglas, confirming the inadequacy of r-AFS in explaining dyspareunia severity.[16] Diagnosis of deeply infiltrating endometriosis is confirmed ultimately by resection of the disease for histology and assessment for depth of infiltration.

In the past, surgical treatment of severe endometriosis consisted of total abdominal hysterectomy and bilateral salpingo-oophorectomy, but this could not obviously be considered the best surgical option in younger patients. Furthermore, female castration without removing the surrounding fibrotic tissue can result, even if infrequently, in persistence of symptoms,[17] probably due to local production of aromatase enzyme, which converts adrenal precursors into estrogen.[18]

Several studies have shown that the degree of pain relief correlates with completeness of disease ablation (Figure 11.3).[19-21] Resection of endometriotic implants by both laparoscopy and laparotomy has been shown to be a highly effective treatment for reduction of pain, with a low rate of recurrence following conservative treatment.[22,23] Donnez et al reported 2-year follow-up success rates of 96.3% and 98.8% in relieving pelvic pain and dyspareunia, respectively, in 242 patients in a large series of 497 women who underwent laparoscopic resection of rectovaginal deep endometriosis.[24]

A previous paper[25] on 23 patients with complete obliteration of posterior cul-de-sac treated laparoscopically reported a pain relief of 89%. Redwine and Wright[26] prospectively evaluated 84 patients with obliterated cul-de-sac through a five-point questionnaire evaluating pre- and postoperative symptoms. Aggressive laparoscopic surgery, consisting of radical treatment of complete obliteration of the cul-de-sac by en bloc resection of endometriosis and bowel resection if required, showed improvement in all symptom categories. Sixty-one patients (73%) required rectal surgery,

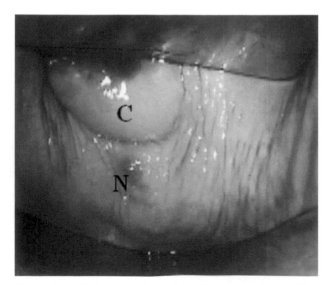

Figure 11.2 Endometriotic nodule of vaginal mucosa. C = cervix; N = nodule.

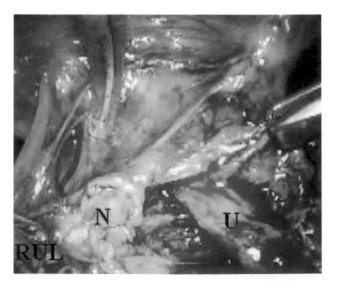

Figure 11.3 Removal of an endometriotic nodule deep infiltrating the right broad ligament, close to the ureter. N = nodule; U = ureter; RUL = right uterosacral ligament.

and rectal endometriosis was confirmed histologically. A very recent paper by Fedele et al on 83 patients who underwent conservative surgery for rectovaginal endometriosis showed a 28% recurrence rate of pain symptoms (dysmenorrhea, pelvic pain, or dyspareunia) at 36 months. The authors found a higher risk of recurrence for younger women and lower risk if surgical excision also included a segmental bowel resection and anastomosis.[27]

Operations specifically for the relief of dysmenorrhea

Treatment of midline pelvic pain or dyspareunia with *resection of the uterosacral ligaments* has recently been advocated during laparoscopic treatment for endometriosis.[16] This is a different procedure than simple division of the nerves of the Lee–Frankenhäuser plexus in the uterosacral ligaments – LUNA (laparoscopic uterosacral nerve ablation) (Figure 11.4). A recent survey has shown that almost half of the gynecologists in the UK perform the LUNA procedure as a part of their treatment for endometriosis.[28,29] Sutton et al,[30] comparing patients who underwent laser ablation of endometriosis together with the LUNA procedure with those who simply underwent diagnostic laparoscopy, found a statistically significant difference in pain reduction or resolution at 6-month follow-up in first group (62.5% vs 22.6%; *p* >0.01). The authors hypothesized that the LUNA was possibly effective in reducing dysmenorrhea and pelvic pain rather than the ablation of endometriosis. A few years later, the same group investigated this by a prospective, double-blind controlled trial and randomized 51 women with pelvic pain and pelvic endometriosis who underwent laser ablation of endometriosis to LUNA or to no further treatment. Their conclusion was that the resulting reduction of dysmenorrhea and chronic nonmenstrual pain at 6-month follow-up was attributable to the laser vaporization of endometriotic lesions rather than to LUNA itself.[31] In a more recent study, Vercellini et al randomized 180 patients with minimal to severe symptomatic endometriosis to laparoscopic conservative treatment with or without uterosacral ligaments resection. At 1-year follow-up, the recurrence rate of dysmenorrhea did not significantly differ in the two groups (29% vs 27%), as long as after 3 years from surgery (36% vs 32%). No significant difference between the two groups was observed in reduction of deep dyspareunia.[32] Furthermore, a recent meta-analysis did not confirm the efficacy of the LUNA procedure in reducing pain symptoms, without histologically proven infiltration of uterosacral ligaments.[33]

(a)

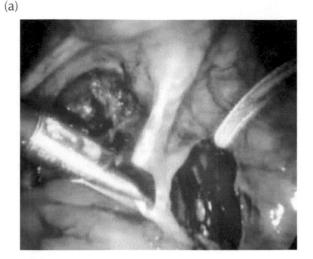

(b)

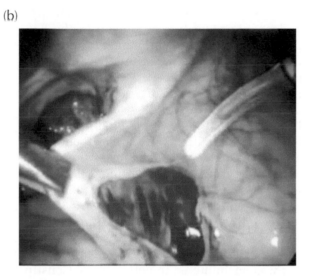

(c)

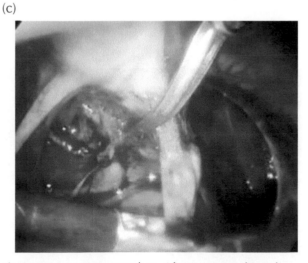

Figure 11.4 LUNA procedure. After exposing the right uterosacral ligament (a), having previously opened a peritoneal window in the broad ligament and thus moving aside the ureter (b), a portion of uterosacral ligament is resected (c).

Midline abdominal dysmenorrheic pain can be also treated with surgical removal of the presacral nerves lying within the interiliac triangle, thus interrupting the majority of the cervical sensory nerve fibers (Figure 11.5). *Presacral neurectomy (PSN)* has been described by many authors as an effective surgical technique to decrease midline pelvic pain in women affected by endometriotic disease. Candiani et al,[34] comparing a group of 71 patients with moderate and severe endometriosis who underwent open PSN combined with surgical treatment of endometriosis vs surgical treatment of endometriosis alone, reported a reduction in pelvic pain at 12-month follow-up, even if not significant ($p = 0.06$), in the group of patients with PSN. Since Perez has shown the feasibility of PSN by laparoscopy,[35] laparoscopic PSN has been recommended for the treatment of midline chronic pelvic pain and dysmenorrhea in selected patients.[36] However, this operation is an advanced endoscopic procedure and, even in the hands of skilled surgeons, the proximity of great vessels, ureter, and lymphatic channels, as well as the extreme vascularity of the presacral tissue, can increase the incidence of serious complications.[37]

In a very recent paper Zullo et al randomized 141 fertile women with r-AFS stage I–IV endometriosis and chronic severe dysmenorrhea to laparoscopic surgical treatment with or without PSN. At 1-year follow-up, the cure rate was significantly higher in patients who received PSN (85.7% vs 57.1%). At a longer follow-up of 24 months, the cure rate was still significantly higher in the same group (83.3% vs 53.3%), whereas an improvement in quality of life was encountered in both groups. Constipation (15%) and urinary urgency (5%) were reported as long-term complications.[38,39]

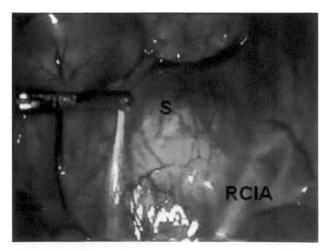

Figure 11.5 Presacral space. S = Sacrum; RCIA = Right Common Iliac Artery.

Chen et al[40] randomly compared laparoscopic presacral neurectomy (LPSN) and laparoscopic uterine nerve ablation in 68 patients with primary dysmenorrhea poorly responsive to medical treatment, showing a more significant efficacy of LPSN at the 12-month follow-up visit (81.8% vs 51.4%).

To decrease major surgical risks related to PSN, maintaining the benefits on pain relief, some authors have recently described a laparoscopic presacral neurolysis on 15 patients with minimal–moderate endometriosis, which consisted in a chemical neurolysis obtained by injecting 10 mL of phenol in the retroperitoneal space overlying the sacral promontory. The authors reported a significant reduction in pelvic symptom score as compared with baseline at 1-year follow-up, with no major complications.[41]

Surgical treatment of endometriosis-associated infertility

According to an Italian multicenter study[42] on 3684 fertile women of reproductive age undergoing surgery for benign gynecologic disease, prevalence of endometriosis ranged between 12% and 45%, with an incidence of 30% in those with the problem of infertility. Higher rates of infertility associated with endometriosis (20–70%) are reported by several authors.[43]

The relationship between endometriosis and infertility appears clearly evident in moderate and severe stages of the disease, when dense adhesions involving the tube and the ovary interfere with tubal motility and oocyte's pick-up, which could contribute to the impairment of potential fertility of the patient. This finding has been supported in a recent Cochrane review by Watson et al,[3] which concluded that infertility is directly related to severity of adhesions.

A different scenario is observed in the patient with minimal and mild endometriosis, in which anatomic relationships between the ovaries and the tubes are normal and the presence of the disease is limited to peritoneal or ovarian implants and to filmy adnexal adhesions (Figure 11.6). In these stages of the disease the correlation with infertility is still debated. A Canadian multicenter study[45] that compared 331 women with minimal or mild endometriosis and women with unexplained infertility undergoing diagnostic laparoscopy did not register significant differ-

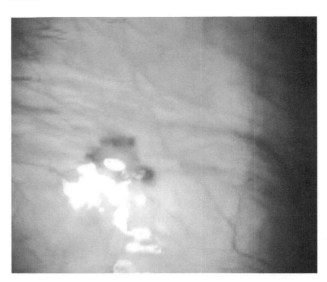

Figure 11.6 Superficial peritoneal implant of red endometriosis.

ences in terms of fecundity between the two groups (18.2% vs 23.7%).

Nevertheless, a recent meta-analysis[46] demonstrated a 54% reduction in pregnancy rate after in vitro fertilization (IVF) (odds ratio (OR), 0.46; confidence interval (CI), 0.28–0.74), compared with women with tubal factor infertility, and a 36% reduction for those with severe endometriosis, compared with those with mild disease (OR, 0.64; CI, 0.35–1.17). A direct negative effect of endometriosis on the oocyte's development, embryogenesis, or implantation, together with an altered inflammatory response mediated by interleukins or other cytokines and with autoimmune factors, has been advocated to somehow explain endometriosis-associated infertility, particularly lower stages of the disease on the r-AFS scale.[47,48]

The role of surgery in endometriosis-associated infertility is to restore normal anatomy through meticulous adhesiolysis, in order to facilitate fecundity. A meta-analysis by Adamson and Pasta,[49] showed that either no treatment or surgery provide a better pregnancy rate (almost 70%) with respect to medical treatment in those patients with minimal and mild endometriosis associated with infertility, whereas for moderate and severe disease, similar results were observed in both groups treated either with laparoscopy or laparotomy, respectively 62% and 44%.

A Canadian randomized multicenter trial,[50] evaluating 341 infertile women with minimal or mild endometriosis undergoing laparoscopic surgery with or without ablations of visible endometriotic lesions, demonstrated a significantly higher preg-

nancy rate (30.7% vs 17.7; $p = 0.006$) in those patients who received resection or ablation of endometriosis. A different and controversial conclusion was achieved by the Gruppo Italiano per lo Studio dell'Endometriosi,[51] who evaluated a group of patients with characteristics similar to the Canadian group trial. In fact, the pregnancy rate observed in the two groups was basically overlapping (24% vs 29%). More recently, Olive and Pritts[52] confirmed the latter findings, concluding that, despite the disparate results from the two trials, when the studies are combined, analysis reveals a significant benefit of surgical treatment (OR for pregnancy, 1.7). Subsequently, a *Cochrane Review* by Jacobson and Barlow[53] supported these conclusions.

Ovarian endometriosis

According to several studies in the literature, laparotomy does not seem to add any advantage in terms of pregnancy rate or recurrence rate in the surgical treatment of ovarian endometrioma;[54–57] thus, laparoscopy can be effectively considered the best surgical approach for ovarian endometriotic cysts (Figure 11.7).[58] Nevertheless, a recent paper by Jones et al, which gathered the answers to a questionnaire of 651 UK specialist gynecologists, still reported a rate of laparotomy of 42.3% in the treatment of ovarian endometrioma.[59] There are several papers in the literature comparing different surgical techniques in order to treat the endometriotic cysts with lower rate of recurrence and a higher pregnancy rate.[60,61]

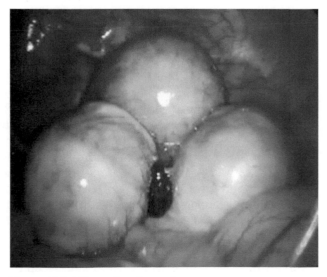

Figure 11.7 Bilateral endometriomas.

Nevertheless, it can be summarized in two schools of thought:

- cystectomy with excision of the endometriotic cyst
- drainage/aspiration of cyst content and ablation of the cyst capsule with laser or electro-coagulation.

The study of Beretta et al is the one and only randomized study[62] in which these two different approaches to the management of chocolate cysts have been compared, showing no statistically significant difference in the rate of disease recurrence between the two groups (6.2% vs 18.8%), but a higher pregnancy rate at 24-month follow-up in the group treated with complete cyst excision. It must be pointed out, however, that the pregnancy rate of the ablation group is one of the lowest in the literature compared to other series, with a pregnancy rate of 57% using the KTP/S32 laser to ablate the capsule.[63] Unfortunately the Beretta et al study[62] is the only randomized controlled trial (RCT) to compare excision vs ablation, but this very low pregnancy rate makes one question the technique used to ablate the endometriosis. These two different surgical techniques were retrospectively compared by another group[63] who concluded that laparoscopic excision of ovarian endometriomas at 42-month follow-up is associated with a lower reoperation rate than that of fenestration and ablation (23.6% vs 57.8%).

Recently, Brosens et al[64] and Donnez et al[65] have questioned the cyst excision technique because of its association with the removal of healthy ovarian tissue along with the wall of ovarian cysts, impairing ovarian reserve. Muzii et al[66] performed a histologic analysis on 26 ovarian endometriomas, showing ovarian tissue removed with the cyst pseudocapsule in 54% of cases. Nevertheless, in none of the specimens examined did the ovarian tissue adjacent to the cyst wall show the follicular pattern that is observed in normal ovaries.

The risk of ovarian recurrence of endometriosis after cystectomy varies among series.[60–62,67] According to a previous study[67] carried out in our department on 366 patients who underwent laparoscopic cystectomy for endometrioma, the cumulative rate of ultrasonographic recurrence over 48 months was 11.7%, whereas the cumulative rate of a reoperation was 8.2%. A recurrence rate of 4.2% (3/72) at a longer follow-up, 10 years, is reported by Marconi et al.[68]

Vercellini et al,[69] reviewing several studies on this topic, showed a three times increase in risk of cyst recurrence after coagulation or laser vaporization with respect to cystectomy (OR, 3.09; 95% CI, 1.78–5.36). Severity of endometriosis and a previous history of endometriosis seem to be bad prognostic factors. Some authors also indicate cyst diameter (>4 cm) as a predictive factor for reoperation.[61,67]

With respect to the advantage of adding medical therapy after surgery, Busacca et al,[70] in a randomized study on 89 patients with symptomatic endometriosis stage III–IV, showed no benefits in terms of symptoms recurrence and pregnancy rate after 3 months of gonadotropin-releasing hormone (GnRH) analogues after surgery. The same group reached the same conclusions in another randomized study using danazol, 600 mg daily for 3 months, after the operation.[71]

Ovarian endometriosis and infertility

The association between endometriosis and infertility is as well known as the mechanism by which a women with endometriosis is infertile is unknown. The finding of endometriosis as only confined to the ovary is rare, about 1%, as reported by Redwine[72] in 1999. Whereas r-AFS stage III/IV endometriosis may impair fertility by mechanical means, it is probable that interleukins or other cytokines, alteration in inflammatory response, or autoimmune factors may affect oocyte development, embryogenesis, or implantation, causing infertility in women with minimal and mild stage disease.[73–77]

As regards the recurrence rate, which is the best surgical technique to achieve a better pregnancy rate is still controversial. In a recent prospective cohort study, Jones and Sutton[78] reported a cumulative pregnancy rate of 39.5% at 12-month follow-up, whereas, according to the only randomized study[79] comparing the two different techniques, a better pregnancy rate is achieved with cyst excision (67% vs 23.5% at 24 months).

Several studies have shown that both surgical approaches, cystectomy and laser ablation, do not impair ovarian response to IVF and embryo transfer (ET), if care is taken in avoiding damage to the remaining ovarian tissue.[80,81]

Furthermore, given the adverse effect of prolonged ovarian stimulation on endometriotic ovaries, which could lead to a progression of the disease,

IVF–ET should be preferred to controlled ovarian hyperstimulation and intrauterine insemination (COH–IUI). Dmowsky et al[82] in a recent study concluded that one cycle of IVF–ET offers a better probability of conception than do six COH–IUI cycles in women with endometriosis, regardless of the woman's age and stage of disease, suggesting that COH–IUI be limited to a maximum of three or four cycles.

Hysterectomy

Women suffering from endometriosis-induced pelvic pain that is unresponsive to conservative, medical, or surgical therapy often undergo hysterectomy, with or without bilateral oophorectomy. Determinants such as age, gravidity, and parity must be carefully considered when deciding whether to perform salpingo-oophorectomy at the time of hysterectomy. Leaving the ovaries allows endogenous hormone production and also provides the option of oocyte transfer to a surrogate carrier for those women in reproductive age. Reoperation for adnexal diseases is relatively low. Nevertheless, repeated surgery after bilateral salpingo-oophorectomy is rare.[83] When proposing a hysterectomy, age is the most important factor to take into account. MacDonald et al reported that women <30 years old who undergo hysterectomy for chronic pelvic pain and endometriosis are more likely to show residual symptoms, to report a sense of loss, and to report more disruption from pain in different aspects of their lives.[84]

The use of laparoscopic-assisted vaginal hysterectomy (LAVH) or total laparoscopic hysterectomy (TLH) has been reported as an alternative to abdominal or vaginal hysterectomy. The laparoscopic approach allows treatment of residual disease at the time of hysterectomy. Furthermore, it allows management of the adnexa, that would otherwise have been difficult to remove via the vaginal route, due to presence of adhesions or endometriomas. Supracervical hysterectomy, even if it is associated with a lower risk of ureteral and vesical injuries,[85] must be avoided because of the frequent involvement of the cervix and of the uterosacral ligaments in the disease.

Nevertheless, even when hysterectomy is performed, not all the endometrial tissue implanted outside the uterus is necessarily removed and thus, in some patients, symptoms may persist. According to several authors, substantial pain relief can be achieved in almost 90% of patients undergoing hysterectomy for chronic pelvic pain.[86,87]

Surgical treatment of recurrence of endometriosis

The real incidence of endometriosis recurrence is not yet well defined, because of the different criteria of evaluation: some authors consider the reappearance of symptoms as disease recurrence despite ultrasonographic or surgical findings. An increasing frequency of recurrence has been observed in the last decades, probably due to a more conservative therapeutic approach.

Nevertheless, the need for a conservative surgery is mandatory even when facing a recurrence, because of the young age of patients affected by this disease and their desire for pregnancy. Several authors have observed a consistent recovery of infertility (crude pregnancy rate from 20% to 47%) after open conservative surgery for recurrent endometriosis.[88,89]

The data in the literature concerning the recurrence of ovarian endometrioma are not sufficiently indicative, depending on the type of surgical technique, the use of medical therapy, and on the length of follow-up.[90,91]

Laparoscopy is to be considered the first-choice technique in the treatment of ovarian endometriomas because of low morbidity, high tolerance, and overall low costs. However, when compared to laparotomy in terms of recurrence and adhesion rates, data are overlapping.[92–94]

A recent study[95] carried out in our department on 81 women with recurrent endometriosis, surgically treated either via laparoscopy (40 patients) or via laparotomy (41 patients), showed no significant differences in terms of recurrence of dysmenorrhea (34% vs 43%), of frequency of recurrence of pelvic pain, dyspareunia, and of clinical findings between the two groups. The cumulative pregnancy rate at 24 months was also comparable (45% in laparotomy and 54% in the laparoscopy group). The conclusion was that laparoscopy was as efficacious as surgery at laparotomy in conservative surgical treatment for recurrent endometriosis.[95]

According to some authors,[96] laparotomy should be performed whenever cleavage planes cannot be identified clearly at laparoscopy and/or optimal conservative surgery is not feasible. Nevertheless, the augmented anatomic vision obtained at laparoscopy allows a detailed visualization of the pelvis, and gentle handling and precise dissection of the tissues (Figure 11.8).

(a)

(b)

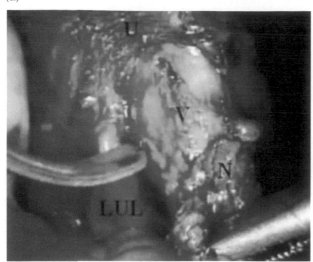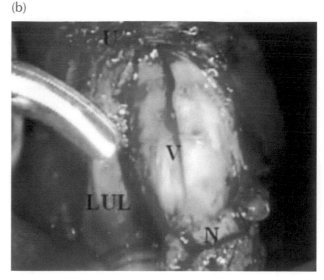

Figure 11.8 (a and b) Removal of deep endometriosis from posterior cul-de-sac. V = vagina; N = nodule; LUL = left uterosacral ligament; and U = uterus.

It is currently believed that infertile patients with recurrent endometriosis should be included in assisted reproduction programs. However, the poor results of these techniques and their cost make operative laparoscopy the treatment of choice in such women. Likewise, operative laparoscopy seems to offer notable advantages with respect to repeated courses of medical therapy, which are necessary for patients with pelvic pain associated with recurrent endometriosis.

REFERENCES

Deep endometriosis

1. Koninckx PR, Martin D. Treatment of deeply infiltrating endometriosis. Curr Opin Obstet Gynecol 1994; 6: 231–241

2. Cornillie FJ, Oosterlynck D, Lauweryns JM, et al. Deeply infiltrating pelvic endometriosis: histology and clinical significance. Fertil Steril 1990; 53: 978–983.

3. Chapron C, Fauconnier A, Vieira M, et al. Anatomic distribution of deeply infiltrating endometrosis: surgical implications and proposition for a classification. Hum Reprod 2003; 18: 157–162.

4. Martin DC, Batt RE. Retrocervical, retrovaginal pouch, and rectovaginal septum endometriosis. J Am Assoc Gynecol Laparosc 2001; 8: 12–17.

5. Koninckx PR, Meuleman C, Demeyere S, et al. Suggestive evidence that pelvic endometriosis is a progressive disease, whereas deeply infiltrating endometriosis is associated with pelvic pain. Fertil Steril 1991; 55: 759–765.

6. Vercellini P. Endometriosis: what a pain it is. Semin Reprod Endocrinol 1997; 15: 251–261.

7. The American Fertility Society. Revised American Fertility Society classification of endometriosis: 1985. Fertil Steril 1985; 43: 351–352.

8. Fedele L, Parazzini F, Bianchi S, et al. Stage and localization of pelvic endometriosis and pain. Fertil Steril 1990; 53: 155–158.

9. Marana R, Muzii L, Caruana P, et al. Evaluation of the correlation between endometriosis extent, age of the patients and associated symptomatology. Acta Eur Fertil 1991; 22: 209–212.

10. Porpora MG, Koninckx PR, Piazze J, et al. Correlation between endometriosis and pelvic pain. J Am Assoc Gynecol Laparosc 1999; 6: 429–434.

11. Buttram VC. Conservative surgery for endometriosis in the infertile female: a study of 206 patients with implications for both medical and surgical therapy. Fertil Steril 1979; 31: 117–123.

12. Fauconnier A, Chapron C, Dubuisson JB, et al. Relation between pain symptoms and the anatomic location of deep infiltrating endometriosis. Fertil Steril 2002; 78: 719–726.

13. Anaf V, Simon P, El Nakadi I, et al. Relationship between endometriotic foci and nerves in rectovaginal endometriotic nodules. Hum Reprod 2000; 15(8): 1744–1750.

14. Redwine DB. Laparoscopic en bloc resection for treatment of the obliterated cul-de-sac in endometriosis. J Reprod Med 1992; 37: 695–698.

15. Vercellini P, Trespidi L, De Giorgi O, et al. Endometriosis and pelvic pain: relation to disease stage and localization. Fertil Steril 1996; 65: 299–304.

16. Chapron C, Fauconnier A, Dubuisson JB, et al. Deep infiltrating endometriosis: relation between severity of dysmenorrhoea and extent of disease. Hum Reprod 2003; 18(4): 760–766.

17. Redwine DB. Endometriosis persisting after castration: clinical characteristics and results of surgical management. Obstet Gynecol 1994; 83: 405–413.

18. Takayama K, Zeitoun K, Gunby RT, et al. Treatment of severe postmenopausal endometriosis with an aromatase inhibitor. Fertil Steril 1998; 69: 709–713.

19. Nezhat C, Nezhat F, Pennington E. Laparoscopic treatment of infiltrative rectosigmoid colon and rectovaginal septum endometriosis by the technique of videolaparoscopy and the CO_2 laser. Br J Obstet Gynaecol 1992; 99: 664–667.

20. Reich H, McGlynn F, Salvat J. Laparoscopic treatment of cul-de-sac obliteration secondary to retrocervical deep fibrotic endometriosis. J Reprod Med 1991; 36: 516–522.

21. Redwine DB. Conservative laparoscopic excision of endometriosis by sharp dissection: life table analysis of reoperation and persistent or recurrent disase. Fertil Steril 1991; 56: 628–634.

22. Crosignani PG, Vercellini P, Biffignandi F, et al. Laparoscopy versus laparotomy in conservative surgical treatment for severe endometriosis. Fertil Steril 1996; 66: 706–711.

23. Wheeler JM, Malinak LR. Recurrent endometriosis. Contrib Gynecol Obstet 1987; 16: 13–21.

24. Donnez J, Nisolle M, Gillerot S, et al. Rectovaginal septum adenomyotic nodules: a series of 500 cases. Br J Obstet Gynaecol 1997; 104: 1014–1018.

25. Reich H, McGlynn F, Salvat J. Laparoscopic treatment of cul-de-sac obliteration secondary to retrocervical deep fibrotic endometriosis. J Reprod Med 1991; 36: 516–522.

26. Redwine DB, Wright JT. Laparoscopic treatment of complete obliteration of the cul-de-sac associated with endometriosis: long-term follow-up of en bloc resection. Fertil Steril 2001; 76: 358–365.

27. Fedele L, Bianchi S, Zanconato G, et al. Long-term follow-up after conservative surgery for rectovaginal endometriosis. Am J Obstet Gynecol 2004; 190: 1020–1024.

28. Khan KS, Khan SF, Nwosu CR, et al. Laparoscopic uterosacral nerve ablation in chronic pelvic pain: an overview. Gynaecol Endosc 1999; 8: 257–265.

29. Daniels J, Gray R, Khan KS, et al. Laparoscopic uterine nerve ablation: a survey of gynecologic practice in UK. Gynaecol Endosc 2000; 9: 157–159.

30. Sutton CJG, Ewen SP, Whitelaw N, et al. Prospective, randomized double-blind controlled trial of laser laparoscopy in the treatment of pelvic pain associated with minimal, mild and moderate endometriosis. Fertil Steril 1994; 62(4): 696–700.

31. Sutton CJG, Pooley AS, Jones KD, et al. A prospective, randomized, double-blind controlled trial of laparoscopic uterine nerve ablation in the treatment of pelvic pain associated with endometriosis. Gynaecol Endosc 2001; 10: 217–222.

32. Vercellini P, Aimi G, Busacca M, et al. Laparoscopic uterosacral ligament resection for dysmenorrhea associated with endometriosis: results of a randomized, controlled trial. Fertil Steril 2003; 80: 310–319.

33. Proctor ML, Farquhar CM, Sinclair OJ, et al. Surgical interruption of pelvic nerve pathways for primary and secondary dysmenorrhoea (Cochrane Review). In: The Cochrane Library. Oxford: Update Software; 2002: Issue 4.

34. Candiani GB, Fedele L, Vercellini P, et al. Presacral neurectomy for the treatment of pelvic pain associated with endometriosis: a controlled study. Am J Obstet Gynecol 1992; 167(1): 100–103.

35. Perez JJ. Laparoscopic presacral neurectomy. Results of the first 25 cases. J Reprod Med 1990; 35: 625–630.

36. Kwok A, Lam A, Ford R. Laparoscopic presacral neurectomy: a review. Obstet Gynecol Surv 2001; 56: 99–104.

37. Chen FP, Soong YK. The efficacy and complications of laparoscopic presacral neurectomy in pelvic pain. Obstet Gynecol 1997; 90: 974–977.

38. Zullo F, Palomba S, Zupi E, et al. Effectiveness of presacral neurectomy in women with severe dysmenorrhea due to endometriosis treated with laparoscopic conservative surgery: a 1-year randomized double-blind controlled trial. Am J Obstet Gynecol 2003; 189: 5–10.

39. Zullo F, Palomba S, Zupi E, et al. Long-term effectiveness of presacral neurectomy for the treatment of severe dysmenorrhea due to endometriosis. J Am Assoc Gynecol Laparosc 2004; 11(1): 23–28.

40. Chen FP, Chang SD, Chu KK, et al. Comparison of laparoscopic presacral neurectomy and laparoscopic uterine nerve ablation for primary dysmenorrhea. J Reprod Med 1996; 41(7): 463–466.

41. Soysal ME, Soysal S, Gurses E, et al. Laparoscopic presacral neurolysis for endometriosis-related pelvic pain. Hum Reprod 2003; 18(3): 588–592.

Surgical treatment of endometriosis-associated infertility

42. Gruppo Italiano per lo Studio dell'Endometriosis. Prevalence and anatomical distribution of endometriosis in women with selected gynecologic conditions: results from a multicenter Italian study. Hum Reprod 1994; 6: 1158–1162.

43. Chapron C, Fritel X, Dubuisson JB. Fertility after laparoscopic management of deep endometriosis infiltrating the uterosacral ligaments. Hum Reprod 1999; 14(2): 329–332.

44. Watson A, Vandekerckhove P, Liford R. Techniques for pelvic surgery in subfertility. Cochrane Database Syst Rev 2001; 2: CD000221.

45. Bérubé S, Marcoux S, Langevin S, et al. Fecundity of

infertile women with minimal or mild endometriosis and women with unexplained infertility. Fertil Steril 1998; 69: 1034–1041.

46. Barnhart K, Dunsmoor-Su R, Coutifaris C. Effect of endometriosis on in vitro fertilization. Fertil Steril 2002; 77: 1148–1155.

47. Pellicer A, Oliveira N, Ruiz A, et al. Exploring the mechanism(s) of endometriosis-related infertility: an analysis of embryo development and implantation in assisted reproduction. Hum Reprod 1995; 10: 91–97.

48. Lucena E, Cubillos J. Immune abnormalities in endometriosis compromising fertility in IVF–ET patients. J Reprod Med 1999; 44: 458–464.

49. Adamson GD, Pasta DJ. Surgical treatment of endometriosis-associated infertility: meta-analysis compared with survival analysis. Am J Obstet Gynecol 1994: 171(6): 1488–1504.

50. Marcoux S, Maheux R, Bèrubè S. Laparoscopic surgery in infertile women with minimal or mild endometriosis. N Engl J Med 1997; 337: 217–222.

51. Parazzini F. Ablation of lesions or no treatment in minimal-mild endometriosis in infertile women: a randomized trial. Hum Reprod 1999; 14: 1332–1334.

52. Olive DL, Pritts EA. Treatment of endometriosis. N Engl J Med 2001; 345(4): 266–275.

53. Jacobson T, Barlow D. Laparoscopic surgery for subfertility associated with endometriosis. Cochrane Database Syst Rev 2001; 4: CD001300.

Ovarian endometrioma

54. Bateman BG, Kolp LA, Mills S. Endoscopic versus laparotomy management of endometriomas. Fertil Steril 1994; 62: 690–695.

55. Catalano GF, Marana R, Caruana P, et al. Laparoscopy versus microsurgery by laparotomy for excision of ovarian cysts in patients with moderate or severe endometriosis. J Am Assoc Gynecol Laparosc 1996; 3: 267–270.

56. Adamson GD, Subak LL, Pasta DJ, et al. Comparison of CO_2 laser laparoscopy with laparotomy for treatment of endometriomata. Fertil Steril 1992; 57: 965–973.

57. Sawada T, Satoshi O, Kawakami S, et al. Laparoscopic surgery versus laparotomy management for infertile patients with ovarian endometriomas. J Gynaecol Endosc 1999; 8: 17–19.

58. Chapron C, Vercellini P, Barakat H, et al. Management of ovarian endometriomas. Hum Reprod Update 2002; 8(6): 591–597.

59. Jones KD, Fan A, Sutton CJ. The ovarian endometrioma: why is it so poorly managed? Indicators from an anonymous survey. Hum Reprod 2002; 17: 845–849.

60. Hemmings R, Bissinnette F, Bouzayen R. Results of laparoscopic treatments of ovarian endometriomas: laparoscopic ovarian fenestration and coagulation. Fertil Steril 1998; 70: 527–529.

61. Saleh A, Tulandi T. Reoperation after laparoscopic treatment of ovarian endometriomas by excision and by fenestration. Fertil Steril 1999; 72: 322–324.

62. Beretta P, Franchi M, Ghezzi F, et al. Randomized clinical trial of two laparoscopic treatments of endometriomas: cystectomy versus drainage and coagulation. Fertil Steril 1998; 70: 1176–1180.

63. Sutton CJG, Ewen SP, Jacobs SA et al. Laser laparoscopic surgery in the treatment of ovarian endometriomas. J Am Assoc Gynecol Laparosc 1997; 4(3): 319–323.

64. Brosens IA, Van Ballaer P, Puttemans P, et al. Reconstruction of the ovary containing large endometriomas by an extraovarian endosurgical technique. Fertil Steril 1996; 66: 517–521.

65. Donnez J, Nisolle M, Gillet N, et al. Large ovarian endometriomas. Hum Reprod 1996; 11: 641–646.

66. Muzii L, Bianchi A, Crocè C, et al. Laparoscopic excision of ovarian cysts: is the stripping technique a tissue-sparing procedure? Fertil Steril 2002; 77: 609–614.

67. Busacca M, Marana R, Caruana P, et al. Recurrence of ovarian endometrioma after laparoscopic excision. Am J Obstet Gynecol 1999; 180: 519–523.

68. Marconi G, Vilela M, Quintana R, et al. Laparoscopic ovarian cystectomy of endometriomas does not affect the ovarian response to gonadotropin stimulation. Fertil Steril 2002; 78(4): 876–878.

69. Vercellini P, Chapron C, De Giorgi O, et al. Coagulation or excision of ovarian endometriomas? Am J Obstet Gynecol 2003; 88: 606–610.

70. Busacca M, Somigliana E, Bianchi S, et al. Post-operative GnRH analogue treatment after conservative surgery for symptomatic endometriosis stage III-IV: a randomized controlled trial. Hum Reprod 2001; 16: 2399–2402.

71. Bianchi S, Busacca M, Agnoli B, et al. Effects of 3 month therapy with danazol after laparoscopic surgery for stage III/IV endometriosis: a randomized study. Hum Reprod 1999; 14(5): 1335–1337.

Ovarian endometriosis and infertility

72. Redwine DB. Ovarian endometriosis: a marker for more extensive pelvic and intestinal disease. Fertil Steril 1999; 72: 310–315.

73. Ayers JWT, Birenbaum DL, Jiaram Menon KM. Luteal phase dysfunction in endometriosis: elevated progesterone levels in peripheral and ovarian veins during the follicular phase. Fertil Steril 1987; 47: 925–929.

74. Hahn DW, Carraher RP, Foldesy RG, et al. Experimental evidence for failure to implant as a mechanism of infertility associated with endometriosis. Am J Obstet Gynecol 1986; 155: 1109–1113.

75. Pellicer A, Oliveira N, Ruiz A, et al. Exploring the mechanism(s) of endometriosis-related infertility: an analysis of embryo development and implantation in assisted reproduction. Hum Reprod 1995; 10: 91–97.

76. Yovitch JL, Matson PL, Richardson PA, et al. Hormonal

profiles and embryo quality in women with severe endometriosis treated by in vitro fertilization and embryo transfer. Fertil Steril 1988; 50: 308–313.

77. Lucena E, Cubillos J. Immune abnormalities in endometriosis compromising fertility in IVF-ET patients. J Reprod Med 1999; 44: 458–464.

78. Jones KD, Sutton CJG. Pregnancy rates following ablative laparoscopic surgery for endometrioma. Hum Reprod 2002; 17: 782–785.

79. Beretta P, Franchi M, Ghezzi F, et al. Randomized clinical trial of two laparoscopic treatments of endometriomas: cystectomy versus drainage and coagulation. Fertil Steril 1998; 70: 1176–1180.

80. Donnez J, Wyns C, Nisolle M. Does ovarian surgery for endometriomas impair the ovarian response to gonadotropin? Fertil Steril 2001; 76: 662–665.

81. Canis M, Pouly JL, Tamburro S, et al. Ovarian response during IVF-embryo transfer cycles after laparoscopic ovarian cystectomy for endometriotic cysts of 43 cm in diameter. Hum Reprod 2001; 16: 2583–2586.

82. Dmowski WP, Pry M, Ding J, et al. Cycle-specific and cumulative fecundity in patients with endometriosis who are undergoing controlled ovarian hyperstimulation–intrauterine insemination or in vitro fertilization–embryo transfer. Fertil Steril 2002; 78(4): 750–756.

Hysterectomy

83. Henderson AF. In: Thomas E, Rock J, eds. Modern approach in endometriosis. Carnfoth: Kluwer Academic; 1991: 275–290.

84. MacDonald SR, Klock SC, Milad MP. Long-term outcome of nonconservative surgery (hysterectomy) for endometriosis-associated pain in women <30 years old. Am J Obstet Gynecol 1999; 180: 1360–1363.

85. Wood C, Maher P, eds. Hysterectomy. In: Laparoscopic hysterectomy. Baillière's Clin Obstet Gynaecol 2001; 11: 111–136.

86. Beard RW, Kennedy RG, Gangar KF, et al. Bilateral oophorectomy and hysterectomy in the treatment of intractable pelvic pain associated with pelvic congestion. Br J Obstet Gynaecol 1991; 98: 988–992.

87. Hillis SD, Marchblanks PA, Peterson HB. The effectiveness of hysterectomy for chronic pelvic pain. Obstet Gynecol 1995; 86: 941–945.

Surgical treatment of recurrence of endometriosis

88. Wheeler JM, Malinak LR. Recurrent endometriosis: incidence, management and prognosis. Am J Obstet Gynecol 1983; 146: 247–253.

89. Wheeler JM, Malinak LR. Recurrent endometriosis. Contrib Gynecol Obstet 1987; 16: 13–21.

90. Donnez J, Nisolle M, Gillet N, et al Large ovarian endometriomas. Hum Reprod 1996; 11: 641–646.

91. Sutton CJG, Ewen SP, Jacobs SA, et al Laser laparoscopic surgery in the treatment of ovarian endometriomas. J Am Assoc Gynecol Laparosc 1997; 4: 319–323.

92. Bateman BG, Kolp LA, Mills S. Endoscopic versus laparotomy management of endometriomas. Fertil Steril 1994; 62: 690–695.

93. Canis M, Mage G, Wattiez A, et al Second look laparoscopy after laparoscopic cystectomy of large ovarian endometriomas. Fertil Steril 1992; 58: 611–619.

94. Redwine DB. Conservative laparoscopic excision of endometriosis by sharp dissection: life table analysis of reoperation and persistent or recurrent disease. Fertil Steril 1991; 56: 628–634.

95. Busacca M, Fedele L, Bianchi S, et al. Surgical treatment of recurrent endometriosis: laparotomy versus laparoscopy. Hum Reprod 1998; 13(8): 2271–2274.

96. Cook AS, Rock JA. The role of laparoscopy in the treatment of endometriosis. Fertil Steril 1991; 55: 663–680.

12 Laparoscopic treatment of superficial peritoneal endometriosis

Christopher Sutton

When I first learned the technique of diagnostic laparoscopy as a resident (USA)/registrar (UK) during my surgical training, the diagnosis of endometriosis was most commonly made after observing the classical black powder-burn lesion associated with a deposit of hemosiderin on the peritoneal surface. Subsequently, although we have not made any great advances in understanding the pathogenesis of this obscure disease, we have progressed considerably in the diagnosis and surgical treatment of this condition. We now accept that there are three different types of endometriosis,[1] which may coexist or may present separately: namely, deep infiltrating endometriosis (DIE) or, more correctly, adenomyosis; ovarian endometriomas; and superficial peritoneal implants. Although the ovarian endometrioma can be detected by an ultrasound examination, deep infiltrating disease is often better felt as tender nodules by clinical examination, preferably performed during the perimenstruum, and often this disease is not strikingly obvious on laparoscopic examination, certainly to those who are unfamiliar with the diagnosis and treatment of DIE. This chapter will deal almost exclusively with peritoneal disease, but it must be realized that, if adequate pain relief and optimal conditions for conception are to be realized, coexisting endometriosis and endometriomas must also be eradicated at the same time.

Etiology and pathogenesis

Numerous theories abound to explain the etiology and pathogenesis of endometriosis since the actual term 'endometriosis' was first coined by Sampson in 1921.[2] In fact he was describing ovarian endometriomas, although that condition had been recognized for many years before this. In 1927 Sampson[3] was the first to suggest that menstrual blood containing fragments of endometrium might pass along the fallopian tubes in a retrograde fashion and implant on the peritoneal surface of organs or tissues in the pelvis and abdomen and during subsequent menstrual cycles would undergo sequential proliferation and bleeding in much the same fashion as the endometrium responds to the ovarian hormones. It has been known for a long time that viable endometrial cells can be obtained from this bloodstained peritoneal fluid that accumulates in the posterior cul-de-sac[4] and also that endometriosis may develop following intraperitoneal injection of menstrual blood in the human being.[5] Nevertheless, it appears that there must be other factors operating because menstrual blood and viable endometrial cells can be found in the cul-de-sac of almost all menstruating women[6] but only a fraction of these women appear to develop the disease. Clearly there are other factors operating, and these are fully discussed in Chapter 3, but retrograde menstruation must play some part in the development of peritoneal endometriosis because women with congenital absence of the uterus do not develop pelvic endometriosis.[7]

Observational studies[8] have shown that endometriosis is more commonly found in sites where endometrial cells from retrograde menstruation may settle undisturbed, such as the ovaries, posterior cul-de-sac, and the back of the broad ligament, whereas it is relatively uncommon on mobile structures such as the small intestine or the fallopian tube. The anatomic distribution of the implants is consistent with retrograde menstruation, and lesions are most common in dependent areas of the pelvis. In a study of 182 patients with endometriosis, Jenkins et al[9] found that 31% of patients had implants on the right ovary, with 14% having adhesions present. The percentages for the left ovary were slightly higher, with 44% having implants and 25% having adhesions. Ample evidence suggests that patients with retrograde menstruation, such as caused by anomalies of Müllerian duct development with outflow obstruction,[10–12] and patients with relative hypotonia of the uterotubal junction are at increased risk of the disease.[13]

For some time it has been appreciated that endometrial tissue is refluxed into the peritoneal cavity to a greater extent and more frequently in women with endometriosis than in women with patent fallopian tubes without endometriosis.[13] There must be other factors, such as an impaired immune response or abnormal response to tissue injury, which result in an inability to remove refluxed menstrual debris, resulting in endometrial tissue implanting and growing. This complicated series of interactions has been comprehensively reviewed recently by Giudice and Kao[14] and is covered in detail elsewhere in this book

Clinical presentation and symptomatology

One of the major complaints of patients with endometriosis is directed at the failure of their general practitioners or primary care physicians to arrive at an early diagnosis. In a survey conducted by Hadfield et al in 1996, the observed mean delay between the onset of symptoms and the arrival at a diagnosis of endometriosis was 12 years in the USA and 8 years in the UK.[15] Other studies from Scandinavia[16] and Brazil[17] have reported delays of diagnosis of 6.7 and 7.0 years, respectively, and the delay was inversely related to the age of the patient at the onset of symptoms, with the mean delay for women under 20 years old being 12.1 years (range 8–17.2 years).

This long delay is often due to the diversity of symptoms and the fact that the main symptom, dysmenorrhea, is a frequent reason for consultation among teenagers. Because it responds reasonably satisfactorily to the oral contraceptive or nonsteroidal anti-inflammatory agents, the background pathology in those patients where it is due to endometriosis is often missed. In addition, there is unfortunately no simple non-invasive test to pick up superficial endometriosis, and transvaginal ultrasound is only of use if there is obvious pathology in the form of an ovarian endometrioma or significant nodules in the uterosacral ligament complex or rectovaginal septum.

The diversity of the symptomatology can be seen in Table 12.1, which represents the results of a lifetime study of endometriosis by Dr Daniel O'Connor, who was impressed by the high incidence of endometriosis in Guildford (Surrey, UK) when he was a senior resident/registrar there in the late 1970s. This awakened an interest in endometriosis, which he has pursued throughout his clinical lifetime and he has recorded in detail the symptoms of all the endometriosis patients that he has treated. It can be seen from Table 12.1 that although the majority of patients have all the leading symptoms of dysmenorrhea, dyspareunia, and noncyclical pelvic pain, with dysmenorrhea

Table 12.1 Endometriosis symptoms* in order of occurrence

Dysmenorrhea	227	Altered menstrual cycle	72
Dyspareunia	188	Pelvic mass	8
Nil	155	Bowel symptoms	3
Infertility	131	Bladder symptoms	2
Pelvic pain	114	Galactorrhea	2
Menorrhagia	105		

Source: Daniel O'Connor (1987).
*155 of 717 patients (22%) had no symptoms at all; 39 of 717 patients (5%) had all cardinal symptoms

by far the most common symptom, nevertheless just over one-fifth of the patients (22.6%) had no symptoms at all and the disease was discovered accidentally during a laparoscopy for another reason. Against this background, it is therefore not surprising that it is difficult for primary care physicians to establish an early diagnosis. Nevertheless, it behoves them to have a high index of suspicion in a young girl who presents with extremely severe dysmenorrhea, especially if the condition does not respond to simple oral analgesics. It is well known that many of the first cycles following the menarche are anovulatory and therefore painless, but there are a group of young girls who have extremely severe dysmenorrhea starting from the very first period and these girls should be referred to a hospital consultant without undue delay. There has been an increase in medicolegal cases recently directed at general practitioners for failing to diagnose the condition until the disease had reached a very advanced stage, resulting in infertility, and the fact that a girl is of a very young age does not mean that dysmenorrhea is not due to endometriosis. It can start

with the very first period and we have had patients as young as 11 years old who after only a few menstrual cycles have already developed very florid peritoneal endometriosis.

Dysmenorrhoea

Dysmenorrhea is without doubt the cardinal symptom of endometriosis, as can be seen from the cover of a very helpful information booklet produced by the American Endometriosis Society (Figure 12.1). The picture clearly shows a woman in great pain and many patients find that even strong analgesics merely take the edge off the pain but they still have to resort to other methods of alleviating the discomfort, such as bending over a pillow clutched to the lower abdomen, or even using hot water bottles on the abdomen; sometimes the heat employed to inflict another source of pain is sufficient to cause burns on the abdomen, as shown in the patient in Figure 12.2. The usual scenario in the consulting room is an

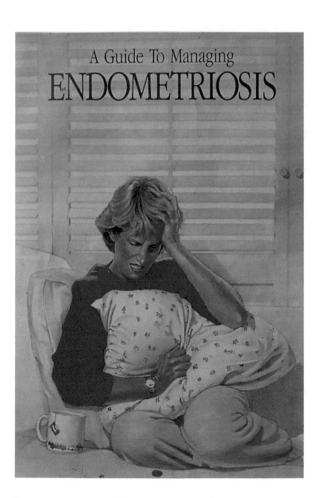

Figure 12.1 Cover of an American Endometriosis Society brochure illustrating the severe pain of dysmenorrhea due to endometriosis.

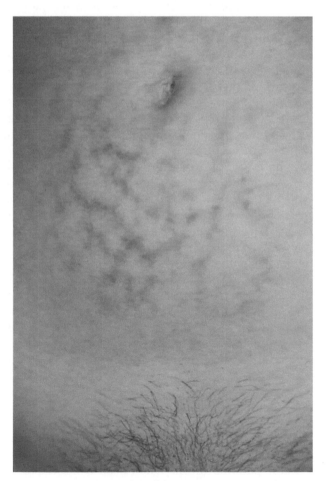

Figure 12.2 Abdominal wall burns in a patient with severe dysmenorrhea. The pain was sufficiently intense to employ a scalding hot water bottle to distract the patient from her period pain, which resulted in these burns.

adolescent or young woman who has had severe dysmenorrhea, often from the very first period. After increasing use of over-the-counter analgesics, she finally consults her GP, only to be told that it is a 'woman's lot' to suffer such pain. She is then usually put on increasingly strong non-steroidal analgesics and, eventually, the oral contraceptive. Initially, the pain seems to be of the spasmodic variety, mainly occurring during menstruation, with severe uterine cramps. As time goes on, a congestive element appears and the pain starts earlier before the menstrual flow, and sometimes patients are in pain from the time of ovulation until the onset of the menses.

A useful way of quantifying the level of discomfort is to present the woman with a linear analogue scale from 0 to 10, with 0 being no pain at all and 10 being the worst pain experienced in her life. This method of evaluating pain severity has been well validated.[18] It has been widely used for evaluating the efficacy of laparoscopic surgery in the alleviation of pain due to endometriosis.[19] It has certain failings because some patients who have had, for example, a fractured femur from a skiing injury will clearly count that as the worst pain in their life, and if that is the case then there should be a note made to that effect to make allowance for this. Additionally, it does give an opportunity to judge the patient's general life attitude; it is sometimes said that if a patient marks the cross of the 'worst pain ever' beyond the end of the scale, there are often psychosomatic or hypochondriacal features present, and equally it allows one to witness the interaction between the woman and her partner. Some of the partners of women with long-term endometriosis can seem overly attentive and this can also lead to attention-seeking on the part of the woman. It is not unusual for the partner to actually answer intimate questions about the patient's symptoms without reference to the woman sitting beside him and I even had one woman hand the pen over to her partner to fill in the linear analogue scale for dysmenorrhea on the grounds that 'he knows what I'm like'. And he actually did it and marked her at 9.8! Nevertheless, the linear analogue scale probably provides the best evaluation of pain we have and certainly in our initial retrospective study on uterine nerve ablation using the laser at laparoscopy we found that before treatment the average score on the visual analogue scale was 9.2, and out of 100 women, 81 (86%) with endometriosis were improved, with an average score among the successful patients of 3.4 when seen 6 months after the operation.[20]

Dyspareunia

Deep dyspareunia becomes an increasing problem in patients with both superficial and deep disease of the cul-de-sac or infiltration of the uterosacral ligaments. It can first present as difficulty in inserting tampons and later becomes more of a problem, especially in association with positions allowing deep penetration. Women often complain of 'something being hit', which can be sufficiently severe to have to stop intercourse, or increasingly to avoid intercourse altogether, which can cause marital disharmony and increasing psychosexual problems that can be extremely complex. With obliteration of the cul-de-sac, deep penetration during intercourse may radiate pain into the rectum.[21]

Dyschezia and rectal bleeding

It is absolutely imperative due to the increased incidence of DIE of the rectovaginal septum and the uterosacral ligaments that questions are asked about bowel movements and whether there is pain when opening the bowels (dyschezia) at the time of menstruation. With increasing involvement of the rectal wall, patients may complain of rectal pain with each bowel movement throughout the month or even complain of rectal pain when passing flatus or even sitting down for long periods of time. Inquiry should also be made about rectal bleeding, especially if it is cyclical and occurs with each menstruation. Patients can easily differentiate between rectal and vaginal bleeding, but it is important to rule out local causes of bleeding, such as hemorrhoids or anal fissures. Rectal bleeding with each menstruation is highly suggestive of endometriotic involvement, going through all layers of the rectal wall. Interestingly, proctoscopy or sigmoidoscopy does not necessarily demonstrate any lesions unless it is carefully timed to coincide with menstruation, and coloproctologists rarely seem to do this or even realize the importance of it. More reliability on localizing these lesions and seeing the extent of penetration is, in our experience, better obtained from an air-contrast barium enema looked at in a lateral view by a radiologist experienced in dealing with DIE (adenomyosis) of the bowel and rectovaginal septum.

Chronic nonmenstrual pain

Many patients complain of pain unrelated either to ovulation or menstruation and one should always be alerted to the possibility that the pain is due to other conditions, such as adenomyosis, or the pain of irritable bowel syndrome and, interestingly, many patients with endometriosis do seem to suffer from this condition in addition to their endometriosis and many report that the pain is remarkably similar. For further information, the reader is referred to Chapter 25. Inquiries should be made about abdominal distention, alternating diarrhea and constipation, increased flatus, borborygmi, and the presence of mucus in the stools. We have found that many of our treatment failures who have been found to have no residual endometriosis at second-look laparoscopy are often found to have irritable bowel syndrome, a disease that can take many forms, and only really get relief when dealt with by an expert in this very common condition. This particular syndrome seems to account for so many referrals to a surgical clinic that most general bowel surgeons have little interest in it. Patients should really be referred to a medical gastroenterologist with a particular interest in this difficult condition.

Ovarian endometriomas

Endometriomas tend to give rise to an unpleasant deep pain, usually located to either the right or left iliac fossa, or both if the chocolate cysts are bilateral. Pain tends to be worse at the time of ovulation, particularly if there are periovarian adhesions; however, pain can be present throughout the month and also may be exacerbated at the time of menstruation. If the ovarian endometrioma is adherent to the pelvic side wall, which occurs in about 90% of cases, patients typically complain of pain radiating round the flank and into the lower back and characteristically to an area over the upper part of the gluteus maximus. This pain results from irritation to nerves running round the pelvic side wall. This referred pain can also go down the front and outside of the thighs, but rarely from this condition does it extend beneath the knee. Occasionally, endometriomas can cause pressure on the ureter. This can also occur with DIE, which often encircles the ureter but rarely actually invades it. Both of these conditions can cause dilatation of the ureter, with backpressure and pain in the flank and also in the loin over the kidney.

Physical examination

Pelvic examination is important in order to try and exclude disease in the rectovaginal septum or vaginal fornices: if this is suspected, examination is best performed at the time of menstruation.[22] Some women find this embarrassing and, although every effort should be made to try to persuade them that this is the best time to examine them – and in certain countries such as Belgium they would only be examined at the time of menstruation – nevertheless, one has to desist if the patient finds it unacceptable. Interestingly, many patients who claim to be having menstruation are not in fact bleeding at all and are merely using this as an excuse to avoid vaginal examination, because they are anticipating the fact that it will almost certainly be painful. It is therefore very important to reassure the patient and to be as tactful and gentle as possible, and clearly if pain is being elicited then the gynecologist should not continue with the examination because he has probably already got sufficient information to arrive at the correct diagnosis. Some patients with superficial peritoneal disease will have quite acute pain, which can clearly be seen in the patient's facial muscles and even by the patient withdrawing up the examining couch when the cervix is rocked anteriorly by an examining finger in the posterior fornix. Careful examination of the fornices and the rectovaginal septum is imperative to make absolutely certain that there are no palpable nodules. If nodules are present, it is important to assess their localization and to note their size. If nodules are present, a rectal examination should be performed to see whether the mucosa will slide over the nodules, since it is important to predict the depth of rectal resection that will be necessary to remove them entirely. Very rarely a nodule may be felt anterior to the uterus, which indicates deep infiltrating disease in the bladder; these patients will almost certainly have urinary symptoms, especially pain, when the bladder is distended. Speculum examination will occasionally show obvious endometriosis in the posterior vaginal fornix with thickening of the adjacent epithelium and often obvious hemorrhage. Characteristic blue domed cysts can also rarely be seen and they contain a variable amount of old blood and hemosiderin.

The diagnosis of adenomyosis can always give rise to diagnostic difficulty and I have seen many patients who have a normal appearance on laparoscopy and no sign of any deep infiltrating endometriosis but nevertheless continue to have pain sometimes throughout the cycle but particularly during menstruation and often associated with menorrhagia and the passage of large clots and often an increased amount of brown or black old blood. These patients almost certainly have adenomyosis of the uterus and the uterus can be extremely tender when it is compressed bimanually.

Diagnosis and staging

The diagnosis of endometriosis can only be made with certainty by laparoscopic examination of the pelvis and abdomen supplemented by a careful vaginal examination, preferably around the time of menstruation[22] or under a general anesthetic to detect any nodularity caused by DIE of the rectovaginal septum and uterosacral ligament complex. The diagnosis of endometriosis carries significant implications for any woman and it is therefore vital that the assessment laparoscopy should be performed by a gynecologist who is aware of the various different appearances of the disease rather than someone who is merely looking for hemosiderin deposits on the peritoneal surface, which often represent burnt-out or inactive disease. There appears to be a relationship between the color and the age of the endometrial implants and, indeed, even with the age of the patient; the nonhemorrhagic lesions are more usually found in young women and the black deposits laden with hemosiderin are more common in the older patients.[23]

These nonpigmented lesions include white opacified peritoneum that resembles vesicles or sago-grains (Figure 12.3), red flame-like telangiectatic lesions (Figure 12.4), and glandular lesions with an appearance similar to that of endometrium (Figure 12.5) seen at hysteroscopy. Jansen and Russell[24] showed that many of these macroscopic appearances are associated with active endometriosis by demonstrating endometrial glands and stroma on histologic examination of peritoneal biopsies in 67–81% of cases. They also described other appearances, such as subovarian adhesions (Figure 12.6), yellow-brown peritoneum (Figure 12.7), and peritoneal defects, (Figure 12.8), which had endometriosis present in

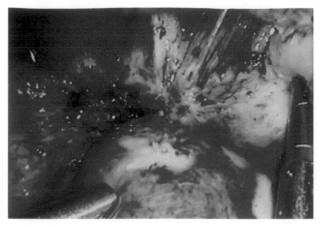

Figure 12.4 Red flame-like lesions overlying a large nodule in the rectovaginal septum invading into the wall of the rectum.

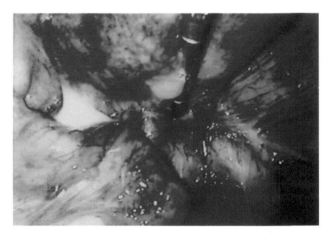

Figure 12.5 Flame-like red active lesions and glandular tissue resembling endometrium at hysteroscopy.

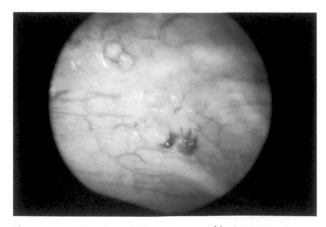

Figure 12.3 The three different types of lesions seen in endometriosis. Sago grains at the top with some vesicles and a red and black lesion. The black is hemosiderin, resulting from a past bleeding episode.

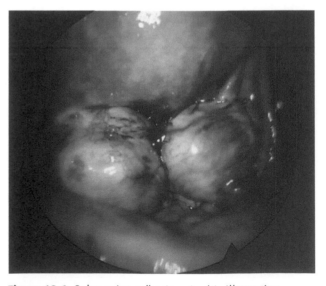

Figure 12.6 Subovarian adhesions in this illustration, resulting in kissing ovaries with bilateral ovarian endometriomas densely adherent to the pelvic sidewall, the cul-de-sac, the rectum, and also to each other.

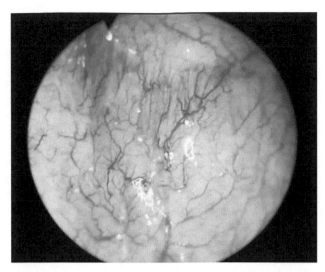

Figure 12.7 Yellow-brown peritoneum with abnormal vessels illustrating neoangiogenesis.

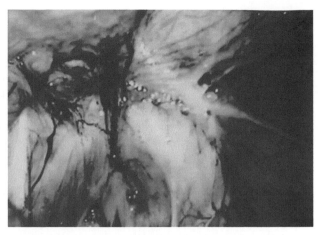

Figure 12.9 Abnormal blood vessels illustrating active neoangiogenesis. Note the differences in caliber of the vessels, which are straight and not arborizing, as in normal peritoneum.

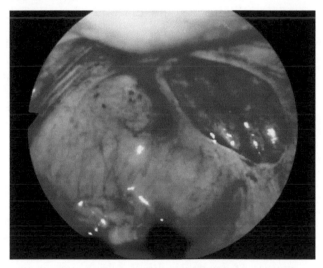

Figure 12.8 Peritoneal pouches (Allen–Masters syndrome). There is active endometriosis in the base of the pouches and the ongoing adhesion formation eventually leads to complete obliteration of the cul-de-sac.

half of the biopsies. More recently, interest has been shown in the abnormal vasculature around the active peritoneal deposits which sometimes almost has the appearance of microinvasive carcinoma of the cervix, as seen at colposcopy (Figure 12.9). Instead of the normal arborizing pattern resembling the branches of a tree, this neoangiogenesis is composed of straight vessels of varying diameter and hairpin capillaries.

In a recent study, Demco has shown that if the diagnostic laparoscopy is enhanced with the aid of green light supplied by a special light source and transmitted via a specially designed laparoscope, the neoangiogenesis is more obvious and spreads much further peripherally than the naked eye

appearances would suggest.[25] This finding probably explains earlier paradoxes when clinicians had demonstrated endometrial glands and stroma in visually normal peritoneum.[26,27] These findings are particularly important when planning a therapeutic approach to the eradication of peritoneal endometriosis.

Systematic and thorough inspection of the peritoneal surfaces of the pelvis and abdomen should be made, employing a double-puncture technique with an aspiration and irrigation cannula inserted suprapubically in the midline. This is used to remove the serosanguinous fluid that is usually present in patients with endometriosis and fills the posterior and sometimes the anterior cul-de-sac to a varying degree. This fluid is laden with breakdown products of blood, together with prostanoids, macrophages, and numerous other substances that are characteristically present in women with active endometriosis.[28,29] Unless this fluid is removed, it is impossible to inspect the cul-de-sac adequately, and for this reason a double-puncture approach is mandatory. A probe or grasping forceps are used to elevate the ovary to check for subovarian adhesions and the presence of endometriosis in the ovarian fossa or on the posterior surface of the ovary.

If an ovarian endometrioma is suspected and the ovary is mobile, needle aspiration can be performed to check for the presence of hemosiderin-laden fluid characteristic of these chocolate cysts. In my experience the vast majority (about 90%) of ovarian endometriomas are not mobile but are firmly adherent to the peritoneum of the ovarian fossa just above the ureter and require careful dissection of the pelvic side wall to avoid damage to the ureter; during this dissection, they inevitably rupture and release the hemosiderin-laden fluid. If the CO_2 laser is to be used to eradicate superficial peritoneal endometriosis, it is suggested that this dissection of an endometrioma is delayed until the peritoneal deposits are dealt with, since this thick fluid absorbs the CO_2 laser energy and can interfere with adequate vaporization of the peritoneal deposits. The superficial peritoneal endometriosis should be treated first; then the endometrioma can either be stripped or coagulated with the KTP laser, electrocoagulation, or the Helica thermal coagulator once biopsies of the pseudocapsule have been taken, because it is now being suggested that these endometriomas have a small but definite chance of progressing to malignancy, particularly as clear cell or endometrioid neoplasms.[30] Having said that, I tend not to alarm patients because in over 800 endometriomas that we have treated in the past 25 years we have not yet had one undergo malignant transformation to the best of our knowledge.

The inspection of the pelvis and abdomen should always be performed in a systematic manner, starting with the upper abdomen to check that there are no endometriotic deposits in the dome of the diaphragm and no violin string adhesions characteristic of the Fitz-Hugh–Curtis syndrome, which is associated with previous gonococcal or chlamydial infection. It is useful at this stage to completely rotate the laparoscope in order to check that no bowel injury has occurred during insertion of the primary trocar. The appendix should be visualized and a careful check on any possible endometriotic implants on the large or small bowel; then the entire pelvis is inspected, usually in a counterclockwise manner, starting with the uterovesical fold, then looking at the right ovary, and under the right ovary and then the posterior cul-de-sac, before working round to the left side, back to the uterovesical fold. The left side is usually more difficult to inspect because the left sigmoid colon is congenitally adherent to the pelvic side wall. It can usually be displaced by a blunt probe in order to see the left ovary clearly. The surgeon should resist any temptation to divide these adhesions, since they are not pathologic and are dangerously close to the large external iliac vessels. All the lesions and vascular appearances should be carefully drawn and it is probably better to do a freestyle drawing than using a rubber-stamp diagram of the pelvis, because the anatomy, particularly the tubo-ovarian relationship can differ widely from one patient to the other, especially if there are a large number of adhesions.

During the initial inspection we always take individual digital photos that can be shown to the patients and stored in the notes. We usually videotape our procedures, but unless particularly requested we do not give these videotapes to the patients. This is because there have been some cases of litigation when adhesions have formed following a laparoscopic procedure that were not present on a previous video recording and can be clearly shown on a subsequent video, providing a cast-iron case of causation for any litigation lawyer. Our tapes are usually recorded on a Super VHS format, which is not usually playable on domestic VHS recorders, and later downloaded onto digital tapes and/or DVDs.[31] In recent months we have started to record directly to digital camcorders and then download selected clips onto our laptops for teaching and conference presentations. We feel more information can be shown to the patient by a full explanation, after full recovery from the anesthetic, with the aid of digital photographic still images and diagrams drawn at the end of the operation.

After the initial inspection, an attempt should be made to grade the severity of the disease using the revised American Fertility Society (r-AFS) scale.[32] Both the patient and the clinician must be aware that the attainment of a high numerical grade on a scoring system does not necessarily correlate with the degree of pain experienced by the woman. Several years ago, studies showed that the pain in endometriosis is linked to some extent to prostaglandin metabolism, particularly prostaglandin F,[33] as well as to numerous other pain-mediating substances secreted by active implants. Even small lesions are capable of producing large amounts of prostaglandin F, which may account for the finding that patients with mild or moderate disease on the AFS scale can often have much more pain than those with extensive disease, whereas massive adhesion formation dominates the appearance of stage IV disease but the active deposits of endometriosis have long ago 'burnt out' and become inactive.

Technical aspects

In our department we tend to use reusable trocars and laparoscopic surgical instruments, where possible, in order to contain costs. We do, however, make an exception with the Veres needle and use disposable Veres needles because they are invariably extremely sharp and thus allow the crucial first entry to be achieved safely in the majority of cases. We tend to adhere to the recommendations of the Middlesborough Consensus Meeting on Safe Entry held in 1998 and reported in an editorial by Professor Ray Garry in *Gynecologic Endoscopy*,[34] and we employ a vertical incision deep inside the umbilicus where all the layers of the abdominal wall come together due to the insertion of the umbilical cord in this area. Even in obese patients, the layers of the abdominal wall are thin at this point and if the needle is introduced vertically two audible clicks can be heard and felt, which usually signifies entry into the peritoneal cavity. This is confirmed by Palmer's test (the 'syringe test'), whereby 5–10 ml of normal saline are injected and if the fluid does not return it can usually be assumed that the tip of the needle is in the correct position.[35]

We are aware that there are deficiencies with these various entry tests but are also uncomfortably aware that, in the case of litigation, proceeding to a court appearance, lawyers will now ask whether such a safeguard was used, and if the surgeon admits to failure to perform this, the judge will tend to infer that he or she has not observed the principles of safe surgical practice. If the patient has had a midline incision and sometimes, even a Pfannenstiel transverse incision, or if there is any worries about the correct positioning of the needle after two attempts at insufflation, we tend increasingly to use Palmer's point, just beneath the left lower rib in the mid-axillary line, for insertion of the Veres needle. Once adequate insufflation has been achieved, the area beneath the umbilicus can be visualized with a 5 mm endoscope, the region beneath the umbilicus can be inspected to make sure that there are no adhesions involving the bowel, and direct entry of the main trocar can be performed under visual control, which is much safer.

Many centers in France preferentially use Palmer's point for first entry, because the area under the left hypochondrium is less likely to be involved in adhesive disease than anywhere else in the peritoneal cavity. Alain Audebert from Bordeaux conducted a highly original study[36] to look at the incidence of adhesions under the umbilicus through a small laparoscope inserted at Palmer's point. The results were interesting and also a cause for serious concern, since, following a midline incision, 51.7% of patients had adhesions underneath the umbilicus and as many as 19.8% following a low transverse incision. In women with a previous laparoscopy, the incidence was 1.6%, and even in those with no history of any surgery at all, 0.68% had adhesions to the under surface of the anterior abdominal wall at the traditional site for first entry with a Veres needle or trocar.

We try to insufflate the abdomen to 25 mmHg, regardless of the volume needed to achieve this.

This provides a sufficiently large volume of gas to increase the distance between the great vessels and the anterior abdominal wall, and should allow entry with the main trocar to be safely achieved without any risk of damaging these large blood vessels, which represents the single biggest hazard during laparoscopy. Once the primary trocar has been satisfactorily inserted, we then tilt the patient into a steep Trendelenburg position and reduce the pressure of the insufflating gas to between 12 and 15 mmHg for the rest of the procedure. At this stage, the full inspection of the abdomen and pelvis is performed, as described above. Depending on the complexity of the procedure, further incisions are planned in the right and left iliac fossa for the insertion of various operating instruments or laser cannulae. All of these ancillary ports are introduced under direct visualization and great care is taken to avoid the inferior epigastric vessels which, apart from in extremely obese patients, can almost invariably be visualized and damage to them be avoided.

Advantages of the CO_2 laser for removal of superficial peritoneal endometriosis

The CO_2 laser is an invisible light laser with a long wavelength of 10.6 μm that produces only excitational and rotational energy in tissue, which results in rapid boiling of cell contents by the process known as vaporization. The laser beam is concentrated at a fine focal point and the high-energy impact produces steam that explodes the intracellular water, resulting in cell debris rising out of the wound that then ignites in the laser beam and is carried off as smoke (the laser plume). This has to be evacuated rapidly with an efficient smoke evacuation system, otherwise the operator's view is obscured. Water in the tissue adjacent to the impact zone absorbs any remaining laser energy and therefore acts as an insulator and limits the zone of irreversible cellular damage to 300–500 μm and the extent of thermal necrosis to only 100 μm,[37] which can be reduced to as little as 50 μm using an ultrapulse laser.

The unique characteristics of this wavelength make this laser ideal for precise incision of human tissue because the thermal effect inherent in the laser–tissue interaction results in sealing of small vessels, lessening the problems associated with capillary oozing. Vessels larger than small arterioles may not be sealed, even with a defocused beam, and the resulting release of blood absorbs the CO_2 laser energy, rendering it ineffective, so it is always essential to have bipolar diathermy instantly available and, because of the unreliability of this energy source when reusable equipment is used, it should always be tried and tested before the laser surgery is commenced.

The main advantage of the CO_2 laser is that it is possible to precisely vaporize abnormal tissue layer by layer, and this is facilitated by the invention of the rotating mirror delivery system (Swiftlase) developed by Sharplan Laser Industries in Tel Aviv, Israel. This allows a higher-power density to be employed and the high-speed rotating mirrors allow the laser beam to transit the implant far more rapidly than would be possible with the human hand. Thus, tissue is vaporized layer by layer, until one can clearly see that one is down to normal retroperitoneal fat and all the endometrial implants and any accompanying fibromuscular hyperplasia have been removed. For the successful treatment of endometriosis, it is essential that the laser is not merely fired at an area, but that vaporization continues to a depth when all the diseased tissue has been vaporized. The precision of the laser using this technique means that implants can be removed, even if they are situated on the ureter (Figure 12.10) or even the bowel (Figures 12.11 and 12.12); however, before attempting this, the operator must have considerable experience of laser tissue interaction. It is also important to employ irrigation intermittently to cool the tissue and to remove any carbon particles and other tissue debris. If this is performed correctly, virtually all tissue debris is evacuated either as smoke in the laser plume or by irrigation of the carbon deposits, so that the

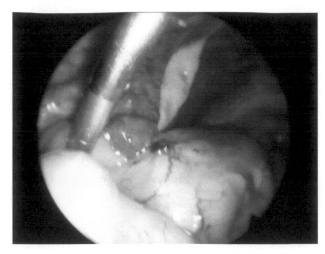

Figure 12.11 Endometriosis on the sigmoid colon. A lesion like this would be difficult and dangerous to remove with electrosurgery.

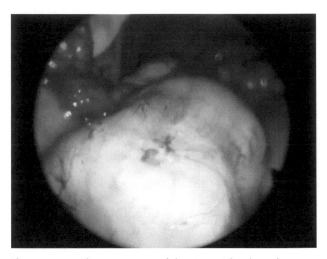

Figure 12.12 The same area of the sigmoid colon after careful vaporization of the lesion, which has been vaporized layer by layer down to normal tissue without perforating the bowel.

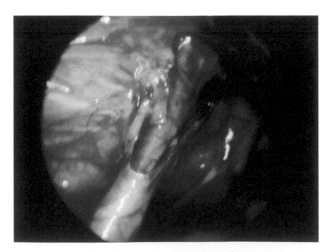

Figure 12.10 This slide shows the ureter after vaporization of deep infiltrating endometriosis around the ureter causing a hydroureter, which would eventually lead to renal failure. Vaporization has continued right down to the serosa of the ureter without damage to the ureter.

wound is able to heal with minimal fibrosis or scar tissue formation and second-look laparoscopy of laser wounds shows that they heal with virtually no contracture or anatomic distortion.[38]

The advantage of the Swiftlase high-speed rotating mirror delivery system is that this device can be attached to a relatively low-power laser, such as one delivering 20–30 W at tissue, and this will provide an almost identical tissue effect to that of lasers delivering 70–100 W in the ultrapulse mode. Such lasers will provide a similar tissue effect but require considerably more caution in their use and inevitably are extremely expensive. The Swiftlase device, however, can be attached to any low-power CO_2 laser generator, many of which are gathering dust in colposcopy suites, since the simpler electrosurgical technology using the large loop excision of the transformation zone has rendered the laser to be unnecessarily complicated and expensive for treatment of cervical intraepithelial neoplasia (CIN). The CO_2 laser, however, has advantages at laparoscopic surgery because it allows endometriotic deposits to be removed by vaporization almost bloodlessly and extremely rapidly; also, in practice, operations using the CO_2 laser take about one-third of the time of electrosurgical or ultrasonic devices.

Initial studies of healing of laser craters

In the early 1980s when we were starting to use the CO_2 laser at laparoscopy, we were interested to check on the healing of the peritoneum after vaporization with the CO_2 laser and felt it was ethically reasonable to perform second-look laparoscopies 6 weeks after the initial treatment on some of our early cases. Figure 12.13 shows a typical peritoneal implant of active endometriosis with a sago grain vesicular appearance in the center and obvious neoangiogenesis radiating to and from the deposit. Figure 12.14 shows the appearance immediately after laser vaporization and some carbon particles can be seen among the retroperitoneal fat. Closer inspection shows that there is neoangiogenesis and atypical vessels further out from the treated area, and particularly a hairpin capillary at the bottom left-hand side of the picture at approximately 5 o'clock. Figure 12.15 shows the same area rotated slightly, and it can be seen that in the area treated, the blood vessels now arborize like the branches of a tree and have the appear-

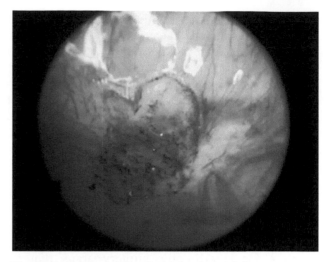

Figure 12.14 The implant has been lasered down to retroperitoneal fat. In recent years we would have lasered much more widely to remove the neoangiogenesis, particularly respresented by the hairpin capillary at 5 o'clock.

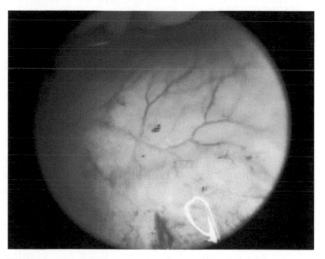

Figure 12.15 The same area at second-look laparoscopy 6 weeks later. The vessels are now arborizing like the branches of a tree, but the hairpin capillary representing neoangiogenesis is still present. This illustrates the importance of lasering widely around each lesion.

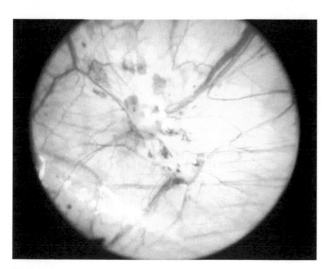

Figure 12.13 Sago grain vesicular implant with radiating neoangiogenesis.

ance of healthy blood vessels. The hairpin capillary can still be seen, although due to rotation of the laparoscope it is now at 6 o'clock; however, clearly the vaporization has not been performed widely enough, and this represents residual disease. The small black deposits are the carbon particles and do not represent recurrent endometriosis. This was proven by the biopsy taken 6 weeks later, which merely showed carbon particles and foreign body giant cells, but there was no evidence of recurrent endometrial glands or stroma. This experience taught us to vaporize more widely than the area visually involved and to try and take out all the neoangiogenesis. It is an example of why vaporization is more easy to perform than excision, because during excision one tends only to remove the implant and its immediate surrounding tissue. Careful examination of the area vaporized shows no fibrosis and contracture or scarring, which is characteristic of the near-perfect healing associated with CO_2 laser surgery.

Disadvantages of CO_2 laser laparoscopy

Critics of the use of the CO_2 laser as an energy source for laparoscopic surgery argue that the vaporization of tissue means that there is no histology. This is really a fatuous argument, because it is perfectly easy to take biopsies with the ovarian biopsy forceps. We always do this when there is any doubt about the lesions and definitely if there is the least suspicion of malignancy. However, the lesions of endometriosis are very characteristic and when there is extensive fibromuscular hyperplasia of the uterosacral ligaments the reality is that the biopsy only shows glands and stroma in about 50% of cases and thus is not necessary for the diagnosis of endometriosis. This was clearly shown by Chapron et al in their study of the efficacy of radical excision of the uterosacral ligament complex.[39] If en bloc excision is required, it is perfectly easy to use the laser in a sharply focused mode with a high-power density employing backstops or fluid to prevent onward transmission of the laser beam. This technique is clearly more time-consuming than vaporization and when one is dealing with a nonmalignant disease it is completely unnecessary and is rather akin to taking a hammer to crack a walnut.

Another criticism of the use of lasers is that it is technically difficult. We find it easier to use a cannula in the right or left iliac fossa, rather than transmitting the laser beam directly down the operating laparoscope. Instead of using the micro manipulator to align the beam, we use a fixed-focus lens, whereby the beam is focused 20 mm beyond the end of the probe (Figure 12.16). For difficult-access lesions under the ovary, we use a mirror that reflects the beam at right angles to the axis of the cannula; for dividing adhesions, we use a backstop to prevent onward transmission of the laser energy. In practice, since laparoscopic scissors are so much more efficient than they used to be, we tend to use laparoscopic scissors with no energy to divide adhesions, particularly if they are close to the bowel and we rely on natural hemostasis or fine bipolar forceps if bleeding is a problem at the end of the procedure.

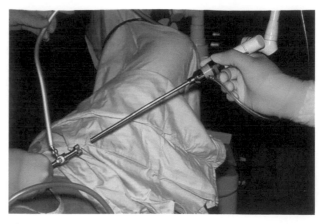

Figure 12.16 Laser energy delivered via a 7 mm cannula in the right or left iliac fossa.

The laser generates a fair amount of smoke and requires high-flow insufflators and efficient smoke extraction, but these technical problems are very easily resolved with modern equipment.

Some people have criticized the use of lasers on the grounds of expense, but the first CO_2 laser we purchased in 1982 for £15 000 ($27 300) was still working effectively after 18 years, had literally never let us down, and only required servicing on an annual basis. The running costs are therefore extremely low and it only had to be replaced because the plastic surgeons required a CO_2 laser with a surface scanner for dealing with crow's feet and other facial wrinkles as part of an increasing need on the part of modern women for cosmetic surgery. I rarely use more than 20 W of power and a 20 W laser now costs about £25 000 ($45 500, €37 500), with an additional £3000 ($5500, €4 500) for the high-speed rotating mirror delivery system (Swiftlase) which allows layer-by-layer vaporization of endometriotic disease. A basic CO_2 laser with a scanning facility for cosmetic surgery probably costs about £75 000 ($136 700, €112 700), but this degree of sophistication is not necessary if it is to be used by the Gynecology Department alone. In our hospital there is no additional fee for the use of the laser, so the long-term use we had from our first laser showed that it was extremely cost-effective and very reliable.

Development of laparoscopic laser surgery for endometriosis

During the 1980s, several centers in Europe and the United States reported the effectiveness of various lasers in relieving the pain of endometriosis in 60–70% of women following vaporization of superficial endometriosis with the CO_2

laser.[40–42] Similar results were achieved with the neodymium-YAG laser[43] the argon laser,[44] and the KTP-532 laser.[45]

When we started using the CO_2 laser down the laparoscope in October 1982 in Guildford, we were mainly concerned with the safety of using such a high-powered energy source within the abdominal cavity. We already had considerable experience using the CO_2 laser on the cervix for the destruction of CIN, but were unaware of any other center using it intraperitoneally via the laparoscope. We later found that it had first been used by Professor Bruhat's group in Clermont Ferrand, France, and the technique was presented in an abstract at the 1st Lasers in Medicine Congress in Japan in 1979.[46] Thinking we were the first to use this technique, we conducted safety experiments firing the laser in an atmosphere of CO_2 at isolated bowel specimens removed by our surgical colleagues. No methane explosions occurred, so we considered it safe. In fact, it turned out to be very safe indeed; during the last 25 years, having treated well over 14 500 women, we have had no accidents with the CO_2 laser. This is partly due to the fact that one has to exercise extreme caution and only activate the laser when the helium–neon aiming beam can be clearly seen and also make absolutely sure that no vital structures are in close proximity.

Our next important goal was to look at the effectiveness of using the laser to ablate peritoneal endometriosis. We therefore followed our first 228 patients over 5 years (Figure 12.17) and at the end of that time 126 of the 187 patients suffering from pain (70%) were pain-free. Thirty-eight patients were not improved, but most of these patients consented to a second-look laparoscopy. There was no sign of any recurrent endometriosis and many of these patients subsequently had different reasons for their pelvic pain, such as irritable bowel syndrome; several also had various psychologic problems, 2 being eventually diagnosed as having Munchausens' syndrome. Seventeen patients suffered a relapse during the 5-year follow-up and second-look laparoscopy showed that endometriosis had recurred, but almost always at different sites; 6 patients were lost to follow-up. Of the 56 patients with infertility due to endometriosis alone, 45 became pregnant, with an 80% pregnancy rate.

Unfortunately, this study was a retrospective one and although it is difficult to argue with the conception rate, the relief of pain is a highly subjective phenomenon. It would be entirely possible for a surgeon to influence the result of the pain relief, particularly when using highly technological equipment such as a laser, which tends to increase the patient's perception of the result: in some instances, the patient will indicate that pain relief has been achieved in order to please the surgeon.

The only way that this issue could be resolved, was to perform a randomized controlled trial

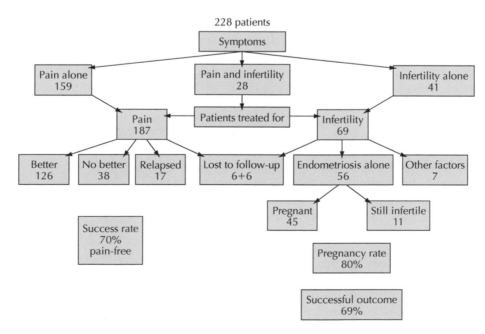

Figure 12.17 Results of a 5-year study of laser laparoscopy in patients with endometriosis.

(RCT), which had to be prospective, and also had to be double-blind so that neither the patient nor the person following up the patient was aware that intervention had occurred in the form of laser surgery or whether the intervention was merely a diagnostic laparoscopy alone. In 1995, we published the results of such a trial, which was the first such trial in the world literature on endometriosis.[19]

Evidence-based medicine – the Guildford laser laparoscopy trial

The aim of this study was to assess the efficacy of laser laparoscopy by the established scientific method of a prospective, double-blind RCT comparing the results of those women with minimal to moderate endometriosis AFS stages I–III who were treated by the laser and those in the sham arm who had diagnostic laparoscopy alone.

This study was approved by the Hospital Ethics Committee, but they reasonably felt that it was unethical to withhold treatment from patients in severe pain due to stage IV disease, particularly because our previous experience had shown 80% pain relief in this group, most of whom had failed to respond to medical therapy.

The study population was recruited from women seen in the gynecologic outpatient clinic with pain suggestive of endometriosis who had been advised to undergo a diagnostic laparoscopy. In order to be included in the study, women were between 18 and 45 years of age, were neither pregnant nor lactating, and had not received any treatment (medical or surgical) for endometriosis in the previous 6 months.

The study was explained in detail and informed consent was obtained. This was particularly difficult because many of these women had been specifically referred for laser surgery by consultants in other hospitals. The research registrars had the unenviable task of having to explain to women that, at this stage of development of laser laparoscopy, we were not entirely sure whether this procedure worked. To offset any inconvenience it was agreed that if, when the code was broken at 6 months, the patient was still experiencing pain and was in the 'no treatment' group, we would expedite her admission for laparoscopic laser surgery. Before the laparoscopy, the patients were asked to record the intensity of their pain on a 10 cm linear analogue scale marked from 0 to 10: 0 represented no pain at all and 10 represented the worst pain they had experienced in their life.

Between March 1990 and February 1993, 74 women were recruited, and at the time of laparoscopy treatment, allocated randomly (computer-generated randomization sequence) to laser treatment or expectant management. The laser treatment included vaporization of all visible endometriotic implants, adhesiolysis, and uterine nerve transection using a triple-puncture technique. The patients in the sham arm had exactly the same incisions but merely had a diagnostic laparoscopy, although during this it was necessary to remove the serosanguinous fluid from the pouch of Douglas in order to perform a thorough inspection of the entire pelvic peritoneum. Patients were not informed which treatment group they had been allocated to and were followed up at 3 months and 6 months after surgery by an independent observer (research nurse), who was also unaware of the treatment that had been carried out.

Results of the study

Of 74 women who entered the study, 63 (32 laser, 31 expectant) completed the study to the 6-month follow-up visit. The 11 patients who were excluded had either become pregnant or been put on the oral contraceptive by their family doctor, although both the patients and the doctors were requested not to do this during the course of the study, and 3 were lost to follow-up. The results can be seen in Figures 12.18 and 12.19; it can clearly be seen that at 3 months post-operation there was very little difference between the two groups, but at 6 months the difference reached statistical significance and 62.5% of the patients who had the laser treatment had sustained pain

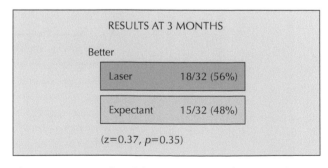

Figure 12.18 Results of the Guildford Birthright Study at 3 months, showing little difference between the laser-treated group and those who had expectant management only.

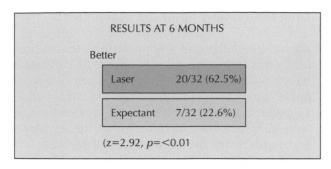

RESULTS AT 6 MONTHS

Better

| Laser | 20/32 (62.5%) |
| Expectant | 7/32 (22.6%) |

(z=2.92, p=<0.01

Figure 12.19 The results of the Guildford Birthright Study at 6 months, showing that the laser group had continued to improve, whereas those undergoing expectant management was less than at 3 months. The differences are statistically significant.

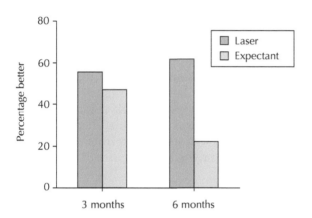

Figure 12.20 Proportion of patients with pain symptom alleviation: stages I–III.

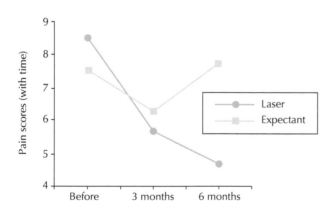

Figure 12.21 The results of the Guildford Birthright Study shown using visual analogue pain scores with time. The treated group continued to improve up to 6 months, but those undergoing expectant management, although slightly improved at 3 months, returned almost to the baseline at 6 months.

relief and only 22.6% of the patients who had no treatment said they were better (z = 2.92, $p < 0.01$, Fisher's exact test) (Figures 12.20 and 12.21). The results were worst for stage I disease (Figure 12.22) and this is probably because some of the minimal changes seen in mild endometriosis could possibly be due to inflammatory changes or Walthard's cell rests or other nonspecific changes in the appearance of the peritoneum. Unfortunately, the disease could not be confirmed by biopsy, because that would have acted as a cytoreductive procedure and could not truly be called expectant management. If the stage I patients were excluded, then 73.7% of patients achieved pain relief, which is very similar to the figure obtained in our retrospective study.

Initial placebo effect

There are several interesting features of this study that merit discussion. We were surprised that the results at 3 months were very similar for the laser group (56%) compared with the expectant group (48%). There was no significant difference between these two figures, and we were surprised to find that almost half of the patients with no treatment claimed that they were better. This placebo effect has been noticed in other studies where dysmenorrhea was reported to have improved: in up to 30% of patients in the placebo arm of an Italian study comparing expectant management with gonadotropin-releasing hormone (GnRH) analogues.[47] They found that this improvement did not last longer than 3 months and that was exactly the same as our finding and in particular the visual analogue scale clearly

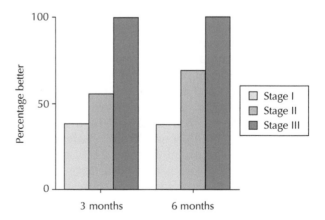

Figure 12.22 Pain symptom alleviation related to the stage of disease. The results were less good for stage I disease, since some of the minimal appearances may not have been endometriosis. This may have a bearing on the poor results for stage I.

shows that at 6 months in the expectant arm the patients had returned to the original score, whereas the laser group had continued to improve. This has also shown us that it can take at least 3 months for the benefit of laparoscopic laser surgery to be noticed, so we now advise patients of this and only see them for follow-up at 6 months.

Natural history of endometriosis

Another benefit of this study was to allow us to look at the natural history of endometriosis, because it had widely been assumed that it was invariably a progressive disease. We had the opportunity to look at a group of patients who had not received any treatment but had an established diagnosis and to report the findings of the second-look laparoscopy and compare the changes in their symptoms.[48] At second-look laparoscopy, 10 cases (42%) had no change in the AFS score, 7 cases (29%) had an increased score with 3 patients moving to a higher stage, but we were surprised to find that 7 women (29%) had a reduced AFS score, with 3 patients moving to a lower stage. Thus, the median change in AFS score was in fact 0 ($p = 0.8$ Wilcoxon signed rank test) and the degree of change in score was not related to the time interval between the procedures (Kendall's tau = 0.5, $p = 0.8$).

Our findings can be compared with three published RCTs of medical therapies that have included a placebo group as well as second-look laparoscopy and comparison of AFS scores. All of these studies are based on relatively small patient numbers, but in the study by Thomas and Cooke,[49] in which 17 asymptomatic infertile patients were followed and had second-look laparoscopies, they showed that in 47% the disease had progressed, 24% were static, and 21% improved. This compared with a slightly smaller study of 11 patients by Mahmood and Templeton,[8] which showed that 64% progressed, 9% were static, and 27% improved. Although there have been five RCTs of placebo medical therapy for the painful symptoms of endometriosis, only one trial had 6 months follow-up of the AFS scores.[50] In that study by Telimaa and colleagues from Finland, of 17 patients with minimal disease, 24% showed progression, 59% were static, and 17% improved. Our results are very similar to those observed in baboons and other higher primates[51] and lead us to conclude that painful endometriosis when left untreated is a dynamic disease which may remain static, or progress, or diminish at varying speeds. As it will progress in 29% of women and since laparoscopic ablation of endometrial implants is a safe procedure, it should be offered at the same time as the diagnostic laparoscopy.

Long-term follow-up of the trial patients

We have recently had an opportunity to conduct a long-term follow-up on this cohort of patients by telephone interview, with a mean time since the operation of 88.6 months (range 77–104).[52] Of the 32 patients who had had a laser laparoscopy, we were able to contact 22 (68.8%); we had to remove 4 patients from the study (12.5%) because they had been taking the oral contraceptive pill, which diminishes the symptoms of endometriosis, and 6 patients (18.8%) were lost to follow-up. Nevertheless, we found that 60% of the patients had continued to have satisfactory symptom relief: 1 patient was menopausal and 4 patients needed mild analgesia only. Three of the patients had repeat laser laparoscopy for new disease in different sites; 5 patients were leading pain-free lives, and 3 of these had had successful pregnancies. Of those patients that continued to have painful symptoms, 6 patients had repeated laser laparoscopy on one or more occasions and two patients had required psychiatric help for Munchausen syndrome and required strong analgesia. Interestingly, of the 6 patients who eventually had a hysterectomy and bilateral salpingo-oophorectomy, all of them had a normal pelvis macroscopically at the time of operation and no histologic evidence of endometriosis was seen, apart from one very small focus of adenomyosis in one uterus.

Denervation operations – laparoscopic uterine nerve ablation (LUNA)

The other aspect of pain relief that our study had not addressed was the role played by the division of the uterosacral ligaments which contain many of the afferent sensory pain fibers to the uterus.[53]

The sensory parasympathetic fibers to the cervix and the sensory sympathetic fibers to the corpus traverse the cervical division of the Lee–Frankenhäuser plexus (Figures 12.23 and 12.24) which lies in, under, and around the attachments of the uterosacral ligaments to the cervix and are concentrated mainly on the medial aspect. Sympathetic fibers that have reached the cervix by accompanying the uterine and ovarian arteries can also be found in this area.

The parasympathetic components originate from the first to the third and fourth sacral nerves, reaching the plexus by the pelvic nerves (nervi erigentes). In a study of 33 cadavers, Campbell in 1950[54] confirmed the findings of earlier workers[55]

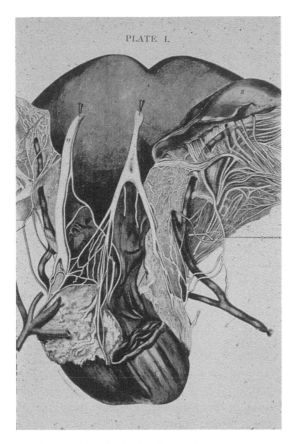

Figure 12.23 Robert Lee's drawing of the Lee–Frankenhäuser plexus.

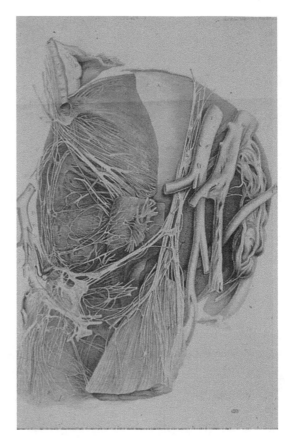

Figure 12.24 Another drawing of the Lee–Frankenhäuser plexus taken from Robert Lee's original drawing.

by identifying parasympathetic fibers in the anterior two-thirds of the uterosacral ligaments and demonstrating the presence of small ganglia around the area where the ligaments attach to the cervix. Theoretically, therefore, division of the uterosacral ligaments at the point of their attachment to the cervix should lead to interruption of most of the cervical sensory fibers and some of the corporal sensory fibers and lead to a diminution in uterine pain at the time of menstruation. This was first performed in 1954 by Joseph Doyle,[56] but required a large abdominal incision and a prolonged hospital stay. Although he had impressive results for complete pain relief in 63 out of 73 cases (86%), the advent of the oral contraceptive pill and powerful nonsteroidal anti-inflammatory drugs reduced the demand for such major surgery and Doyle's procedure lapsed into obscurity as have many other operations in the relatively short history of gynecologic surgery. Later, Doyle modified the approach and suggested that gynecologists would be more comfortable with the vaginal approach. A suture was placed through the posterior lip of the cervix at the apex of the vagina and traction on this suture increased the distance of

the cervix from the ureter, which is clearly demonstrated in his article by a very convincing cervico-ureterogram. The attachments of the uterosacral ligaments to the cervix were then divided between two Heaney clamps and, to prevent regrowth of the bisected nerve trunks, the posterior leaf of the peritoneal incision was interposed between them.

With the advent of laparoscopic surgery, it rapidly became evident that uterine nerve ablation performed laparoscopically with electrosurgery, or with the laser, could be easily achieved in a few minutes (Figure 12.25) and it was particularly effective in patients where the uterosacral ligaments were infiltrated by deep deposits of endometriosis and white scar tissue (fibromuscular hyperplasia) (Figure 12.26). In our first 100 patients with endometriosis, 6 patients were lost to follow-up; but of the remainder, 13 patients remained the same and 81 patients (86%) were markedly improved (Table 12.2). On a linear analogue pain scale, the initial score was 9.2 on average, went down to 3.4 on average, and the majority of patients were satisfied with the proce-

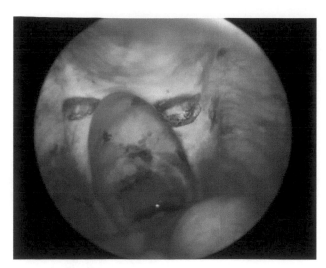

Figure 12.25 Ablation of the nerves in the Lee-Frankenhäuser plexus in the uterosacral ligaments.

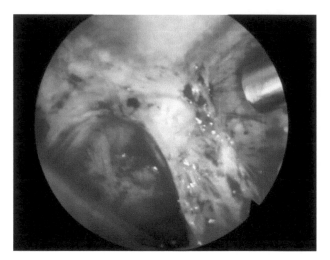

Figure 12.26 Fibromuscular hyperplasia due to deep infiltrating endometriosis in the uterosacral ligaments. The removal of this tissue by a large LUNA procedure may have explained some of the initial good results.

dure. It is important to counsel the patient that the relief is not necessarily apparent in the first 3 months and it often takes the following 3 months before the benefits are noticeable. We have not found that any of our patients have been made worse, but James Daniell from Nashville, Tennessee[57] did counsel his patients that some might be made worse: sure enough, out of 80 patients, 60 (75%) were improved, 17 (21%) were the same, and 3 (4%) were made worse. In this study, the results were not so good with primary dysmenorrhea, with an improvement rate of 60%, and 10% being made worse, and we also found that the numbers that improved were less satisfactory than if endometriosis was infiltrating the uterosacral ligaments. In our hands, this procedure has been extremely safe, but it is possible to have bleeding from deep inside the uterosacral ligaments or from the plexus of veins that run just lateral to it. It is therefore necessary to have effective bipolar coagulating equipment immediately available, as well as a good irrigator and sucker, and also one must take great care to identify the ureters close to the pelvic brim and follow them forward to make sure that they are well clear of the uterosacral ligaments. About 5% of patients have double ureters and, in that case, they are often situated even closer to the uterosacral ligaments and the ablation should be concentrated mainly on the anterior and medial aspects of the uterosacral ligaments. Some surgeons even link up the two ablated areas in order to destroy the central cross-over fibers and also to avoid any damage laterally, which could include the ureter.

Interestingly, the division of uterine nerves has been subject to a small RCT by Lichten and Bombard employing electrosurgery in 1987,[58] and we thought it would be interesting in a larger

Table 12.2 LUNA results with CO_2 laser				
	LFU*	Improved	Same	Worse
Endometriosis 100 patients	6	81 (86%)	13	—
Primary dysmenorrhea 26 patients	4	16 (73%)	6	—
Total 126 patients	10	97 (84%)	19	—
* LFU = Lost to follow-up.				

series to know what effect the uterine nerve ablation has as an additional treatment to vaporization of the endometriotic implants. We conducted such a trial, which was published in 2001.[59]

A randomized controlled trial of laser laparoscopy for pelvic pain associated with endometriosis with and without uterine nerve ablation

One of the criticisms of the original Guildford RCT was that we had routinely used the LUNA procedure as an adjunct to vaporization of the endometriotic implants. We did this in the belief that it would improve patients, particularly with central dysmenorrhea. For many years it had formed a basis of our practice, because in an early retrospective study reported above, 86% of patients obtained considerable relief from this simple laparoscopic operation. I was firmly of the opinion that the LUNA procedure was responsible for most of the benefit, but we needed to do a prospective, double-blind RCT in order to find out the contribution, if any, of division of the nerves in the uterosacral ligament. The study was similar to the original trial, except on this occasion there was no requirement for a no treatment arm and one group had laser vaporization of all visible endometriotic implants on the peritoneum and reproductive organs, whereas the other group had the same operation but additionally had a LUNA procedure. We recruited 51 patients who had pelvic pain due to endometriosis. Ethical approval was obtained from the Hospital Ethics Committee and all patients were fully informed and consented and knew that they would not know whether they had had a uterine nerve ablation or not and neither would the research nurse who followed them up. The main outcome measures were dysmenorrhea, dyspareunia, and chronic nonmenstrual pelvic pain, which were assessed by visual analogue scales and structured questionnaires preoperatively and at 3 and 6 months postoperatively. Randomization occurred intraoperatively by a computer-generated randomization sequence in sealed envelopes in the operating theater; the envelopes were only opened at the time of randomization.

We recruited 51 women and the exclusion criteria were similar to the previous study: 24 patients were randomized to receive laser vaporization alone and 27 to receive a LUNA procedure in addition. The mean age of patients involved was 28 years old (range 20–41), with no differences between the groups for stages of endometriosis. Comparisons were made between the two treatment groups at 3 and 6 months. Significant differ-

ences in favor of the non-LUNA group occurred at 3 months ($p = 0.003$), and at 6 months ($p = 0.022$) for dysmenorrhea. A significant difference in favor of the non-LUNA group also occurred at 6 months for chronic nonmenstrual pain ($p = 0.323$). There were no significant differences recorded for dyspareunia. Bonferroni's adjustment was applied, and the only difference remaining significant was for dysmenorrhea at 3 months ($p = 0.033$) in favor of the nonLUNA group. The preoperative and 6-month pain scores for all the patients were combined. There was a significant improvement in the pain scores recorded at 6 months ($p < 0.0001$).

The conclusion of this study was that laparoscopic laser ablation of endometriosis is confirmed as an effective treatment, since the results in terms of pain relief were almost exactly the same as the previous study, but I was surprised to find that LUNA with the laser added no benefit. This result was exactly the opposite to what I had anticipated, which shows the value of a prospective double-blind study where the surgeon has really no influence at all on the outcome and is therefore completely unbiased.

These results have been confirmed by a larger study by Paolo Vercellini et al in Milan[60] who also showed that LUNA added no additional benefit to the good results obtained by ablation of peritoneal implants. Their study was slightly larger than ours, but was not double-blind, and it would be useful to have some further studies in order to increase the numbers available for study. A large multicenter study is being conducted in the UK at the Women's Hospital in Birmingham but it is looking at the role of LUNA in the treatment of chronic pelvic pain rather than dysmenorrhea, which it was originally designed for.

In order to explain why we had such good results from our original retrospective LUNA study, I looked at some of the patients who had second-look procedures as part of a separate adhesion second-look study we were performing many years later. The size of the uterine nerve ablation crater in some of the patients showed that there was a huge amount of the uterosacral complex removed and, as can be seen from Figure 12.27, this very large crater is removing a huge amount of fibromuscular hyperplasia and DIE and almost amounts to a radical vaporization of the uterosacral complex. It is probably for this reason that the result in terms of dysmenorrhea relief of 86% was obtained and is in fact very similar to the results of radical excision of the uterosacral complex reported by Chapron et al from Paris.[39] In other words, it is the removal of the white areas of fibromuscular hyperplasia (which we originally thought were nerve fibers)

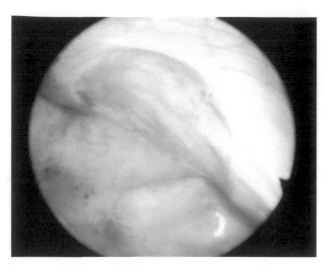

Figure 12.27 Large LUNA crater seen at second-look laparoscopy may explain why the removal of a large amount of deep infiltrating endometriosis was the reason for the pain relief rather than the division of the nerves.

that was the key to our original success when we mistakenly thought we were performing a denervation procedure.[61]

Electrocoagulation of endometriosis

Electrocoagulation of endometriosis can only be used for superficial peritoneal disease and can be an alternative to the KTP laser for coagulation of the capsule of an ovarian endometrioma. Bipolar electrosurgery, although excellent for achieving hemostasis in laparoscopic surgery, suffers from the basic physical problem that it is not easy to assess the depth of penetration of the energy and there is always a risk that deeper deposits of endometriosis will remain untreated. The other electrosurgical coagulators, such as the argon beam coagulator, the helica thermo coagulator, or the cold plasma coagulator, will only treat superficial peritoneal deposits and are not suitable and, indeed, are not designed for the treatment of DIE.

Bipolar electrosurgery

In the bipolar system, the current from the electrosurgical generator flows through the active electrode, which is one of the blades of the forceps, through the intervening tissue to the other blade, which acts as the inactive electrode, and thence back to the electrosurgical unit. This is an inherently safe system, because only the tissue grasped between the blades of the forceps is coagulated

and ultimately desiccated, and no ground plate is required. The effect is therefore focused and, although damage to adjacent tissue is minimized, it must be understood that there is a considerable build-up of temperature in the adjacent tissue.[62] Phipps plotted a graph showing the amount of irreversible damage that can occur to tissue, plotted against the distance from the bipolar forceps. This is particularly important when using bipolar current to desiccate uterine arteries during a laparoscopic hysterectomy and also deposits of endometriosis which are in close proximity to the ureter. The white area lateral to the forceps will be irreversibly damaged and it is important to realize that irreversible damage can occur at a temperature as low as 60°C.

Argon beam coagulator

Because of the way it has been marketed, with a bright blue light coming from the end of the generator and impinging on tissue some distance away, many people think the argon beam coagulator is a laser (Figure 12.28). In fact, it is merely a way of delivering monopolar current via an electron channel, consisting of a flow of argon gas, which has the effect of blowing off the blood, char, and debris from the target zone, and thus allowing the unipolar current to directly impinge on a bleeding vessel. It is an excellent hemostatic energy source and is useful during vascular procedures, such as a myomectomy and a presacral neurectomy.[63] The surgeons also find it particularly useful for highly vascular procedures, such as liver surgery.

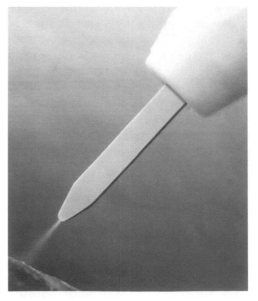

Figure 12.28 Argon beam coagulator. An electric current (monopolar) is delivered down a gas channel of argon, directly impinging on the tissue.

It produces less smoke than other similar energy sources, but it is absolutely vital to have an adequate suction system to siphon off the gas, because there have been reports of deaths from argon gas embolism, both in animal studies[64] and also in human subjects.[65] Accidents are due to a combination of high intraperitoneal pressures and open blood vessels and can be avoided when using a high-flow automatic insufflator that shuts off when the intraperitoneal pressure is greater than 20 mmHg; just before firing the ABC, a suction irrigation probe is placed close to the point of impact to aspirate the argon gas when the device is fired. This eliminates the accumulation of argon gas within the peritoneum and helps to reduce the intraperitoneal pressure.

Although electrosurgical energy is invisible, when the electrons flow through the argon gas channel, there is an arcing effect, which is visible and is similar to the glow seen with neon lights. This allows the surgeon to see the actual diameter of the beam when firing it laparoscopically and, because there is a reduction in smoke with coagulation compared with electrosurgery and various lasers, it allows excellent visibility of the tissue effects. The tip of the probe should be allowed to touch the planned impact site and then is backed away to a distance of 2–3 mm. After initial suction aspiration of the gas in the vicinity, the device is then activated and the distance from the tip of the probe to the tissue is adjusted, depending on the visible tissue effect. The 4 L/min plume of argon gas begins to flow just before the electrode is energized, allowing any excessive blood or irrigation fluids to be blown away from the impact site, and thus facilitating rapid hemostasis by direct coagulation of the exposed vessel. Since the spot size is 3 mm, fine cutting is difficult with this device: it does allow superficial coagulation of endometriotic implants but is not suitable for excisional techniques aimed to remove DIE. Because of its excellent hemostatic properties, the argon beam coagulator is an excellent device for presacral neurectomy, but care must be taken because accidents have been reported due to the electron channel of gas being deflected off the shiny surface of the peritoneum over the sacral promontory and causing serious injury to the pelvic side-wall vessels.

Helica thermal coagulator

The Helica thermal coagulator (Helica Instruments, Broxburn, Lothian, UK) produces a similar effect to the argon beam coagulator but employs helium gas. When the foot switch is operated, a corona-type flame issues from the end of the nozzle with a high electron temperature but low molecular temperature, typically about 20°C, until such time as the flame is brought close to the surface, when it is capacitively coupled or directly connected to earth. The corona-type flame then changes to an arc discharge flame, which has a higher molecular temperature, typically in the order of 800°C. The flame takes place in an atmosphere provided by the flowing helium gas, which, being inert, minimizes oxidation at the tissue.

The Helica thermal coagulator is a power-controlled device and the voltage is reduced along the length of the flame, so that only low electrical power is passed to the tissue. The power delivered to the surface can be controlled to a few watts. The depth of penetration is easily controlled by the power setting and the distance of the probe from the tissue. The device is extremely versatile, easy to use, and appears to be very safe;[66] it is particularly effective for peritoneal surface endometriotic implants because it can cauterize soft tissue to a depth of one cell, allowing the diseased tissue to be removed layer by layer, as with the CO_2 laser at rapid fluence. As with the argon beam coagulator, this device is really mainly used for superficial peritoneal endometriosis because of its very limited depth of penetration, but by removing the eschar it is possible to vaporize layer by layer or by using the recently introduced cutting device to excise deep infiltrating disease. It has the advantage that it is cheaper than a laser, but unlike the CO_2 laser, which uses reusable delivery channels for the transmission of energy, the Helica devices are single use only and thus an ongoing expense. It is, however, a much cheaper alternative than the KTP laser, which uses disposable fibers for coagulating the capsule of an endometrioma of the ovary.

Cold plasma coagulation

The latest type of coagulator is the cold plasma coagulator (CPC) (Soring, Quickborn, Germany) which has an even more superficial penetration than the argon beam coagulator or the Helica thermal coagulator. It has an advantage that it does not require an earth plate and would appear to be extremely safe, although we await the results of clinical trials, which at the moment are being conducted in Russia.

Conclusion

There is really little to choose, in terms of clinical outcome, between the various surgical power sources. Operative laparoscopy is safe and effective, whether using sharp scissor dissection, the ultrasonic scalpel, electrosurgery, or laser energy, as long as the surgeon is familiar with the physics of the modality used, is aware of the complications that can occur with misuse, and takes every possible step to avoid them. The newer surgical modalities, such as the Helica thermal coagulator and the cold plasma coagulator require further evaluation and comparison with more established power sources, preferably in double-blind, prospective clinical trials. At this moment in time, electrosurgery is by far the most popular and cheapest power source in endoscopic surgery, but only the laser has been subjected to prospective, randomized clinical studies which have also been double-blind. In the final analysis, the skill and experience of surgeons, together with their preference of the technique employed, and careful patient selection play more important roles than the energy source in the clinical outcome of laparoscopic surgery.[67]

REFERENCES

1. Nisolle M, Donnez J. Peritoneal endometriosis, ovarian endometriosis and adenomyotic nodules of the rectovaginal septum are three different entities. Fertil Steril 1997; 68: 585–596.

2. Sampson JA. Perforating haemorrhage cysts of the ovary. Arch Surg 1921; 3: 245–261.

3. Sampson JA. Peritoneal endometriosis due to menstrual dissemination of endometrial tissue into the peritoneal cavity. Am J Obstet Gynecol 1927; 14: 422–469.

4. Ridley JH. The histogenesis of endometriosis. Obstet Gynaecol Surv 1968; 23: 1–35.

5. Ridley JH, Edwards IK. Experimental endometriosis in the human. Obstet Gynaecol Surv 1958; 76: 783–790.

6. Halme J, Hammond MG, Hulka JF, et al. Retrograde menstruation in healthy women and in patients with endometriosis. Obstet Gynaecol 1984; 64: 151–154.

7. Edmonds DK. Endometriosis. In: Edmonds DK, ed. Dewhursts textbook of obstetrics & gynaecology for postgraduates, 6th edn. Oxford: Blackwell Science; 1999: 420–431.

8. Mahmood TA, Templeton JF. Prevalence and genesis of endometriosis. Hum Reprod 1991; 1: 544–549.

9. Jenkins S, Olive DL, Haney AF. Endometriosis: pathogenic implications of the anatomic distribution. Obstet Gynaecol 1986; 67: 335–338.

10. Golan A, Langer R, Bukofsky I, et al. Congenital anomalies of the müllerian system. Fertil Steril 1989; 51: 747–755.

11. Olive DL, Henderson DY. Endometriosis and müllerian anomalies. Obstet Gynaecol 1987; 69: 412–415.

12. Ansbacher R. Uterine anomalies in future pregnancies. Clin Perinatol 1983; 10: 295–304.

13. Bartosik D, Jacobs SL, Kelley LJ. Endometrial tissue in peritoneal fluid. Fertil Steril 1986; 46: 796–800.

14. Giudice LC, Kao LC. Endometriosis. Lancet 2004; 364: 1789–1799.

15. Hadfield R, Mardon H, Barlow D, et al. Delay in diagnosis of endometriosis: a survey of women from the USA and the UK. Hum Reprod 1996; 11: 878–880.

16. Husby GK, Haugen RS, Moen MH. Diagnostic delay in women with pain and endometriosis. Acta Obstetrica Gynecologica Scandinavica 2003; 82: 649–653.

17. Arruda MS, Petta CA, Abrao MS, et al. Time elapsed from onset of symptoms to diagnosis of endometriosis in a cohort study of Brazilian women. Hum Reprod 2003; 18: 756–759.

18. Revill SI, Robinson JO, Rosen M, et al. The reliability of a linear analogue scale for evaluating pain. Anaesthesia 1976; 31: 1191–1198.

19. Sutton CJG, Ewen SP, Whitelaw N, et al. Prospective, randomised, double-blind, controlled trial of laser laparoscopy in the treatment of pelvic pain associated with minimal, mild and moderate endometriosis. Fertil Steril 1994; 62: 696–700.

20. Sutton CJG. Laser uterine nerve ablation. In: Donnez J, Nisolle M, eds. An atlas of laser operative laparoscopy and hysteroscopy. London: Parthenon; 1994; 47–52.

21. Redwine DB. Patient preparation. In: Redwine DB, ed. Surgical management of endometriosis. New York: Martin Dunitz; 2004; 47–59.

22. Koninckx PR, Meuleman C, Oosterlynk D, et al. Diagnosis of deep endometriosis by clinical examination during menstruation and plasma Ca-125 concentration. Fertil Steril 1996; 65: 280–287.

23. Redwine DB. Age-related evolution in colour appearance of endometriosis. Fertil Steril 1987; 48(6): 1062–1065.

24. Jansen R, Russell P. Non-pigmented endometriosis: clinical, laparoscopic and pathological definition. Am J Obstet Gynecol 1986; 155: 1154–1159.

25. Demco L. Photospectrometry in the diagnosis of peritoneal endometriosis. J Amer Assoc Gynecol Laparosc May 2004.

26. Nisolle M, Paindaveine B, Boudon A, et al. Histologic study of peritoneal endometriosis in infertile women. Fertil Steril 1990; 53: 984–988.

27. Murphy A, Green WR, Bobbie D, et al. Unsuspected endometriosis documented by scanning electron microscopy in visually normal peritoneum. Fertil Steril 1986; 46: 522–524.

28. Khoo SK, Brodie A, Mackay EV. Peritoneal fluid biochemistry in infertile women with mild pelvic endometriosis: prognostic value of prostaglandin F2 alpha concentrations to subsequent pregnancy. Aust N Z J Obstet Gynaecol 1986; 26: 210–215.

29. Hurst DS, Rock JA. The peritoneal environment in endometriosis. In: Thomas E, Rock JA, eds. Modern approaches to endometriosis. Lancaster, UK: Kluwer Academic Publishers; 1991: 79–96.

30. Stern RC, Dash R, Bentley RC, et al. Malignancy in endometriosis: frequency and comparison of ovarian and extra-ovarian types. Int J Gynaecol Pathol 2001; 20: 133–139.

31. Sutton CJG, Scott M. Minimal access surgery: image display and archiving. In: Maxwell DJ, ed. Surgical techniques in obstetrics & gynaecology. Edinburgh: Churchill Livingstone; 2004: 167–174.

32. American Fertility Society. Classification of endometriosis. Fertil Steril 1985; 43: 351–352.

33. Vernon MW, Beard JS, Graves K, et al. Classification of endometriotic implants by morphological appearance and capacity to synthesise prostaglandin F. Fertil Steril 1986; 46: 801–806.

34. Garry R. Editorial. Towards evidence-based laparoscopic entry techniques. Clinical problems and dilemmas. Gynecol Endosc 1999; 8: 315–326.

35. Harding SG, McMillan DL. Laparoscopic complications and how to avoid them. In: Lower A, Sutton C, Grudzinskas G, eds. Introduction to gynecologic endoscopy. Oxford: Isis; 1996: 73–97.

36. Audebert AJM. The role of microlaparoscopy for safer wall entry: incidence of umbilical adhesions according to past surgical history. Gynaecol Endosc 1999; 8: 363–367.

37. Bellina JH, Hemmings R, Voros IJ, et al. Carbon dioxide laser and electrosurgical wound study with an animal model. A comparison of tissue damage and healing patterns in peritoneal tissue. Am J Obstet Gynecol 1984; 148: 327–330.

38. Allen JM, Stein DS, Shingleton HM. Regeneration of cervical epithelium after laser vaporisation. Obstet Gynaecol 1983; 62: 700–704.

39. Chapron C, Dubuisson JB, Fritel X, et al. Operative management of deep endometriosis infiltrating the uterosacral ligaments. J Am Assoc Gynecol Laparosc 1999; 1: 31–37.

40. Daniell JF. Operative laparoscopy for endometriosis. Semin Reprod Endocrinol 1985; 3(4): 353–359.

41. Donnez J. Carbon dioxide laser laparoscopy in infertile women with adhesions or endometriosis. Fertil Steril 1987; 48: 390–394.

42. Nezhat C, Crowgey SR, Garrison CP. Surgical treatment of endometriosis via laser laparoscopy. Fertil Steril 1986; 45: 778–783.

43. Lomano JM. Laparoscopic ablation of endometriosis with the YAG laser. Lasers Surg Med 1983; 3: 179–183.

44. Keye WR, Matson GA, Dixon J. The use of the argon laser in the treatment of experimental endometriosis. Fertil Steril 1983; 39: 26–31.

45. Daniell JF. Laparoscopic evaluation of the KTP/532 laser for treating endometriosis – initial report. Fertil Steril 1986; 46: 373–377.

46. Bruhat M, Mage C, Manhes M. Use of carbon dioxide laser via laparoscopy. In: Kaplan E, ed. Laser surgery III. Proceedings of the Third Congress for the International Society for Laser Surgery. Tel Aviv: International Society for Laser Surgery; 1979: 275–282.

47. Fedele L, Bianci S, Bocciolone I, et al. Buserelin acetate in the treatment of pelvic pain associated with minimal and mild endometriosis: a controlled study. Fertil Steril 1983; 59: 516–521.

48. Sutton CJG, Pooley AS, Ewen SP, et al. Follow-up report on a randomised, controlled trial of laser laparoscopy in the treatment of pelvic pain associated with minimal to moderate endometriosis. Fertil Steril 1997; 68: 1070–1074.

49. Thomas EJ, Cooke I. Impact of Gestrinone on the course of asymptomatic endometriosis. BMJ 1987; 294: 272–274.

50. Telimaa S, Puolakka J, Ronnberg I, et al. Placebo controlled comparison of danazol and high-dose medroxyprogesterone acetate in the treatment of endometriosis. Gynecol Endocrinol 1987; 1: 13–23.

51. D'Hooghe TM. Natural history of endometriosis in baboons: is endometriosis an intermittent and/or progressive disease? In: Venturini PL, Evers JLH, eds. Endometriosis: basic research and clinical practice. London: Parthenon; 1997.

52. Jones KD, Haines P, Sutton CJ. Long-term follow-up on a controlled trial of laser laparoscopy for pelvic pain. J Soc Laparos Endosc Surg 2001; 5: 111–115.

53. Frankenhauser G. Die Bewegungenerven der Gebarmutter. Z Med Nat Wiss 1864; 1: 35–39.

54. Campbell RM. Anatomy and physiology of sacro-uterine ligaments. Am J Obstet Gynecol 1950; 59: 1–5.

55. Latarjet A, Roget P. Le plexus hypogastrique chez la femme. Gynecol Obstet 1922; 6: 225–228.

56. Doyle JB. Paracervical uterine denervation of dysmenorrhoea. Trans N Engl Obstet Gynaecol Soc 1954; 8: 143–146.

57. Daniell JF, Lalonde CJ. Advanced laparoscopic procedures for pelvic pain and dysmenorrhoea. In: Sutton CJG, ed. Baillière's Clin Obstet Gynaecol Adv Laparosc Surg 1995; 9: 795–807.

58. Lichten EM, Bombard J. Surgical treatment of primary dysmenorrhoea with laparoscopic uterine nerve ablation. J Reprod Med 1987; 32: 37–41.

59. Sutton CJG, Pooley A, Jones KD, et al. Prospective, randomised double-blind controlled trial of laparoscopic laser uterine nerve ablation in the treatment of pelvic pain associated with minimal, mild and moderate endometriosis. Gynaecol Endosc 2001; 10: 1–8.

60. Vercellini P, Aimi G, Busacca M, et al. Laparoscopic uterosacral ligament resection for dysmenorrhoea associated with endometriosis: results of a randomised controlled trial. Fertil Steril 1997; 68 (Suppl 1): 3.

61. Jones KD, Sutton CJG. Arcus taurinus: the mother and father of all LUNAs. Gynaecol Endosc 2001; 10: 83–89.

62. Phipps J. Thermometry studies with bipolar diathermy during hysterectomy. Gynaecol Endosc 1993; 3: 5–7.

63. Daniell JF. Laparoscopic use of the argon beam coagulator. In: Sutton CJG, Diamond M, eds. Endoscopic surgery for gynaecologists. London: WB Saunders; 1993: 71–76.

64. Palmer M, Miller CW, van Way CW, et al. Venous gas embolism associated with argon-inhanced coagulation of the liver. J Invest Surg 1993; 6(5): 391–399.

65. Anonymous. Fatal gas embolism caused by over pressurisation during laparoscopic use of argon-enhanced coagulation. Health Devices 1994; 23(6): 257–259.

66. Hill NCW, Erian J, Chandakas S. A series of 250 patients treated with 'Helica' for endometriosis: a new and safe thermal energy. Presented at the Int Soc Gynaecol Endosc Meeting in London, April 2005.

67. Tulandi T, Bugnah M. Operative laparoscopy: surgical modalities. Fertil Steril 1995; 63: 237–245.

13 Surgical management of ovarian endometrioma: cystectomy by stripping of the capsule

Abdul Aziz Al-Shahrani and Togas Tulandi

The ovary is a common site of endometriotic cyst or endometrioma. Perhaps, the irregular surface of the ovary allows endometrial tissue to burrow into its substance, predisposing to the development of ovarian endometrioma. Sampson in 1927[1] first described the term 'chocolate' cyst for ovarian endometrioma. Similar to that of endometriotic implants, the left ovary is more commonly affected than the right.[2]

Pathogenesis

The exact pathophysiology of ovarian endometrioma remains unclear.[3–5] Hughesdon[6] and Brosens et al[7] postulated that endometrioma develops by progressive invagination of the endometriosis-affected ovarian cortex. Endometrial cells spilling from the fallopian tube implant on the ovarian surface. Since the blood from the endometrial implants is unable to escape, the result is an expanding sphere of old blood invaginating the ovarian cortex (Figure 13.1). Other theories include metaplasia of the coelomic epithelium covering the ovary[8,9] or secondary involvement of the functional ovarian cyst.[10]

Endometrioma is often associated with pelvic pain and infertility. The diagnosis is suspected on pelvic examination or ultrasound examination. It is confirmed at the time of surgery and established by histopathologic examination. Bilateral and large endometriomas tend to adhere to each other and are frequently called 'kissing ovaries' (See Figure 13.1).

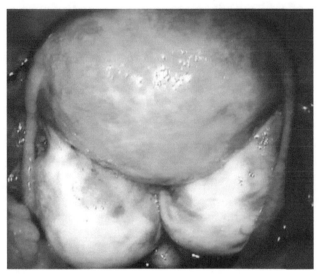

Figure 13.1 Bilateral endometriomas. The ovaries are adherent to each other ('kissing ovaries').

Endometrioma and malignancy

In a study of 20 686 women with endometriosis and followed for a mean of 11.4 years, the authors found an increased risk for ovarian cancer among those patients with ovarian endometriosis.[11] However, malignancy rarely arises from endometriosis. The incidence is between 0.3% and 0.8%.[12]

Studying over 1000 cases of endometriosis, Stern et al[13] found that malignancies were more commonly found in endometriosis-containing ovaries

151

(5%) than at the extraovarian sites (1%).

The histopathology commonly linked with ovarian endometriosis is clear cell and endometrioid carcinoma, whereas clear cell adenosarcoma is most frequently associated with extraovarian endometriosis. An actual transition from endometriosis to endometrioid carcinoma can be demonstrated in only 5–10% of cases.[14–16] The relationship between endometriosis and cancer remains unclear.

Medical treatment

The use of medical treatment for endometrioma is limited. Ovarian endometrioma larger than 1 cm do not respond favorably to medical treatment with hormonal suppression.[17] Also, Muzii et al[18] reported that the preoperative use of gonadotropin-releasing hormone agonist (GnRH-a) offered no advantage to surgery or to the recurrence rate. Medical treatment is associated with symptomatic improvement in 50% of the patients but the symptoms tend to recur 6–12 months following cessation of therapy.[16–21] It also has no effect on pregnancy or on recurrence rates.

Laparotomy or laparoscopy?

Traditionally, endometrioma was removed by the laparotomy approach. With advances in laparoscopic techniques, most endometrioma can be treated by laparoscopy.[24–33] In fact, the laparoscopic approach is more effective than the laparotomy approach.[22,33]

Laparoscopic aspiration of endometrioma

Compared with the ultrasound approach, aspiration of endometrioma by laparoscopy allows the surgeon to perform a thorough irrigation and removal of the contents of the endometrioma. Furthermore, evaluation of the whole abdominal cavity can be performed. The diagnosis is more accurate, and the endometriosis can be staged and excised. However, as with ultrasound drainage of ovarian endometrioma, laparoscopic aspiration is associated with a high recurrence rate. The reported recurrence rate is 21–88% at 6-month follow-up.[29–31]

Donnez et al[33] studied the effect of GnRH-a following laparoscopic fenestration and drainage of endometrioma. At second-look laparoscopy 12 weeks later, the size of the endometrioma was reduced by 50%. However, all patients subsequently required further surgery for ablation of the cyst wall.

Two-step eversion technique

Based on the hypothesis that ovarian endometrioma develops as a consequence of invagination of the ovarian cortex and that active endometriosis is often found on the ovarian surface, a two-step laparoscopic technique was proposed.[34] In most cases, the site of the invagination or inversion can be seen as a dimple on the surface of the endometrioma.

The first step is biopsy of the endometriotic lesion, adhesiolysis, wide opening of the inversion site, and excision of the endometriotic rings. The second step is performed 2–3 months after the first laparoscopy. Laparoscopic adhesiolysis and coagulation of the neovascularization and the endometriotic implants are then performed. In 18 patients, Brosens reported no recurrence.[34] The drawback of this technique is the need for two laparoscopic procedures.

Laparoscopic fenestration and ablation of the cyst wall

Several studies have shown that laparoscopic treatment of ovarian endometrioma is as effective or better than that by laparotomy.[23,25,35] However, the choice of laparoscopic techniques remains controversial. In general, endometrioma is removed by excising the endometriotic cyst. Some authors prefer fenestration followed by ablation of the cyst wall using laser or electrocoagulation. The proponents of this technique believe that this procedure is associated with minimal loss of viable ovarian cortex and less adhesion formation.

Laparoscopic stripping or excision of the endometriotic cyst wall

Mettler and Semm[36] first performed laparoscopic treatment of endometrioma by removal of the endometriotic cyst wall. First the contents of the endometrioma are drained. The cyst wall is then stripped from the normal ovarian tissue. The recurrence rate after this procedure is 5–12%. All the procedures are done in a single laparoscopic setting.

In our practice, we try to enucleate the whole endometrioma intact[30] (Figures 13.2 and 13.3). However, it often ruptures. In this case, stripping of the cyst wall is performed (Figure 13.4). If endometriosis is found on the vermiform appendix, the appendix should be removed at the time of laparoscopy. Occasionally, the appendix is adherent to the ovary (Figure 13.5 and Figure 13.6).

Results of laparoscopic fenestration and ablation, and excision

There have been several studies on the results of different laparoscopic treatments of endometrioma (Table 13.1). Most were observational studies; confounding factors of postoperative medical treatment were not taken into consideration and the follow-up period was short.

In a retrospective study, Hemmings et al concluded that laparoscopic ablation is as effective as excision of the cyst wall.[29] Contrary to their findings, we found[30] that the recurrence rate after excision is significantly lower than that after ablation. This could be attributed to several factors. We studied a large number of patients and one laparoscopic surgeon performed excision. Furthermore, instead of using a crude rate, our results are reported using life table analysis. This analysis takes into account patients who already have reoperation and who are lost from follow-up at a given time.

Our findings support a randomized prospective study[28] that demonstrates the superiority of excision to fenestration and coagulation. It was found that the recurrence rates of dysmenorrhea, dyspareunia, and pelvic pain were lower and the pregnancy rate was higher in the excision group

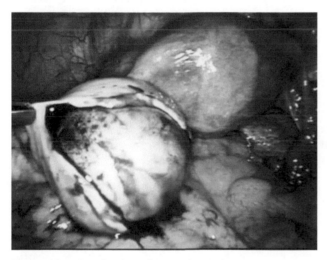

Figure 13.2 Enucleation of an endometrioma.

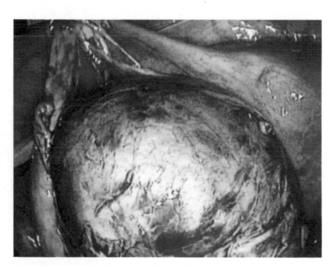

Figure 13.3 Enucleation of an endometrioma.

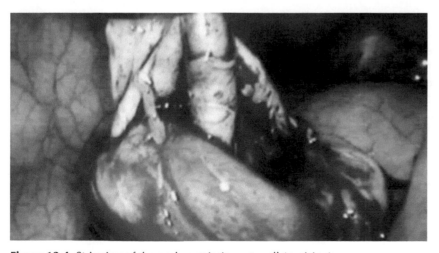

Figure 13.4 Stripping of the endometriotic cyst wall (excision).

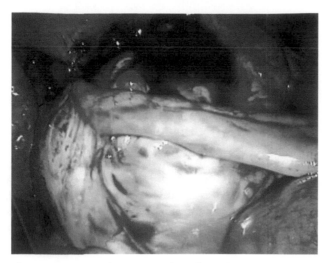

Figure 13.5 Vermiform appendix adhered to an ovarian endometrioma.

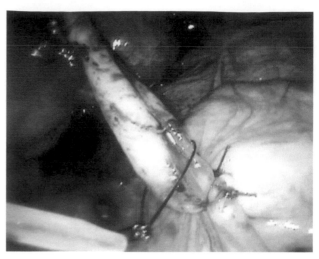

Figure 13.6 Removal of endometriosis containing appendix.

Table 13.1 Results of laparoscopic excision of ovarian endometrioma versus ablation of the cyst wall

Authors	Type of study	No. of patients	Type of treatment	Diameter (cm)	Length of follow-up (months)	No. of recurrences (%)
Fayez and Vogel (1991)[26]	Prospective, non-randomized	56	Ablation (n = 30) Excision (n = 26)	1–9	2–12	8 (26.7) 0
Hemmings et al (1998)[29]	Retrospective	103	Ablation (n = 80) Excision (n = 23)	4.6 4.8	36	10 (12.5) 2 (8.7)
Beretta et al (1998)[28]	Randomized trial	64	Ablation (n = 32) Excision (n = 32)	4.5 5.0	24	6 (18.8) 2 (6.2)
Saleh and Tulandi (1999)[30]	Retrospective	231	Ablation (n = 70) Excision (n = 161)	4.0 4.0	12–48	15 (21.4) 10 (6.2)

than in the fenestration group. The recurrence rate of endometrioma was 6.2% in the excision group and 18.8% in the fenestration group. This is in agreement with our reoperation rate at 18 months follow-up.[30] The concern of loss of viable ovarian tissue with excision is unfounded. Histopathology of the excised tissue in our series revealed absence of follicles in all specimens.

In a review, Vercellini et al[32] reported a threefold increased risk of cyst recurrence after coagulation or laser vaporization compared to excision: odds ratio (OR), 3.09; 95% confidence interval (CI), 1.78–5.36.

Ovarian response after conservative laparoscopic surgery

Some investigators feel that ovarian surgery might have a deleterious effect on the residual normal ovarian cortex. In a histopathologic study of 26 ovarian endometrioma, 54% of the endometriomas removed contained ovarian tissue.[31] However, the ovarian tissues adjacent to the cyst wall did not show the normal follicular pattern.

Clinically, in a retrospective study of 820 cycles,[33] the outcome of in vitro fertilization and embryo transfer (IVF-ET) after ablation of ovarian endometrioma was similar to that of tubal factors. The clinical pregnancy rate was 37.4% in the endometrioma group and 34.6% in the tubal factor group. The number of follicles and the number of mature oocytes were similar between the two groups. More importantly, the previously operated ovary had a similar response to the nonoperated contralateral ovary. In a smaller series, Marconi et al[37] reported similar findings.

Conclusions

Ovarian endometrioma larger than 1 cm do not respond favorably to medical treatment. Aspiration of endometrioma either by ultrasound or laparoscopy leads to a high recurrence rate in a short time. However, endometrioma aspiration before IVF might be beneficial to the IVF outcome.[38]

The best surgical treatment of ovarian endometrioma is laparoscopic excision of the cyst wall. The procedure is technically more demanding than laparoscopic fenestration and ablation of the cyst wall, but is associated with prolonged symptomatic improvement, a lower recurrence of pelvic pain, and a lower reoperation rate. The pregnancy rate after excision is also higher. Concerns that excision of the endometrioma will result in more adhesion formation and the loss of ovarian follicles are not supported by the results of a randomized study.

Studies to date have shown that laparoscopic excision of ovarian endometrioma results in a lower reoperation rate, a lower recurrence of symptoms, and a better improvement of pain compared with the ablation technique.

REFERENCES

1. Sampson JA. Peritoneal endometriosis due to menstrual dissemination of endometrial tissue into the peritoneal cavity. Am J Obstet Gynecol 1927; 14: 422–469.

2. Al-Fozan H, Tulandi T. Left lateral predisposition of endometriosis and endometrioma. Obstet Gynecol 2003; 101: 164–166.

3. Ajossa S, Mais V, Guerriero S, et al. The prevalence of endometriosis in premenopausal women undergoing gynecological surgery. Clin Exp Obstet Gynecol 1994; 21: 195–197.

4. Redwine DB. Ovarian endometriosis: a marker for more extensive pelvic and intestinal disease. Fertil Steril 1999; 72: 310–315.

5. Shaw RT. The role of GnRH analogues in the treatment of endometriosis. Br J Obstet Gynaecol 1992; 99: 9–12.

6. Hughesdon PE. The structure of endometriosis cysts of the ovary. J Obstet Gynaecol Br Emp 1957; 44: 69–84.

7. Brosens IA, Puttemans PJ, Deprest J. The endoscopic localization of endometrial implants in the ovarian chocolate cyst. Fertil Steril 1994; 61: 1034–1038.

8. Busacca M, Vigano P, Magri B, et al. The adhesion molecules on human endometrial stromal cells. Ann N Y Acad Sci 1994; 734: 43–46.

9. Vignali M, Infantino M, Matrone R, et al. Endometriosis: novel etiopathogenetic concepts and clinical perspectives. Fertil Steril 2002; 78: 665–678.

10. Jain S, Dalton ME. Chocolate cysts from ovarian follicles. Fertil Steril 1999; 72: 852–856.

11. Brinton LA, Gridley G, Persson I, et al. Cancer risk after a hospital discharge diagnosis of endometriosis. Am J Obstet Gynecol 1997; 176: 572–579.

12. Czeknobilsky B, Silverman BB, Mikuta JJ. Endometrioid carcinoma of the ovary: a clinicopathologic study of 75 cases. Cancer 1970; 26: 1141–1152.

13. Stern RC, Dash R, Bentley RC, et al. Malignancy in endometriosis: frequency and comparison of ovarian and extraovarian types. Int J Gynecol Pathol 2001; 20: 133–139.

14. Moll UM, Chumas JC, Chalas E, et al. Ovarian carcinoma arising in atypical endometrium. Obstet Gynecol 1990; 75: 537–539.

15. Romanini C, Ciavattini A, Cignitti M, et al. Endometrioid carcinoma arising in endometriosis: case report. Eur J Gynaecol Oncol 1992; 13: 228–230.

16. Sainz de la Cuesta R, Eichhorn JH, Rice LW, et al. Histologic transformation of benign endometriosis to early epithelial ovarian cancer. Gynecol Oncol 1996; 60: 238–244.

17. Buttram V, Reiter R, Ward S. Treatment of endometriosis with danazol: report of a 6-year prospective study. Fertil Steril 1985; 43: 353–360.

18. Muzii L, Marana R, Caruna P, et al. The impact of preoperative gonadotropin-releasing hormone agonist treatment on laparoscopic excision of ovarian endometriotic cysts. Fertil Steril 1996; 65: 1235–1237.

19. Donnez J, Nisolle M, Gillet N, et al. Large ovarian endometrioma. Hum Reprod 1996; 11: 641–646.

20. Schenken RS. Gonadotropin-releasing hormone analogs in the treatment of endometrioma. Am J Obstet Gynecol 1990; 162: 579–581.

21. Shaw RT. Treatment of endometriosis. Lancet 1992; 340: 1267–1271.

22. Bateman BG, Kolp LA, Mills S. Endoscopic versus laparotomy management of endometriomas. Fertil Steril 1994; 62: 690–695.

23. Catalano GF, Marana R, Caruona P. Laparoscopy versus microsurgery by laparotomy for excision of ovarian cyst in patients with moderate or severe endometriosis. J Am Assoc Gynecol Laparosc 1996; 3: 267–270.

24. Garry R. Laparoscopic excision of endometrioma: the treatment of choice? Br J Obstet Gynaecol 1997; 104: 513–515.

25. Crosignani G, Vercellini P, Biffignandi F, et al. Laparoscopy versus laparotomy in conservative surgical treatment for severe endometriosis. Fertil Steril 1996; 66: 706–711.

26. Fayez JA, Vogel MF. Comparison of different treatment methods of endometrioma by laparoscopy. Obstet Gynecol 1991; 78: 660–665.

27. Vercellini P, Vendola N, Bocciolone L, et al. Laparoscopic aspiration of ovarian endometriomas. Effect with postoperative gonadotropin releasing hormone agonist treatment. J Reprod Med 1992; 37: 577–580.

28. Beretta P, Franchi M, Ghezzi F, et al. Randomized clinical trial of two laparoscopic treatments of endometriomas: cystectomy versus drainage and coagulation. Fertil Steril 1998; 70: 1176–1180.

29. Hemmings R, Bissonnette F, Bouzayen R. Results of laparoscopic treatments of ovarian endometriomas: laparoscopic ovarian fenestration and coagulation. Fertil Steril 1998; 70: 527–529.

30. Saleh A, Tulandi T. Reoperation after laparoscopic treatment of ovarian endometriomas by excision and by fenestration. Fertil Steril 1999; 72: 322–324.

31. Muzii L, Bianchi A, Croce C, et al. Laparoscopic excision of ovarian cysts: is the stripping technique a tissue-sparing procedure? Fertil Steril 2002; 77: 609–614.

32. Vercellini P, Chapron C, De Giorgi O, et al. Coagulation or excision of ovarian endometrioma? Am J Obstet Gynecol 2003; 188: 606–610.

33. Donnez J, Wyns C, Nisolle M. Does ovarian surgery for endometriomas impair the ovarian response to gonadotropin? Fertil Steril 2001; 76: 662–665.

34. Brosens I. Management of ovarian endometriomas and pregnancy. Fertil Steril 1999; 71: 1166–1167.

35. Milingos S, Loutradis D, Kallipolitis G, et al. Comparison of laparoscopy with laparotomy for the treatment of extensive endometriosis with large endometriomata. J Gynecol Surg 1999; 15: 131–136.

36. Mettler L, Semm K. Three step medical and surgical treatment of endometriosis. Ir J Med Sci 1983; 152: 26–28.

37. Marconi G, Vilela M, Quintana R, et al. Laparoscopic ovarian cystectomy of endometriomas does not affect the ovarian response to gonadotropin stimulation. Fertil Steril 2002; 78: 876–878.

38. Aboulghar MA, Mansour RT, Serour GI, et al. Ultrasonic transvaginal aspiration of endometriotic cysts: an optional line of treatment in selected cases of endometriosis. Hum Reprod 1991; 6: 1408–1410.

14 KTP laser photocoagulation of ovarian endometriosis

Kevin Jones

Introduction

There is considerable controversy over the pathogenesis as well as the surgical management of ovarian endometriomas.[1] In 1957 Hughesdon suggested that bleeding from endometriotic implants on the posterior surface of the ovary caused the ovary to adhere to the peritoneum of the ovarian fossa.[2] Subsequent bleeding into the space enclosed by the adhesions prevents the escape of the blood and results in the invagination of the ovarian cortex as the endometrioma enlarges (Figures 14.1 and 14.2). If this hypothesis is correct, the endometrioma is a pseudocyst which can be mobilized, fenestrated, and then the pseudo-

cyst capsule ablated using a KTP (potassium titanyl phosphate) laser. The KTP laser penetrates tissue to a depth of between 70 and 200 µm and therefore does not damage the underlying follicles in the ovarian cortex.

The aim of ablative surgery is to relieve painful symptoms, improve fertility, and achieve a low cyst recurrence rate. It is also important to treat

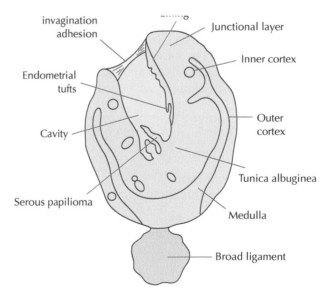

Figure 14.2 Sagittal section of an endometrioma showing invagination of the cortex due to bleeding from the ovarian fossa. The inside of the chocolate cyst is therefore the outside of the ovarian cortex. Reproduced from *BJOG*, Volume 64, Hughesdon PE, The structure of endometrial cysts of the ovary, with permission of the Royal College of Obstetricians and Gynaecologists.

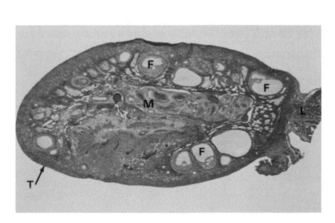

Figure 14.1 Monkey ovary. The outer connective tissue capsule (T), the outer cortex containing follicles (F), and the central vascular medulla zone (M), the broad ligament (L). Reprinted from *Whealer's Functional Histology*, 4th edn, Young & Heath, 2000, with permission from Elsevier.

other endometriotic deposits at the same time if the patient is to benefit from the operation, and this is discussed elsewhere in this book.

Patient selection

The indications and contraindications for a laparoscopic KTP laser ablation of an endometriotic cyst are set out in Table 14.1. Patients typically have a tender mass in the pelvis adherent to the pelvic side wall or, if it is a large cyst, it often fills the pouch of Douglas. Many cysts are bilateral and are often adherent to the back of the uterus, or small or large bowel, and sometimes even to each other (kissing ovaries). Endometriotic cysts are often associated with deeply infiltrating disease in the rectovaginal septum and patients may have palpable nodules in the posterior fornix of the vagina. To achieve complete symptom relief, all this disease must be eradicated, as described in other chapters in this book.

The severity of chronic nonmenstrual pelvic pain, dysmenorrhea, dyspareunia, and dyschezia, may be assessed using a linear analogue score (0 is no pain, and 10 is the worst pain imaginable), or quality of life indicators may also be applied. If infertility is an issue, the patient should have undergone tests to confirm that ovulation is occurring. Her rubella status should be known, and she should have been tested and, if necessary, treated for *Chlamydia* infection. If indicated, her serum gonadotropin levels (follicle-stimulating hormone (FSH) and luteinizing hormone (LH)), prolactin level, and testosterone and sex hormone binding globulin (SHBG) levels should also be measured. A test of tubal patency can be carried out during the laser laparoscopy. To complete the fertility investigations, the patient's partner should have undergone a seminal fluid analysis.

A transvaginal ultrasound scan (TVS) should be carried out to measure the dimensions of the cyst and to exclude other pathologic causes for the pelvic pain. If there is any doubt about the nature of the cyst, a magnetic resonance imaging (MRI) scan may be helpful. Cancer antigen CA-125 levels are sometimes measured, but these can be raised in patients with endometriosis, particularly if an endometrioma is present, as well as epithelial cancers of the ovary.

Perioperative management

KTP laser laparoscopy may be carried out in an ambulatory day surgical hospital or as an inpatient. Potential complications must be discussed, including the need for conversion to a laparotomy for visceral injury, especially bowel injury, and informed consent for laparotomy must be obtained. Bowel preparation using a bowel cleansing solution is carried out: e.g. Citramag (Bioglan Labratories, Herts, UK) 1 sachet dissolved in 200 ml of water and taken during the evening before the procedure. In addition, a rectal washout may be undertaken immediately prior to the operation using chlorhexidine solution.

Operating room set-up

The patient is asked to void before coming into the operating suite or a urinary catheter is passed once

---

Table 14.1 Indications and contraindications for a KTP laser ablation of an endometrioma

General indications
Pelvic pain, particularly dyspareunia and dysmenorrhea, and subfertility associated with endometriosis

Specific indications
Endometriotic cyst identified
To assist conception or prior to assisted conception (IVF)

Contraindication(s)
Laparoscopic surgery contraindicated for medical reasons
Surgeon not trained in the use of the KTP laser
Ovarian cyst suspicious of malignancy on ultrasound and/or MRI

Relative contraindication(s)
Medical therapy effective, with minimal side effects/no desire to conceive

IVF = in vitro fertilization; KTP = potassium titanyl phosphate; MRI = magnetic resonance imaging.

the operative field has been cleaned and draped. The procedure is carried out under general anesthetic. The patient wears flowtron (or graduated compression stockings) boots to prevent deep vein thrombosis. If she is at particular risk of thromboembolism, subcutaneous heparin is administered preoperatively. She is then placed in the lithotomy position (Lloyd-Davis poles for the legs), with her arms secured in a position parallel to her sides. A pneumoperitonium is induced and ports are inserted according to the Middlesbrough consensus guidelines.[3] A KTP laser is then set up, according to local guidelines for the safe use of lasers.

Technical description

The capsule wall is vaporized with a KTP laser (Laserscope, Cwymbran, UK; San Jose, CA, USA) at a power setting of 18 W. The energy is generated from an Nd:YAG laser and the beam is then passed through a crystal of potassium titanyl phosphate (KTP). This results in doubling the frequency and halving the wavelength from 1064 nm to 532 nm, which is in the visible part of the electromagnetic spectrum and produces an emerald green light (Figure 14.3) and avoids the need for an aiming beam.

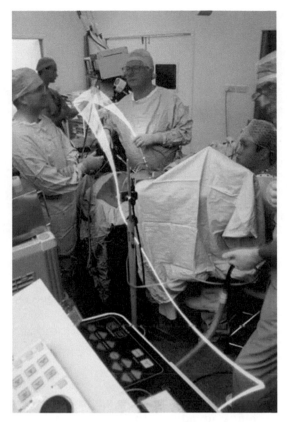

Figure 14.3 The emerald green light of the KTP laser. Reprinted from *Endoscopic Surgery for Gynaecologists*, edited by Chris Sutton and Michael Diamond, 1993, with permission from Elsevier.

The KTP laser penetrates soft tissue to a depth of between 70 and 200 μm with minimal lateral scatter, making it much safer to use within the abdominal cavity than the bare fiber of an Nd:YAG laser. In addition, because there is no need for sapphire tips or sculpted fibers, the surgeon can get a great many uses out of a single fiber since it can be resterilized. The wavelength at which the KTP laser operates is close to the absorption peak for hemosiderin and hemoglobin and it is selectively taken up by tissue of this color, making it particularly useful for the ablation of endometriomas by a photoactive effect. The CO_2 laser is absorbed by fluid and it is unsuited to use in a wet environment. Surgeons who use the CO_2 laser to treat endometriomas generally carry out a two-stage procedure for this reason: aspirating the endometrioma and treating peritoneal disease at the initial laparoscopy, and then administering a gonadotropin-releasing hormone (GnRH) analogue for 3–6 months prior to ablating the pseudocapsule with the CO_2 laser at a second laparoscopy. The KTP laser does not become contaminated with charred blood and hemosiderin during the ablation, which frequently happens with a bipolar electrosurgical device, but it does need to be recleaved at intervals. This is an important advantage the KTP laser has to maintain effec-

tive power-density over electrosurgery for ablation of endometriomas.

Operation

The cervix is grasped by a vulsellum forceps attached to the anterior lip and the uterine cavity is then cannulated with a dilator to manipulate the pelvic organs during the procedure. The KTP laser is charged up, and the laser fibers inserted through the suction irrigation device so that the fiber tip can be extended or retracted at will (Figure 14.4). A safety shutter must be incorporated between the eyepiece of the laparoscope and the camera, and this is activated whenever the laser is fired. This avoids the need for operating room personnel to have to wear safety goggles.

The ovary is mobilized from the pelvic side wall using a combination of blunt and sharp dissection with a strong stainless steel probe. Dense adhesions need to be divided by laparoscopic scissors, taking great care to avoid the ureter, which runs

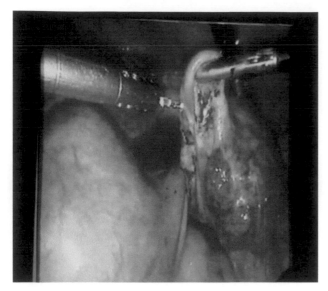

Figure 14.4 The KTP laser being used inside the pelvis. Reproduced from *Endometriosis*, 2004, with permission of the Royal College of Obstetricians and Gynaecologists.

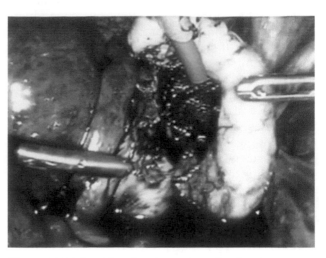

Figure 14.6 The ablated endometrioma healing by secondary intention. Reproduced from *Endometriosis*, 2004, with permission of the Royal College of Obstetricians and Gynaecologists.

directly underneath the area where the endometrioma tends to adhere to the ovarian fossa. The ovary is gradually levered upwards and away from the ovarian fossa. Where possible, the endometrioma is opened at the site of invagination during mobilization. During this process, the cyst may rupture; if it does not, it is fenestrated with laparoscopic scissors (Figure 14.5), and the chocolate fluid is then aspirated using the suction irrigation device. Prior to activating the KTP laser, the pelvis is irrigated with heparinized Hartmann's solution until all the hemosiderin has been removed, and

then the cyst wall is inspected. If there are any features suspicious of additional pathology, it is biopsied. The capsule wall is then vaporized with a KTP laser at a power setting of 18 W. The KTP laser will photovaporize tissue if it is held in contact with the surface, and photocoagulate tissue if it is pulled slightly away from the tissue. Hemostasis is achieved, and the ovary is then left to heal by secondary intention (Figure 14.6). Any coexisting endometriosis is ablated, and at the end of the operation the pelvic organs are aquafloated with heparinized Hartmann's solution or an adhesion barrier.

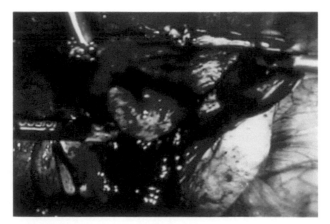

Figure 14.5 The endometrioma being fenestrated and the hemosiderin being drained. Reproduced from *Endometriosis*, 2004, with permission of the Royal College of Obstetricians and Gynaecologists.

Postoperative course

Patients generally recover quickly from laser laparoscopies and they can be discharged home the same day. Patients who do not want to conceive are prescribed a GnRH analogue or the combined oral contraceptive pill for 3 months following the procedure. Those patients who initially presented with infertility are encouraged to try and get pregnant as soon as possible after the operation. Patients are offered a postoperative TVS at 3, 6, and 12 months, and a detailed medical history is recorded using a structured questionnaire at each clinic visit. This enables the surgeon to detect recurrent cysts at an early stage, and it also avoids the routine use of second-look laparoscopies.

Clinical evidence

The KTP laser has been used for many years to ablate endometriotic cysts. The outcomes following surgery have been reported in a retrospective study[4] and most recently in a large prospective cohort series.[5–7] The objectives of the prospective study were to determine:

- the recurrence rate of chocolate cysts
- the need for a repeat surgical procedure
- the change in pain scores
- patient satisfaction
- the cumulative pregnancy rate over 12 months.

There were 96 cysts (23 bilateral) in the 73 women (1 patient underwent a two-stage procedure). The mean age of the women was 33.4 years (range 20–43) and the mean diameter of the endometrioma was 4.79 cm (range 2–25). The median revised American Fertility Society (r-AFS) score was 56 (range 22–128), and 55 (75.3%) patients had stage IV disease. At 12 months, 5 (6.9%) patients have been lost to follow-up and 12 patients had a recurrent cyst. Therefore, the cyst recurrence rate/patient was 12/73 (16.4%) and the cyst recurrence rate/cyst was 12/96 (12.5%). Eighteen patients had repeat operations (including operations on recurrent cysts): therefore, the reoperation rate was 18/73 (24.6%) per patient.[5] There were no major surgical complications.

Pre- and postoperative visual analogue scores for pelvic pain were completed. Patient satisfaction was scored from 1 to 10, with 10 being most satisfied. At 12 months, the mean temporal decrease in pain score for dyspareunia was 2.14 ± 0.41 ($p < 0.001$), for dysmenorrhea 1.52 ± 0.38 ($p < 0.001$), and for chronic nonmenstrual pain 2.37 ± 0.43 ($p < 0.001$). Sixty-four (87.7%) patients were satisfied or very satisfied with the treatment.[6]

A subgroup of 39 women (38 intention to treat as a single procedure) who had been trying to conceive for >12 months was also followed up. Seven patients (18%) had previously had a live birth, and 17 (43.6%) had undergone assisted conception in the past. The cumulative pregnancy rate was 15/38 (39.5%).[7]

The results of this study[5–7] compare favorably with other cohort studies where ablation has been carried out to treat endometriomas (Tables 14.2 and 14.3). However, these results also need to be compared to the results following excisional surgery. In order to do this, a logistic regression analysis was carried out to compare laparoscopic excision with ablation for endometriotic cysts.[17] Four comparative studies were identified. Cyst recurrence (%, ± SE) was twice as likely for the ablation treatment (26.6%, ± 0.032) than for the excision treatment (13.2%, ± 0.019), ($p < 0.005$, relative risk, 1.9). Two comparative studies were identified where post-procedure pregnancy rates were an outcome measure. Postoperative pregnancy rates (%, ± SE) were not significantly different for the ablation treatment (41.6%, ± 0.138) than for the excision treatment (56.9%, ± 0.23). There is only one comparative study to investigate symptom relief; therefore, logistic regression analysis is not possible. Three studies have compared excisional surgery and perioperative medication with excisional surgery only. Cyst recurrence rates (%, ± SE) were not significantly different for the group who received medication (10.3%, ± 0.033) than for those that did not (4.0%, ± 0.02). Although this study demonstrates that ablation (in general) compares less favorably with

Table 14.2 Recurrence rates following the laparoscopic ablation of the endometriomas

Main author	Year	N	Follow-up (months)	Medication	Recurrence rate (%)
Marrs[8]	1991	31	6	Yes	3.2
Fayez[9]	1991	30	2	Yes	33
Donnez[10]	1996	814	2–11 years	Yes	8
Brosens[11]	1996	18	30.5	Nil	0
Sutton[4]	1997	165	6	Nil	12.5–30
Hemmings[12]	1998	80	36	Nil	8
Beretta[13]	1998	64	24	Nil	6.2
Saleh[14]	1999	70	18	Nil	21.9

N = Number of patients reported on.

Table 14.3 Pregnancy rates following the laparoscopic ablation of the endometriomas

Main author (%)	Year	N	Intervention	Pregnancy rate
Daniell[15]	1991	32	Laser ablation and cyst stripping	44
Marrs[8]	1991	23	KTP laser ablation	30.4
Montanino[16]	1996	13	Cyst stripping + GnRH-a	45
Donnez[10]	1996	814	CO_2 laser ablation + GnRH-a	51
Sutton[4]	1995	24	CO_2 + KTP laser vaporization	57
Hemmings[12]	1998	84	Cyst stripping vs electrocoagulation	50–60
Beretta[13]	1998	26	Cyst stripping vs electrocoagulation	66.7–23.5

N = number of infertile patients reported on; GnRH-a = gonadotropin-releasing hormone agonist; KTP = potassium titanyl phosphate.

cyst excision, in terms of cyst recurrence, ablation with the KTP laser (12.5%)[5] is as effective as cyst excision (13.2%).[17]

Discussion

General considerations

The main reasons for using an ablative technique rather than cyst excision to treat endometriomas focus on the nature of the endometriotic cyst and the potential damage to ovarian follicles. If endometriotic cysts originate by implantation,[2] then the disease is superficial and the pseudocyst capsule can be ablated with minimal loss of normal tissue. The lack of the cleavage plane of the 'true' endometrioma and the effect that resection may have on follicular reserve reinforces the argument that the cyst should be left in situ and the wall ablated.

There are several studies which suggest that excision may be harmful to the follicular reserve, which lies close to the cleavage plane of the cyst.[10] Loh et al demonstrated that the follicular response in natural and clomiphene citrate stimulated cycles for women <35 years old was reduced after laparoscopic ovarian cystectomy.[18] The effect endometriomas have on in vitro fertilization and embryo transfer (IVF–ET) cycle outcome also suggests that excision is harmful. Seventeen patients with endometriomas were compared to 44 patients who had undergone ovarian cystectomy. The patients with endometriomas had higher ongoing pregnancy rates per IVF cycle (50%; confidence interval (CI), 24–75%) compared with controls (25%; CI, 17–35%). There was also a consistent reduction in oocyte yields from postcystectomy ovaries com-

pared with intact ovaries, despite different ovarian stimulation protocols.[19] Adverse changes in ovarian artery blood flow have also been reported following laparoscopic stripping.[20]

There are a number of potential limitations inherent in the management strategy described in this chapter:

1. The diagnosis of an endometrioma depends on a combination of visual inspection and selective biopsy.

- The main concern is that a malignancy will be missed. The frequency of a malignant tumor arising in ovarian endometriosis ranges from 0.3 to 0.8%, and most of these tumors are well-differentiated endometrioid carcinomas.[21]
- Histologic confirmation of a suspected endometrioma may vary from 0 to 100%.[1]
- The visual diagnosis of an endometrioma (96%) is sufficiently accurate to rely on it in most clinical situations.[22]

Because of this, ovarian biopsy, although desirable in some cases, is often dispensable for a correct laparoscopic diagnosis.

2. TVS is the most widely used noninvasive method for identifying endometriomas. The sensitivity varies between 83 and 88.9%, the specificity between 89 and 99.1%, the positive predictive values range from 78 to 94%, and the negative predictive values range from 92.8 to 98.2%.[23] On the basis of these data, TVS is a reliable method of identifying endometriotic cysts in clinical practice.

3. A 3-month course of GnRH-a has been shown to significantly improve pelvic pain, as well as

quality of life.[24] Furthermore, 3–6 months of post-operative treatment with a GnRH-a has been shown to prolong the pain-free interval after conservative surgery for endometriosis, and this effect can persist for up to 12 months.[25,26] Therefore, the beneficial effects of KTP laser ablation can be improved by adopting a management strategy that combines surgery and medical therapy.

Recurrence rates

A retrospective review of patients with endometriomas who were treated with the KTP laser has been reported.[4] The cyst recurrence rate per patient was 12.5%. In the prospective series from the same unit, similar cyst recurrence rates (12.5%/cyst vs 16.4%/patient) were observed.[5] The data have also been plotted as a survival analysis (Figure 14.7). This type of analysis takes into account patients who have already undergone a repeat operation and those who have been lost to follow-up at any given time. Eighteen patients, 18/73 (24.7%) in the prospective series had repeat operations (including operations on recurrent cysts) at 12 months. Therefore, it appears that the reoperation rates following a KTP ablation are high compared to other groups. This may be explained by examining a prospective, multicenter cohort study of 366 patients who had a minimum of 6 months follow-up.[27] Six risk factors were evaluated to assess their effect on two separate outcomes. The cumulative rate of cyst recurrence over 48 months was 11.7% and of second surgery was 8.2%. In this study, ultrasonographic cyst recurrence was not associated with pain recurrence in 27.5% of cases. This suggests that if patients are not followed up with serial TVS or a second-look laparoscopy, the recurrence rates will be under-reported. Because serial postoperative TVS was performed on every patient in the prospective series, the reported recurrence rates are comparatively higher. The stage of the disease and previous surgery for endometriosis were also shown to be unfavorable prognostic factors.[27] Of the patients who had a cyst recurrence following KTP ablation, 50% had a previous laparotomy, whereas 37.7% patients who did not have a cyst recurrence had a previous laparotomy. These data suggest that previous open surgery may be a risk factor for cyst recurrence, which is likely to be due to surgical adhesions.

Pain relief

The major decreases in pain occurred during the first 3 months, and these effects persist at 12 months following surgery (Figure 14.8).[6] There are a number of other papers reporting pain relief following laparoscopic surgery for endometriomas.[28] Unfortunately, all of these studies lack an objective measurement of pain such as a visual analogue score; nor do they analyze individual symptoms. It could be argued that these authors are reporting an expression of 'patient satisfaction' with the procedure, rather than quantifiable, objective measurements of change. In a prospective series, 64 (87.7%) patients[6] who were treated with a KTP laser were satisfied or very satisfied with the treatment at 12 months, and this compares favorably with other studies.[28]

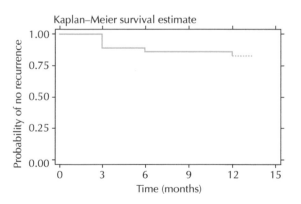

Figure 14.7 A 'survival' plot for cyst recurrence with time (Kaplan–Meier method for censored data). Reprinted from *AAGL*, Volume 9, Jones KD and Sutton CJ, Recurrence of chocolate cysts after laparoscopic ablation, 315–320, 2002, with permission from the American Association of Gynecologic Laparoscopists.

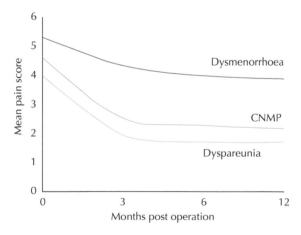

Figure 14.8 The temporal changes in pain scores. CNMP = chronic non-menstral pain. Reprinted from *Fertility and Sterility*, Volume 79, Jones KD et al, Patient satisfaction and changes in pain scores, after ablative laparoscopic surgery for stage III-IV endometriosis and endometriomas, 1086–1090, 2003, with permission from the American Society for Reproductive Medicine.

Fertility

The fertility outcome following KTP ablation has been documented in a retrospective review of 66 infertile patients with endometriomas.[4] The cumulative pregnancy rate was 35% at 12 months, and 45% at 36 months. The interval between laparoscopy and conception was 12 months for 77% of the women. These beneficial effects on fer-

tility following KTP laser ablation have been supported by prospective studies which demonstrate similar cumulative pregnancy rates at 12 months (35% vs 39%) (Figure 14.9).[7] There are only three other prospective studies in the literature where pregnancy rates following ablative laparoscopic surgery are reported (Table 14.3) and only one of these authors carried out the ablation with a KTP laser (pregnancy rate 30.4%).[8]

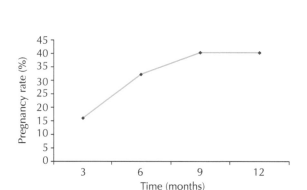

Figure 14.9 The cumulative pregnancy rate over 12 months. Reproduced from Jones KD, Sutton CJG, Pregnancy rates following ablative laparoscopic surgery for endometriomas. *Human Reproduction* 2002; 17(3): 782–785, with permission of European Society of Human Reproduction and Embryology.

Conclusion

There are plausible histologic arguments suggesting that ablation of the endometriotic pseudocyst capsule is a better operative technique than excision or electrosurgical ablation. These arguments are supported by large retrospective and prospective cohort studies which have demonstrated that a management strategy based on KTP laser ablation is clinically effective and safe. Compared to excision, cyst recurrence was on average twice as likely in patients undergoing ablative surgery. However, the favorable cyst recurrence rate after excision was similar to the recurrence rate following ablation with the KTP laser. There was no demonstrable difference between excision and ablation for postoperative pregnancy rates or for pain relief.

REFERENCES

1. Jones KD, Sutton CJG. Endometriotic cysts: the case for ablative laparoscopic surgery. Gynaecolog Endosc 2002; 10: 281–287.
2. Hughesdon PE. The structure of endometrial cysts of the ovary. J Obstet Gynaecol Br Emp 1957; 44: 481–487.
3. Garry R. A consensus document concerning laparoscopic entry techniques: Middlesbrough, March 19–20, 1999. Gynaecol Endosc 1999; 8: 327–334.
4. Sutton CJG, Ewen SP, Jacobs SA, et al. Laser laparoscopic surgery in the treatment of ovarian endometriomas. J Am Assoc Gynecol Laparosc 1997; 4(3): 319–323.
5. Jones KD, Sutton CJG. Recurrence of chocolate cysts after laparoscopic ablation. J Am Assoc Gynecol Laparosc 2002; 9(3): 27–32.
6. Jones KD, Sutton CJG. Patient satisfaction and changes in pain scores, after ablative laparoscopic surgery for stage III-IV endometriosis and endometriomas. Fertil Steril 2003; 79: 1086–1090.
7. Jones KD, Sutton CJG. Pregnancy rates following ablative laparoscopic surgery for endometriomas. Hum Reprod 2002; 17(3): 782–785.
8. Marrs RP. The use of potassium-titanyl-phosphate laser for laparoscopic removal of ovarian endometrioma. Am J Obstet Gynecol 1991; 164: 1622–1628.
9. Fayez JA, Vogel MF. Comparison of different treatment methods of endometriomas by laparoscopy. Obstet Gynecol 1991; 78: 660–665.
10. Donnez, J, Nisolle M, Gillet N, et al. Large ovarian endometriomas. Hum Reprod 1996; 11(3): 641–646.
11. Brosens IA, Van Ballaer P, Puttemans P, et al. Reconstruction of the ovary containing large endometriomas by an extraovarian endosurgical technique. Fertil Steril 1996; 66: 517–521.
12. Hemmings R, Bissonnette F, Bouzayen R. Result of laparoscopic treatments of ovarian endometriomas:

laparoscopic ovarian fenestration and coagulation. Fertil Steril 1998; 70: 527–529.

13. Beretta P, Franchi M, Ghezzi F, et al. Randomized clinical trial of two laparoscopic treatments of endometriomas: cystectomy versus drainage and coagulation. Fertil Steril 1998; 70(6): 1176–1180.

14. Saleh A, Tulandi T. Reoperation after laparoscopic treatment of endometriomas by excision and fenestration. Fertil Steril 1999; 72: 322–324.

15. Daniell JF, Kurtz BR, Gurley LD. Laser laparoscopic management of large endometriomas. Fertil Steril 1991; 55(4): 692–695.

16. Montanino G, Porpora MG, Montanino Oliva M, et al. Laparoscopic treatment of ovarian endometrioma. One year follow-up. Clin Exp Obstet Gynecol 1996; 23: 70–72.

17. Jones KD, Wright JT. Ablative or excisional laparoscopic surgery for endometriotic cysts: resolving the issue. J Am Assoc Gynecol Laparosc 2004: 11: 293–296.

18. Loh FH, Tan A, Kumar J, et al. Ovarian response after laparoscopic ovarian cystectomy for endometriotic cysts in 132 monitored cycles. Fertil Steril 1999; 72: 316–321.

19. Nargund G, Cheng WC, Parsons J. The impact of ovarian cystectomy on ovarian response to stimulation during in-vitro fertilisation cycles. Hum Reprod 1996; 11: 81–83.

20. La Torre R, Montanino-Oliva M, Marchiani E, et al. Ovarian blood flow before and after conservative laparoscopic treatment for endometrioma. Clin Exp Obstet Gynecol 1998; 25(1–2): 12–14.

21. Heaps JM, Nieberg RK, Berek JS. Malignant neoplasms arising in endometriosis. Obstet Gynecol 1990; 75: 1023–1028.

22. Vercellini P, Vendola N, Bocciolone L, et al. Reliability of the visual diagnosis of ovarian endometriosis. Fertil Steril 1991; 56: 1198–1200.

23. Jones KD, Sutton CJG. Laparoscopic management of ovarian endometriomas: a critical review of current practice. Curr Opin Obstet Gynecol 2000; 12: 309–315.

24. Vercellini P, De Giorgi O, Mosconi P, et al. Cyproterone acetate versus a continuous monophasic oral contraceptive in the treatment of recurrent pelvic pain after conservative surgery for symptomatic endometriosis. Fertil Steril 2002; 77(1): 52–61.

25. Vercellini P, Crosignani PG, Fadini R, et al. A gonadotrophin-releasing hormone agonist compared with expectant management after conservative surgery for symptomatic endometriosis. Br J Obstet Gynaecol 1999; 106(7): 672–677.

26. Hornstein MD, Yuzpe AA, Burry KA, et al. Prospective randomized double-blind trial of 3 versus 6 months of nafarelin therapy for endometriosis associated pelvic pain. Fertil Steril 1995; 65(5): 955–962.

27. Busacca M, Marana R, Caruana et al. Recurrence of ovarian endometrioma after laparoscopic excision. Am J Obstet Gynecol 1999; 180: 519–523.

28. Jones KD, Sutton CJG. Does laparoscopic surgery for endometriomas really relieve painful symptoms ? Gynaecol Surg 2002; 18(2): 39–43.

15 Pelvic denervation procedures as surgical management of pelvic pain due to endometriosis

Stefano Palomba and Fulvio Zullo

Introduction

Most primary care physicians consider pelvic pain as a common clinical problem which accounts for as much as 25% of routine gynecologic office visits.[1] About 15% of cases of pelvic pain are due to endometriosis.[2] Endometriosis is frequently associated with several types of pelvic pain such as dysmenorrhea, chronic pelvic pain, deep dyspareunia, and, occasionally, painful defecation. Specifically, endometriosis was found in 37–74% of women undergoing laparoscopy for chronic pelvic pain.[3–5]

The endometriosis-related pelvic pain has no relation with the localization of the lesions[3–5] and with the stage of the disease, as categorized according to the revised American Fertility Society (r-AFS) classification.[6] In fact, the r-AFS classification system is inadequate to express the severity of the symptomatology because it does not reflect the disease in terms of cellular mass or activity.[5,7–9]

Several medical treatments have been proposed to treat secondary chronic pelvic pain due to endometriosis,[2] but little data are available regarding the effectiveness of these treatments on quality of life of women with endometriosis,[2] which seems to be deeply impaired.[9,10]

About 20% of women with chronic pelvic pain due to endometriosis are unresponsive to medical treatment.[2] In these selected cases, surgery represents the final diagnostic and therapeutic option.[2,11,12] Several procedures have been described to treat medically untreatable pelvic pain.[13] Furthermore, nonconservative procedures such as hysterectomy[14,15] are questionably effective in terms of pain relief, can even be associated with a decrease in quality of life,[16] and are unacceptable to many woman who wish to preserve intact their reproductive organs.

Several publications show that conservative surgical treatment of endometriosis is effective, and sometimes even curative, in terms of pain relief[17–19] and quality of life[20] in women with secondary pelvic pain. Based on these considerations, other surgical procedures can be primarily utilized or added to surgical endometriosis treatment[21] such as the interruption of a majority of cervical and uterine sensory nerve fibers. These procedures are known as pelvic denervations and consist essentially in two specific surgical interventions: the uterosacral ligaments resection (USR), also called uterine nerve ablation (UNA), and the presacral neurectomy (PSN).

In this chapter we shall first illustrate briefly the anatomy of the autonomic nerves of the pelvis and then describe both pelvic denervation procedures with particular regard to surgical technique, safety, and effectiveness.

Anatomy of the autonomic nerves of the pelvis

The anatomy of the autonomic nerves of the pelvis has been well described by Curtis et al[22] more than

60 years ago in a series of 30 cadaveric dissections. In Figure 15.1 are shown the major anatomic structures involved in the pelvic denervation procedures. The lumbar and lower thoracic sympathetic ganglia, and the superior, middle, and inferior hypogastric plexus provide the afferent pathways for the pelvic viscera.[22] The pain afferent fibers from the ovaries and distal fallopian tubes travel to the aortic and renal plexus via the infundibulopelvic ligaments.[22] The sigmoid colon also sends visceral afferents to the inferior mesenteric plexus.[22] Pain afferents from the uterus, cervix, and proximal fallopian tubes travel with the sympathetic nerves via the uterosacral and cardinal ligaments to join with the pelvic plexus (Lee–Frankenhäuser plexus).[22]

The fibers from the pelvic plexus course proximally to become the inferior, the middle hypogastric plexus, and then the superior hypogastric plexus.[22] Over the sacral promontory there is only the middle hypogastric plexus. Instead, the superior hypogastric plexus is in front of the fifth lumbar vertebrae.[22] The presacral nerve is a direct extension of the aortic plexus below the aortic bifurcation. This plexus spreads out behind the peritoneum in loose areolar tissue lying over the fourth and fifth lumbar vertebrae.[22]

Between the vertebrae and the presacral nerve lies the middle sacral artery. The superior and middle hypogastric plexus lie on the left and in the midline in about 75 and 25% of cases, respectively.[22] In no cases has this plexus been observed on the right.[22] The right ureter and common iliac vessels are on the right of the presacral nerve, whereas on the left lies the sigmoid colon, inferior mesenteric vessels, and left ureter.[22] The left ureter is frequently obscured by the sigmoid colon.[22]

Uterosacral ligament resection

USR consists of the resection or ablation of a segment of at least 1 cm in depth and length of the uterosacral ligaments at their uterine junction. Clear identification of uterosacral ligaments is a prerequisite for the use of diathermy or lasers; in fact, the posterior leaf of the broad ligament should be carefully inspected to identify the course of ureters, which on rare occasions can be particularly close to the uterosacral ligaments. The excision of uterosacral ligaments at their attachment to the cervix interrupts most of the sympathetic fibers deriving from the superior hypogastric plexus and the parasympathetic fibers from S2, S3, and S4,

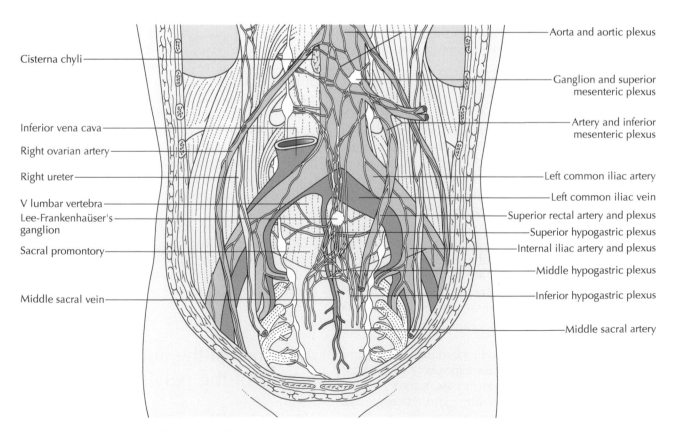

Figure 15.1 Anatomy of pelvic innervation

resulting in a reduction of pelvic pain. In fact, the uterosacral ligaments carry many of the afferent sensory nerve fibers to the lower parts of the uterus by way of the Lee–Frankenhäuser plexus, which lies in and around the uterosacral ligaments as they insert into the posterior cervix.

USR may be more effective if accompanied by resection also of the connective fiber tissues bridging the posterior aspect of the cervix from left to right uterosacral ligament and lower isthmic region where the nerve fibers coalesce.[23] In these cases, care should be taken to identify thin-walled pelvic veins, which often lie lateral to the uterosacral ligaments.

Finally, if endometriotic lesions are localized on the uterosacral ligament, the ligaments should be excised along with the endometriotic glands and stroma and any associated fibromuscular hyperplasia. This then becomes a radical excision of the uterosacral complex and is fully described in Chapter 21.

Safety

The USR is a simple and feasible surgical procedure associated with no specific intraoperative complications.[20] Rare complications reported are ureter injury and bleeding from the veins that lie just medial to the uterosacral ligament.

Although the precise role of the uterosacral ligaments in supporting the uterus has not been completely clarified, there is concern that USR may results in rare cases of uterine prolapse.[24]

Effectiveness

In his original paper, Doyle[25] demonstrated that by transecting the uterosacral ligaments close to their point of origin on the cervix it was possible to achieve complete pain relief in 86.0% of women with primary dysmenorrhea and in 86.8% of cases of secondary dysmenorrhea.

Few papers have been produced throughout the years on this surgical procedure, specifically with regard to the endometriosis-related pelvic pain.

The advent of laparoscopy has simplified the surgical procedure, making this technique mini-invasive. A survey of gynecologic practice in the UK has, in fact, shown that 45% of laparoscopic surgeons perform laparoscopic UNA (LUNA) routinely during the surgical treatment of endometriosis.[26]

The efficacy of the procedure has been initially evaluated in uncontrolled studies.[27,28] In a series of 100 patients who were treated with LUNA using the CO_2 laser and were followed up for more than 12 months, 50% experienced complete relief of symptoms and 41% experienced a mild or moderate decrease.[27] Also, Corson et al[28] showed a significant improvement of dysmenorrhea in about 70% of patients with endometriosis-related pelvic pain treated with LUNA.

Only recently has the effectiveness of USR and LUNA been studied in randomized controlled trials (RCTs).[29–32] In particular, Vercellini et al[29] have evaluated the efficacy of laparoscopic USR in 81 women with moderate and severe midline endometriosis-related dysmenorrhea treated with conservative surgery consisting of the simple excision of the endometriotic lesions. After a mean follow-up of 9 months, the USR addition did not produce any benefit in terms of frequency and severity of postoperative recurrence of dysmenorrhea. In fact, according to the Kaplan–Meier method, the 12-month cumulative probability of recurrence of moderate/severe dysmenorrhea was 33.7% and 27.5% in the groups treated with laparoscopic conservative surgery plus USR and with laparoscopic conservative surgery alone, respectively. The same authors, in a more complete paper,[30] have confirmed their previous results,[29] concluding that addition of LUNA to conservative laparoscopic surgery for endometriosis did not reduce the medium- or long-term frequency and severity of recurrence of dysmenorrhea.

Also, in a well-designed RCT on 51 women affected by pelvic pain and endometriosis at stages I–III, Sutton et al[32] have confirmed that the laparoscopic laser ablation of endometriotic lesions is effective, and that the addition of LUNA is not related to a significant improvement in pain symptomatology. Specifically, after 3- and 6-month follow-up, the improvement in chronic dysmenorrhea and nonmenstrual pain was significantly higher in the women who did not receive LUNA as an additive procedure. More recently, in another RCT, Johnson et al[31] have shown that LUNA was effective in terms of dysmenorrhea relief in women with primary chronic pelvic pain, whereas no benefit in any pain outcomes was observed in patients with endometriosis-related pelvic pain when the procedure was added to conservative treatment of endometriosis.

About 1 year ago, a multicenter RCT on a large sample, having as objectives to test the efficacy in terms of quality of life assessment of LUNA in women with primary and secondary (mild endometriosis with r-AFS score <5) pelvic pain, has been started[33] and the results are awaited with interest.

For ethical reasons, no study has evaluated the efficacy of URS alone vs the conservative treatment of endometriosis alone, whereas only one study has evaluated the effectiveness of USR as an additive procedure to PSN in women with pelvic pain and has shown, furthermore, no significant benefit.[34]

Presacral neurectomy

PSN involves the total transection of the presacral nerves lying within the boundaries of the Cotte's interiliac triangle.

We feel that the surgical steps should not differ between the laparoscopic and laparotomic access. The first step consists in the retraction of the sigmoid colon and the identification of the major vessels (aortic bifurcation, bilateral common iliac arteries, inferior mesentery artery, and superior hemorrhoidal vessels). A vasopressin infiltration of the sacral promontory area is performed. In order to have access to the retroperitoneal space, the peritoneum overlying the sacral promontory is elevated about 1 cm caudally to the aortic bifurcation and incised transversally from major vessels or the ureter on the right to the mesentery of the sigmoid on the left. As described before, the left ureter is frequently not seen because it is often covered by the sigmoid colon.[17] The incision on the retroperitoneum is extended caudally. The excised edges of the presacral area should be cauterized by bipolar forceps to reduce the risk of chylous ascites. The presacral area is exposed with blunt dissection of the underlying adipose tissues. To reduce the bleedings, the blunt dissection should be performed transversally, avoiding an axial way parallel to major vessels.[35] Bleeding is generally controlled with the use of electrocautery (i.e. monopolar scissors and bipolar forceps). The great vessels are again visualized and identified. A semilunar piece of retroperitoneal tissue should be dissected away and sent routinely to confirm the presence of nerve fibers pathologically. In the region near the aortic bifurcation, two or three large continuous nerve bundles will constitute the superior hypogastric plexus, whereas in the area more caudal of the sacral promontory the nerve fibers are less distinct and 12–15 individual fibers will be present. All underlying tissue layers down to the periosteum should be cauterized with bipolar coagulation or transected with unipolar

scissors. At the end of the procedure, all the presacral nerves lying within the boundaries of the interiliac triangle should be totally removed or destroyed.

Safety

Since the operative field is in close proximity to major vessels and the right ureter, the anatomy and its variability presents the possibility of significant complications. Nevertheless, major operative complications are generally rare. On the contrary, the long-term adverse events are significantly more common when PSN is associated with standard conservative surgery.

Probably, the only possible serious intraoperative complication of the PSN is venous sacral hemorrhage. Although the middle sacral vein should be routinely identified and isolated, it is possible that several branches of the presacral venous plexus coming from the sacral surface are lacerated during attempted blunt dissection of the presacral area. This complication is more frequent when the dissection is performed over the S1–S2 space. The valveless intrasacral venous plexus, in fact, has an extensive collateral venous circulation and numerous perforating vessels that exit onto the anterior sacrum. Conventional measures to treat the venous sacral hemorrhage include the use of cautery. Furthermore, when the bleeding is significant, it is sometimes necessary to use a suture ligation. It is also possible that, when the presacral fascia is open, they retract into the bone. In these cases, it can be useful to place stainless steel thumbtacks into each foramen.[36] In our series,[37,38] heavy bleeding from the middle sacral vein was observed in about 0.5% of cases and was always successfully treated by bipolar electrocauterization during laparoscopy.

Another rare intraoperative complication, with an incidence of 0.6%, is the division of the presacral lymphatic vessels or plexus with leakage of milky chyle.[39–41] The surgeon can diagnose this complication intra- or postoperatively.[40,41] In the first case, the lymphatic vessels should be sealed using bipolar coagulation; a drain tube should be placed in the pelvic cavity and removed on the second postoperative day after no further chylous drainage.[40,41] In the second case, the patient presents, after a few days following hospital discharge, with progressive abdominal distention, tenderness, and rebound pain. The diagnosis of chylous ascites is made on the basis of a milky fluid aspirated by culdocentesis.[39] If the chylous ascites is not severe (or if the lymphatic repair during surgery is inadequate), it is necessary to perform percutaneous external drainage, and bed rest and a high-protein, low-fat, medium-chain triglyceride diet recommended to decrease chyle production.[40,41] Particular attention should be give for electrolyte imbalance, hypoproteinemia, and risk of infection. The hospitalization is generally prolonged. If this conservative treatment does not resolve the chylous ascites, the surgical repair of lymphatic vessels is still indicated.[40,41]

Postoperative complications consist essentially in short-term retention of urine, long-term urinary urgency, constipation, and alterations of uterine contractions in labor.[17] These postoperative consequences regard, in fact, about one-fifth of patients who undergo PSN.[35,42] Alterations of labor[34,42–45] and vaginal dryness[44] have also been reported, affecting about 2–3% of patients. Furthermore, about 60% of patients had painless labor in one report alone.[34] Backache is another rare complication reported in same papers, with an incidence of about 1%.[34,44] No data are available on sexual function.[17,35]

About 1–10% of patients treated surgically with PSN have urinary urgency.[26,37,38,43,46] This percentage is unchanged throughout the long-term follow-up of 2 years in our series,[37,38] whereas in another study a spontaneous improvement was noted.[47] Tolterodine tartate treatment, 2 mg twice daily, was used, but unfortunately only a light improvement was observed.[38]

Constipation was reported in about 4–74% of subjects.[37–39,43,44,46]

In our series, 30% of subjects reported constipation after 6 months from surgery. Furthermore, about half of these patients were spontaneously free of this symptom after 12 and 24 months of follow-up. Medical treatment with laxatives is effective in the majority of symptomatic patients.[38]

In conclusion, there are great differences in the incidence of long-term consequences between different studies, probably due to the major or minor extension of the neurectomy, the anatomic heterogeneity of the pelvic innervation, and the various capacities of reinnervation after surgery.

Effectiveness

Presacral neurectomy performed by laparotomy was first introduced by Jouboulay[48] and Ruggi[49] in 1899, but only Cotte[50] used this procedure routinely. Successively, other authors in the United States have described this procedure in retrospective or open studies, with an efficacy in pain relief varying from 37% to 89%.[42,45,51–54] Until then, the pelvic pain surgically treated in these studies[42,45,51–54] had not been well differentiated. In particular, no clear data are available specifically on endometriosis-related pelvic pain.

Few data are available during the 1970s on the surgical treatment of pelvic pain because of the widespread use of oral contraceptives and nonsteroidal anti-inflammatory drugs (NSAIDs). Furthermore, after this period, the limited possibilities of medical treatment for pelvic pain due to endometriosis gave new interest to pelvic denervation and these surgical procedures were re-evaluated as an option for treating selectively primary and/or secondary chronic pelvic pain initially in prospective nonrandomized uncontrolled studies and then in RCTs. At the end of the 1970s, in fact, two retrospective studies[55,56] reanalyzed the efficacy of PSN performed by laparotomy for the treatment of endometriosis-related pelvic pain in women treated with conservative surgery. The former analysis[55] showed a significant difference in dysmenorrhea (97% vs 72%) and in dyspareunia (74% vs 58%) when PNS was added to conservative surgery. The latter study[56] noted that the pain symptoms were resolved or markedly attenuated in 80% and in 90% of women treated with laparotomic conservative surgery alone and in laparotomic conservative surgery plus PSN, respectively.

Two prospective uncontrolled studies[34,57] have demonstrated the effectiveness of laparotomic PSN for the treatment of organic pelvic pain. Furthermore, both studies[34,57] included unselected patients with different causes of pelvic pain.

More recently, Tjaden et al,[47] in an RCT, demonstrated a complete relief of midline pelvic pain in all women who underwent laparotomic PSN, whereas no variation was observed in those women who underwent laparotomy for conservative resection of endometriosis. Furthermore, in this last study, only 8 women were randomized, since the ethical committee stopped enrolment due to the consideration that depriving patients with midline dysmenorrhea of the benefits of PSN was unethical.

With the rapid development of laparoscopic techniques, interest in PSN was revised. The use of the laparoscopic approach provides, in fact, a magnification of the operating field with a better exposure and results in a selective and a more complete ablation of nerve pathways, decreasing morbidity and shortening hospital stay and recovery.

In a retrospective analysis,[58] Zullo et al have shown that laparoscopic PSN (LPSN) is highly effective for pelvic pain relief when used alone or in combination with the classic ablative surgery for endometriosis. The same surgical strategy is effective in the treatment of midline pelvic pain and improves dysmenorrhea scores significantly rather than a LUNA.

Other observational and/or uncontrolled studies[39,44,46,59] have also suggested that LPSN is effective in the treatment of midline endometriosis-related dysmenorrhea and/or chronic pelvic pain in women treated with laparoscopic conservative surgery.

Many authors[43,46] have emphasized the importance of carefully selecting patients exclusively with endometriosis-related severe midline dysmenorrhea and/or chronic pelvic pain. In routine clinical practice, this selection is more difficult because only a small percentage of patients have these characteristics. Many women with endometriosis primarily report a strong lateral dysmenorrhea and/or chronic pelvic pain associated with a central component.

Based on these considerations, in our department a prospective, randomized, double-blind, controlled trial was performed in order to evaluate the effectiveness of the laparoscopic conservative surgery plus LPSN in a group of women with endometriosis-related pelvic pain who were not specifically selected with regard to the type of pelvic pain (midline or lateral) and to endometriosis stage.[37] In particular, the exclusive presence of midline pelvic pain was not an inclusion criteria, whereas the absence of a midline component was considered an exclusion criteria. The two groups of women had a midline component of dysmenorrhea with a lateral component associated in similar percentages of cases. Our findings have shown that the surgical treatment of endometrial implants plus LPSN induces a significantly higher cure rate compared to surgical treatment of endometriosis alone. The 6- and 12-month follow-ups revealed improved relief with regards to the severity of dysmenorrhea, dyspareunia, and chronic pelvic pain in patients treated with LPSN in comparison with conservative surgery alone (Table 15.1). In this last study[37] the bilateral LUNA was not performed as a single treatment option but only as part of the deep endometriosis treatment.

Our data are in contrast to a previous RCT[43] available in the literature.[18,19,43] In fact, Candiani et al[43] have shown no significant difference in the cure rate between the experimental and control groups. Furthermore, when only midline dysmenorrhea is considered, they have stated that this type of pain responds better to PSN; however, the difference did not reach statistical significance. Unfortunately, the major problem in this trial was the sample size consisting of only 71 women with a power of 80% to detect differences greater than 30%, whereas the difference in pain relief between the two groups was only 5%.[21]

We agree that the presence of chronic pelvic pain with a marked lateral component may be considered a negative predictive factor for the effectiveness of PSN[60] and that PSN does not significantly relieve adnexal pain.[44,47,61] Moreover, the laparoscopic conservative surgery (enucleation of endometriomas and lysis of pelvic adhesions) could specifically attenuate the lateral component of pelvic pain in subjects with endometriosis[37]. Alternatively, PSN has a greater effect of relief on the midline component. Thus, the association of both techniques may be beneficial for pelvic pain relief[37].

Our results are similar to that obtained by Sutton et al[18,19] in a prospective, double-blind RCT. In this trial,[18,19] the use of laparoscopic conservative surgery plus UNA resulted in an improvement of the symptomatology in 62.5% of the subjects. When successful outcomes are analyzed by stage, the results were poorest for stage I and best for stage III, with a significant trend between pain relief and stage of disease in Sutton et al's study, whereas no difference was observed in Zullo et al's study.[18,19,37,38]

After conservative treatment of endometriosis alone, pain relief was significantly lower in patients with deep rectovaginal septum endometriosis, whereas this difference was not observed in women treated with LPSN addition, suggesting that this last surgical procedure could avoid the suboptimal results obtained with ablation of endometriotic lesions (see Table 15.1).[37] A concrete conclusion on this issue cannot be drawn, since this study[37] was not powered with this intention. Indeed, it is possible to hypothesize that in women with deep rectovaginal septum endometriosis, the LPSN addition to standard surgery could be an additive procedure to make the surgical approach less aggressive, reducing the rate of bowel and/or rectosigmoid resection.[62]

The association of the LPSN to laparoscopic con-

Table 15.1 Number and percentage of women cured of pain according to the endometriosis stage (based on r-AFS classification of endometriosis) and deep rectovaginal septum endometriosis in patients who do not receive (group A) or receive (group B) PSN[37] . Reprinted from *Am J Obstet Gynecol*, 189, Zullo F et al. Effectiveness of presacral neurectomy in women with severe dysmenorrhea caused by endometriosis who were treated with laparoscopic conservative surgery: a 1-year prospective randomized double-blind controlled trial. pp 5–10, 2003, with permission from Elsevier.[37]

Endometriosis stage	Group A ($n = 63$)	Group B ($n = 63$)
Stage I (%)	18 (28.6)	16 (25.4)
Cure rate (%)		
6-month follow-up	11 (61.1)	14 (87.5)*
12-month follow-up	11 (61.1)	14 (87.5)*
Stage II (%)	21 (33.3)	22 (34.9)
Cure rate (%)		
6-month follow-up	13 (61.9)	19 (86.4)*
12-month follow-up	12 (57.1)	19 (86.4)*
Stage III (%)	17 (27.0)	17 (27.0)
Cure rate (%)		
6-month follow-up	10 (58.8)	15 (88.2)*
12-month follow-up	10 (58.8)	15 (88.2)*
Stage IV (%)	7 (11.1)	8 (12.7)
Cure rate (%)		
6-month follow-up	4 (57.1)	7 (87.5)*
12-month follow-up	3 (42.9)	6 (75.0)*
Deep rectovaginal septum endometriosis	6 (9.5)	7 (11.1)
Cure rate (%)		
6-month follow-up	2 (33.3)†	5 (71.4)*
12-month follow-up	1 (16.7)**	4 (57.1)*

*$p < 0.05$ vs group A; †$p < 0.05$ vs stages I–III; **$p < 0.05$ vs stages I–IV.
r-AFS = revised American Fertility Society.

servative treatment for endometriosis maintains its efficacy even after long-term follow-up.[19,38,46] These data partially eliminate the criticisms regarding the poor long-term effectiveness of PSN due to reinnervation, which should be usually completed within 12–18 months or less.[35] The inappropriate selection of the cases to treat, the neurologic variability, and failure to ablate all nerve fibers within the Cotte's triangle are the three main reasons for the less than absolute short-term effectiveness of PSN.

Finally, the long-term efficacy of LPSN in women with endometriosis-related pelvic pain has been evaluated also in terms of improvement in quality of life.[38] Specifically, after 2 years following surgery, a significant difference in quality of life, as evaluated with the Short-Form Health Survey,[63] has been demonstrated when the LPSN was added to laparoscopic conservative surgery.[38]

As with URS, no study is available for PSN with regard to its efficacy alone vs the conservative treatment of endometriosis alone.

Conclusions

The efficacy of pelvic denervations for the treatment of secondary pelvic pain due to endometriosis is difficult to extrapolate. The majority of the papers published are retrospective and uncontrolled. In addition, the severity of the pain and the cure rates have been evaluated in several ways. Finally, the procedures are often performed in association with others, such as adhesiolysis or ablation of endometriosis, and it is difficult to discern which is the main contributing factor to the pain relief. For example, the USR is a procedure frequently performed during the treatment of endometriosis when the uterosacral ligaments are macro- or microscopically involved.[64]

Notwithstanding the dearth of long-term follow-up data, we feel that the LPSN in women with endometriosis-related dysmenorrhea and chronic pelvic pain, if performed by an experienced surgical team, can be considered an effective and minimally invasive procedure to add to the conservative treatment of endometriosis in order to improve the cure rate at each stage of the disease.

However, it is essential to carefully select patients. Specifically, the patient with endometriosis should be affected by severe chronic pelvic pain and/or dysmenorrhea for at least 6 months unresponsive to medical treatment.[65] At the moment, a pivotal prerequisite is, probably, the presence of a midline component of pain. Because pelvic denervation is related to alterations of colon and bladder motility, we maintain that, in patients affected by or with history of severe constipation and/or urinary dysfunction, these procedures should be avoided or performed only after a well-detailed informed consent.

REFERENCES

1. Hurd WW. Criteria that indicate endometriosis is the cause of chronic pelvic pain. Obstet Gynecol 1998; 92: 1029–1032.
2. Olive DL, Pritts EA. Treatment of endometriosis. N Engl J Med 2001; 345: 266–275.
3. Demco L. Mapping the source and character of pain due to endometriosis by patient-assisted laparoscopy. J Am Assoc Gynecol Laparosc 1998; 5: 241–245.
4. Porpora MG, Gomel V. The role of laparoscopy in the management of pelvic pain in women of reproductive age. Fertil Steril 1997; 68: 765–779.
5. Gruppo Italiano per lo Studio dell'Endometriosi. Relationship between stage, site and morphological characteristics of pelvic endometriosis and pain. Hum Reprod 2001; 16: 2668–2671.
6. The American Fertility Society. Revised American Fertility Society classification of endometriosis: 1985. Fertil Steril 1985; 43: 351–355.
7. Fedele L, Parazzini F, Bianchi S, et al. Stage and localization of pelvic endometriosis and pain. Fertil Steril 1990; 53: 155–158.
8. Vercellini P, Trespidi L, De Giorgi O, et al. Endometriosis and pelvic pain: relation to disease stage and localization. Fertil Steril 1996; 65: 299–304.
9. Colwell HH, Mathias SD, Pasta DJ, et al. A health-related quality-of-life instrument for symptomatic patients with endometriosis: a validation study. Am J Obstet Gynecol 1998; 179: 47–55.
10. Jones GL, Kennedy SH, Jenkinson C. Health-related quality of life measurement in women with common benign gynaecologic conditions: a systematic review. Am J Obstet Gynecol 2002; 187: 501–511.
11. Prentice A. Endometriosis. Br Med J 2001; 323: 93–95.
12. Stones RW, Mountfield J. Interventions for treating chronic pelvic pain in women (Cochrane Review). In: The Cochrane Library, Issue 2, 2002. Oxford: Update Software.
13. Carter JE. Surgical treatment for chronic pelvic pain. JSLS 1998; 2: 129–139.
14. Rannestad T, Eikeland OJ, Helland H, et al. The quality of life in women suffering from gynecological disorders is improved by means of hysterectomy. Absolute and relative differences between pre- and postoperative measures. Acta Obstet Gynecol Scand 2001; 80: 46–51.
15. Lefebvre G, Allaire C, Jeffrey J, et al. Clinical Practice Gynaecology Committee and Executive Committee and Council, Society of Obstetricians and Gynaecologists of Canada. SOGC clinical guidelines. Hysterectomy. J Obstet Gynaecol Can 2002; 24: 37–61.
16. MacDonald SR, Klock SC, Milad MP. Long-term outcome of nonconservative surgery (hysterectomy) for endometriosis-associated pain in women <30 years old. Am J Obstet Gynecol 1999; 180: 1360–1363.
17. Zullo F, Palomba S, Marconi D, et al. Presacral neurectomy for the surgical management of pelvic pain due to endometriosis. Acta Obstet Gynecol Scand 2005 (in press).
18. Sutton CJ, Ewen SP, Whitelaw N, et al. Prospective, randomized double-blind controlled trial of laser laparoscopy in the treatment of pelvic pain associated with minimal, mild and moderate endometriosis. Fertil Steril 1994; 62: 696–700.
19. Sutton CJ, Pooley AS, Ewen SP, et al. Follow-up report on a randomised controlled trial of laser laparoscopy in the treatment of pelvic pain associated with minimal to moderate endometriosis. Fertil Steril 1997; 68: 1070–1074.
20. Garry R, Clayton R, Hawe J. The effect of endometriosis and its radical laparoscopic excision on quality of life indicators. BJOG 2000; 107: 44–54.
21. Proctor ML, Farquhar CM, Sinclair OJ, et al. Surgical interruption of pelvic nerve pathways for primary and secondary dysmenorrhea (Cochrane Review). In: The Cochrane Library, Issue 2, 2002. Oxford: Update Software.
22. Curtis AH, Anson BJ, Ashley FL, et al. The anatomy of the pelvic autonomic nerves in relation to gynecology. Surg Gynecol Obstet 1942; 73: 743–750.
23. Sutton CJG. Laser uterine nerve ablation. In: Donnez J, ed. Laser operative laparoscopy and hysteroscopy. Leuven, Belgium: Nouwelaerts Printing; 1989: 43–52.
24. Davis GD. Uterine prolapse after laparoscopic uterosacral transection in nulliparous airborne trainees: a report of three cases. J Reprod Med 1996; 41: 279–282.
25. Doyle JB. Paracervical uterine denervation by transection of the cervical plexus for the relief of dysmenorrhea. Am J Obstet Gynecol 1955; 70: 1–16.
26. Daniels J, Garry R, Khan KS, et al. Laparoscopic uterine

nerve ablation: a survey of gynaecological practice in UK. Gynecol Endosc 2000; 9: 157–159.

27. Donnez J, Nisolle M. Carbon-dioxide laser laparoscopy in pelvic pain and infertility. Baillières Clin Obstet Gynecol 1989; 3: 525–544.

28. Corson SL, Unger M, Kwa D, et al. Laparoscopic laser treatment of endometriosis with the Nd:YAG sapphire probe. Am J Obstet Gynecol 1989; 160: 718–723.

29. Vercellini P, Aimi G, Busacca M, et al. Laparoscopic uterosacral ligament resection for dysmenorrhea associated with endometriosis: results of a randomized controlled trial. Fertil Steril 1997; 68: 3.

30. Vercellini P, Aimi G, Busacca M, et al. Laparoscopic uterosacral ligament resection for dysmenorrhea associated with endometriosis: results of a randomized, controlled trial. Fertil Steril 2003; 80: 310–319.

31. Johnson NP, Farquar CM, Crossley S, et al. A double-blind randomized controlled trial of laparoscopic uterine nerve ablation for women with chronic pelvic pain. BJOG 2004; 111: 950–959.

32. Sutton CJG, Pooley A, Jones KD, et al. Prospective, randomized, double-blind controlled trial of laparoscopic uterine nerve ablation in the treatment of pelvic pain associated with endometriosis. Gynecol Endosc 2001; 10: 217–222.

33. The LUNA Trial Collaboration. A randomized controlled trial to assess the efficacy of laparoscopic uterosacral nerve ablation (LUNA) in the treatment of chronic pelvic pain: the trial protocol [ISRCTN41196151]. BMC Women's Health 2003; 3: 1–6.

34. Lee RB, Stone K, Magelssen D, et al. Presacral neurectomy for chronic pelvic pain. Obstet Gynecol 1986; 68: 517–521.

35. Steege JF. Presacral neurectomy. In: Nichols DH, Clarke-Pearson DL eds, Gynecologic and obstetric, and related surgery, 2nd edn. St. Louis: Mosby; 2002: 610–614.

36. Patsner B, Orr JW Jr. Intractable venous sacral hemorrhage: use of stainless steel thumbtacks to obtain hemostasis. Am J Obstet Gynecol 1990; 162: 452.

37. Zullo F, Palomba S, Zupi E, et al. Effectiveness of presacral neurectomy in women with severe dysmenorrhea caused by endometriosis who were treated with laparoscopic conservative surgery: a 1-year prospective randomized double-blind controlled trial. Am J Obstet Gynecol 2003; 189: 5–10.

38. Zullo F, Palomba S, Zupi E, et al. Long-term effectiveness of presacral neurectomy for the treatment of severe dysmenorrhea due to endometriosis. J Am Assoc Gynecol Laparosc 2004; 11: 23–28.

39. Chen FP, Soong YK. The efficacy and complications of laparoscopic presacral neurectomy in pelvic pain. Obstet Gynecol 1997; 90: 974–977.

40. Chen FP, Lo TS, Soong YK. Management of chylous ascites following laparoscopic presacral neurectomy. Hum Reprod 1998; 13: 880–883.

41. Lo T-S, Chen F-P, Chu K-K, et al. Successful management of chylous ascites after laparoscopic presacral neurectomy. J Am Assoc Gynecol Laparosc 1998; 5: 431–433.

42. Ingersoll FM, Meigs JV. Presacral neurectomy for dysmenorrhea. N Engl J Med 1948; 238: 357–350.

43. Candiani GB, Fedele L, Vercellini P, et al. Presacral neurectomy for the treatment of pelvic pain associated with endometriosis: a controlled study. Am J Obstet Gynecol 1992; 167: 100–103.

44. Nezhat C, Nezhat F. A simplified method of laparoscopic presacral neurectomy for the treatment of central pelvic pain due to endometriosis. Br J Obstet Gynaecol 1996; 99: 659–663.

45. Meigs JV. Excision of the superior hypogastric plexus (presacral nerve) for primary dysmenorrhoea. Surg Gynecol Obstet 1939; 68: 723–728.

46. Nezhat CH, Seidman DS, Nezhat FR, et al. Long-term outcome of laparoscopic presacral neurectomy for the treatment of central pelvic pain attributed to endometriosis. Obstet Gynecol 1998; 91: 701–704.

47. Tjaden B, Schlaff WD, Kimball A, et al. The efficacy of presacral neurectomy for the relief of midline dysmenorrhoea. Obstet Gynecol 1990; 76: 89–91.

48. Jouboulay M. Le traitement de la névralgie pelvienne par la paralysie du sympathique sacre. Lyon Med 1899; 90: 102–108.

49. Ruggi C. La simpatectomia addominale utero-ovarica come mezzo di cura di alcune lesioni interne degli organi genitali della donna. Bologna: Zanichelli; 1899.

50. Cotte G. La sympathectomie hypogastrique: a-t-elle sa place dans la thérapeutique gynécologique? Presse Med 1925; 33: 98–102.

51. Counseller VS, Craig WM. The treatment of dysmenorrhea by resection of the presacral sympathetic nerves: evaluation of end-results. Am J Obstet Gynecol 1934; 29: 161–170.

52. Tucker AW Jr, Mass N. An evaluation of presacral neurectomy in the treatment of dysmenorrhea. Am J Obstet Gynecol 1947; 53: 226–232.

53. Black JrWT. Use of presacral sympathectomy in the treatment of dysmenorrhea – a second look after 25 years. Am J Obstet Gynecol 1964; 89: 16–22.

54. Frier A. Pelvic neurectomy in gynecology. Obstet Gynecol 1965; 25: 48–52.

55. Garcia CR, David SS. Pelvic endometriosis: infertility and pelvic pain. Am J Obstet Gynecol 1977; 129: 740–747.

56. Puolakka J, Kauppila A, Ronnberg L. Results in the operative treatment of pelvic endometriosis. Acta Obstet Gynecol Scand 1980; 59: 429–431.

57. Polan ML, DeCherney A. Presacral neurectomy for pelvic pain in infertility. Fertil Steril 1980; 34: 557–560.

58. Zullo F, Pellicano M, De Stefano R, et al. Efficacy of laparoscopic pelvic denervation in central-type chronic pelvic pain: a multicenter study. J Gynecol Surg 1996; 12: 35–40.

59. Chen FP, Chang SD, Chu KK, et al. Comparison of laparoscopic presacral neurectomy and laparoscopic uterine nerve ablation for primary dysmenorrhea. J Reprod Med 1996; 41: 463–466.

60. Temple JL, Bradshaw HB, Wood E, et al. Effects of hypogastric neurectomy on escape responses to uterine distention in the rat. Pain 1999; Suppl 6: 13–20.

61. Perez JJ. Laparoscopic presacral neurectomy. Results of the first 25 cases. J Reprod Med 1993; 35: 625–630.

62. Redwine DB, Wright JT. Laparoscopic treatment of complete obliteration of the cul-de-sac associated with endometriosis: long-term follow-up of en bloc resection. Fertil Steril 2001; 76: 358–365.

63. Ware JE Jr, Sherbourne CD. The MOS 36-item short-form health survey (SF-36). I. Conceptual framework and item selection. Med Care 1992; 30: 473–483.

64. Bonte H, Chapron C, Vieira M, et al. Histologic appearance of endometriosis infiltrating uterosacral ligaments in women with painful symptoms. J Am Assoc Gynecol Laparosc 2002; 9: 519–524.

65. Gambone JC, Mittman BS, Munro MG, et al. Chronic Pelvic Pain/Endometriosis Working Group. Consensus statement for the management of chronic pelvic pain and endometriosis: proceeding of an expert-panel consensus process. Fertil Steril 2002; 78: 961–972.

16 The laparoscopic treatment of intestinal endometriosis

Jöerg Keckstein and Hubert Wiesinger

Introduction

The incidence of intestinal endometriosis is reported to range from 3 to 37% of the patients suffering from endometriosis.

The most frequent localization of this extragenital endometriosis is the rectosigmoid colon, followed by the sigmoid colon, the cecum, the appendix, and the small intestine (Figure 16.1 and Table 16.1). The extent may range from a microscopically small nodule to a big, tumor-like infiltrate of the entire bowel wall, with consecutive narrow-

Table 16.1 Localization of intestinal endometriosis
Deep endometriosis (rectum, rectosigmoidal passage)
Upper sigmoid loop
Cecum
Appendix
Small intestine

ing. Consequently, symptoms differ. The diagnosis can be impeded by the localization, extent, and different activity of the nodules.

Patients with severe symptoms and signs and ineffective medical therapy must undergo surgery. The access through the vagina especially serves the exposure when the diagnostic findings are deeply seated. Access through the abdomen enables the surgeon to see the entire pelvis and, thus, to treat further endometriotic nodules, e.g. at the uterus, the pelvic side wall, and the ovaries. According to the localization and the size of the diagnostic findings, both surgical methods can, if applicable, be combined. Due to the enormous development of endoscopic surgical techniques over the past few years, it is now also possible to remove the intestinal endometriosis laparoscopically and/or with laparoscopic assistance.

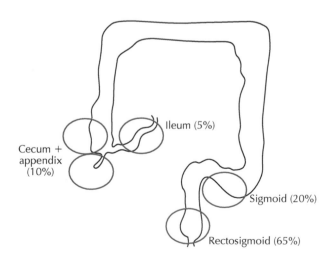

Cecum + appendix (10%)

Ileum (5%)

Sigmoid (20%)

Rectosigmoid (65%)

Figure 16.1 Localization of the intestinal endometriosis.

Symptoms of intestinal endometriosis

In Table 16.2, the typical symptoms of intestinal endometriosis are listed.

Small endometriosis nodules on the serosal surface and/or the muscular coat of the bowel are often irrelevant to the patient. More widespread nodules, which are especially intramuscular, result in a stenosis of the bowel's lumen and a stiffness of the bowel wall. Nodules in the recto-vaginal septum also infiltrate (apart from the bowel wall) the holding apparatus (paraproctia) as well as the adjacent organs (uterus, cardinal ligament, sacrouterine ligament, ureter, etc.).

With all these symptoms, the dependency on the menstrual cycle is especially of vital diagnostic importance. Although rectal bleeding is a typical indication of intestinal endometriosis, its absence does not eliminate the possibility of intestinal endometriosis. Crampy abdominal pain and pressure on the coccyx, perimenstrual flatulence, as well as ileus may also be clues as to the presence of intestinal endometriosis.

Diagnostics

The diagnosis of intestinal endometriosis (Table 16.3) begins with an evaluation of the patient's medical history as well as with an extensive clinical examination, particularly by palpation and ultrasound (Figures 16.2 and 16.3). In cases of doubt, an additional intestinal endoscopy as well

---

Table 16.2 Symptoms of intestinal endometriosis

Severe dysmenorrhea
Severe dyspareunia
Dysfunctions of the bowel (depending on the menstruation):
    Pressure on the rectum – extending to the coccyx
    Bleedings
    Discharge of mucus
    Obstipation/diarrhea
    Painful defecation
    Flatulence
    Subileus phenomena

Table 16.3 Pre-operative methods to diagnose intestinal endometriosis

Medical history
Clinical examination
Ultrasound (transvaginal, transrectal)
Colon – contrast enema
Magnetic resonance imaging (MRI)
Colonoscopy

---

as a double-contrast examination of the colon and a magnetic resonance imaging (MRI) examination may help. However, in most cases, the only way a definite diagnosis can be made is by diagnostic laparoscopy (Table 16.4).

Staging

Intestinal endometriosis is only indirectly considered in the revised American Fertility Society (r-AFS) system (score for endometriosis), which does not quantify the disease's extent and its relation to the adjacent organs and/or structures. There is no correlation between r-AFS classification and endometriosis-related pain. In our department, out of 95 patients with diagnosed intestinal endometriosis, only 50 had stage IV according to r-AFS.[1] Complementary to the r-AFS classification, a new classification system (Enzian)[2] serves to completely include the entire extraperitoneal endometriosis nodules. Following the tumor–node–metastasis (TNM) classification, the proliferative (infiltrative) character of deep endometriosis is included and topographically classified. This score considers the infiltration of the vagina, the rectovaginal septum, and the bowel, but also the adjacent structures such as cardinal ligaments, pelvic wall, urinary tract, and also endometriosis nodules outside the pelvis. By means of this score, the extent of deep endometriosis can easily be stated and, thus, compared with findings from other studies (Figure 16.4).

Therapy

The objective in treating intestinal endometriosis is pain relief and/or a normal functioning of the organs. The choice of the therapy is primarily dependent on the extent of the diagnostic findings, the symptoms and signs, and the expected therapy results.

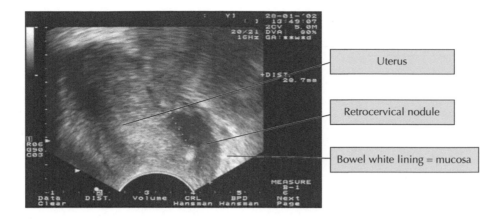

Figure 16.2 Ultrasound image of a deep endometriosis in the rectovaginal septum (vaginal ultrasound). The nonechogenic crescent-shaped structure behind the cervix infiltrates the front rectum wall. Behind the node, there are the two bowel walls that have a C-shaped curvature.

Surgical techniques

Surgical techniques are shown in Figures 16.5, 16.6, and 16.7.

Pre-surgery preparation

Preoperatively, the surgery's extent is discussed with the patient in detail, particularly the weighing of physical and psychologic strain and the operative risks. The possibility of interdisciplinary cooperation is planned with the abdominal surgeon or urologist (if necessary). Because of the risk of a perforation of the bowel, but also because of the possible resection of a bowel segment, each patient should be pretreated with a colonic

irrigation (e.g. Fleet©). A perioperative antibiotics prophylaxis is recommendable.

Surgery strategy

Surgical access (vaginal, abdominal, laparoscopic, or combined) is determined by the location of the endometriotic deposits found during diagnostic tests and the surgeon's training.

Vaginal access offers several advantages. Palpation facilitates a radical removal and, at the same time, the care of the intestinal structures. Lesions on the bowel's surface can be dealt with without any problems. However, when the vagina is extremely narrow (for the most part, where young nulliparae

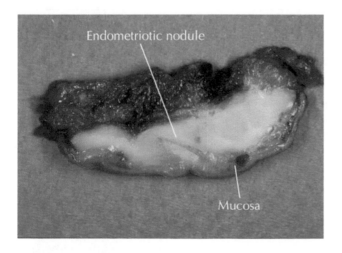

Figure 16.3 Macroscopic image of a deep endometriotic nodule in the rectovaginal septum after a segment resection by laparoscopy. The muscular layer is raised; the mucous membrane seems to be intact.

Table 16.4 Characteristics of severe (deep) intestinal endometriosis

Sturdy node, retrocervical
Deep pain (pressure, etc.)
Detectable by ultrasound
Submucous, located in the muscle layer (*not* depictable by endoscopy)
Involvement of adjacent organs (uterus, parametria, ureter, etc.)
r-AFS score *does not* correlate with the disease's extent

r-AFS = (revised American Fertility Society)

Enzian Score

| a
* cul-de-sac
* vagina | b
* uterosacral ligament
* cardinal ligament | | c
* bowel, rectum
* rectosigmoid |

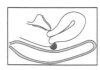 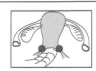 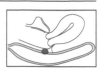

| E1a = isolated nodule the pouch of Douglas | E1b = isolated nodule <1 cm from the uterine sacral ligament (USL) | E1bb = bilateral infiltration of the USL | E1c = isolated nodule in the rectovaginal space |

| E2a = infiltration of the upper third of the vagina | E2b = infiltration of the USL >1 cm | E2bb = bilateral | E2c = infiltration of rectum <1 cm |

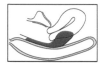

| E3a = infiltration of the middle part of the vagina | E3b = infiltration of the cardinal ligament (without ureterohydronephrosis) | E3bb = bilateral | E3c = infiltration of the rectum 1–3 cm without stenosis |

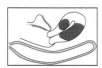

| E4a = infiltration of uterus and/or lower third of the vagina | E4b = infiltration of the cardinal ligament to pelvic side wall and/or ureterohydronephrosis | E4bb = bilateral | E4c = infiltration of the rectum >3 cm and/or rectal stenosis |

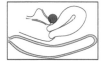

| FA = adenomyosis uteri | FB = deep infiltration of the bladder | FU = ureteral infiltration (intrinsic) | FI = intestinal infiltration (other side than rectum or sigmoid) |

FO = other locations

Figure 16.4 Enzian score – staging system to classify the deep endometriosis of the SEF (Stiftung Endometriose-Forschung, Germany).

are concerned), the access can be difficult; therefore, the necessary extent of the surgery can be judged only with difficulty.

Nodules that are located higher up or more complex findings indicate that abdominal access is necessary;[3] primarily by laparoscopy. Without opening the bowel lumen, small, superficial endometriotic nodules can be resected from the bowel wall with scissors or a monopolar needle. Afterwards, the muscular coat's defect is secured by reaching interrupted button sutures.

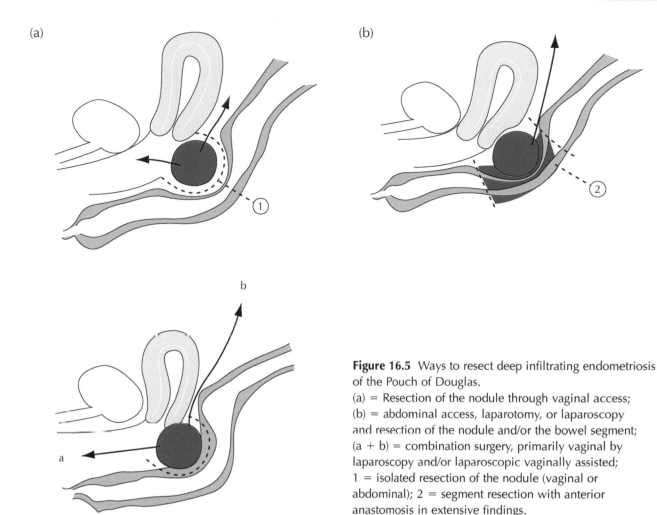

(a)

(b)

b

a

Figure 16.5 Ways to resect deep infiltrating endometriosis of the Pouch of Douglas.
(a) = Resection of the nodule through vaginal access;
(b) = abdominal access, laparotomy, or laparoscopy and resection of the nodule and/or the bowel segment;
(a + b) = combination surgery, primarily vaginal by laparoscopy and/or laparoscopic vaginally assisted;
1 = isolated resection of the nodule (vaginal or abdominal); 2 = segment resection with anterior anastomosis in extensive findings.

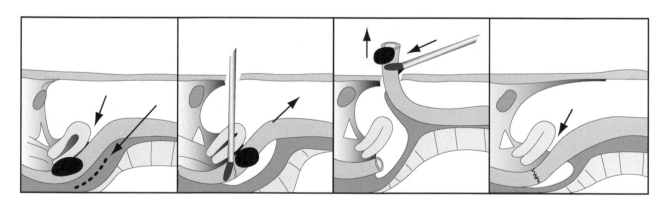

Figure 16.6 Technique for a laparoscopically assisted anterior resection with intestinal endometriosis.

Extensive findings, possibly involving other pelvic structures, call for a different surgical technique. As a majority of the patients suffer from infertility, it is necessary to remove the endometrioic nodules, and also to act in an organ-sparing and/or organ-reconstructing way. Adhesions often obscure a complete view into the true pelvis. An extremely retroflexed uterus or a uterus fixed in the rectouterine pouch has first to be loosened and tipped into its correct position. The presence of a deep endometriotic nodule becomes apparent when there is fibrotic obliteration of the cul-de-sac.

The objective of surgery is to mobilize the node by exposing the adjacent healthy structures in order to

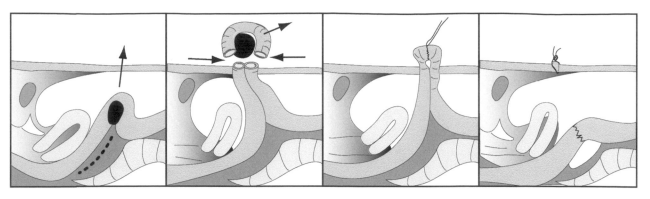

Figure 16.7 Resection of the intestinal endometriosis on the sigma with hand-sewn anastomosis, laparoscopically assisted.

be able to assess if, and to what extent, the lesion has spread to one or more organs (Figure 16.8). In the course of surgery, the adhesiolysis is carried out first and, if necessary, the bowel has to be freed from the adhesions. Substantial adhesions between the sigmoid colon and the left adnex can be caused by infiltrative endometriosis in the sigmoid colon (the endometriotic nodule cannot be visualized without extensive adhesiolysis).

The preparation starts with dissecting around the peritoneum of the nodules visible in the abdominal cavity. Here, the uterosacral ligaments from near the uterus up to the pelvic wall are divided. The dissection should start lateral to this ligament, after identifying the ureter. Occasionally, the parametria and/or the paraproctia also have to be exposed up to the pelvis wall. Then, the nodule itself has to be removed from the cervix; if necessary, the fornix of the vagina has to be opened in order to do this. After opening the pararectal areas, it is possible to better mobilize the bowel and to locate the corresponding nodule by means of a blunt dissection technique. In case of deep preparation, the course of the splanchnic nerves has to be identified in order to avoid postoperative urinary

problems. The dissection of the posterior fornix of the vagina can be facilitated by using a manipulator placed in the vagina and/or by a corresponding manipulator placed in the rectum. Without opening the bowel lumen, the nodule can be removed from the bowel wall by lifting the nodule with grasping forceps and, simultaneously, resecting the nodule with scissors, laser, or monopolar needle, or with the Endo GIA. If the musculature of the bowel is also resected, the defect is secured by interrupted knot sutures or a stapling device.[4–6] If the bowel lumen is also completely opened, the bowel has to be closed by a double suture. To facilitate the closing of the bowel, two holding sutures at the lateral corners of the wound's edges are used. Using an all-layered suture with Vicryl 30 and round needle, the wound can be secured watertight. A larger defect (more than 1 cm) or a long denudation of the bowel's musculature involves the risk of a postoperative perforation of the bowel. Then, a segmental bowel resection becomes necessary (Figures 16.6 and 16.7). This necessity also arises if the endometriosis nodule is located in higher bowel segments. In our series of more than 200 patients, 25% had a multifocal involvement of the bowel wall. The principle of

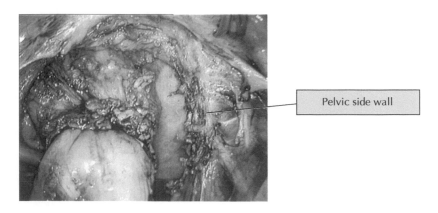

Pelvic side wall

Figure 16.8 Presentation of an infiltration of the front rectum wall with consecutive pulling-in of the musculature and/or stenosis of the bowel section.

the endoscopic segment resection with anterior anastomosis corresponds to a laparoscopically assisted abdominal procedure. As the anastomosis is mostly deeply located, stapler systems (Endo GIA or CEEA) are used[5,7–10] (Figures 16.9–16.11).

After the nodule is mobilized from the posterior fornix of the vagina, the bowel is removed from its holding structures via the sacral cavity. The blood vessels, which are exposed in the course of this, are coagulated with bipolar and cut divided. In doing so, the sigmoidal colon is gradually

removed from the transversalis fascia. The further mobilization of the sigmoidal colon and/or the descending colon has to be adapted depending on the length of the resected part of bowel. The exposed bowel is transected caudal to the pathologic finding using Endo GIA (Figure 16.9). The midline trocar puncture site is expanded to a mini-laparotomy (5 cm) and, then, the bowel stump, which includes the endometriosis, is brought through the wound onto the abdominal wall (Figures 16.12 and 16.13). The affected bowel segment is resected (Figure 16.11). The anvil of the

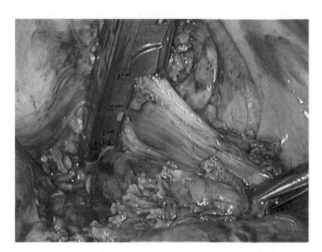

Figure 16.9 Resection of deep endometriosis involving the anterior rectum wall. After skeletization of the rectosigmoid and delineation of the endometriotic nodule, the bowel is stapled with an Endo GIA and cut through.

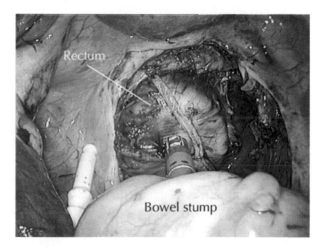

Figure 16.11 After the insertion of the transanal stapler device and its connection with the bowel stump, the bowel stumps are approximated and the anastomosis is performed. The tightness of the bowel lumen can be checked by a rectoscopy and/or by injection of methylene blue solution into the rectum.

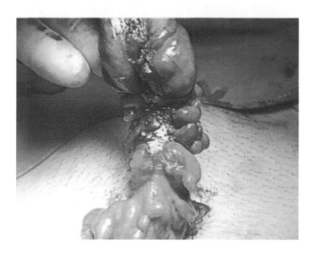

Figure 16.10 After the expansion of the middle trocar puncture to a mini-laparotomy, the cranial bowel stump, which includes the pathologic lesion, is drawn in front of the abdominal wall in order to be conventionally resected. After the insertion of the pressure plate of the transanal stapler device CEEA, the bowel stump is replaced into the abdominal cavity.

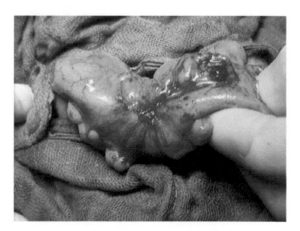

Figure 16.12 Presentation of a mobilized sigmoid loop with included endometriotic nodule that is drawn in front of the abdominal wall by a mini-laparotomy.

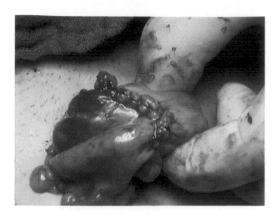

Figure 16.13 After the conventional removal of the nodule, the anastomosis is performed by two semicircular sutures.

stapler device is inserted into the proximal bowel stump and fixed by a purse-string suture.

The bowel stump is replaced into the abdominal cavity, and the mini-laparotomy is closed. The pressure plate is coupled with the transanal inserted CEEA stapler device, and the anastomosis is performed by closing the device. After the removal of the instrument from the bowel, the tightness of the anastomosis is checked by air insufflation under water.

In case the nodule is located high up in the sigmoid a different technique can be used. The whole sigmoid loop is mobilized laparoscopically and brought in front of the abdominal wall through a small incision (3–5 cm). The segmental resection of the bowel including the endometriosis is done in a conventional way (Figures 16.7, 16.12 and 16.13).

Advantages of laparoscopic access

Advantages of laparoscopic access are shown in Table 16.5. Combined with vaginal access, deep endometriosis can be mobilized and removed.[1,4,8,9,11–19]

Table 16.5 Advantages of laparoscopic surgery regarding intestinal endometriosis

No drying effect
Permanent lavage
Image enlargement
Minimal tissue trauma
Minimal bleeding tendency
Combinable with vaginal access

If necessary, additional intra-abdominal pathological changes on the bowel (endometriosis on the appendix, cecum, ileum) can also be seen and removed by endoscopic surgery.

Results

Between 1996 and 2004, 202 patients (Table 16.6) with severe endometriosis involving the bowel wall were successfully treated by laparoscopy. Over that period, only one patient underwent laparotomy in order to simultaneously carry out a reconstruction of the ureter with psoas bladder hitch.

In a prospective study of 142 patients with deep endometriosis and simultaneous involvement of the bowel wall with consecutive segment resection, it was possible to eliminate or significantly improve pelvic pain (96%), dyschezia (88%), and dyspareunia (87%) (Figure 16.14).

It was remarkable that, due to the surgery, preoperative sexual disorders could be eliminated or improved in 75% of cases. Postoperative dysmenorrhea was only observed in patients suspected of suffering from adenomyosis uteri.

Crucial to the relief of symptoms is the extent of the endometriosis resection, which is supported by the data provided by Redwine and Wright.[21]

In patients undergoing laparotomy with bowel resection, Egger et al[3] state that pelvic pain vanished and/or improved in 60–70% of cases and the cohabitation complaints in 60–83% of cases.

Fertility

Among the 36 patients wishing to conceive, 18 (50%) became pregnant. Two patients bore two children. Egger et al describe a pregnancy rate of 61%, quoting an observation period of up to 9 years.[3]

Recurrent disease

In cases of severe endometriosis, the rates of recurrence after laparoscopy range from 18% to 29% and after laparotomy 14% to 22%.[11] In our series, there were 7% of cases of residual endometriosis found in the pouch of Douglas (max. stage II), uterosacral ligaments, and/or the vagina wall. A recurrance infiltration of the bowel was not observed during an observation period of up to

Table 16.6 A total of 202 patients with intestinal endometriosis were operated on laparoscopically (several with multiple involvement of the digestive tract)

Number of patients operated on	202
Bowel resection, laparoscopically assisted (stapler anastomosis), rectum, rectosigmoid	142
Sigmoid resection, laparoscopically assisted (hand-sewn anastomosis)	32
Small intestine resection, laparoscopically assisted (hand-sewn anastomosis)	8
Appendectomy (stapler technique)	14
Resection of the cecum pole (laparoscopically assisted)	6

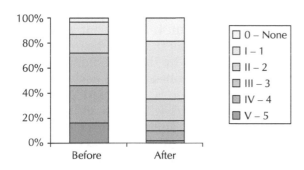

Figure 16.14 Pain before and after surgery with intestinal endometriosis (study on 142 patients in a prospective study). 0–V: score of pain in a visual analogue scoring system/VAS.

96 months. In 3 cases, endometriosis reappeared in another part of the bowel (e.g. small intestine and/or cecum). After the surgery, two patients developed deep infiltrative bladder wall endometriosis. As deep endometriosis is a disease that spreads to different organs, a complete relief of pain cannot really be expected since the organs are not removed. The surgery is undertaken to minimize the symptoms (debulking).

Quality of life

In our cohort, the quality of life was improved in 93% of cases. Bailey et al describe a satisfaction rate of 88% following laparotomy.[21]

In addition, an improvement of sexual life can be expected due to the relief of pain.

Complications

The complication rate is determined by the size and the extent of the tissue removed. Small nodes

can be removed quite easily, with low risk attributed to laparoscopic access. An involvement of the adjacent organs and a similar fibrosis of the peritoneum of the Pouch of Douglas may complicate a layer-upon-layer dissection.

The isolated removal of large nodules involving the bowel musculature makes it necessary to open the bowel lumen, which has a greater risk of complication.[15] Unnoticed and/or insufficiently treated bowel complications involve the highest risk of fistula development and peritonitis.

In our series of 202 patients, a leakage of the anastomosis occurred in 6 cases (3%). The postoperative defecation can be particularly disturbing in cases of deep resection. During an observation period of more than 8 years, no severe long-term problems of intestinal function were observed in our series (Table 16.7).

Table 16.7 Patients and surgery data concerning 202 patients with intestinal endometriosis (laparoscopically assisted)

Number of patients	202
Age	22–54 years (33.0)
Duration of surgery	181 minutes (45–260)
Complications:	
Leakage of the anastomosis	6 (3%)
Pararectal abscess	2 (1%)
Blood transfusion	1 (0.5%)
Severe stenosis of the anastomosis (dilation)	6 (3%)

Extensive nodules in the rectovaginal septum, which extend over the pararectal area on both sides and/or to the pelvis wall, may include the parasympathetic nerve fibers, particularly those for the bladder. A radical dissection of the nodule involves the risk of a severe dysfunction of the motor and sensory activity of the bladder.

If the holding structures (cardinal ligament, parametria, paracolpium) are involved, the additional risk of ureter damage has to be taken into account.

Pre- and postoperative therapies

Pre-operative therapy

Medication can prevent surgery only in cases of mild to moderate symptoms.

Here, a low-dose progesterone has proved its worth, since, owing to the side effects, danazol and/or GnRH (gonadotropin-releasing hormone) analogues can only be administered for a short time.

However, there are several reasons for not using a medication alone:

1. The endometriotic nodules 'flourish' again very quickly after the therapy.
2. The improvement of fertility is not proven.
3. Medication cannot remove adhesions.
4. Side effects of the hormone therapy are often severe and limiting.

If surgery is planned, the following should be taken into consideration before medication is administered: long-term medical therapies can cause inactive nodules to be missed during surgery which are then left behind. Necrosis and/or avascularity and fibrosis that result from hormone therapy may significantly hinder the dissection during surgery.

Postoperative therapy

At present, opinions on the usefulness of a postoperative follow-up after treatment differ. For a long time, it was thought that an incomplete surgical excision was the main reason to follow patients up. In comparative studies, Busacca et al[22] showed that the application of GnRH analogues immediately after the surgical therapy of endometriosis (stage III/IV) did not have any advantages. However, it seems to be practical and justifiable to wait 2–4 months after the surgery in order to be able to review the result of surgical intervention.

If there are still symptoms, the residual endometriosis may be present; then, the long-term administration of an ovulation inhibitor or of progestins is helpful. If the patient suffered from severe endometriosis and had a desire for children and if a follow-up by the reproductive medicine specialists was planned, GnRH analogues should be used. In our series, we could prove adenomyosis of the uterus with deep endometriosis in more than 80% of patients. In this case, the fertility impairment might be caused by a distinct change of the anatomy and/or physiology of the uterus. Then, remaining internal endometriosis nodules (adenomyosis) can be inactivated by GnRH analogues (short- or long-term protocol). Afterwards, ovulation induction therapy follows in order to treat the fertility impairment.

Summary

The operative therapy of endometriosis with intestinal involvement leads to a significant improvement of the symptoms and the patient's quality of life. Combining surgical techniques makes the radical removal of this severe form of endometriosis possible. The advantages of laparoscopic access are evident.

Because of the frequent coincidence of intestinal endometriosis and adenomyosis, postoperative therapy may be necessary in patients with fertility impairment.

REFERENCES

1. Koninckx PR, Meuleman C, Demeyere S, et al. Suggestive evidence that pelvic endometriosis is a progressive disease, whereas deeply infiltrating endometriosis is associated with pelvic pain. Fertil Steril 1991; 56: 590–591.

2. Keckstein J, Ulrich U, Possover M, et al. ENZIAN-Klassifikation der tief infiltrierenden Endometriose. Zentralbl Gynakol 2003; 125: 291–309.

3. Egger H, Turnwald W, Weiß S. Radikale operative Behandlung der Endometriose mit Darmteilresektion. Geburtshilfe Frauenheilkunde 1998; 58: 415–419.

4. Nezhat C, Pennington E, Nezhat F, et al. Laparoscopically assisted anterior rectal wall resection and reanastomosis for deeply infiltrating endometriosis. Surg Laparosc Endosc 1991; 1: 106–108.

5. Gordon SJ, Maher PJ, Woods R. Use of the CEEA stapler to avoid ultra-low segmental resection of a full-thickness rectal anometriotic nodule. J Am Assoc Gynecol Laparosc 2001; 8: 312–316.

6. Donnez J, Nisolle M. Advanced laparoscopic surgery for the removal of rectovaginal septum endometriotic or adenomyotic nodules: a series of 500 cases. Baillière's Clin Obstet Gynaecol 1995; 9: 769–774.

7. Jerby BL, Kessler H, Falcone T, et al. Laparoscopic management of colorectal endometriosis. Surg Endosc 1999; 13: 1125–1128.

8. Keckstein J, Wiesinger H, Schwarzer U. Endometriose. In: Keckstein J, Hucke J, eds. Die endoskopischen Operationen in der Gynäkologie. München: Urban & Fischer, 2000: 188–213.

9. Possover M, Diebolder H, Plaul K, et al. Laparoscopically assisted vaginal resection of rectovaginal endometriosis. Obstet Gynecol 2000; 96: 304–307.

10. Sharpe DR, Redwine D. Laparoscopic segmental resection of the sigmoid and rectosigmoid colon for endometriosis. Surg Laparosc Endosc 1992; 2: 120–124.

11. Keckstein J. Die chirurgische Therapie der Endometriose. WMW 1999; 13: 366–371.

12. Keckstein J, Tuttlies F. Die laparoskopische Therapie der Endometriose. Gynäkologe 1997; 30: 473–482.

13. Keckstein J, Wiesinger H, Kandolf O. Laparoscopic bowel resection in severe endometriosis in 35 patients. Meeting of the European Society of Gynecological Endoscopy; 1999.

14. Koninckx PR, Martin D. Treatment of deeply infiltrating endometriosis. Curr Opin Obstet Gynecol 1994; 6: 231–241.

15. Koninckx PR, Timmermans B, Meuleman C, et al. Complications of CO_2-laser endoscopic excision of deep endometriosis. Hum Reprod 1996; 11: 2263–2268.

16. Maher P, Wood C, Hill D. Excision of endometriosis in the pouch of Douglas by combined laparovaginal surgery using the Maher abdominal elevator. J Am Assoc Gynecol Laparosc 1995; 2: 199–202.

17. Nezhat F, Nezhat C, Pennington E, et al. Laparoscopic segmental resection for infiltrating endometriosis of the rectosigmoid colon: a preliminary report. Surg Laparosc Endosc 1992; 2: 212–216.

18. Nezhat C, Pennington E, Nezhat CH, et al. Laparoscopic disk excision and primary repair of the anterior rectal wall for the treatment of full-thickness bowel endometriosis. Surg Endosc 1994; 8: 682–685.

19. Redwine D, Sharpe DR. Laparoscopic segmental resection of the sigmoid colon for endometriosis. Laparoendosc Surg 1991; 1: 217–220.

20. Redwine D, Wright J. Laparoscopic treatment of complete obliteration of the cul-de-sac with endometriosis: long-term follow-up of en bloc resection. Fertil Steril 2001; 76: 358–365.

21. Bailey HR, Ott MT, Hartendorp P. Aggressive surgical management for advanced colorectal endometriosis. Dis Colon Rectum 1994; 37: 747–753.

22. Busacca M, Bianchi S, Agnoli B, et al. Follow-up of laparoscopic treatment of stage III-IV endometriosis. J Am Assoc Gynecol Laparosc 1999; 6: 55–58.

17 Severe endometriosis involving the bowel – a colo-rectal surgeon's approach

Angela J Skull and Timothy A Rockall

Introduction

Endometriosis affects up to 10% of the female population, and the bowel is involved in up to 30% of those cases.[1] The affected areas tend to be localized to the pelvic parts of the bowel, with sigmoid colon involvement in up to 73% of cases, and the rectovaginal septum containing deposits in 13% of affected patients.[2] Surgery is used in severe cases that have not responded to medical treatment, such as those with deep-seated invasive disease, endometriomas, and cul-de-sac obliteration. The latter is defined as 'extensive adhesions in the cul-de-sac, obliterating its lower portion and uniting the cervix or the lower portion of the uterus to the rectum'.[3] The posterior vaginal wall is frequently involved in cul-de-sac obliteration, too. There is some evidence to suggest that rectovaginal septum endometriosis may initially originate from adenomyotic lesions of the uterus which invade the anterior wall of the rectum.[4]

Colorectal surgery in these circumstances abides by the same principles used in treating other endometriotic lesions throughout the pelvis. All visible disease should be eradicated by excision or destruction, normal anatomy should be restored, and an attempt to minimize adhesions made while doing so. Complete excision or destruction is required to prevent recurrence. These techniques aim to increase fertility and decrease pelvic pain. Laparoscopic resection of bowel lesions is ideal, as tissue manipulation is minimal and post-operative recovery is short. It can also be easily combined with laser vaporization of any accompanying implants to ensure complete obliteration of endometrial disease.

Symptoms suggesting bowel involvement

The majority of patients with rectovaginal septum endometriosis present with pelvic pain, severe dysmenorrhea, and deep dyspareunia. Up to 25% of these patients also suffer infertility.[5] Menstrually related bowel dysfunction is reported, but the subjectivivity of the symptoms make them difficult to quantify. A change in bowel habit that precedes menstruation by 1 or 2 days is suggestive of endometriosis affecting the bowel. This may manifest by diarrhoea or constipation, and may be associated with abdominal distention, abdominal colic, and tenesmus. Perimenopausal rectal bleeding is reported in about 5% of patients, and there have been accounts of rectal endometriosis mimicking solitary rectal ulcer syndrome.[6] Bowel involvement is usually established at diagnostic laparoscopy, but can also be assessed pre-operatively with several imaging modalities.

Radiologic assessment of bowel involvement

The accuracy of detecting cul-de-sac disease by rectovaginal examination under general anesthesia is known to be poor. Sensitivity and positive predictive value for detecting rectal disease is 34% and 55.6%, respectively, in the hands of even the most experienced surgeons. Assessment of uterosacral ligament involvement is even more inaccurate.[7] More information can be obtained by performing a vaginal examination to feel for painful nodules, in the posterior and lateral vaginal fornices, which is particularly obvious if the examination is performed during menstruation.[8] Radiologic investigation is used to delineate the extent of rectal involvement prior to laparoscopy and to predict the likelihood of bowel resection. The best assessment is by an air-contrast barium enema with or without a vaginogram looked at in a lateral view by a radiologist experienced in dealing with deep infiltrating endometriosis.[9]

Transrectal ultrasound

Since 1997 there have been several studies that have assessed ultrasound imaging of the rectal wall. For accurate transrectal ultrasound, a higher-frequency 7.5 MHz probe is used. Although there is a limited field of view, there is improved resolution of close structures, enabling assessment of the rectal and vaginal walls and uterosacral ligaments. The lesions are detected as hypoechoic irregular areas surrounded by a hyperechoic rim. A study comparing these ultrasonographic findings with histology suggests that the hypoechoic area corresponds to a layer of hypertrophic mus-

cularis propria of the lesion, and the hyperechoic rim represents the mucosa, submucosa, and serosa of the bowel wall.[10] The accuracy of diagnosis with transrectal ultrasound is consistently good in the published studies, with sensitivity and specificity of 97% and 96%, respectively, for diagnosis of rectovaginal involvement in the largest series, and 80% and 97%, respectively, for uterosacral involvement (Table 17.1). Doniec et al report a histologically proven 76% sensitivity for demonstrating involvement of the muscularis propria, and 66% sensitivity to submucosal infiltration of the bowel wall.[11] Transrectal ultrasound, which is a simple and noninvasive technique, can provide a reliable indicator of deep bowel infiltration. The results obtained can be an effective aid to predict the nature of any surgery that may be necessary.

Transvaginal ultrasound

Transvaginal ultrasound is used frequently in the diagnosis of pelvic disease, and is recommended for the diagnosis of ovarian and bladder endometriosis. A wide-band 5–9 MHz transducer is used and the patient has an empty bladder. Only recently has it been evaluated for the diagnosis of rectosigmoid and uterosacral endometriosis. Bazot et al prospectively studied 30 patients and showed that the transvaginal approach was as efficient as transrectal imaging in detecting posterior pelvic endometriosis.[12] Transvaginal examination may suffice when medical treatment is being insti-

Table 17.1 Rectal endometriosis. Diagnostic accuracy of transrectal ultrasound – summary of studies

Main author	No. of patients	Sensitivity (%)	Specificity (%)	Comments
Schroeder 1997	16			6 with rectal wall involvement, 8 excluded, confirmed at laparoscopy
Fedele 1998	140	97 80	96 97	Rectovaginal septum involvement Uterosacral involvement
Chapron 1998	38			Rectovaginal septum and uterosacrals. 100% histologic confirmation
Doniec 2003	85	97 76 66	97	Rectal wall involvement Muscularis propria involvement Submucosa involvement
Abrao 2004	32	100	67	With colonoscopy

gated; however, transrectal ultrasound also determines the distance of lesions from the anal margin, which is more pertinent when surgical resection is being considered.

Magnetic resonance imaging

Magnetic resonance imaging (MRI) is an important technique in assessment of pelvic disease. It gives high soft tissue contrast resolution and discrimination in multiple planes. The T2-weighted images show zonal anatomy, and vascular structures can be identified with the T1 images. Compared with abdominal MRI, there is no motion artifact.

Endometriomas of 1 cm or more appear as homogeneously hyperintense masses on T1-weighted MR images, and as low-signal intensity masses with areas of high signal intensity on T2-weighted images. It may also be seen as multiple, homogeneously hyperintense cysts on T1-weighted images.

Studies investigating MRI in deeply invasive endometriosis have shown success in diagnosing deep endometriosis involving the uterosacral ligaments and the pouch of Douglas, but less success in detecting rectal involvement.[13] More recently, a study aimed at assessing the accuracy of rectal ultrasound and MRI prediction of rectal wall involvement in patients with already proven deeply infiltrating endometriosis has shown a higher sensitivity and negative predictive value with ultrasound.[14] This was a relatively small retrospective study and needs validation with larger prospective studies.

MRI is a useful complementary tool in the assessment of endometriosis. Used in conjunction with laparoscopy, it can depict lesions hidden by dense adhesions. However, rectovaginal septum disease is often fibrotic and does not contain blood-filled cysts that can be picked up by MRI. Rectal wall involvement is also, poorly defined.

Other imaging

Other methods of imaging have been used to investigate pelvic endometriosis, such as computed tomography (CT) colonoscopy and barium enema. CT colonoscopy may show stenotic lesions and submucosal masses. Double-contrast barium enema often shows a mass effect with crenelation of the bowel wall, which although not pathognomonic, appears to be characteristic of endometriotic bowel wall involvement.

Surgical excision of endometriosis

Surgical excision of endometriosis is considered when medical management has failed either to control pain or achieve pregnancy. Surgery attempts to excise completely any disease, in order to abate symptoms and reduce the risk of recurrence. Patients considered for excision of implants involving the colon or rectum will already have had laparoscopic assessment and any appropriate imaging to aid planning of the procedure. However thorough the preoperative investigation, it is only at the time of operation that the full extent of disease is known, and only then that the exact procedure to be performed is known. Only after dissecting down into the rectovaginal space can the decision about the extent of rectal surgery be made. A colorectal surgeon should be involved in any case where preoperative imaging has suggested involvement of the colon or rectum, which includes cul-de-sac obliteration. Any patient undergoing this surgery should be fully informed of the possible range of procedures that may be performed, and warned of the possibility of temporary stoma formation. Suitable stoma sites should be marked preoperatively. Bowel preparation with an osmotic laxative on the day prior to operation is advisable.

At the beginning of the operation, examination under anesthetic can reveal vaginal nodules, and sigmoidoscopy may help in determining any rectal mucosal abnormalities. The surgeon requires two assistants, one of whom is positioned between the legs for rectal and vaginal instrumentation. A cannula is inserted into the endometrial cavity to antevert the uterus, or a sponge on a ring forceps is inserted to aid visualization of the rectovaginal septum, and a sigmoidoscope may be used to help in defining the relative anatomy. A Hegar dilator or other rectal probe inserted into the rectum may be more manageable once the procedure is under way. After the procedure is completed, the sigmoidoscope is used to inflate air into the rectum while the pelvis is filled with warmed isotonic saline to exclude air leaks of any anastomosis. Destruction of any further endometriotic implants within the pelvis can be performed after bowel surgery by vaporization with a laser.

The surgical options for removal of endometriotic implants are as follows:

- anterior resection of the rectum
- shave excision
- rectal disk excision
- stapled excision.

Anterior resection of the rectum

A 12 mm umbilical port is used in laparoscopic resections, with a lateral 5 mm port, a lateral 12 mm port, and a 10 mm suprapubic port. Carbon dioxide is insufflated to 14 mmHg. A cannula is inserted into the uterus, and a Hegar dilator into the rectum. Commencing at the pelvic brim, the ureters are identified and ureterolysis performed as necessary so that these retract upwards and laterally, out of the operative field. It is most important that the ureters are identified in all cases at the beginning of the operation, as fibrosis often displaces them medially, leaving them susceptible to iatrogenic damage. The endometriotic lesion is removed, as described by Redwine and Wright,[15] commencing dissection in a non-involved portion of peritoneum, starting at the left pelvic side wall, just lateral to the deposit. The incision extends medially towards the uterus, taking the uterosacral ligaments with the specimen if they are involved. The incision is continued across the back of the uterus, transecting the uterosacral ligaments, along the right pelvic side wall until clear of any endometriotic deposits. The dissection continues back to come across the rectum and join up with the starting point of dissection. A rectangle of tissue is excised, tethered by the underlying structures, being the rectum, rectovaginal septum, and prerectal tissues down to the pelvic floor. A combination of sharp and blunt dissection is used to separate the structures. Dissection beyond the nodule into normal distal rectovaginal septum frees the lesion so that it is only the rectum that is attached. It is often necessary to excise part of the vaginal wall in order to fully excise the affected tissue. Once the part of rectum to be removed is identified, the mesentery is incised at the sacral promontory and the inferior mesenteric artery isolated, ligated, and divided. The proximal sigmoid is mobilized adequately, and the distal rectum transected using an endoscopic stapler. The divided rectum is delivered through a small suprapubic incision. The well-vascularized sigmoid or left colon is identified, divided, and a purse-string suture applied and the anvil of the circular stapler is inserted. Once returned to the abdomen, an intracorporeal circular end-to-end stapled anastamosis is performed.

The diseased bowel can be removed through the vaginal opening if this has been created during dissection.[16] The proximal bowel is then pulled through this opening and the purse-string suture applied before returning to the abdomen, to complete the anastamosis with a standard circular stapler. The vagina can subsequently be repaired transvaginally or laparoscopically. The integrity of the anastamosis is tested as previously described.

Shave excision

Shave excision of endometriosis is used for the superficial excision of serosal implants on the bowel wall. If the endometriotic nodules in the prerectal fascia are mobile, shave excision is usually possible. This is performed laparascopically, using an harmonic scalpel to excise the implant. Diathermy excision is not advisable, as depth of tissue injury is greater and the risk of a full-thickness burn is much higher. It is advisable to visualize the bowel lumen after excision by proctosigmoidoscopy if possible, and ensure against any rectosigmoid injury by filling the pelvis with warmed isotonic fluid to observe any air leakage.

Rectal disk excision

After full laparoscopic dissection of the rectovaginal septum, it is sometimes apparent that the endometriotic nodule, although adherent to the anterior rectal wall, encompasses less than 50% of the circumference of the rectal wall. In these cases, rectal disk excision can be performed. The affected tissue is excised en bloc, and the anterior rectal wall is repaired transversely using interrupted absorbable intracorporeal sutures. This technique has been effective, and there is no discernible increase in stricture formation as a result of this method.[17]

Stapled excision

Since 2001, disk excision of endometriosis affecting the anterior rectal wall has been performed using a circular stapling device in limited cases. Initially, this method was used in a case where complete excision would have resulted in an ultra low rectal resection and anastamosis. Subsequently, this procedure has been used in selected circumstances. Stapled excision is effective where the disease is less than 2 cm in diameter and does not involve more than one-third of the total circumference of the rectum.[18] Laboratory studies performed by Harris and Rieger testing the efficacy of the anastamotic join shows that its competence equals that of an end-on stapled anastamosis.[19] This has been borne out by the patient outcomes.[18]

To perform the stapled excision, the rectum must be fully mobilized around the disease present on the anterior rectal wall. Importantly, the vagina must be mobilized from the rectum by a sufficient length to avoid imbrication into the stapling device. Stay sutures are placed either side of the affected area, and the circular stapler inserted per anus. The staple gun is opened fully, and then, with guidance by the stay sutures, the gun is closed while incorporating the affected bowel. The staple gun is fired as recommended by the manufacturer, which results in simultaneous excision and closure of the anterior rectal wall. The device is removed from the anus. On inspection of the excised disk, a full-thickness circle of tissue should be present.

These are the different variations in surgical procedures commonly performed for rectovaginal endometriosis. Of course, the chosen procedure varies with individual surgeons as well as with patients, but there are three series that give a representation of the type of surgery to be expected when undertaking this procedure (Table 17.2). Ford[20] reports that of 60 radical resections, 48 patients underwent a prerectal shave, 2 had disk excisions, and 10 had anterior resections performed. When following up patients with stage IV endometriosis and bowel involvement at the Cleveland Clinic, Duepree et al noted that 26 had superficial shave excisions, 18 had bowel resections, and 5 underwent disk excisions.[21] A retrospective study of 169 patients undergoing rectal dissection or excision for endometriosis at the Mercy Hospital for Women in Melbourne recorded 132 patients undergoing a superficial shave dissection, 12 having a disk excision and 25 undergoing a segmental resection.[16]

Evidence for aggressive treatment of endometriosis

Treatment aims in endometriosis are to stop pelvic pain and enhance fertility. Treatment is also preventive, especially in younger patients, as halting this progressive disease can avoid massive distortion of the pelvis, which may affect future fertility. Although gonadotropin releasing hormone analogues help dysmenorrhea and possibly control disease progression, they do not control dyspareu-

nia. They have side effects including bone loss, which may take years to replace, and currently they should not be taken for long periods of time. Laparoscopic colorectal and pelvic surgery has been called 'aggressive but conservative surgery',[16] as the aim is to maintain gynecologic function while facilitating a cure of disease. The factors of utmost import in determining the future of this surgery are whether there is an acceptable complication rate and whether the quality of life improves after surgery.

Complication rates

In 1992 Nehzat published a series of 16 rectal resections for endometriosis, and reported no major complications.[22] Subsequently, Duepree retrospectively analyzed 50 patients who underwent laparoscopic resection of rectal endometriosis. He reported an average 2 day hospital stay, and 10.3% complication rate.[21] In 2003 Varol reported a series of 169 women who underwent similar procedures, and reported an overall morbidity of 12.4% – half of which was urinary tract infection.[16] The most recently reported cohort study of 60 radical resections of endometriosis recorded the mean duration of surgery being 146 minutes, with a mean estimated blood loss of 400 ml and average 4.6 days hospital stay. Five of the patients needed blood transfusions, and two required a temporary colostomy. Two patients required ureteric stents because of extensive ureterolysis, and two patients have had subsequent anastamotic dilatation.[20]

Quality of life after surgery

There have been several studies investigating symptoms following surgery to resect endometriosis in the pouch of Douglas,[4,5,23] but these have not included bowel resection. In 1993 Wood et al reported marked reduction in coital and rectal pain in 92% of patients.[23] Donnez et al followed up 242 patients for over 2 years following surgery, and reported only a 3.7% rate of continued severe

Table 17.2 Frequency of surgical procedures

Main author	Number of patients	Shave	Bowel resection	Disk excision
Duepree 2002[21]	51	26 (50%)	18 (35%)	5 (10%)
Varol 2003[16]	169	132 (78%)	25 (15%)	12 (7%)
Ford 2004[19]	60	48 (80%)	10 (17%)	2 (3%)

pain, and 1.2% dyspareunia.[4] Garry et al analyzed 57 patients who were severely ill with impaired quality of life and sexual activity, and found there was a significant improvement in all measured parameters, including quality of life 4 months after surgery.[5]

Surgery, including bowel resections has been reported, but not yet in such numbers: 29 patients who underwent open bowel resection for endometriosis had a 100% subjective improvement, with 48% 'cured', with no reported symptoms.[24] It was noted that the most successful operations tended to include hysterectomy and oophorectomy. Fedele analyzed the cases of 83 women, some of whom underwent rectal resection.[25] At 12 months, 28% had pain recurrence. The younger patients were at higher risk of recurrence and those who underwent bowel resection had the lowest risk.

In a follow-up study of 169 patients,[16] 36% required further laparoscopy for pain, although mostly this was due to filmy adhesions, and was successfully treated, whereas 15% had evidence of recurrence. Ford et al's review of 60 resections found that 70% had a good response at 12 months.[19] Those who had a disk or segmental resection, reported a good response and a normal quality of life. Overall, the quality of life scores in the study group were lower than in the background population.

Conclusions

Rectovaginal septum endometriosis is at the more severe end of the spectrum of the disease. When complete cul-de-sac obliteration is present, it is a debilitating and painful condition associated with poor quality of life scores. Laparoscopic equipment and techniques are now advanced enough to offer safe, radical excision of endometriotic implants, including bowel resection if necessary. These procedures must be planned so that a colorectal surgeon is involved, and all cases should be fully prepared for bowel resection as the extent of surgery is only known at the time of the operation. Although stoma sites should be marked, data suggest that the risk of temporary stoma formation is 4%. Most procedures involve a rectal shave (50–80%); diskectomy is the least performed, in 3–10% of cases; and resection of the bowel is performed in 15–35% of procedures.

This surgery may involve technically challenging dissection, but can be accomplished effectively with short recovery times and low postoperative morbidity. Aggressive laparoscopic excision should be performed by specialists. Although only small numbers of retrospective studies are available, it seems that bowel resection seems to be associated with better symptom control. With this in mind, radical surgery excising all endometriosis should be planned, and bowel resection should be actively pursued.

REFERENCES

1. Regenet N, Metairie S, Cousin GM, et al. [Colorectal endometriosis. Diagnosis and management]. Ann Chir 2001; 126(8): 734–742. [in French]
2. Bartkowiak R, Zieniewicz K, Kaminski P, et al. Diagnosis and treatment of sigmoidal endometriosis – a case report. Med Sci Monit 2000; 6(4): 787–790.
3. Sampson JA. The life history of ovarian haematomas (haemorrhagic cysts of endometrial (Mullerian) type. Am J Obstet Gynecol 1922; 4: 451–456.
4. Donnez J, Nisolle M, Gillerot S, et al. Rectovaginal septum adenomyotic nodules: a series of 500 cases. Br J Obstet Gynaecol 1997; 104(9): 1014–1018.
5. Garry R, Clayton R, Hawe J. The effect of endometriosis and its radical laparoscopic excision on quality of life indicators. BJOG 2000; 107(1): 44–54.
6. Daya D, O'Connell G, DeNardi F. Rectal endometriosis mimicking solitary rectal ulcer syndrome. Mod Pathol 1995; 8(6): 599–602.
7. Dragisic KG, Padilla LA, Milad MP. The accuracy of the rectovaginal examination in detecting cul-de-sac disease in patients under general anaesthesia. Hum Reprod 2003; 18(8): 1712–1715.
8. Koninckx PR, Meuleman C, Oosterlynk D, et al. Diagnosis of deep endometriosis by clinical examination during menstruation and plasma CA-125 concentration. Fertil Steril 1996; 65: 280–287.
9. Walker W. Personal communication.
10. Koga K, Osuga Y, Yano T, et al. Characteristic images of deeply infiltrating rectosigmoid endometriosis on transvaginal and transrectal ultrasonography. Hum Reprod 2003; 18(6): 1328–1333.
11. Doniec JM, Kahlke V, Peetz F, et al. Rectal endometriosis: high sensitivity and specificity of endorectal ultrasound with an impact for the operative management. Dis Colon Rectum 2003; 46(12): 1667–1673.
12. Bazot M, Detchev R, Cortez A, et al. Transvaginal sonography and rectal endoscopic sonography for the

assessment of pelvic endometriosis: a preliminary comparison. Hum Reprod 2003; 18(8): 1686–1692.

13. Kinkel K, Chapron C, Balleyguier C, et al. Magnetic resonance imaging characteristics of deep endometriosis. Hum Reprod 1999; 14(4): 1080–1086.

14. Chapron C, Vieira M, Chopin N, et al. Accuracy of rectal endoscopic ultrasonography and magnetic resonance imaging in the diagnosis of rectal involvement for patients presenting with deeply infiltrating endometriosis. Ultrasound Obstet Gynecol 2004; 24(2): 175–179.

15. Redwine DB, Wright JT. Laparoscopic treatment of complete obliteration of the cul-de-sac associated with endometriosis: long-term follow-up of en bloc resection. Fertil Steril 2001; 76(2): 358–365.

16. Varol N, Maher P, Healey M, et al. Rectal surgery for endometriosis – should we be aggressive? J Am Assoc Gynecol Laparosc 2003; 10(2): 182–189.

17. Nezhat C, Nezhat F, Pennington E, et al. Laparoscopic disk excision and primary repair of the anterior rectal wall for the treatment of full-thickness bowel endometriosis. Surg Endosc 1994; 8(6): 682–685.

18. Woods RJ, Heriot AG, Chen FC. Anterior rectal wall excision for endometriosis using the circular stapler. ANZ J Surg 2003; 73(8): 647–648.

19. Harris GJC, Ringer N. Personal communication.

20. Ford J, English J, Miles WA, et al. Pain, quality of life and complications following the radical resection of rectovaginal endometriosis. BJOG 2004; 111(4): 353–356.

21. Duepree HJ, Senagore AJ, Delaney CP, et al. Laparoscopic resection of deep pelvic endometriosis with rectosigmoid involvement. J Am Coll Surg 2002; 195(6): 754–758.

22. Nezhat F, Nezhat C, Pennington E, et al. Laparoscopic segmental resection for infiltrating endometriosis of the rectosigmoid colon: a preliminary report. Surg Laparosc Endosc 1992; 2(3): 212–216.

23. Wood C, Maher P, Hill D. Laparoscopic removal of endometriosis in the pouch of Douglas. Aust N Z J Obstet Gynaecol 199; 33(3): 295–299.

24. Urbach DR, Reedijk M, Richard CS, et al. Bowel resection for intestinal endometriosis. Dis Colon Rectum 1998; 41(9): 1158–1164.

25. Fedele L, Bianchi S, Zanconato G, et al. Long-term follow-up after conservative surgery for rectovaginal endometriosis. Am J Obstet Gynecol 2004; 190(4): 1020–1024.

18 Bowel resection

Marc Possover and David Adamson

Anatomic considerations required for the 'parasympathetic nerve-sparing technique'

Parasympathetic innervation of the pelvis

The nervus vagus, also the nervus pneumogastricus, is generally called the bowel nerve and functions as a combination of two counterparts. The right nervus vagus mainly innervates the bowel channel up to the colon flexor, whereas the left nervus vagus is primarily for the nervous regulation of the epigastric region and the liver.

The nervi splanchnici pelvini, which are the preganglion fibers leading out of the parasympathetic heartland of the spinal sacral vertebra S2–4 and S5, provide the parasympathetic innervation of the pelvis. These nerves run in the pars nervosa of the ligamentum cardinale, medial to the musculus ischiococcygeus and then directly to the rectum, the internal anal sphincter, and the bladder. In the neural part of the cardinal ligament, the more mediodorsal parasympathetic fibers proceed to the rectum, whereas the more lateroventral fibers supply the bladder.

The parasympathetic fibers anastomose medial to the musculus ischiococcygeus with the homolateral distal part of the plexus pelvicus, or the plexus hypogastricus inferior. The plexus pelvicus expands to the side of the rectum in the rectovaginal ligament.

The parasympathetic nerves in the pelvis are responsible for bladder micturition, sensation in the rectum and defecation, which is accomplished by the process of contracting the bowel wall of the rectum and subsequently relaxing the internal anal sphincter.

From a surgical perspective, the cranial nerves of the plexus pelvicus contain mainly sympathetic fibers, whereas the caudal nerves contain sympathetic and parasympathetic fibers, such as the ligamenti rectovaginales. The more radical the surgical removal of the ligamenti rectovaginales, the higher is the rate of postoperative functional morbidity, including problems with chronic obstipation and the elimination of bladder sensation, which results in the need to empty the bladder hourly by pressing on the stomach. Similar morbidity can be expected when the nervi splanchnici are transected during removal of the pars nervosa of the cardinal ligament directly after its exit from the plexus sacralis.

The sympathetic innervation of the pelvis

The sympathetic innervation of the pelvis is effected by two different sympathetic systems: the hypogastric nervous system and the truncus sympathicus.

The hypogastric nervous system

As different plexi emanate from the vegetative plexus solaris, they orientate themselves along the various collaterals of the aorta and innervate all the abdominal organs. One of them is the plexus intermesentericus, which runs ventrolaterally to the aorta, between both arteriae mesentericae, and forms the plexus mesentericus inferior. This plexus dispatches branches, which partially accompany the arteria mesenterica and branches that run between the arteria mesenterica inferior and the aorta to form the roots of both the nervi hypogastrici inferiores.

In order to avoid injury to these nerves during a left-sided para-aortic lymphadenectomy, it is recommended that the mesosigmoid be prepared dorsal to the arteria mesenterica inferior along the arteria iliaca communis sinstra. This way, one reaches an anatomic level dorsal to the plexus hypogastricus superior or mesentericus inferior. At the level of the fifth lumbar vertebrae or ventral to the promontory, both the nervis hypogastrici divide laterally, run caudal dorsally to the rectosigmoid, ventrally to the Waldeyer's fascia and anastomose with the plexus hypogastricus inferior.

The plexus hypogastricus inferior von Hovelacque (Knot from Lee, hypogastric knots, or plexus pelvicus) lies deep in the pelvis in the spatium pelvorectal superior von Gregoire lateral to the rectum and the craniodorsal part of the vagina. The plexus shows itself as a net of fibers that form a 'sacrouterine ligament', also called a 'rectovaginal pillar'.

Two groups of terminal fibers come out of the plexus hypogastricus inferior:

1 A craniomedial pelvic group that forms four further plexi:

  • The uterine plexus: coming from the front part of the plexus hypogastricus inferior and running along the plexus uterinus in the ventral and cranial part of the ligamentum sacrouterinum and reaching the uterus in the area of the isthmus.
  • The vaginal plexus.
  • The ureteral plexus along the terminal ureters, about 1 cm from the vesicoureteral mouth. The periureteral tissue at this point should be preserved to prevent a ureteral stenosis.
  • The vesical plexus that is anastomosed with the ureteral plexus and lies on the crossing of the lateral to the dorsocaudal part of the bladder.

2 A perineopelvic group, which also innervates the ureter, the bladder, the plexus rectalis, and the plexus hemorrhoidalis medial.

The plexus hypogastricus connects dorsally to the truncus sympathicus and caudally to the nervis planchnici pelvici. The stimulation of the nervi hypogastrici inferior has a sympathetic effect – relaxation of the flat musculature of the rectum and contraction of the sphincter ani internus – and is certainly involved in the sexual lubrication of the patient.

The truncus sympathicus

The truncus sympathicus stretches on both sides of the spine as a uniform nerve fiber–ganglion cord. The trunk part of the truncus sympathicus is proximal to the lumbal and sacral part. Both trunci lumbales run directly along the medial insertion of the musculus iliopsoas, ventral to the venae lumbales and leave about four ganglia neuralgia.

From a surgical perspective, the left truncus sympathicus can be identified beside the aorta, whereas the right truncus sympathicus remains hidden behind the vena cava inferior and can only be damaged by a retrocaval lymphadenectomy. Damage to the truncus sympathicus typically leads to homolateral peripheral vasodilation and consequential warming of the homolateral foot.

The sacral part of the truncus sympathicus runs along the SWS, medial to the anterior foramina sacralia. It normally consists of three ganglia sacralia, which form fibers ventral to the os sacrum of the opposite ganglion and show anastomosis to the plexus hypogastricus inferior. This anastomosis seems to be responsible for the sensation of fullness in the bladder and rectum.

Surgery

Preparation of the patient

The classical bowel lavage with a few liters of fluid has been abandoned and is no longer performed, even when a rectum resection/anastomosis must be accomplished. The new protocol instructs the patient to take two or four bisacodyl tablets, depending on her weight the day before surgery.

The operation

The surgical procedure must always begin with a rectovaginal examination of the patient under anesthesia in order to explore the relation between the vagina and the rectum. Infiltration of the rectum and stenosis should be felt, as endometriosis mainly infiltrates the rectum about 5–7 cm above the linea dentata.

Part 1: the vaginal part

After disinfection of the vagina, the posterior fornix of the vagina is exposed by two Breisky specula and the cervix is pulled ventrally by two tenacula. The vagina as well as the posterior cervix are infiltrated with about 5–10 ml of lidocaine hydrochloride 1% with epinephrine. The vasoconstrictor effect of the epinephrine is of great importance, as dissection of the rectovaginal septum and the Denonvilliers' fascia requires optimal vision and blood-free incisions.

After waiting for the injection puncture to stop bleeding, which takes from 2 to 3 minutes, the vagina is incised around the endometriotic nodule with adequate free margin; direct digital palpation allows for optimal control of the limit between the lesion and the surrounding healthy tissue.

The lesion is transected from the cervix using monopolar needle electrosurgery upwards over 2–3 cm. If photodocumentation from previous surgery demonstrates that no intestinal adhesions are attached to the cervix and/or pouch of Douglas, dissection of the lesion from the cervix is carried on upwards with scissors and the pouch of Douglas is opened.

This dissection saves a lot of time during the subsequent laparoscopic component of the surgical procedure, as laparoscopic dissection of the lesion from the cervix is not easy. When this dissection is performed ventrally, a large resection of the cervix is perfomed. A dorsal dissection risks potential damage to the bowel. Vaginal dissection permits the surgeon to follow the dorsal wall of the cervix and to optimally control potential bleeding.

If no documentation can prove that the pouch of Douglas is free, the dissection of the posterior cervix is stopped, before opening the pouch of Douglas, so that injury associated with any attached intestinal adhesions may be avoided. The dissection of the cervix is performed lateral to the rectovaginal ligament and is stopped at that point to prevent endangering the ureter. The dissection of the rest of the vagina and of the rectovaginal space is performed with scissors. After placing a finger in the rectum, the Denonvilliers' fascia, just caudal to the lesion, is exposed and divided.

The Denonvilliers' fascia is an extremely important anatomical stucture; this fascia builds an anatomical fence against infiltration by endometriosis. In many cases, dissection of the space dorsal to it shows an infiltration of the fascia without infiltration of the prerectal space, so bowel resection is not required. The dissection vaginally saves time because it is much easier than the laparoscopic approach. Concomitant digital rectal palpation allows for the surgeon to know exactly the limit of the rectum and to control minor bleeding, which could potentially obscure optimal sight and exposure of the dissection area.

The rectovaginal space caudal to the nodule is expanded by blunt dissection to expose the rectal wall, where the transection will be performed laparoscopically. Lateral to the rectum, both pararectal spaces are dissected and extended dorsally to the coccygeal bone and as close to the rectal wall as possible.

The insertion of a finger in the rectum allows for the dissection of both pararectal spaces close to the rectum, so that the space medial to the pelvic splanchnic nerves may be opened with a lower risk of injuring the rectum.

The excised portion of the vagina is left on the rectum and the vagina is sutured to the posterior cervix by interrupted sutures. No manipulator is used on the uterus because uterine manipulation could pull out the vaginal sutures.

In the situation where there is anastomotic leakage, the opening of the vagina is the best natural drainage for early diagnosis, before the patient develops pelvic peritonitis. For circumstances involving postoperative hematoma of the pelvis, removal of one or two sutures will allow for spontaneous flow and evacuation of any residual blood through the vagina.

Part 2: the laparoscopic 'en bloc dissection'

For the laparoscopic part of the procedure, the patient is placed in the Trendelenburg position with straight legs, as no further rectovaginal examination or uterine manipulation is required during this phase of the procedure. A 10 mm trocar is passed through the umbilicus to hold the laparoscope with the mounted camera. Additionally, three 5 mm trocars are placed in the lower abdomen, with the lateral trocars positioned lateral to the epigastric vessels. For the dissection, only scissors, two forceps, and a 3 mm bipolar coagulation forceps are utilized.

The principle of this dissection is not primarily removal of the nodule from the surrounding tissue, but exposure of the surrounding anatomic structures. During excision of a nodule from the rectovaginal septum, some neural structures must be resected. Part of the rectovaginal ligament and the cranial part of the inferior hypogastric plexus are mainly involved. To reduce functional complications postoperatively, the nerve at the level of the nodule must be saved. At the pelvic wall, the anatomy is respected and left intact, at least on one side. It is easier to expose the parasympathetic nerves as they exit with the sacral roots (S2–S3) and then dissect them by following them. The resection of the nodule, or of the rectum, is not difficult with the surrounding anatomic structures exposed and the rectosigmoid freed.

On the right side, the retroperitoneal space is opened at the promontory between the sigmoid and the right ureter. The right pararectal and retro-sigmoid-rectal spaces are extended by blunt dissection directly along the sacrum and more caudally to the coccygeal bone, strictly on the medial line. An identical dissection is performed on the opposite side medial to the left ureter and unification with the right dissection is performed dorsal to the rectosigmoid. Both pararectal gutters are transected caudal to the level of both recto-vaginal ligaments, whereas both ureters are dissected to the level of their crossing with the uterine arteries. The rectosigmoid is completely freed from the pelvic floor.

This dissection is continued laterally and ventrally in the direction of the dorsal aspect of the cardinal ligament by absolute smooth and gentle dissection. The third sacral root is identified lateral to the fascia hypogastric sacralis. Confirmation is acquired by using laparoscopic electrostimulation: the S3 nerves are responsible for levator movement, or bellow movement, of the peritoneum. Visually, this is apparent as a deepening and flattening of the buttock groove as well as plantar flexion of the large toe and, to a lesser extent, the smaller toes. Identification of S3 is performed because S3 and S4 are the roots responsible for bladder function. By maximal use of the endoscope's magnification, dissection of S3 is extended ventrally and the parasympathetic nerves, which emanate mediocaudally from this root, are identified and their function is confirmed using laparoscopic neuro-navigation – LANN.[1,2] The nerves are followed ventrally by extremely gentle dissection to their anastomosis with the homolateral inferior hypogastric plexus. If it is possible, depending on the extent of the endometriosis, this dissection of the parasympathetic nerves is performed on both sides.

It is normally not feasible to preserve the cranial part of the inferior hypogastric plexus, as endometriosis usually infiltrates this area of the rectovaginal ligament. However, the parasympathetic nerves anastomose to this pelvic plexus much more caudally and can be preserved for the most part, at least on one side. Postoperative functional morbidities are generally not due to infiltration or destruction of these nerves by endometriosis, but due to their transection during the dissection.

Dissection is continued dorsally and Waldeyer's fascia is opened just caudal to the endometriotic nodule. Both pararectal spaces that have been opened vaginally are exposed.

Finally, transection of the rest of the rectocervico-vaginal ligament is performed close to the cervix, allowing development of the rectovaginal space caudal to the lesion that had been vaginally opened.

The endometriotic nodule is completely mobilized en bloc and remains on the anterior wall of the rectum covered by the excised portion of the vagina. The rectum below the lesion is free and mobile enough for this transection. The middle 5 mm suprapubic trocar is removed and is replaced by a 12 mm trocar and the rectum is transected caudal to the endometriotic lesion using a laparoscopic stapling device Endo-GIA manufactured by Ethicon Endosurgery Cincinati, OH.

Complete laparoscopic mobilization of the recto-sigmoid allows extraction of its cephalad portion through a suprapubic minilaparotomy, 2–3 cm wide. If mobilization of the pelvic connective tissue is not sufficient, the mesosigmoid is mobilized by incision of the peritoneum in the left paracolic gutter and the left colonic flexure. Particular attention is paid to avoid uretal injury.

To check if the deep anterior colorectal anastomosis is free of tension, the endometriotic lesion is grasped and pulled up to the suprapubic trocar. If there is tension caused by this maneuver, there is a risk of tension on the anastomosis and transection of the superior rectal artery is required. A transection of the inferior mesenteric artery or the sigmoidal artery is normally not necessary because with endometriosis of the rectovaginal space, the tension on the anastomosis is normally not due to the shortness of the rectosigmoid, but to the tension of the meso rectosigmoid. Transection of the superior rectal artery can be performed as the blood supply to the terminal rectum is assured by the arcade of Drummond, the prolongation of Riolan's arch, and, consequently, of the arteria colica sinistra.

Part 3: the deep anterior colorectal anastomosis
After removal of the 12 mm trocar, this incision is enlarged to a length of about 2–3 cm. Complete

laparoscopic mobilization of the rectosigmoid allows extraction of the cephalad portion of the rectum through this suprapubic minilaparotomy. The best area for the bowel transection cranial to the endometriotic lesion is selected by extra-abdominal inspection and palpation. This transection is performed with a purse-string suture. After dilatation of the bowel, the tilt-top anvil of a transanal circular stapler is introduced and the purse-string suture is knotted.

To reduce the risk of the anastomosis stenosing, the size of the circular stapler chosen must be as large as possible. At the level of the lower rectum, size 33/34, and 31 at least, can usually be used.

The bowel is reintroduced into the abdomen and the minilaparotomy incision is closed. The stapler is then inserted into the rectal stump transanally and the connector is pushed just lateral to the existing staple line (Figure 18.1).

Transanal colorectal anastomosis is performed by connecting the stapling device with the anvil and firing the stapler. The anastomosis is controlled laparoscopically by transanal air insufflation while compressing the sigmoid to confirm integrity of the anastomosis.

At the end of the procedure, a drainage Charrière 16–18 is placed in the pelvis, but direct contact with the anastomosis must be avoided.

When rectal resection with deep anterior colorectal anastomosis less than 6 cm from the linea dentata is performed, even with the 'parasympathetic nerve-sparing technique', a suprapubic catheter is placed at the end of the procedure for two reasons:

1. to avoid filling of the bladder before spontaneous defecation, which could disturb the healing process of the deep anterior colorectal anastomosis
2. because dissection of the nerve, even gentle dissection, can produce a neuropraxy for a few days and, consequently, temporary bladder atony.

Postoperative management

During the first 6 days following the procedure, no rectovaginal manipulation should be performed and no solid foods are given to avoid stimulating bowel movement. The patient receives an intravenous infusion program of about 2.5 L/day and 0.5 L of oral liquid is permitted.

To make the postoperative follow-up as safe as possible, the bladder is drained for the first 6 postoperative days, during which time the risk of anastomosis leakage is the highest. Bladder training begins after sponataneous defecation, generally between the 6th and 8th postoperative day. The suprapubic catheter is removed when the post-micturition residual urine volume is measured to be consistently less than 70 ml. After spontaneous defecation, the patient is allowed to resume eating, starting with a bland diet.

Laparoscopic-assisted vaginal 'parasympathetic nerve-sparing' technique – why this technique?

Radical pelvic surgery is usually restricted to malignant diseases. Thus, retroperitoneal dissection with bowel resection and anastomosis might appear too drastic, with a high risk of adverse postoperative symptoms such as anastomotic leakage and bladder atony.

(a)   (b)   (c)

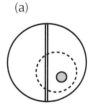 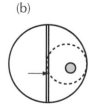 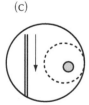

Figure 18.1 The transfixion of the rectal stump does not have to be performed through the staple line because the risk of separation is high. (a) The transfixion does not have to be performed more than 2 cm away from this staple line. (b) Superposition of both staple lines exposes the anastomosis to an increased risk of leakage. (c) When a bridge of tissue occurs between both staple lines, the risk of a fistula and ischemia of this tissue is extremely high.

Why rectum resection/anastomosis?

Submucosal excision of bowel endometriosis can only be used with limited lesions, and in-situ resection is uncertain because deep endometriosis of the bowel is characterized by multifocal disease in the muscularis of the intestinal wall. This dissection is tedious and time-consuming in large lesions; intraoperative bowel perforation or extended coagulation with ischemia of the remaining wall can occur, and the risk of post-operative bowel perforation/fistula is high. Thus, with endometriosis infiltrating an area of the rectum wall more than 3 cm in diameter, resection with anastomosis is safer than local excision.

Why laparoscopic-assisted vaginal technique?

For treatment of deep rectovaginal endometriosis, several surgical approaches have been described.[3-8] Regardless of approach, two specific conditions must be met during the surgery to remove rectovaginal endometriosis completely. First, the ureter and uterine artery must be dissected from surrounding tissue because endometriosis infiltrates the tissue along the uterine artery quite frequently.[4] Secondly, digital palpation of the tissue, first of all the vagina, the cervix, and the rectum, is mandatory to select the optimal resection plane for complete removal of all endometriotic tissue.

Table 18.1 shows the advantages and disadvantages of the different techniques. All 'one-way' approaches have their own benefits and drawbacks and no one of these approaches presents all of the necessary advantages at once. With our 'three-way' approach we have all the advantages together:

1. Vaginal:
   - Transvaginal identification of adequate levels of the caudal resection margins

Table 18.1 Advantages and disadvantages of the different techniques

Surgical approach	Advantages	Disadvantages
Vaginal approach	Resection of the vagina adapted to the size of the lesion Optimal dissection of the lower part of the lesion Optimal dissection of the space dorsal to Denonvilliers' fascia Optimal resection of the nodule from the dorsal cervix Time-saving	No dissection of the uterine arteries and of the ureters No approach to the entire pelvic cavity No mobilization of the rectosigmoid Risk of intestinal injury in frozen pelvis Partial rectum resection depends on the view and the technical approach
Laparoscopic approach	Optimal view of the entire pelvic cavity Optimal access to all regions of the pelvis Possibility of 'nerve-sparing' technique Blood-free/fewer adhesions Optimal mobilization of the recto-sigmoid	Difficult to find the right plane to the dorsal cervix Difficulties in adapting the colpectomy to the exact degree of infiltration Time-consuming
Laparotomy approach	Digital palpation of the tissue	Techniques of macrosurgery Difficulties of access to the depth of the pelvis by preservation of the uterus Postoperative adhesions Difficulties of view and dissection dorsal to the rectum

becomes possible by direct digital exploration of the rectovaginal and pararectal spaces.

- Since the space of Denonvillier is a barrier to the dorsal progression of the endometriosis to the rectum, dissection dorsal to this fascia can be performed with optimal view and saves dissection of the rectum. If a lesion of the lower rectum appears or if a circular rectum excision has to be performed, suturing may be used extraperitoneally and under optimal conditions.
- Dissection of the rectum, at the level where the stapler transection will be performed, as close as possible to the rectal wall, avoids injury to the splanchnic pelvic nerves.

2. Laparoscopic:

- All intrapelvic lesions can be removed and further associated urologic or intestinal procedures can be performed.
- Laparoscopic magnification and the possibility of dissection in all parts of the retroperitoneal space are the basis for the 'parasympathetic nerve-sparing technique'.
- A retroperitoneal approach and mobilization of the lesion en bloc with the rectosigmoid minimizes blood loss and shortens operating time.

3. Minilaparotomy:

- Exenteration of the rectosigmoid through a minilaparotomy allows in-situ resection of the infiltrated segment by direct palpation and inspection of the bowel wall and its lumen.
- Digital palpation of the pelvis and part of the abdomen is possible through minilaparotomy.
- When further partial bladder resection or ureter resection is performed by laparoscopy, suturing of the bladder or uretero-cystoneostomy can be performed more easily and quickly through minilaparotomy than laparoscopy.

Our technique is to be differentiated from the other described techniques, as the endometriotic nodule is not dissected from the surrounding tissue, but instead the retroperitoneal space is first dissected at the pelvic wall where the normal anatomy allows for exposure of all anatomic structures, primarily the parasympathetic nerves.

Why the 'parasympathetic nerve-sparing technique'?

In our series of consecutive patients following 'parasympathetic nerve-sparing' major surgery for deep infiltrating endometriosis ($n = 91$), the suprapubic catheter could be removed after an average of 2 days of bladder training. It was always possible to intraoperatively preserve at least one side of the parasympathetic nerves. All of these patients were able to void their bladders normally, spontaneously, and continuously.

Our technique of laparoscopic-assisted vaginal nerve-sparing resection of the rectum, with deep anterior colorectal anastomosis in extended endometriosis, is based on the principle of primary systematic identification, dissection, and preservation of the parasympathetic nerves before dissection of the endometriotic nodule because exposure of the nerves close to the nodule is technically not possible. The only chance of identifying the pelvic parasympathetic nerves is near the pelvic wall, where the tissue is normally not invaded by endometriosis and consequently the anatomy has remained normal. Our results show a significantly lower rate of reduced bladder function after deep anterior colorectal anastomosis, even in comparison to the nerve-sparing mesorectal excision technique, which is about 20–40%. To date, we have performed laparoscopic rectum resection with deep anterior colorectal anastomosis on 91 consecutive patients. No patient in our series had to use self-catheterization but in comparison to our first series, the mean duration of bladder training was reduced from 11.3 to 2.0 days. The preservation of the sympathetic part of the inferior hypogastric plexus is, for the most part, impossible as endometriosis infiltrates the rectovaginal space, generally lateral to the pelvic plexus itself. The risk of destruction to the vesical splanchnic nerves occurs primarily by the transection of the rectovaginal ligament lateroventral to the rectum. When the rectum is mobilized dorsal to Waldeyer's fascia and its mobilization continues laterally following this fascia and more ventral to the space of Denonvilliers, the parasympathetic nerves for the bladder are almost always destroyed. When the parasympathetic nerves are ventrally dissected, it is systematically found that these nerves transfix this fascia in its dorsolateral portion. Thus, dissection of the rectum at a level deeper than 6 cm from the linea dentata must be performed medial to the perirectal fascia and as close as possible to the rectum. This is much easier when the dissection of the pararectal spaces has been previously performed vaginally by simultaneous endorectal palpation.

These techniques to expose the autonomic pelvic nerves can be performed by laparotomy as well as by laparoscopy, but exposure dorsal to the rectum is much easier by laparoscopy due to the magnification of the endoscope's optics and to the possiblity of good access to all parts of the pelvis, inluding the deep retrorectal space. The 'nerve-sparing techniques' should change the surgeon's philosophy and cause him to change his surgical technique from 'macrosurgery' with clamp/section to the technique of minute and blood-free dissection. This new knowledge about the functional pelvic neuroanatomy not only changes our surgical concepts, but also the classical nomenclature of 'cardinal ligament' and 'uterosacral ligament', which is no longer acceptable, as these structures do not exist as ligaments. The classical concept of pelvic support by ligaments should be reviewed.

REFERENCES

1. Possover M, Rhiem K. Influence of "parasympathetic-nerve-sparing" technique in laparoscopic radical pelvic surgery for cervical cancer and for deep infiltrating endometriosis on postoperative bladder dysfunction. Submitted for pulication in 2004.

2. Possover M, Rhiem K, Chiantera V. The "Laparoscopic Neuro-Navigation" – LANN: from a new field of laparoscopic surgery to a functional cartography of the pelvic autonomous neurosystem. Minim Invasiv Ther 2004; 5–6: 362–367.

3. Tuson JR, Everett WG. A retrospective study of colostomies, leaks and strictures after colorectal anastomosis. Int J Colorectal Dis 1990; 5: 44–48.

4. Candiani GB, Vercellini P, Fedele L, et al. Conservative surgical treatment of rectovaginal septum endometriosis. J Gynecol Surg 1992; 8: 177–182.

5. Nezhat C, Nezhat F, Pennington E. Laparoscopic treatment of infiltrative rectosigmoid colon and rectovaginal septum endometriosis by the technique of videolaparoscopy and the CO_2 laser. Br J Obstet Gynaecol 1992; 99: 664–667.

6. Reich H, McGlynn F, Salvat J. Laparoscopic treatment of cul-de-sac obliteration secondary to retrocervical deep fibrotic endometriosis. J Reprod Med 1991; 36: 516–522.

7. Martin DC. Laparoscopic and vaginal colpotomy for the excision of infiltrating cul-de-sac endometriosis. J Reprod Med 1988; 33: 806–808.

8. Redwine DB, Koning M, Sharpe DR. Laparoscopically assisted transvaginal segmental resection of the rectosigmoid colon for endometriosis. Fertil Steril 1996; 65: 193–197.

19 Severe endometriosis involving the urogenital system

Jacques Donnez, Jean Squifflet, Mireille Smets, and Pascale Jadoul

This chapter describes two forms of endometriosis involving the urogenital system. It should be pointed out that the prevalence of both ureteral and bladder endometriosis has dramatically and significantly increased in recent years. According to the findings of one of our last studies, environmental toxins could be responsible for this increase.[1]

Ureteral endometriosis

Despite thousands of scientific reports in the literature on endometriosis, its prevalence in the general population is unknown. In women with pelvic pain and/or infertility, a highly variable prevalence, ranging from 20 to 90%, has been reported.[2–5]

Endometriosis usually involves the peritoneum, the ovaries, or the rectovaginal septum, and three distinct entities have been described.[5] Ureteral endometriosis is relatively uncommon and is estimated to occur in about 0.08–1% of patients with endometriosis.[6,7] The prevalence of 1% observed in the study by Nezhat and colleagues[7] was considered to be somewhat overestimated according to Donnez and Brosens, who observed only 6 cases in a series of 6285 patients (0.1%).[8] It was suggested, in 1997, that there was a more frequent association of obstructive uropathy with rectovaginal adenomyosis.[8]

A distinction must be made between extrinsic and intrinsic ureteral endometriosis.[9,10] Indeed, intrinsic ureteral endometriosis, characterized by the presence of endometriotic glands and stroma in the ureteral wall, is a very rare entity. However, extrinsic ureteral endometriosis, caused by extra-ureteral disease, is more frequent.

The late consequence of ureteral endometriosis is the silent loss of renal function caused by the progressive 'enclosure' of the lower part of the ureter by adenomyosis.

Prevalence of ureteral endometriosis in women with rectovaginal nodules

The prevalence of ureteral lesions in a series of 306 patients treated for rectovaginal adenomyotic nodules was evaluated between March 1998 and July 2000, and published in *Fertility and Sterility*.[11] The patients were classified according to the size of the nodule (<2 cm, >2 cm but <3 cm, and >3 cm). The size of the nodule was evaluated by palpation of the posterior fornix of the vagina during vaginal examination and vaginal echography. Intravenous pyelography (IVP) was performed in all patients prior to surgery. Care was taken to analyze the lower segment of the ureter. Stenosis was judged to be partial or complete (Figure 19.1). The degree of ureterohydronephrosis was evaluated according to ureteral diameter. In case of cortical atrophy, kidney scintigraphy (Tc-99m DMSA) was performed preoperatively and postoperatively in order to evaluate renal function.

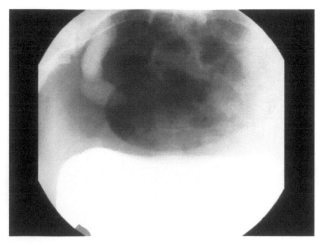

Figure 19.1 Intravenous pyelogram (IVP): complete stenosis with subsequent cortical atrophy.

In this series of 306 cases of rectovaginal adenomyosis, ureteral endometriosis was encountered in 14 cases. The prevalence was thus 4.5% in our prospective study.[11]

In the study group, severe dysmenorrhea and deep dyspareunia were experienced by all patients, but only 1 patient, with ureterohydronephrosis, complained of typical pain due to obstructive uropathy.

Isolated ureteral endometriosis was never noted; it was associated with rectovaginal adenomyosis in all cases. Ovarian endometriomas were observed in three cases on the ipsilateral side of ureteral endometriosis but they were always associated with rectovaginal adenomyosis. Ureteral stenosis was not localized where the ovarian endometriomas adhered to the broad ligament.

Classification of patients was carried out according to the size of the rectovaginal adenomyotic nodule (Table 19.1). A significantly (p <0.05)

higher prevalence of ureteral endometriosis (11.2%) was observed in patients with rectovaginal adenomyotic nodules of more than 3 cm in size than in patients with smaller nodules (<2 cm, 0%; >2 but <3 cm, 0.8%).

Unilateral stenosis (partial or complete) and ureterohydronephrosis were detected in 13 cases (right $n = 5$; left $n = 8$) and bilaterally in 1 case. Ureteral stenosis was thus right-sided in six cases and left-sided in 9 cases. The prevalence of right-sided and left-sided lesions was thus 2% (6/306) and 3% (9/306) respectively. In 4 cases, ureterohydronephrosis was severe (ureteral dilatation >1.5 cm) and associated with cortical atrophy diagnosed by kidney scintigraphy (Tc-99m DMSA).

Operative surgery

So far, 52 cases of ureteral endometriosis have been operated on in our department: in all cases but one, conservative surgery without ureteral resection was performed by laparoscopy. Three suprapubic trocars (5 mm; Karl Storz, Tuttlingen, Germany) were placed to insert instruments for the laparoscopic procedure. A CO_2 laser was used for dissection of the bowel and removal of the adenomyotic lesion and vaginal pouch in case of rectovaginal adenomyotic nodules, as previously described.[12,13] In all cases, ureterolysis was performed before adenomyotic nodule resection. The peritoneum covering the ureter was opened with the CO_2 laser, where the ureter was free of adhesions and clearly visible. The dissection was progressively made in the direction of the uterosacral ligament. The ureter was freed from surrounding tissue using CO_2 laser section and vaporization. To facilitate this step of the procedure, a JJ stent was inserted retrogradely by cystoscopy, immediately

Table 19.1 Incidence of ureteral endometriosis according to the size of the rectovaginal adenomyotic nodule (in the prospective study of 306 patients)

Rectovaginal adenomyotic nodule size (cm)	Number of patients	Number of patients with ureteral endometriosis (%)	Prevalence of ureteral endometriosis
<2	71	0	0
>2 but <3	119	1	0.8
>3	116	13	11.2*
Total	306	14	4.5

*The prevalence of ureteral endometriosis is significantly higher in this group of patients than in the other groups (p <0.05).

prior to surgery in 28 cases (55%). After ureterolysis, the fibrotic stenotic ring responsible for the ureteral stricture was removed without opening the ureteral lumen. The adventitial sheath could be cut but the medial muscular layer was preserved as far as possible. Ureteral opening or resection occurred in 2 cases (4%) during the laparoscopic procedure.

In 29 cases (58%), deliberate division of the uterine artery was performed on at least one side, using titanium clips, which were placed on the uterine artery crossing the lowest part of the ureter (Figure 19.2). This procedure allowed us to free the ureter down to its lowest point. At the end of the procedure, the ureter was free of disease in all cases (Figure 19.3).

When partial ureteral resection was required (because of the presence of complete stenosis of more than 3 cm in length), laparotomy with ureteroureterostomy and bladder surgery was carried out. From 1992 to 2004, this occurred in just 4 cases. This means that, in total, 52 cases (93%) of ureteral endometriosis were treated by laparoscopy and 6 cases (7%) by laparotomy.

All the women underwent rectovaginal adenomyotic nodule removal during the same procedure, without segmental bowel resection. In 1 patient, ureteral endometriosis was found to be associated with bladder endometriosis and a rectovaginal adenomyotic nodule.

In patients who underwent preoperative or intraoperative retrograde stent placement, the catheter was left in place for 3 months. After that period, the JJ stent was removed and IVP demonstrated the absence of any ureteral stricture.

Kidney scintigraphy (Tc-99m DMSA) was performed pre- and postoperatively in seven patients with severe pyelic dilatation and cortical atrophy. The association of complete ureterolysis and administration of gonadotropin-releasing hormone analogue (GnRH-a) therapy for 3 months led to a significant recovery of ureteral diameter, but the postoperative kidney scintigraphy revealed only a slight improvement (from 2 to 5%) in renal function, so laparoscopic nephrectomy was carried out in all 7 cases. Now, laparoscopic nephrectomy is routinely proposed in these cases.

Histology

Histologic study of periureteral resection specimens revealed the presence of endometriotic glands in contact with the uterine artery and the ureter itself. Serial sections demonstrated hyperplasia of the smooth muscle, invading the retroperitoneal space. Scanty stroma and

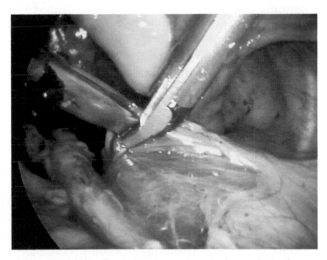

Figure 19.2 The dissection is progressively made in the direction of the uterosacral ligament. Ligation of the uterine artery is performed.

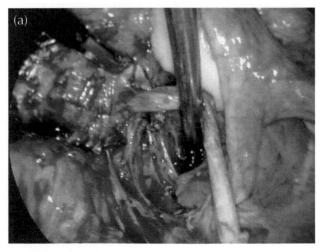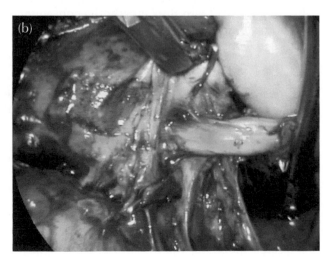

Figure 19.3 (a) and (b) At the end of the dissection, the ureter is free of disease.

glandular epithelium were observed. Periarterial invasion by the retroperitoneal adenomyotic disease was histologically demonstrated in all cases where the uterine artery was resected.

Prevalence

Ureteral endometriosis is infrequent, accounting for less than 0.3% of all endometriotic lesions. Ureteral lesions are relatively rare but they are a very serious condition because they may cause silent loss of renal function. There are two types of ureteral endometriosis, extrinsic and intrinsic.[8–10] Intrinsic ureteral obstruction is characterized by the presence of endometriotic glands and stroma in the ureteral wall due to primary endometriotic involvement of the ureteral wall. This type of ureteral endometriosis is less common, however, than ureteral obstruction, caused by external compression by surrounding endometriosis, which is known as extrinsic ureteral endometriosis. According to Stanley and colleagues,[14] endometriosis of the ureter usually arises by extension from pelvic foci, and ovarian endometriosis is a prerequisite for ureteral involvement.

In a retrospective study from 1988 to 1997, the prevalence of ureteral endometriosis was estimated to be less than 0.1% in case of endometriosis.[8] In women suffering from rectovaginal adenomyosis, it was found to be 0.9% (6/711). In a prospective study, however, the prevalence was 4.5% in a series of 306 cases of rectovaginal endometriosis or adenomyosis. The increasing prevalence of ureteral endometriosis, probably related to the increasing prevalence of deep endometriosis, must be emphasized.

Surrounding endometriotic lesions responsible for external ureteral compression, without histologic evidence of endometriotic glands and stroma in the ureteral wall, are thus mostly the consequence of lateral extension of rectovaginal adenomyotic nodules. These patients also showed other localizations of endometriosis, but ovarian endometriomas were rarely considered to be solely responsible for ureteral endometriosis because they were always associated with rectovaginal adenomyosis.

The concept of adenomyosis of the retroperitoneal space should therefore cover not only the rectovaginal space and the uterovesical space but also the area extending laterally in the direction of the cardinal ligaments.[10,12,13,15,16]

In a large review of the literature on retrospective series of ureteral endometriosis, the proportion of lesions located on the left was found to be significantly higher than on the right.[17] In our study, a higher proportion was also found on the left (9 cases vs 6 cases), but the difference was not significant, the prevalence being, respectively, 3% and 2%. In the series of Nezhat and colleagues, a nonsignificant difference in the prevalence of ureteral endometriosis was also observed between the left and right sides.[7]

In a recent publication by Vercellini and colleagues,[17] 6 cases of ureteral endometriosis were described as being associated with ovarian endometriomas. In the opinion of the authors, however, neither the coelomic metaplasia theory nor the embryonic cell rests theory could explain such a clear-cut difference in the frequency of distribution of ovarian and ureteral lesions between the two pelvic sites. On the contrary, in our study, adenomyotic disease of the retroperitoneal space, originating from metaplasia of müllerian remnants, was most likely to be the cause of extrinsic ureteral endometriosis in our opinion, proved by clinical examination and histologic serial sections.

The management of ureteral endometriosis is controversial. Successful medical therapy (progestin or danazol) of ureteral obstruction secondary to pelvic endometriosis has been reported in the literature.[18,19] Conservative surgery with relief of ureteral obstruction and removal of adenomyosis or endometriosis should be the management of choice. In 1996, Nezhat and colleagues described a series of 17 cases of partial ureteral obstruction.[7] Laparoscopic ureterolysis was performed in 10 women, but 7 of the 17 women (41%) required partial wall resection. More recently, Nezhat and colleagues reported the laparoscopic vesicopsoas hitch for infiltrative ureteral endometriosis to obtain tension-free anastomosis of the bladder.[20] The case report described 1 case of 'recurrent ureteral endometriosis' after partial laparoscopic ureteral resection and ureteroneocystectomy. This approach should be considered only in case of intrinsic ureteral endometriosis involving a long segment of the ureter, to avoid laparotomy.

According to our results, conservative surgery should be proposed in the majority of patients. Indeed, we recommend performing laparoscopic ureterolysis and removal of the adenomyotic lesions responsible for ureteral stenosis, even in case of moderate or severe pyelic dilatation. In the majority of cases, ureteral dissection, with or without uterine artery ligation, is sufficient to free the ureter. In all cases, ureterohydronephrosis was found to be decreased after this procedure. Resection of part of the ureter should only be performed in exceptional cases.

In conclusion, obstructive uropathy is more frequently provoked by 'extrinsic' rather than 'intrinsic' endometriosis. The approximate ratio of 4 cases of extrinsic to 1 case of intrinsic disease, as previously described, has to be re-evaluated according to our study.[7] Obstructive uropathy should be suspected in patients with a rectovaginal adenomyotic nodule of more than 3 cm, because of its high prevalence (11.2%) in such cases. In this group of patients, there is a need to perform noninvasive urinary tract exploration to detect obstructive uropathy and prevent silent loss of renal function.

Bladder endometriosis

Although endometriosis is frequently encountered in females of reproductive age,[5] bladder endometriosis is relatively rare, representing less than 1% of all endometriosis cases. One must take particular care, however, to define bladder endometriosis clearly, as full-thickness detrusor lesions. Indeed, small implants and small nodules of the vesicouterine fornix cannot be considered as bladder endometriosis. The condition was first described by Judd[21] in 1921 and a review of 200 cases was published in 1980.[22] In the literature, two distinct forms appear to exist: one is found in women without any medical history of uterine surgery (primary), whereas the other develops after cesarean section (iatrogenic or secondary).[23]

Prevalence

Between January 1995 and June 2004, 37 women aged 22–46 years underwent laparoscopy for bladder endometriosis. The prevalence of this type of lesion has increased in recent years. The significant increase in the prevalence of vesical adenomyotic nodules is probably due to environmental toxicants, as has been observed for rectovaginal nodules.[1] During the last two years, only 6% of women with bladder endometriosis have previously undergone cesarean section, a much lower rate than that formerly published, which was 25%.[15]

It is important to underline the fact that only full-thickness detrusor lesions (Figure 19.4) were taken into consideration and small subperitoneal nodules or implants of the anterior cul-de-sac were excluded.

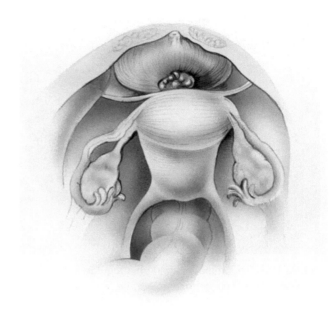

Figure 19.4 Schema of laparoscopic view: note the attachment of the round ligaments to the bladder nodule.

Symptoms and diagnosis

Women suffering from bladder endometriosis (adenomyotic nodules) present with a variety of symptoms, most frequently (76%) menstrual mictalgia and pollakiuria, usually limited to the menstrual period. In our series, no pathogens could be isolated from the urine culture, even after several days. Dysmenorrhea and dyspareunia were also experienced by 88% of women. Only 6% reported gross hematuria during menstruation, which was confirmed by microscopic analysis that failed to determine hematuria in all other cases.

The diagnosis of bladder endometriosis can often be made by vaginal examination. In fact, in our series, a tender nodule could be palpated in the anterior fornix of the vagina in all cases and abdominal ultrasonography confirmed the presence of a regular heterogeneous hypoechogenic nodule of the uterovesical septum (Figure 19.5), showing an association between the endometriotic nodule and the anterior uterine wall.

Cystoscopy was performed in all cases as part of the preoperative assessment. In all patients, a protruded mass of the posterior bladder wall was visible at the level of the fundus or the trigone. It showed a typical bluish or brownish nodule, sometimes with papular lesions (Figure 19.6a and 19.6b).

IVP demonstrated the typical aspect of an extravesical nodule in all cases, revealed by a filling

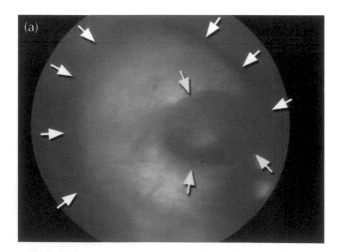

Figure 19.5 Abdominal echography: regular heterogeneous, hypoechogenic nodule (arrows) is clearly visible in the vesical muscularis protruding into the bladder cavity. In the majority of cases, there is no mucosal involvement.

defect in the upper part of the bladder. The vesical filling defect was more obvious on the profile picture.

Magnetic resonance imaging (MRI) should be performed in all patients. In our series, MRI excluded the presence of associated uterine adenomyosis and clearly revealed the presence of a nodular mass in the anterior fornix adjacent to the uterine wall, provoking extensive compression of the posterior bladder wall (Figure 19.7).

Surgical technique

After classic transumbilical insufflation with a Veress needle, the peritoneal cavity was entered by means of one 12 mm umbilical trocar connected to a 12 mm laser laparoscope (Karl Stotz, Tuttlingen, Germany) using a coupler system equipped with the Swiftlase (Model 757, ESC-Sharplan, Needham, MA).[24] Three other suprapubic trocars of 5 mm were also introduced. The first step was to check the uterus, the pouch of Douglas, and the peritoneum for other endometriotic lesions. If minimal peritoneal or ovarian endometriosis was found, it was immediately vaporized. If it was associated with numerous other ovarian lesions (cysts more than 3 cm in size; $n = 4$; 23%), medical therapy (3 months of GnRH-a; Zoladex (goserelin acetate), AstraZeneca, Cambridge, UK) was given after drainage of the ovarian cyst, as previously described. This was followed by surgical treatment, including ovarian cyst wall vaporization and segmental bladder resection, carried out by laparoscopy. In 41% of cases, a rectovaginal adenomyotic nodule was found to be associated. In these cases, the rectovaginal adenomyotic nodule was removed and the associated peritoneal and/or ovarian lesions were vaporized during the first laparoscopy.

The second step was to check the vesicouterine fornix to confirm the presence of a bladder adenomyotic nodule by retroflexing the uterus with a uterine cannula. Grasping forceps were then introduced through the suprapubic trocars to expose the lesion correctly for dissection with the CO_2 laser.

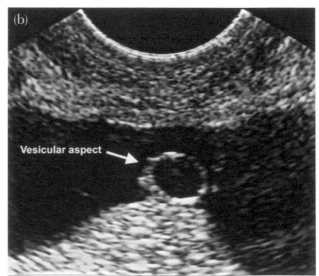

Figure 19.6 (a) Cystoscopy: protruding bluish vesicular nodule (yellow arrows) is clearly visible in the posterior bladder wall (white arrow) with an intact vesical mucosa. (b) In this case, the nodule is clearly visible in the bladder muscularis but, in the bladder, a vesicle was detected on the bladder mucosa.

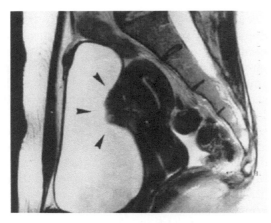

Figure 19.7 Magnetic resonance imaging shows a nodular mass in the anterior fornix adjacent to the uterine wall (arrowheads), causing extensive compression of the posterior bladder wall (note the absence of concomitant uterine adenomyosis): sagittal image.

Both round ligaments were systematically medially attached (Figure 19.8).

Deep nodular lesions involving the vesical muscularis required excision of the nodular tissue from the anterior uterine wall. Attention was first directed towards achieving complete dissection of the uterine wall throughout its area of attachment or involvement until the loose tissue of the vesical space was reached.

This could be done by cutting this area of attachment with the CO_2 laser, while the uterus was retroflexed and the bladder pulled up by grasping forceps. The peritoneum covering the bladder was opened. By gentle traction, the plane of dissection between the fibrotic nodular tissue and the normal vesical muscularis was exposed, and resection of the nodule was easily carried out, as far as possible from the ureteral insertions (Figure 19.9).

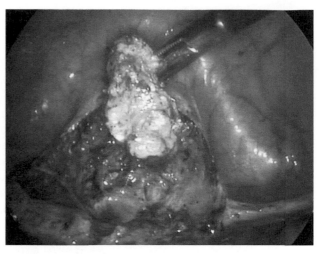

Figure 19.9 Complete extramucosal excision of the nodule; the bladder has not been entered.

At the end of surgery, the vesical muscularis was closed with stitches (Vicryl 2-0), depending on the size of the muscularis defect, either separate stitches or a running suture were performed (Figure 19.10). Finally, a diluted methylene blue solution was injected to ensure the sutures were watertight.

In some cases, a control cystoscopy was carried out to check the bladder defect closure. In all cases, retrograde cystography was performed 10 days postoperatively to confirm the complete recovery of the bladder wall and to exclude any liquid leakage.

The bladder catheter was left in place for 10 days.

Histology

Serial sections were obtained and colored by hematoxylin–eosin or analyzed to evaluate steroid

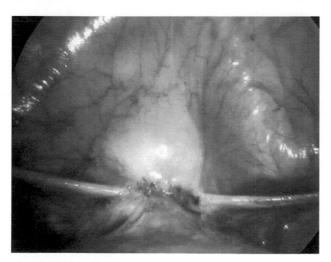

Figure 19.8 First laparoscopic view of the bladder adenomyotic nodule.

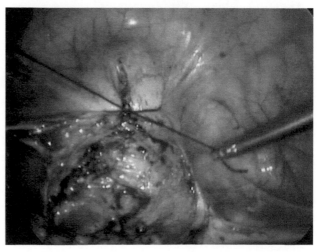

Figure 19.10 Extramucosal vesical suture by separate or continuous stiches of Vicryl 2-0.

receptor (estrogen and progestogen) content according to a previously described method.[25] On microscopic examination (Figure 19.11a and 11.b), the lesion was characterized by the presence of scarce glands, with active endometrial-type epithelium and scanty stroma. No secretory changes were observed, even when the patient was under progestogen therapy or during the luteal phase. More than 90% of the lesion consisted of smooth muscle hyperplasia. The bladder nodule was localized throughout the whole thickness of the bladder wall. By serial section, we were able to demonstrate that endometrial glands were not connected to the peritoneal serosa but were almost all in the subperitoneal space.

Results and discussion

Several authors have recently described two types of bladder endometriosis: the first type occurs in women who have not previously undergone any uterine surgery (primary) and the second type follows cesarean section (iatrogenic or secondary).[26,27] Koninckx and Martin[28] suggested that extraperitoneal endometriosis derives from endoperitoneal disease. In the opinion of Vercellini et al,[26] peritoneal lesions are able to penetrate under the peritoneum and develop into deep-infiltrating endometriosis. If this were

the case, we would have found peritoneal endometriosis in all cases. In our series, 35% of patients had no associated endometriotic lesions, whereas 35% of women had associated rectovaginal adenomyotic nodules, which we clearly described as a distinct retroperitoneal entity.[5,29] Indeed, the rectovaginal septum nodule was described, like the adenomyoma, as a circumscribed nodular aggregate of smooth muscle and endometrial glands surrounded by scanty stroma. We have previously suggested that the rectovaginal nodule may be the consequence of the metaplasia of müllerian remnants. Not surprisingly, the bladder nodule looked exactly the same as the rectovaginal nodule when viewed microscopically.

Not only the frequent association but also the similar histologic findings observed in our study strongly lead us to propose that bladder endometriosis is actually bladder adenomyosis, and also the consequence of metaplasia of müllerian remnants, which can be found in the rectovaginal septum as well as the vesicovaginal septum.

One of the hypotheses advanced by Fedele and colleagues,[23] claiming that detrusor endometriosis could result from the extension of adenomyotic lesions from the anterior uterine wall to the bladder, is not supported by our study. Indeed, although the adenomyotic vesical nodule was systematically found to be adherent to the uterine wall, no adenomyotic nodules of the anterior uterine wall were found. These data, observed at surgery, were corroborated by the absence of uterine adenomyosis at echography and MRI, when available.

Concerning the therapy, although medical therapy has proven effective in relieving symptoms, the quick recurrence of irritative urinary symptoms after cessation of therapy indicates that surgery is required. So far in the literature, partial cystectomy (or segmental bladder resection) has been considered the treatment of choice.[27,30,31]

In conclusion, so-called primary bladder endometriosis must be considered as retroperitoneal adenomyotic disease which is the consequence of metaplasia of müllerian rests and can be resected using a laparoscopic approach.[15]

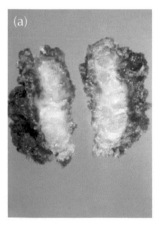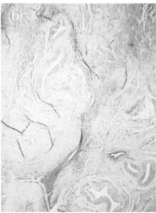

Figure 19.11 Vesical adenomyosis: (a) 90% of the lesion consists of smooth muscle hyperplasia; (b) scarce glands with active endometrial-type epithelium and scanty stroma are visible.

REFERENCES

1. Heilier JF, Ha A-T, Lison D, et al. Increased serum PCB levels in Belgian women with adenomyotic nodules of the rectovaginal septum. Fertil Steril 2004; 81: 456–458.

2. Donnez J, Thomas K. Incidence of the luteinized unruptured follicle syndrome in fertile women and in women with endometriosis. Eur J Obstet Gynecol Reprod Biol 1982; 14: 187–190.

3. Strathy JH, Molgaard GA, Coulam CB, et al. Endometriosis and infertility: a laparoscopic study of endometriosis among fertile and infertile women. Fertil Steril 1982; 38: 667–672.

4. Haney AF. Endometriosis: pathogenesis and pathophysiology. In: Wilson EA, ed. Endometriosis. New York: Alan R Liss; 1987: 23–51.

5. Nisolle M, Donnez J. Peritoneal endometriosis, ovarian endometriosis and adenomyotic nodules of the rectovaginal septum are three different entities. Fertil Steril 1997; 68: 585–596

6. Stillwell TJ, Kramer SAZ, Lee RA. Endometriosis of the ureter. Urology 1986; 26: 81–85.

7. Nezhat C, Nezhat F, Nezhat C, et al. Urinary tract endometriosis treated by laparoscopy. Fertil Steril 1996; 66: 920–924.

8. Donnez J, Brosens I. Definition of ureteral endometriosis? Fertil Steril 1997; 68: 178–179.

9. Donnez J, Nisolle M, Casanas-Roux F. Endometriosis: rationale for surgery. In Donnez J, Nisolle M, eds. An atlas of laser operative laparoscopy and hysteroscopy. Carnforth, UK: Parthenon; 1994: 53–62.

10. Clement PB. Disease of the peritoneum. In: Kurman RJ, ed. Blaustein's pathology of the female genital tract. New York: Springer-Verlag; 1994: 647–703.

11. Donnez J, Nisolle M, Squifflet J. Ureteral endometriosis: a complication of rectovaginal endometriotic (adenomyotic) nodules. Fertil Steril 2002; 77: 32–37.

12. Donnez J, Nisolle M, Casanas-Roux F, et al. Rectovaginal septum endometriosis or adenomyosis: laparoscopic management in a series of 231 patients. Hum Reprod 1995; 10: 630–635.

13. Donnez J, Nisolle M, Gillerot S, et al. Rectovaginal septum adenomyotic nodules: a series of 500 cases. Br J Obstet Gynaecol 1997; 104: 1014–1018.

14. Stanley KE Jr, Utz DC, Dockerty MB. Clinically significant endometriosis of the urinary tract. Surg Gynecol Obstet 1965; 120: 491–502.

15. Donnez J, Spada F, Squifflet J, et al. Bladder endometriosis must be considered as bladder adenomyosis. Fertil Steril 2000; 74: 1175–1181.

16. Donnez J, Nisolle M, Casanas-Roux F, et al. Endometriosis: rationale for surgery. In: Brosens I, Donnez J, eds. The current status of endometriosis and management. Carnforth, UK: Parthenon Publishing, 1993: 385–395.

17. Vercellini P, Pisacreta A, Pesole A, et al. Is ureteral endometriosis an asymmetric disease? Br J Obstet Gynaecol 2000; 107: 559–561.

18. Gantt PA, Hunt JB, McDonough PG. Progestin reversal of ureteral endometriosis. Obstet Gynecol 1981; 57: 665–667.

19. Rivlin ME, Krueger RP, Wiser WL. Danazol in the management of ureteral obstruction secondary to endometriosis. Fertil Steril 1985; 44: 274–276.

20. Nezhat C, Nezhat F, Freiha F, et al. Laparoscopic vesicopsoas hitch for infiltrative ureteral endometriosis. Fertil Steril 1999; 71: 376–379.

21. Judd ES. Adenomyomata presenting as a tumor of the bladder. Surg Clin North Am 1921; 1: 1271–1278.

22. Fianu S, Ingelman-Sundberg A, Nasiell K, et al. Surgical treatment of post abortum endometriosis of the bladder and postoperative bladder function. Scand J Urol Nephrol 1980; 14: 151–155.

23. Fedele L, Piazzola E, Raffaeli R, et al. Bladder endometriosis: deep infiltrating endometriosis or adenomyosis? Fertil Steril 1998; 69: 972–975.

24. Donnez J, Nisolle M, Anaf V, et al. Endoscopic management of peritoneal and ovarian endometriosis. In: Donnez J, Nisolle M, eds. An atlas of laser operative laparoscopy and hysteroscopy. Carnforth, UK: Parthenon Publishing; 1994: 63–74.

25. Nisolle M, Casanas-Roux F, Wyns Ch, et al. Immunohistochemical analysis of estrogen and progesterone receptors in endometrium and peritoneal endometriosis: a new quantitive method. Fertil Steril 1994; 62: 751–759.

26. Vercellini P, Meschia M, De Giorgi O, et al. Bladder detrusor endometriosis: clinical and pathogenetic implication. J Urol 1996; 155: 84–86.

27. Brosens IA, Puttemans P, Deprest J, et al. The endometriosis cycle and its derailments. Hum Reprod 1994; 9: 770–771.

28. Koninckx PR, Martin D. Deep endometriosis: a consequence of infiltration or retraction or possible adenomyosis externa. Fertil Steril 1992; 85: 924–928.

29. Donnez J, Nisolle M, Smoes P, et al. Peritoneal endometriosis and 'endometriotic' nodules of the rectovaginal septum are two different entities. Fertil Steril 1996; 66: 362–368.

30. Zaloudek C, Norris HJ. Mesenchymal tumors of the uterus. In: Kurman R, ed. Blaustein's pathology of the female genital tract. New York: Springer-Verlag; 1987: 373–408

31. Nezhat C, Nehzat F. Laparoscopic segmental bladder resection for endometriosis: a report of two cases. Obstet Gynecol 1993; 81: 882–884.

20 Combined colposcopic and laparoscopic approach to endometriosis in the rectovaginal septum

Kevin Jones and Christopher Sutton

Introduction

The surgical treatment of endometriotic nodules behind the cervix and in the rectovaginal septum is aimed at removing the deeply infiltrating fibromuscular and abnormal glandular tissue in order to relieve pelvic pain, particularly dyspareunia and perimenstrual dyschezia. The laparoscopic approach to the rectovaginal septum is difficult and potentially dangerous. We describe a new mode of access to the rectovaginal septum using a combination of colposcopy and laparoscopy that is potentially quicker and safer to carry out.

Carbon dioxide laser laparoscopy is used in the traditional manner to open up a plane between the back of the cervix and/or vagina and the rectum. Probes are placed in the posterior fornix of the vagina and the rectum to facilitate the dissection and lessen the risk of damage to the rectum.

Once the rectum has been displaced posteriorly by the dissection, the CO_2 laser is attached to a colposcope and is used to ablate rectovaginal nodules in the upper part of the vagina. During the ablation of the nodule in the posterior vaginal wall, hemosiderin 'chocolate fluid' spills from the lesion and the entire nodule can be vaporized until normal tissue is reached. At the end of the procedure, a test of rectal mucosal integrity is carried out and any other deposits of pelvic endometriosis can be ablated laparoscopically.

Patient selection

The indications and contraindications for a combined colposcopic and laparoscopic approach to rectovaginal nodules are set out in Table 20.1. Patients who are suitable for this combined procedure typically have tender nodules in the posterior vaginal wall. The endometriotic deposits are usually positioned at the top of the rectovaginal septum and extend into the posterior vaginal fornix. Patients will also have undergone a radiologic investigation to exclude a lesion that has penetrated the full thickness of the rectal wall. Ideally, they should have a magnetic resonance imaging (MRI) scan to detect any other deep infiltrating endometriosis (DIE) lesions and an air-contrast barium enema and vaginogram (lateral view) to ensure that the disease does not penetrate into the rectum. In addition, all patients should undergo a transvaginal ultrasound scan to exclude other pathologic causes of the pelvic pain such as adenomyosis of the uterus and to measure the dimensions of the gynecologic organs.

The severity of chronic nonmenstrual pelvic pain, dysmenorrhea, dyspareunia, and dyschezia may be assessed individually using a linear analogue score, where 0 is no pain, and 10 is the worst pain imaginable, or quality of life indicators such as the European quality of life (EuroQol) index and sexual activity questionnaire (SAQ) and SF12.

Table 20.1 Indications and contraindications for a combined colposcopic and laparoscopic approach to rectovaginal nodules

General indications
Pelvic pain associated with endometriosis: especially chronic nonmenstrual pelvic pain, dyspareunia, and dyschezia (pain during defecation during menstruation)

Specific indications
Palpable nodules of endometriosis in the posterior wall of the vagina and behind the cervix

Contraindication(s)
Laparoscopic surgery contraindicated
Uterosacral ligaments, ureters, and pelvic blood vessels cannot be identified
Nodules of endometriosis penetrating the full thickness of the rectovaginal septum

Relative contraindication(s)
Medical therapy effective, with minimal side effects
Endometriosis in the pouch of Douglas involving the bowel superficially (serosal layer)

Perioperative management

The procedure may be carried out in an ambulatory day surgical hospital or as an inpatient. Potential complications must be discussed, including the conversion to a laparotomy for visceral injury, especially bowel injury, and informed consent for the procedure must be obtained. Patients should be checked for any allergy to antibiotics, since 1 g of Kefzol (cefazolin) is usually administered intravenously during the procedure, and also any allergy to peanut oil or sulfonamides, which are present in the Sultrin cream (triple sulfa) inserted vaginally at the end of the procedure. Bowel preparation using a bowel cleansing solution is carried out: e.g. 1 sachet of Citramag (Bioglan Laboratories, Herts, UK) dissolved in 200 ml water and taken during the evening before the procedure. In addition, a rectal washout may be undertaken immediately prior to the operation using a disposable Fleet enema.

Operating room set-up

The patient is asked to void before coming into the operating suite or a urinary catheter is passed once the operative field has been cleaned with organic iodine solution (Betadine, UK) and draped. The procedure is carried out under general anesthetic. The patient wears flowtron boots (or graduated compression stockings) to prevent deep vein thrombosis and those at increased risk of thromboembolism are given subcutaneous heparin 1 hour preoperatively. She is then placed in the lithotomy position (Lloyd-Davis stirrups for the legs), with the arms secured in a position parallel to her sides.

Technological description

We use a CO_2 laser (ESC-Sharplan, Needham, MA) at a power setting of 20 W in continuous mode (Figure 20.1) with the helium–neon aiming beam focused to the smallest spot 20 mm from the end of the cannula. We usually use 10 W for superficial lesions; to cut into the hard nodular tissue, 30 W is quicker but generates a large amount of smoke that has to be efficiently evacuated. This provides precise cutting though the dense fibromuscular hyperplasia, which is a characteristic of DIE (Figure 20.2). For more superficial lesions, and

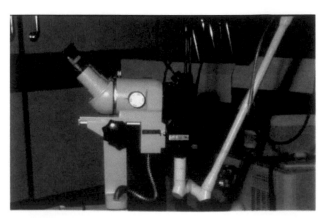

Figure 20.1 A carbon dioxide laser at a power setting of 20 W in continuous mode connected to a colposcope.

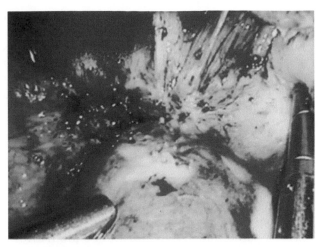

Figure 20.2 Deep nodule of fibromuscular hyperplasia infiltrating between the rectum and vagina.

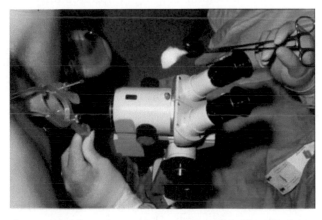

Figure 20.3 The colposcope is used to direct the CO_2 laser into the vagina in order to ablate the rectovaginal nodule.

particularly for those over 'high-risk' structures such as the bowel, bladder, or ureter, the high-speed rotating mirror delivery system (Swiftlase, ESC-Sharplan, Needham, MA) is used to vaporise endometriotic implants layer by layer.

For the vaginal surgery the laser was connected to the colposcope by a laser manipulator, Microslad 719 (ESC-Sharplan, Needham, MA). The colposcope (Carl Zeiss, Hamburg, Germany) is then used to direct the laser beam into the vagina (Figure 20.3) to vaporize all the visible endometriotic lesions in the vaginal fornices.

Operation

A pneumoperitoneum is induced and ports are inserted according to the Middlesborough consensus guidelines.[1] The abdominal cavity is insufflated with a disposable Veress needle to a

pressure of 20–25 mmHg, regardless of the volume used. The pressure and volume are recorded by a nurse prior to insertion of the primary trochar and cannula. Once the laparoscope is inserted (Figure 20.4), a quick circumferential inspection of the entire abdominopelvic cavity is carried out to check that no bowel injury has occurred during entry. A CO_2 laser is introduced via a cannula to the right or left iliac fossa and the laser is powered up according to local and national guidelines for the safe use of lasers. Carbon dioxide laser laparoscopy is used to open up a plane between the vagina and rectum and vaporize any DIE encountered during the dissection. After the rectum has been displaced posteriorly, the pelvis is inspected for adhesions and endometriosis and then filled with normal saline. The pouch of Douglas is visualized throughout the procedure by performing an 'under water inspection' with the laparoscope; Ringer's lactate solution is used as a safety device to absorb laser energy if the vagina has to be opened in order to vaporize lesions that have penetrated the full thickness of the vaginal wall. A blackened Cuscos speculum with an attachment for a smoke extractor is placed in the vagina to expose the upper, posterior wall of the vagina. The cervix is grasped by a vulsellum forceps attached to the anterior lip and the uterine cavity is then cannulated with a dilator to manipulate the pelvic organs during the procedure.

The CO_2 laser is attached to the colposcope, and the aiming beam focused on the nodule. The laser is activated in continuous mode, and 20 W of energy are delivered until hemosiderin, the so-called 'chocolate fluid', spills from the lesion, and the entire nodule is vaporized until normal tissue is seen. If there is a copious amount of 'chocolate fluid', the CO_2 laser energy is absorbed and it is preferable to use the green KTP532 laser (Figure

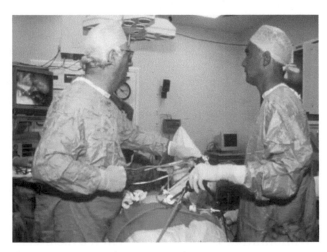

Figure 20.4 Set-up for operating laparoscopy.

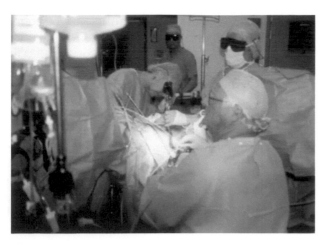

Figure 20.5 If there is a large amount of hemosiderin, the green KTP laser is used.

20.5). Any additional pelvic endometriosis is ablated using a standard technique described previously.[2]

Postoperative course

Patients generally recover quickly from the procedure and can usually be discharged home the same day. An antibiotic cream, usually Sultrin, may be inserted into the vagina and the remainder of the tube plus applicator are prescribed twice daily for 10 days. Patients are given the standard instructions after a large loop excision of the cervical transformation zone and advised to refrain from sexual intercourse for 3 weeks and to use pads rather than tampons for the next menstruation. During the initial 3 weeks, patients may complain of an offensive vaginal discharge, and high vaginal swabs for aerobes, anaerobes, and cervical swabs for *Chlamydia trachomatis* should be carried out; patients should attend their family physician for broad-spectrum antibiotics and metronidazole. At 6 months following the operation, patients are reviewed and, hopefully, the initial symptoms should have resolved and the vaginal mucosa healed without scarring or stenosis. In cases with a good postoperative outcome, there is no evidence of residual or recurrent endometriosis in the septum.

Clinical evidence

We have carried out a retrospective analysis of a cohort of 36 patients treated over 1 year presenting with infiltrating endometriosis in the rectovaginal septum with marked involvement of the vagina in

the posterior fornix, where it was considered technically easier to complete the operation using the CO_2 laser via the colposcope. All the procedures were performed as day cases when the operation took place in the morning or the patient had an overnight stay if the operation took place in the afternoon.

The majority of the patients were tertiary referrals, having failed to respond to medical or surgical treatment at other hospitals. All 36 patients had undergone previous laparoscopic treatment for endometriosis and 5 patients (15%) had more than one previous laparoscopy. Three patients had prior laparotomies for treatment of endometriosis: 1 patient for removal of an endometrioma, 1 patient for anterior resection of rectal endometriosis, and 1 patient had a total abdominal hysterectomy and bilateral salpingo-oophorectomy. Five patients were lost to follow-up and they were excluded from analysis of the subsequent results. The average age of patients was 32 years old (range 20–51 years old). All 31 patients had pelvic pain as the leading complaint: dysmenorrhea in 21 patients (68%); dyspareunia in 20 patients (65%); and dyschezia in 13 patients (42%). Rectal bleeding during menstruation occurred in 5 patients (16%), but the air-contrast barium enemas were all negative for any rectosigmoid involvement or evidence of full-thickness penetrating lesions.

The mean operating time was 48 minutes (range 32–80 minutes). The follow-up period ranged from 6 to 15 months: 15 of the 21 patients (71%) with dysmenorrhea, 14 of the 20 patients (70%) with dyspareunia, and 10 of the 13 patients (77%) with dyschezia indicated improvement of their symptoms. There were 3 patients requiring further laparoscopic CO_2 laser vaporization at 7, 9, and 12 months after the initial treatment, respectively. Two patients are being scheduled for total abdominal hysterectomy and bilateral salpingo-oophorectomy because of suspected adenomyosis. No complications occurred related to laparoscopy or CO_2 laser vaporization.

Discussion

Deep endometriosis is a proliferative lesion composed of fibromuscular tissue with sparse finger-like extensions of glandular and stromal tissue. The endometrial component varies considerably and it may resemble adenomyosis histologically or there may be fibromuscular hyperplasia, which seems to be responsible for the severe pain, with or without evidence of hemosiderin. This pathologic process can involve the rectovaginal septum, producing painful nodules in the posterior fornix and sometimes extending well down the length of the vagina. These patients classically complain of severe dyspareunia and dyschezia, particularly during the menstruation. If the lesion extends through all the layers of the rectal wall, there may be cyclical rectal bleeding. In advanced cases, stricture formation at one or more sites in the rectum or rectosigmoid colon can occur, which may require segmental resection of the affected area.

It is important to note that the laparoscopic inspection of the pelvis may not demonstrate obvious endometriotic lesions, particularly if the endometriosis is low in the septum. These lesions can often be felt rather than seen. Drug therapy is virtually ineffective in this situation and the abnormal tissue needs to be removed surgically. Recent reports by Garry et al[3] and Kwok et al[4] using a laparoscopic electrosurgical excision technique for patients with infiltrating endometriosis of the rectovaginal septum indicate significant improvement of painful symptoms. Proponents of the excision technique have suggested that laser vaporization alone is less effective;[5–7] however, there are no randomized trials to support these claims. The laparoscopic approach to this area can be difficult and dangerous[3,4,8–10] because the pouch of Douglas may be obliterated, and the anterior rectum adherent to the uterus. There is a risk that pelvic blood vessels, bowel, or the ureters may be damaged during the procedure.

During the laparoscopic procedure the rectovaginal septum is opened from above and the excision of abnormal tissue is continued downwards using a variety of techniques and instruments.[3–9,11,12] When the majority of the nodule lies within the pelvis, this is the preferred approach. However, when the major part of the nodule projects into the vagina, the colposcopic route may be preferred. In our series there were no serious complications. A mean operating time of 110 minutes for laparoscopic excision was reported by Garry et al,[3] whereas the mean time using our technique was 48 minutes (range: 32–80 minutes). Furthermore, all the patients were discharged home within 24 hours.

The technique of using the CO_2 laser through the operative channel of laparoscopes to treat endometriosis is now well described.[13] The CO_2 laser has also been used in conjunction with the colposcope to perform laser ablations of the squamocolumnar junction in patients with cervical intraepithelial neoplasia.[14] We have adapted the technique and used the equipment in combination with laparoscopy for ablating nodules of endometriosis in the rectovaginal septum, particu- larly if most of the lesion is on the vaginal side presenting clinically as 'blue domed' cysts that are easily recognized on speculum examination. The colposcope magnifies the nodule in the vagina, and the CO_2 laser is able to ablate the abnormal tissue, precisely, layer by layer.[15] The main advantage of doing this is that it seems to offer a lower operative morbidity and a rapid procedure time without diminishing clinical effectiveness. However, it must be acknowledged that careful patient selection is the key to applying the technique successfully. An air-contrast barium enema was used to exclude patients with nodules that had penetrated the rectal wall. Although this investigation helps to locate the position of the nodule in relation to the bowel lumen, an MRI scan may provide more information about the size and exact position of the nodule in the pelvis. If complete penetration of the bowel wall is suspected, or the nodule is predominately in the pelvis, this technique is unsuitable.

Where the pouch of Douglas is also obliterated with adhesions and endometriotic deposits, a combined laparoscopic and colposcopic approach with the laser may be considered. In order to carry out the procedure safely, the pouch of Douglas is filled with saline, which the CO_2 laser cannot penetrate, since energy at this wavelength is almost totally absorbed by water; this protects the bowel from accidental injury should the laser beam penetrate the vaginal wall accidentally. Direct visualization of the pouch of Douglas during the procedure provides additional reassurance that the vaginal wall has not been breached. The addition of saline into the pouch of Douglas does not protect the lowest part of the rectum from accidental laser damage during the procedure, and this is a potential problem if the nodule is located in the lower parts of the rectovaginal septum. In these cases, it is advisable to carry out a direct inspection of the rectal mucosa after the procedure is complete. A simple test of rectal mucosal integrity is to inject air via a sigmoidoscope through the anus into the rectum and observe for gas bubbles in the fluid filling the pouch of Douglas. Clearly, this will not exclude delayed perforation due to coagulative necrosis, which may occur days later.

Conclusion

We have found the combination of the colposcopic and laparoscopic approach to rectovaginal nodules to be a useful technique in selected patients where the endometrioic deposit projects into the vagina rather than the pouch of Douglas.

REFERENCES

1. Garry R. A consensus document concerning laparoscopic entry techniques: Middlesbrough, March 19–20, 1999. Gynaecol Endosc 1999; 8: 327–334.

2. Sutton C, Hill D. Laser laparoscopy in the treatment of endometriosis. A 5-year study. Br J Obstet Gynaecol 1990; 97: 181–185.

3. Garry R, Clayton R, Hawe J. The effect of endometriosis and its radical laparoscopic excision on quality of life indicators. Br J Obstet Gynaecol 2000; 107(1): 44–54.

4. Kwok A, Lam A, Ford R. Laparoscopic resection of deeply infiltrating endometriosis of the rectovaginal septum: effect on pelvic pain. Gynecol Endosc 2001; 10: 7–10.

5. Redwine DB. Laparoscopic en bloc resection for treatment of the obliterated cul-de-sac in endometriosis. J Reprod Med 1992; 37: 695–698.

6. Wright JT, Shafik A. Quality of life following radical excision of the rectovaginal endometriosis associated with complete obliteration of the posterior cul de sac. Gynecol Endosc 2001; 10: 107–110.

7. Koninckx PR, Martin D. Treatment of deeply infiltrating endometriosis. Gynecol Surg Endosc 1994; 6: 231–241.

8. Donnez J, Nisolle M, Gillerot S, et al. Rectovaginal septum adenomyotic nodules: a series of 500 cases. Br J Obstet Gynaecol 1997; 104: 1014–1018.

9. Nezhat C, Nezhat F, Pennington E. Laparoscopic treatment of infiltrating rectosigmoid colon and rectovaginal septum endometriosis by the technique of videolaparoscopy and CO_2 laser. Br J Obstet Gynaecol 1992; 99: 664–667.

10. Koninckx PR, Timmermans B, Meuleman C, et al. Complications of CO_2 laser endoscopic excision of deep endometriosis. Human Reprod 1996; 11: 1396–1398.

11. Chapron C, Dubuisson JB. Laparoscopic treatment of deep endometriosis located on the uterosacral ligaments. Hum Reprod 1996; 11: 868–873.

12. Wright JT. The diagnosis and management of infiltrating nodular recto-vaginal endometriosis. Curr Opin Obstet Gynaecol 2000; 12: 283–287.

13. Donnez J. CO_2 laser laparoscopy in endometriosis. In: Sutton C, ed. Lasers in gynaecology. London: Chapman & Hall; 1992: 73–91.

14. Saunders N, Sharp F, Jordan JA. Laser treatment of cervical and vaginal intraepithelial neoplasia. In: Sutton C, ed. Lasers in gynaecology. London: Chapman & Hall; 1992: 195–207.

15. Sutton C. Power sources in endoscopic surgery. Curr Opin Obstet Gynecol 1995; 7: 248–256.

21 Radical excision of the uterosacral ligament complex

Charles Chapron, Nicolas Chopin, Bruno Borghese, Cécile Malartic, and Hervé Foulot

Introduction

Three types of endometriosis have been described: superficial endometriosis, ovarian endometriomas, and deeply infiltrating endometriosis (DIE). The definition used for DIE in the international literature is histologic. DIE is defined as an endometriotic lesion penetrating to a depth of at least 5 mm.[1] The main symptom where DIE is involved is pelvic pain, the intensity of which is significantly correlated with the depth to which the lesions penetrate.[1-3]

It is essential to know exactly where deep endometriosis lesions are located because the efficacy of surgical treatment depends on how radical the surgical excision has to be.[4] Magnetic resonance imaging (MRI) results help to pinpoint the location of DIE lesions better. DIE lesions are initially located retrocervically above the upper border of the rectovaginal septum.[5] A retrocervical location is very frequent for DIE lesions and involvement of the rectovaginal septum is not systematic.[6] DIE originates from the retrocervical area and the rectovaginal septum does not appear to be the initial location for DIE lesions.[7]

The uterosacral ligaments (USL) are the most frequent location found for DIE lesions.[8,9] This chapter has a double goal:

- to describe the surgical technique for operative laparoscopic resection of DIE lesions infiltrating the USL
- to clarify the strategy for diagnosis and treatment of patients presenting with DIE lesions infiltrating the USL.

Deeply infiltrating endometriosis infiltrating the uterosacral ligaments

Operative procedure

The procedure of choice for resection of DIE lesions located in the USL is operative laparoscopy. The following are the main points concerning this laparoscopic surgery technique:[10]

- Bowel preparation is systematically performed before the operation. The protocol we use is as follows: low-residue diet for 8 days prior to entering hospital; 1 sachet of X-Prep (sennosides A and B; Laboratoires Plantier, Mérignac, France) for 2 days and the day before entering hospital; a Normacol enema (Laboratoire Norgan, Paris, France) (1 adult dose of 130 ml) the evening of entering hospital, i.e. the day before the operation.

- The way the patient is positioned is important. She is placed under general anesthesia with endotracheal intubation, with the lower limbs very slightly bent, thighs spread, and the buttocks slightly over the edge of the table. A urinary catheter is systematically installed. Exposure is a particular feature of the operation. A smooth curette (gauge 10) is used, fixed to two tenaculum forceps on the anterior and posterior lips of the cervix. This allows the uterus to be mobilized in all directions. The rectum and vagina are mobilized using large-caliber probes.

• Three 5 mm suprapubic ports are essential. The two lateral trocars are inserted under visual control, outside the epigastric pedicles that are first identified using the endoscope.

• The phases in the operation are as follows. In order to obtain trouble-free access to the pelvis, the first step is to push the loops of bowel above the sacral promontory. If adhesions restrict the mobilization of the bowel, they should first be freed. Because the route of the ureter may be modified due to retroperitoneal infiltration of the endometriotic lesions, it is necessary to locate it systematically prior to starting dissection. If there are extensive lesions, the ureter should be carefully dissected (ureterolysis). The lateral pelvic peritoneum should be incised in an area of healthy tissue. The more extensive the retroperitoneal lesions appear to be, the closer to the sacral promontory the initial incision is made. Using laparoscopic scissors after preventive bipolar coagulation, the incision runs under the line taken by the ureter, parallel and above the USL, and towards the point of insertion of the latter in the uterus. Using a grasping forceps inserted in the suprapubic trocar on the contralateral side to the USL in question, the peritoneum and USL are pulled strongly towards the midline of the pelvis. The ureter is freed very gradually. How much retroperitoneal dissection and ureterolysis are needed depends on the depth to which the endometriotic lesions penetrate, and their extent. In the presence of considerable retroperitoneal infiltration, it can sometimes be necessary to take the ureterolysis right up to the point where it crosses the uterine vessels. Once the lateral external surface of the USL has been entirely freed, the ligament is then pulled outwards using a grasping forceps inserted in the homolateral suprapubic trocar. The rectovaginal space is exposed by inserting a large probe in the rectum. After preventive bipolar coagulation, the rectovaginal space is opened using the laparoscopic scissors. Similarly to before, the more retroperitoneal fibrosis there is and the greater the extent of the endometriotic lesions, the more extensive the dissection must be towards the middle part of the pelvis. Once the USL has been totally freed laterally, it is then removed from the posterior surface of the cervix and vagina. The USL is coagulated level with its point of insertion into the uterus, then cut using the laparoscopic scissors. After this, the ligament is freed from the pelvic floor using the same procedure. The excised tissues are

sent for histologic examination. We systematically check hemostasis at the end of the operation, together with inspection of the ureters, and we always check that the rectum is intact by transanal injection of a solution of methylene blue. The operation finishes with copious abdominopelvic washing. We do not reperitonealize and we never leave a drain in place.

• All the other endometriotic lesions (adhesions, ovarian endometriomas, superficial peritoneal implants, etc.) are treated during the same session of laparoscopic surgery.

Strategy

When deciding on the best surgical strategy it is essential to bear in mind that one of the main characteristics of DIE lesions is their multifocal nature[9] (Table 21.1). The mean number of lesions is correlated in a statistically significant manner with the location of the main lesion[9] (Table 21.2). The percentage of isolated DIE lesions, i.e. those located on a single organ (USL; upper third of the posterior vaginal wall; bladder; intestine) varies between 29 and 83%[8] (see Table 21.2). Eighty-three percent of DIE lesions infiltrating the USL are isolated and affect the USL(s) alone.

The multifocal nature of DIE lesions means a very accurate preoperative work-up is necessary in order to obtain a precise map of the DIE lesions prior to the operation. The goal of this work-up is to check whether the DIE lesions infiltrating the USL are isolated or, on the contrary, are associated with DIE in other locations (upper third of the posterior vaginal wall, bladder, or intestine).

Preoperative work-up

The main symptom in cases of DIE is pelvic pain, sometimes associated with infertility. The clinical signs (dysmenorrhea, deep dyspareunia, non-cyclic chronic pelvic pain, and urinary and gastrointestinal symptoms) are significantly correlated with the location of the lesions.[11] In a clinical context suggesting DIE, the presence of deep dyspareunia suggests disease affecting the USL (Table 21.3).

The results of clinical examination vary according to the location of the lesions[12] (Table 21.4). It is very rare to see bluish lesions during speculum inspection in case of isolated lesions of the USL (see Table 21.4). In cases where infiltration of the USL by DIE lesions is histologically proven, vaginal palpation is negative in 17% of these cases. Although painful functional symptoms do

Table 21.1 Deeply infiltrating endometriosis: anatomic distribution

Main lesion	Number of patients	Locations						
		USL			V	B	I	Total*
		R	L	Bl				
Anterior location:								
Bladder	18	0	1	3	3	18		28 (8.1)
Posterior locations:								
USL	158	41	77	40				198 (57.6)
Vaginal	42	4	3	7	42			63 (18.3)
Intestinal	23	2	2	4	5	4	34	55 (16.0)
Total	**241**	**47**	**83**	**54****	**50**	**22**	**34**	**344**

B = bladder; USL = uterosacral ligament; V = vaginal; I = intestinal; R = right; L = left; Bl = bilateral
* Values in parentheses are percentages.
** Each lesion of bilateral pairs is counted as part of a pair, so total number of individual lesions = 108
Source: Adapted from Chapron et al.[9]

Table 21.2 Deeply infiltrating endometriosis (DIE): total number and proportion of isolated DIE lesions

DIE location	Number of locations	Total number of DIE lesions*	Isolated DIE lesion[†]	
			n	%
Bladder	22	1.56 ± 1.04 (1–4)**	13	59.0
USL	238	1.25 ± 0.44 (1–2)**	198	83.2
Vaginal	50	1.50 ± 0.77 (1–3)**	28	56.0
Intestinal	34	2.39 ± 1.37 (1–6)**	10	29.4

USL = uterosacral ligament.
* Data are presented as mean ± standard deviation.
[†] Without any other associated DIE lesions.
** $p < 0.0001$ (Kruskal–Wallis test).
Source: Adapted from Chapron et al.[9]

suggest the diagnosis, a normal clinical examination does not eliminate the possibility of DIE infiltrating the USL. This discrepancy between the results of questioning and routine clinical examination is due to the fact that lesions located on the USL are high up in the pelvis and, therefore, are not always accessible at vaginal examination. When clinical examination reveals positive results during vaginal examination, a nodular lesion is the classic observation but this is not an absolute rule. In certain cases, only the most obvious signs will be evident: lateral deviation of the cervix, asymmetry of the uterosacral ligaments with instead of a nodule a hardened, irregular appearance (see Table 21.4). The essential diagnostic factor is that firm palpation of these lesions causes pain. The accuracy of clinical examination can be increased by carrying out the examination during menstruation.

The limitations of history taking and clinical examination mean that additional investigations are needed to obtain an accurate map of the DIE lesions preoperatively. Transrectal ultrasonography (TRUS) is reliable for the diagnosis of infiltration of the bowel wall.[13–16] If infiltration of the USL is suspected, TRUS should be used systematically in the following situations:

Table 21.3 Deeply infiltrating endometriosis: presenting symptoms

Symptoms	Location		OR adjusted	95%CI
Dyspareunia	USL	No	1	ref
		Yes	3.4	1.4 – 8.2
Menstrual painful defecation	Vagina	No	1	ref
		Yes	2.9	1.5 – 5.7
Noncyclic CPP	Intestine	No	1	ref
		Yes	10.6	3.6 – 30.8
Urinary tract symptoms	Bladder	No	1	ref
		Yes	51.8	13.6–197.7
Gastrointestinal symptoms	Intestine	No	1	ref
		Yes	4.4	1.7 – 11.4
	Vagina	No	1	ref
		Yes	3.1	1.4 – 6.7

OR = odds ratio; CI = confidence interval; CPP = chronic pelvic pain; USL = uterosacral ligaments.
Source: Adapted from Fauconnier et al.[11]

Table 21.4 Deeply infiltrating endometriosis: results of routine clinical examination

Clinical examination	Posterior DIE			p
	USL (n = 102)	Vaginal (n = 30)	Intestine (n = 17)	
Positive speculum inspection	3 (2.9)	16 (53.3)	4 (23.5)	p <0.0001
Positive vaginal touch	85 (83.3)	30 (100.0)	16 (94.1)	p = 0.03
+ Painful nodules	34 (33.3)	24 (80.0)	6 (35.3)	p <0.0001
+ Painful induration	51 (50.0)	6 (20.0)	10 (58.8)	p = 0.005

Values in parentheses are percentages
DIE = deeply infiltrating endometriosis; USL = uterosacral ligaments
Source: Adapted from Chapron et al.[12]

- painful bowel functional symptoms that recur during menstruation, even if there is no rectal bleeding
- the existence of rectal bleeding
- suspicions concerning possible bowel infiltration at clinical examination
- large posterior lesion (3 cm or more).

MRI is a particularly useful means of examination insofar as it allows a complete pelvic work-up with just one investigation. Although MRI allows the diagnosis of deep endometriosis infiltrating the uterosacral ligaments,[17] it appears to be less sensitive than TRUS for the diagnosis of bowel infiltration.[18] In this context of suspected USL involvement, a check should be made on whether the ureter is affected, even though this is a rare occurrence. Involvement of the ureter is frequently asymptomatic,[19] but should be suspected if there are large lesions infiltrating one or both of the USL.[20] In this case it is possible to make URO–MRI (urologic MRI) shots[21–23] during MRI investigation in order to look for ureter involvement without having to carry out an intravenous pyelogram. Cystoscopy will only be necessary if there is any doubt as to the presence of bladder endometriosis associated with the infiltration of the USL. Recent work on DIE has demonstrated the possibilities of transvaginal ultrasonography (TVUS).[24] These encouraging preliminary results need to be confirmed to establish whether TVUS should be carried out systematically at first intention in this context. The goal for the years to come is to map the DIE lesions as accurately as possible preoperatively, with the minimum number of additional means of investigation, while favoring the least-invasive and least-costly methods.[7]

Surgical management

The goal of surgical treatment of DIE is to achieve complete resection of all the DIE lesions giving rise to symptoms in a single operation. It is the location of the DIE lesions that dictates the operating technique to be used. The multifocal character of deep endometriosis has to be taken into account and, if there are multiple lesions, several different surgical procedures may need to be performed. Two recent studies,[25,26] with a very large number of patients and satisfactory postoperative follow-up, showed that complete surgical excision of DIE lesions results in a statistically significant reduction in painful symptoms.

In practical terms, two clinical situations need to be distinguished, because they require totally different surgical management:

Isolated DIE infiltration of USL. In this case, surgical treatment can be by operative laparoscopy exclusively.[10] It is necessary in most cases to carry out ureterolysis in order to be able to achieve complete excision of the USL nodule without any risk of damaging the ureter. Depending on how far the lesions extend, dissection of the lateral rectal fossa may sometimes be required. Laparoscopic surgical resection of the USL should be bilateral only if the nodule invades both USL. When the USL lesion is unilateral, and this is most frequently found on the left side,[27] the healthy contralateral ligament should not be resected. By definition, with this location there is no infiltration of the upper third of the vagina, so laparoscopic surgical resection of the USL can be carried out without any colpectomy or vaginal excision.[28]

DIE infiltration of the USL is associated with other DIE lesions. In this case, resection of the DIE lesions infiltrating the USL must be associated with excision of all the other DIE lesions. Depending on the number and type of associated DIE lesions (vaginal, intestinal, ureteral, etc.) the operation will be carried out using various methods: operative laparoscopy, laparoscopically assisted vaginal surgery, laparotomy. The essential point is that all the lesions must be excised. Excision must never be incomplete due to a desire to carry out a procedure by operative laparoscopy at all costs. Incomplete excision would leave the patient with

the risk of continuing to experience painful symptoms, not forgetting the risk of a repeat operation. In our experience, many patients present a past history of repeated surgery for DIE not because of any true recurrence but because of incomplete excision during previous operations.

The fact that the anatomic distribution of DIE lesions is the main criterion to be taken into account when deciding on the method for surgical treatment prompted us to propose a 'surgical classification' for deep endometriosis[9] based precisely on the location of the lesions (Table 21.5). The advantage of this classification that we propose is that for each location there is a properly standardized operative technique, of proven efficiency. These techniques, shown in the right-hand column of Table 21.5, naturally need to be associated with each other when DIE is found in several locations. The multifocal nature of the lesions may require the surgeon to use laparotomy in order to achieve complete excision in one procedure. In certain cases DIE of the USL can be very voluminous, with infiltration of neighboring organs, notably the rectum and ureter. These associated lesions require bowel resection, and in some cases associated ureteral resection and anastomosis. It would be unreasonable to claim that excision of such a large lesion involving three structures (USL resection, resection with intestinal anastomosis, resection with end-to-end ureteral anastomosis) is possible in a single operative laparoscopy.

Although in this context the treatment of choice should be surgical, that does not mean to say that there is no place for medical treatment. In our opinion, main indications for medical treatment for deep pelvic endometriosis are the following:

1. It is not appropriate to propose this type of radical surgery if there is any doubt about the diagnosis.
2. Patient refusal to undergo a difficult surgical operation with risks that are by no means negligible.
3. Painful recurrence after complete initial surgical treatment: this is a formal indication for prescription of medical treatment rather than recommending repeat pelvic surgery.

In the context of pelvic pain, nothing has been published to date that indicates whether or not preoperative medical treatment should be prescribed. After the operation, it would seem that prescribing postoperative medical treatment is beneficial.[29] All the treatments seem to be of comparable efficiency[29,30] with respect to pain. The choice depends on whether there are any contraindications, the side effects, and the cost,

Table 21.5 Proposition for surgical procedure according to the classification

Classification	Operative procedure
A: Anterior DIE	
A1: Bladder	Laparoscopic partial cystectomy
P: Posterior DIE	
P1: Uterosacral ligament	Laparoscopic resection of USL
P2: Vaginal	Laparoscopically assisted vaginal resection of DIE infiltrating the posterior fornix
P3: Intestinal	
P3a: Solely intestinal location	
– without vaginal infiltration (V−)	Intestinal resection by laparoscopy or by laparotomy
– with vaginal infiltration (V+)	Laparoscopically assisted vaginal intestinal resection or exeresis by laparotomy
P3b: Multiple intestinal location	Intestinal resection by laparotomy

DIE = deeply infiltrating endometriosis; USL = uterosacral ligament.
Source: Adapted from Chapron et al.[9]

which depends on the length of time in the operating room (with long and complex surgery, this can be considerable).[30]

Conclusion

Endometriosis is defined as ectopic implantation of endometrial tissue (glands and stroma) outside the uterine cavity. The endometriotic lesions can penetrate deep into the retroperitoneal space and/or into the walls of the pelvic organs, thus constituting what is called DIE. The uterosacral ligaments are the most frequent location for DIE lesions. DIE appears to originate in the retrocervical area and the rectovaginal septum does not appear to be the initial location for DIE lesions.

Deep pelvic endometriosis is revealed mainly by painful symptoms that flare up with the monthly cycle, with symptomatology that varies according to the location of the lesions. The intensity of pain is significantly correlated with the depth to which the lesions penetrate. A work-up to establish the extent of the disease is indispensable in order to map the DIE lesions precisely, which is the only way to achieve complete excision. Normal clinical examination can in no way be considered as ruling out the diagnosis of DIE infiltrating the USL.

Transrectal ultrasonography is a reliable means of investigation for diagnosis of associated bowel infiltration. Nuclear magnetic resonance is useful in that it allows a complete work-up for the pelvis in one session.

The treatment of choice is surgery, because medical treatments are only palliative in the majority of cases. How successful treatment is depends on how radical the surgical excision is. The principle for surgical treatment is to achieve complete removal of all the DIE lesions that give rise to symptoms in a one-step surgical procedure. The methods used for surgery are dictated by the location and extent of the lesions. In case of isolated infiltrations of the USL, complete excision can be achieved using operative laparoscopy exclusively. In cases of DIE lesions associated with infiltration of the USL, excision of the USL must be accompanied with that of all the other locations (vagina, bladder, ureter, intestine). For certain patients presenting with very extensive lesions infiltrating several organs, it may be necessary to carry out a laparotomy in order to achieve complete treatment.

DIE must be considered as a pelvic pathology that is liable to involve all the organs in the pelvis and not as a pathology situated on a single organ (USL, vagina, bladder, ureter, intestine).

REFERENCES

1. Koninckx PR, Meuleman C, Demeyere S, et al. Suggestive evidence that pelvic endometriosis is a progressive disease, whereas deeply infiltrating endometriosis is associated with pelvic pain. Fertil Steril 1991; 55: 759–765.

2. Porpora MG, Koninckx P, Piazze J, et al. Correlation between endometriosis and pelvic pain. J Am Assoc Gynecol Laparosc 1999; 6: 429–434.

3. Chapron C, Fauconnier A, Dubuisson JB, et al. Deeply infiltrating endometriosis: relation between severity of dysmenorrhoea and extent of the disease. Hum Reprod 2003; 18: 760–766.

4. Garry R. Laparoscopic excision of endometriosis: the treatment of choice? Br J Obstet Gynaecol 1997; 104: 513–515.

5. Chapron C, Liaras E, Fayet P, et al. Magnetic resonance imaging and endometriosis: deeply infiltrating endometriosis does not originate from the rectovaginal septum. Gynecol Obstet Invest 2002; 53: 204–208.

6. Martin DC, Batt RE. Retrocervical, rectovaginal pouch and rectovaginal septum endometriosis. J Am Assoc Gynecol Laparosc 2001; 8: 12–17.

7. Chapron C, Chopin N, Borghese B, et al. Deeply infiltrating endometriosis originates from the retrocervical area. J Am Assoc Gynecol Laparosc 2004; 11 (3): 440–441.

8. Cornillie FJ, Oosterlynck D, Lauweryns JM, et al. Deeply infiltrating pelvic endometriosis: histology and clinical significance. Fertil Steril 1990; 53: 978–983.

9. Chapron C, Fauconnier A, Vieira M, et al. Anatomic distribution of deeply infiltrating endometriosis: surgical implications and proposition for a classification. Hum Reprod 2003; 18: 157–161.

10. Chapron C, Dubuisson JB. Laparoscopic treatment of deep endometriosis located on the uterosacral ligaments. Hum Reprod 1996; 11: 868–873.

11. Fauconnier A, Chapron C, Dubuisson JB, et al. Relation between pain symptoms and the anatomic location of deep infiltrating endometriosis. Fertil Steril 2002; 78: 719–726.

12. Chapron C, Dubuisson JB, Pansini V, et al. Routine clinical examination is not sufficient for the diagnosis and establishing the location of deeply infiltrating endometriosis. J Am Assoc Gynecol Laparosc 2002; 9: 115–119.

13. Chapron C, Dumontier I, Dousset B, et al. Results and role of rectal endoscopic ultrasonography for patients with deep pelvic endometriosis. Hum Reprod 1998; 13: 2266–2270.

14. Fedele L, Bianchi S, Portuese A, et al. Transrectal ultrasonography in the assessment of rectovaginal endometriosis. Obstet Gynecol 1998; 91: 444–448.

15. Schröder J, Löhnert M, Doniec JM, et al. Endoluminal ultrasound diagnosis and operative management of rectal endometriosis. Dis Colon Rectum 1997; 40: 614–617.

16. Abrao MS, Neme RM, Averbach M, et al. Rectal endoscopic ultrasound with radial probe in the assessment of rectovaginal endometriosis. J Am Assoc Gynecol Laparosc 2004; 11: 50–54.

17. Kinkel K, Chapron C, Balleyguier C, et al. Magnetic resonance imaging characteristics of deep endometriosis. Hum Reprod 1999; 14: 1080–1086.

18. Chapron C, Vieira M, Chopin N, et al. Accuracy of rectal endoscopic ultrasonography and magnetic resonance imaging in the diagnosis of rectal involvement for patients presenting with deeply infiltrating endometriosis. Ultrasound Obstet Gynecol 2004; 24: 175–179.

19. Brough RJ, O'Flynn K. Recurrent pelvic endometriosis and bilateral ureteric obstruction associated with hormone replacement therapy. Br Med J 1996; 312: 1221–1222.

20. Donnez J, Nisolle M, Squifflet J. Ureteral endometriosis: a complication of rectovaginal endometriotic (adenomyotic) nodules. Fertil Steril 2002; 77: 32–37.

21. Deprest J, Marchal G, Brosens I. Obstructive uropathy secondary to endometriosis. N Engl J Med 1997; 337: 1174–1175.

22. Harada M, Kase T, Tajima M, et al. [A case of ureteral endometriosis; the usefulness of MRI for preoperative diagnosis]. Hinyokika Kiyo 1992; 38: 207–211 [in Japanese].

23. Balleyguier C, Roupret M, Nguyen T, et al. Ureteral endometriosis: the role of magnetic resonance imaging. J Am Assoc Gynecol Laparosc 2004; 11: 530–536.

24. Bazot M, Detchev R, Cortez A, et al. Transvaginal sonography and rectal endoscopic sonography for the assessment of pelvic endometriosis: a preliminary comparison. Hum Reprod 2003; 18: 1686–1692.

25. Chopin N, Vieira M, Borghese B, et al. Operative management of deeply infiltrating endometriosis: results on pelvic pain symptoms according to a surgical classification. J Minim Invasive Gynecol 2005; 12: 106–112.

26. Abott JA, Hawe J, Clayton RD, et al. The effects and effectiveness of laparoscopic excision of endometriosis: a prospective study with 2–5 year follow-up. Hum Reprod 2003; 9: 1922–1927.

27. Chapron C, Fauconnier A, Dubuisson JB, et al. Does deep endometriosis infiltrating the uterosacral ligaments present an asymmetric lateral distribution? Br J Obstet Gynaecol 2001; 108: 1021–1024.

28. Chapron C, Jacob S, Dubuisson JB, et al. Laparoscopically assisted vaginal management of deep endometriosis infiltrating the rectovaginal septum. Acta Obstet Gynecol Scand 2001; 80: 349–354.

29. Olive DL, Pritts EA. Treatment of endometriosis. N Engl J Med 2001; 345: 266–275.

30. Vercellini P, Cortesi I, Crosignani PG. Progestins for symptomatic endometriosis: a critical analysis of the evidence. Fertil Steril 1997; 68: 393–401.

SECTION IV

Different Power Sources in Laparoscopic Surgery

22 Laparoscopic treatment of endometriosis by electrosurgery

Jeremy T Wright and Saikat Banerjee

Introduction

The surgical management of endometriosis involves the removal of identifiable endometriotic deposits. This may be carried out either by excision or ablation.[1] Although it is debatable as to which method is considered to be superior, both require the use of cutting and coagulation. In order to perform such surgery an energy source is required.

The literature contains advice of the best possible modalities[2,3] but at the end of the day 'a Watt is a Watt is a Watt'.[4] Currently available energy modalities use:

- diathermy[5,6]
- laser (*l*ight *a*mplification by *s*timulated *e*mission of *r*adiation) (from Star Wars technology)[7]
- electrosurgery applied through an electrode or through ionized gas particles, such as the argon beam or helium beam coagulator which use ionised gas to transmit the electron beam[6]
- ultrasound/motion energy.[8]

The foregoing all have one thing in common: they are all energy transfer modalities and thus all have their own dangers.

The widely stated dogma surrounding monopolar diathermy is that it is dangerous,[9] yet there are still many surgeons experienced in its use who appear to get the desired effect, if not superior results, compared to other energy sources.[10] There is no objective evidence outside conjecture of any increases in complication rate, and costs are low.

To date, despite the dogma 'never use monopolar diathermy in the abdomen'[2] and 'lasers cause less scarring'[11] and despite attempted instrument company incentives for alternative modalities, there is still no evidence to support these statements. The authors believe that the training before being allowed to use such advanced energy sources requires the surgeon to demonstrate a thorough knowledge in the energy source, but in fact we are all allowed to pick up a diathermy forceps on our first working day and often by the end of a successful career still have no idea how to use this tool effectively and safely.[12]

The aim of this chapter is to let the surgeon know about electrosurgery using basic principles, as is done for the other energy modalities, so that the dangers can be equally identified and avoided. The advantages should be fully exploited so that the capabilities of this, still the most versatile and cheapest of the energy sources, can be fully harnessed. The second part of the chapter describes the use of diathermy in the treatment of endometriosis.

Principles of electrosurgery

Electrosurgical generators produce a radiofrequency (RF) alternating current where the circuit traverses the patient for the surgical cutting and/or coagulation of tissues. In monopolar diathermy this is between the point electrode and the return plate whereas in bipolar diathermy the current is passed between the two electrodes. This completes the electrical circuit every time the diathermy is engaged.

The frequency of current used is in the region of 500 kHz. The logic for this is to avoid electrocution. Electrocution is the destruction of cells by cell depolarization, which can occur at current frequencies below 100 kHz. Above this frequency, the current direction (remember alternating current) is too rapid to give the cells time to depolarize. Electrocution does not, therefore, occur when the current frequency is very high (diathermy). All surgeons are, however, aware that the application of current can result in muscle twitching/contraction. This is as a result of impurities in the current, with the presence of lower-frequency harmonics in the signal (i.e. some of the current flow is below 100 kHz – demodulation). Electricity companies transport their electricity at the lethal 50 Hz compared to our cotton soft 500 kHz since at these higher frequencies there is a greater rate of energy loss (loss of efficiency), which is significant over the billions of miles of cabling wrapping around our planet compared to the few meters in the operating theater.

Like all domestic electrical appliances, electricity will follow the path of least resistance, which, if grounded to earth, may be through the surgeon or metal in contact with the patient. In the past this has resulted in alternative site burns. Historically, such burns (Figure 22.1) have accounted for 70% of the injuries reported during the use of electrosurgery, according to data collected by Valleylab (Boulder, CO: www.valleylab.com).

Modern diathermy is grounded to the machine rather than the planet; thus, in order to complete an electrical circuit, the electricity must pass via the electrode used and the return plate. These systems are termed grounded electrosurgical systems.

Monopolar diathermy

Monopolar is the most common electrosurgical modality used because of its versatility and clinical effectiveness. The active electrode is in the surgical site, whereas return electrode is via the return plate elsewhere on the patient's body (Figure 22.2).

The current is required to pass through the patient from one electrode to another. The area of contact of the electrode at the surgical site is many times smaller than the area of contact at the return plate. The net result is all the electrons flowing in the circuit have to pass through the narrow point at the active site, resulting in a high current density compared to the large contact area at the return plate, giving a low current density. The high current density results in a concentration of energy, with the area of highest power and effect, from the electricity. At low current densities, the electrons are too diluted to produce an effect. The result is that the return electrode must be applied correctly and completely. Incomplete contact will result in high rather than low current densities and plate site burns (Figure 22.3).

The more concentrated the energy, the greater the thermodynamic effect

Modern diathermy using localized circuits within the plate will check for correct application. Also, the use of wet spirits under the plate will result in combustion, as the current will ignite the spirit cleaner if allowed to pass through the spirits. Therefore, either spirits should be avoided or

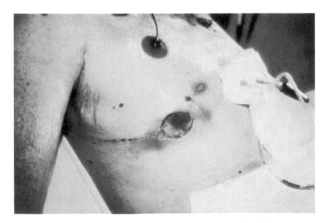

Figure 22.1 Diathermy burn. Courtesy of Valleylab (Boulder, CO). Copyright © 2003, 2004, 2005 Valleylab, a division of Tyco Healthcare Group LP. All rights reserved.

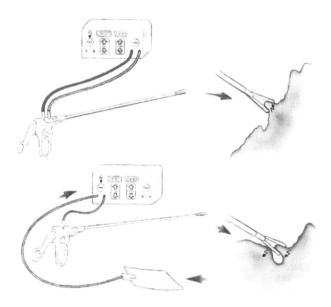

Figure 22.2 (a) Bipolar and (b) monopolar current flow. (Courtesy of Lower, Sutton and Grudzinskas, Isis Medical Media, Oxford)

(a)

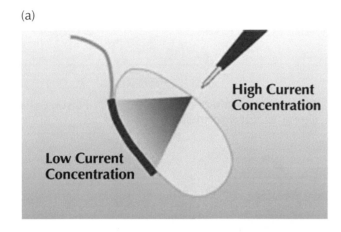

(b)

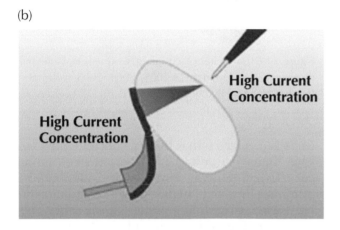

Figure 22.3 (a) High current density at the active electrode compared to the return plate. (b) The effect of incorrect return plate application. Courtesy of Valleylab (Boulder, CO). Copyright © 2003, 2004, 2005 Valleylab, a division of Tyco Healthcare Group LP. All rights reserved.

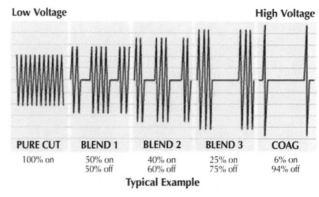

Figure 22.4 Various waveforms used for each type of current effect produced. Courtesy of Valleylab (Boulder, CO). Copyright © 2003, 2004, 2005 Valleylab, a division of Tyco Healthcare Group LP. All rights reserved.

allowed to evaporate and not allowed to pool when draping a patient for surgery where diathermy is used.

The difference in the effect of cutting or coagulation is as a result of the difference in the waveform used. Figure 22.4 represents the various waveforms used: the *x*-axis represents time and the *y*-axis voltage.

Current flow in tissue that acts as a resistor results in heat production. The biologic effect is the irreversible destruction of cells by the denaturation of proteins and desiccation.

- *Cutting current* vaporizes or cuts tissue. The current density is sufficiently high at the point of contact to cause a very rapid rise in temperature to the extent as to vaporize the cut tissue, i.e. a cutting effect.
- *Coagulation currents* use an intermittent more complex waveform that varies between machines. The essential effect is an on–off cur-

rent that is of a high voltage in the 'on phase'. The 'on phase' covers about 4% of the time. The result is that the tissue is allowed to cool between 'on phases', which produces less heat by allowing thermal spread, so that instead of tissue vaporization, a coagulum is produced.
- *Blended current* is an alteration of the time that the current is applied, producing progressively less heat as the time the current is on is reduced and allowing more coagulation to occur.

The higher the cutting current used, the quicker the temperature rise and the less the thermal spread. Also, the smaller the contact area, the higher the current density at the contact point. The result is that using a needle-tip point contact instrument at a suitably high power setting, a cutting effect with minimal thermal spread can be achieved that is identical to that found when using carbon dioxide lasers as an alternative energy source for cutting. Eschar is relatively high in resistance to current, and a tissue build-up can result in a preferential unwanted flow of current to adjacent structures down the path of least resistance, a classic example being the arcing of current to adjacent bowel that can occur when pelvic structures such as the fallopian tubes are cauterized with monopolar diathermy. This is called direct coupling and can be avoided by avoiding the formation of eschar by using a high power, pure cut (rather than coagulation waveform) setting (Figure 22.5).

It is also beneficial to keep electrodes clean and free of eschar. This will enhance performance by maintaining lower resistance within the surgical circuit.

Coagulation currents require a considerably higher voltage than pure cutting current, and this

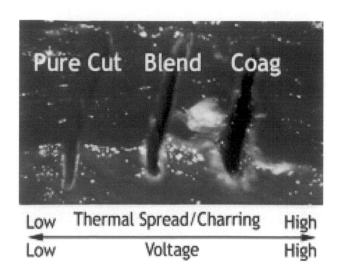

Low **Thermal Spread/Charring** High

Low **Voltage** High

Figure 22.5 Use of various diathermy waveforms and the resultant thermal spread. Courtesy of Valleylab (Boulder, CO). Copyright © 2003, 2004, 2005 Valleylab, a division of Tyco Healthcare Group LP. All rights reserved.

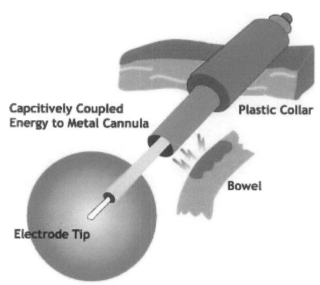

Figure 22.6 Capacitance coupling. Courtesy of Valleylab (Boulder, CO). Copyright © 2003, 2004, 2005 Valleylab, a division of Tyco Healthcare Group LP. All rights reserved.

can increase the risks of the procedure, particularly in relation to minimal access surgery. These higher voltages increase the risk of capacitive coupling; an inadvertent capacitor is created by the surgical instruments, a conductive active electrode being surrounded by nonconductive insulation, which is in turn surrounded by conductive metal cannulas. An electrostatic field is created between the two conductors and, as a result, the current in one conductor can, through the electrostatic field, produce a current in the second conductor. In the context of minimal access surgery, this may be the metal cannula through which the instrument is passed; the cannulas will be in contact with the abdominal wall and may lie against visceral structures such as the small or large bowel, which may then be subjected to heat injury (Figure 22.6).

In order to avoid capacitive coupling, either all-metal or all-plastic cannula systems should be used rather than a hybrid system. If a metal cannula is used, it must be with a metal collar so that any charge induced in the metal cannula can be harmlessly dispersed to the anterior abdominal wall. It is also important never to activate the diathermy under an open-circuit condition such as when the electrode is just sitting within the cannula. Such activation will result in very high voltages, which can result in the forcing of a larger capacitive current flow, the build-up of charge on the metal cannula resulting in capacitive coupling burns.

Electrical energy should be applied for the minimum amount of time and never when the electrode is in space rather than in contact with tissue. This limits the voltages usable with cutting and coagulation. Cutting currents are often used to minimize the use of higher-power coagulation currents when coagulating tissue. This is achieved by increasing the contact area of the electrode (e.g. using the back rather than the tip of the scissors) with the tissue, thus decreasing the current density at the contact point and giving a slower temperature rise and a coagulation effect.

It is important that the current used also does not exceed the insulation effect of the insulator used by the instrument (dielectric strength). This also limits the power of the diathermy used. Use of long electrosurgical instruments also increases the risk of insulation failure along the length of the instruments, which can 'short out' against the metal cannulas. Some modern electrosurgical generators now incorporate safety devices that will detect current leakage (active electrode monitor).

Direct coupling is achieved if the active electrode is not located near to the tissue to be cut. Electricity takes the path of least resistance and may stray to the adjacent bowel, resulting in a bowel burn. This is avoided by only activating the current when the electrode is close to the tissue that is being cut. The electrode should always be under direct vision while in the abdomen and, ideally, should be removed when not in use. This can be easily achieved by just retracting the active electrode within a sheath or cannula.

The other major consideration for electrosurgery in minimal access surgery is the size of the electrode. Smaller electrodes have a higher power density and therefore vaporization of tissue rather than coagulation is concomitantly greater. The spread of destructive thermal energy to underlying structures is proportionally less. It is important to identify tissue desiccation when it occurs. When tissue is desiccated with the electrode in direct contact (touching) with tissue using a cutting current, the tissue's electrical resistance rises as the cells dry out and thus the current concentration falls. The result is a fall in the cutting effect. It is therefore useful to avoid tissue desiccation when cutting. This is done by having a high current density using a small contact area (such as the point of a scissor) and high power settings. The avoidance of dessication during cutting also improves electrical safety by avoiding current straying and minimising the current activation time and thus unwanted tissue heating effect/thermal spread.[13] In desiccation the cells dry out and form a coagulum rather than vaporize and explode. This may be used to the surgeon's advantage if wishing to coagulate using a cutting current. This is achieved by increasing the electrode contact area (such as contact using the flat surface of the scissors) and by keeping the electrode in contact with the tissue, rather than by using the spark.

Fulguration, which is sparking with a coagulation waveform, coagulates and chars the tissue over a wide area. However, because of the high impedance of air, higher voltages are required. Fulguration using argon or neon beams reduces the voltage and increases the safety of these techniques.[8] They should not, however, be used in the presence of significant hemorrhage, as the pressure of gas used is quite high and fatalities from gas embolism have been reported.[14]

The diathermy is used for short bursts at a time to limit heat build-up on the electrode, and tissues are continuously being cooled by use of a laparoscopic saline irrigation system: this is especially important, since adjacent tissue heating can result in tissue hyperthermia. In this instance, tissue may be heated to above 62°C for a prolonged period of time, causing irreversible cell damage. The immediate effects are subtle and not macroscopically evident, leading to an overestimate of safety. The result is the subsequent postoperative delayed presentation of bowel injury.

For the reasons stated above, the authors' preference is the use of a 3 mm sharp-tip electrode using a high-power (75–90 W) setting to produce tissue vaporization with minimal thermal effect.

We use 3 mm scissors, which have a sharp tip for electrosurgical cutting and the back of blades or jaws to increase the contact area for grasping and then coagulating. The instrument is then passed down the operating channel of a 12 mm operating laparoscope (Figure 22.7).

As well as giving better access for the electrode to the rectovaginal septum, this ensures that the active electrode always remains in view when in use and is easy to retract back into the laparoscope when not in use. It is thus ideal for excision work. It is able to produce a cutting signature identical to that of a carbon dioxide laser, but has the added advantage of allowing continuous tactile sensation while operating in order to identify endometriotic and fibrotic tissue from normal tissue. This is not possible and is a limitation with lasers. It is, however, important to appreciate the above physics in order to apply safe techniques when operating using diathermy, particularly in this minimal access setting. The use of this method is a long learning curve,[15] but the result is the most versatile energy source currently available, which is the most easily available and relatively cheap. It is ideal for laparoscopic excisional techniques

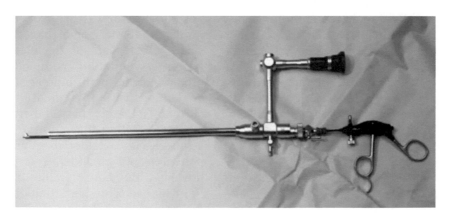

Figure 22.7 Operating laparoscope.

throughout the pelvis, including over vital structures such as the ureters, major blood vessels, and bowel serosa. There is nothing that can be achieved in gynecologic endoscopic surgery using lasers that cannot be achieved using diathermy if the underlying principles are understood and used to the surgeon's benefit rather than detriment.

Bipolar diathermy

So far, our discussions have been exclusively about monopolar diathermy, as this is the most useful electrical modality for the laparoscopic resection of endometriosis. Bipolar diathermy, however, is a useful addition which is often considered safer than monopolar diathermy. To some extent it is true, as both sides of the electrical circuit are through the arms of the instrument (usually grasping forceps). Because the return function is performed by one tine of the forceps, no patient return plate is needed, which therefore limits the flow of current to any tissue between the grasping forceps and the surgical field rather than the whole of the patient (see Figure 22.2).

The advantage is the avoidance of many of the hazards already discussed. There are, however, some qualifications which result in the continuing use of monopolar systems:

1. The jaws of the graspers can become 'live' with respect to the surrounding tissue if the system is activated with no tissues interposed between the blades of the two electrodes. This can result in inadvertent diathermy burns to adjacent structures. It is therefore important that any diathermy or energy source *should never be activated inside the patient without good electrical contact with the target tissue and should ideally be removed from the abdomen when not in active usage.*
2. The effect of passing a current across the tissue in this way is heating. Bipolar diathermy is largely confined to coagulation and thus lacks flexibility. There are hysteroscopic bipolar cutting instruments, such as the Versapoint system (Gynecare, Ascot, UK), which cut by creating a plasma in saline distention medium and vaporizing the tissues. Such bipolar cutting systems for use in laparoscopy are limited in efficiency for the present time.
3. It is important to remember that tissues heated with bipolar systems become very hot – around 340°C at the point of maximal current flow. This makes them very efficient as a coagulator compared to monopolar systems but gives rise to a thermal gradient and greater

thermal spread to surrounding tissues. After 8 seconds of application, tissues at a distance of 15 mm may be heated to histotoxic levels, i.e. above 62°C.[16] It is the authors' belief that this thermal spread can limit the use of bipolar diathermy and may explain some of the higher incidences of ureteric injuries when ligating the uterine artery at laparoscopic hysterectomy.[17] To overcome this problem of thermal spread, there are newer bipolar systems on the market such as the LigaSure vessel sealing system (Valleylab, Boulder, CO). This system works by applying a unique form of bipolar electrosurgery in combination with optimal pressure delivery to fuse the vessel walls and create a permanent seal, which is achieved by reforming the collagen and elastin in vessel walls to form an autologous clip. The output is feedback-controlled so that a reliable seal is achieved in minimal time, independent of the type or amount of tissue in the jaws. Vessels up to and including 7 mm in diameter, such as the uterine and ovarian arteries, can be sealed with the LigaSure system.

Importantly, it is often overlooked that the smoke plume produced during the use of any energy source during surgery contains toxic gases and vapors such as benzene, hydrogen cyanide, and formaldehyde; bioaerosols; dead and live cellular material (including blood fragments); and viruses.[18] In laparoscopic surgery, this is contained within the abdomen. It is, however, a peritoneal irritant and also results in an obscured view of the pelvic organs, so that a smoke filter and evacuation system is recommended.[19]

Treatment of endometriosis by excision or ablation

Electrosurgery is widely used for treating endometriotic lesions as it is easily available. For superficial disease, i.e. shallow peritoneal implants, flame hemorrhages, sago grains, and small white scars of the classic red and black lesions, coagulation using either monopolar or bipolar current, with bipolar electricity, is considered effective.[1] Bipolar diathermy, when the current is merely passed between two adjacent electrodes rather than from a point to a common electrode is considered safer by some, as the patient is not considered as part of the circuit; however, the considerable thermal spread can limit its use. This is particularly so in the pelvis, where adjacent vital structures are prone to injury secondary to their close proximity. Theoretical advantages of ablative techniques are that they are technically easier to perform, treatment is as effective as excision, and widespread areas of endometriosis such as extensive vascular change can be treated by superficial fulguration. However, treatment may be incomplete because of a natural reluctance to treat areas over vital structures such as the ureter or great vessels. Coagulation at the tip of the lesion may conceal the bulk of the lesion below, also resulting in incomplete treatment.

Excision treatment involves using the diathermy as a cutting tool to excise the affected areas of endometriosis and areas of peritoneum, together with a margin of normal tissue; the excision is carried out by a combination of sharp and blunt dissection, although by staying in normal tissue and away from the endometriotic areas, the majority of the dissection can be carried out using blunt dissection.

The affected peritoneum is grasped and traction applied medially; the side-wall tissues are dissected away laterally, safely displacing any vital structures. This can be carried out very safely using a combination of cutting current, coagulation current, and blunt dissection. A pair of 3 mm hook scissors is ideal for this procedure as it can act as point electrode, a forceps for coagulation, a dissecting instrument, and a grasping instrument for removing dissected tissue.

Various other forms of scissors are in use, as are diathermy hooks, but standard laparoscopic scissors have the disadvantage of a large electrode surface, reduced power density, and also increased inadvertent direct coupling with adjacent tissues. A major advantage of excisional treatment is that it allows confirmation of disease by histologic examination. It is particularly important as, frequently, the clinical diagnosis of endometriosis both in individual samples, and indeed patients, is not confirmed by histologic examination, especially where there is previous treatment and there is carbonization of the tissues which can mimic endometriotic lesions. Failure to confirm the diagnosis histologically may lead to the patient being advised to undergo a course of hormone manipulation, with all its associated unpleasant side effects, in the absence of any observable endometriotic disease.[20] A meta-analysis of the literature[21] collaborates this concern, demonstrating that even in expert hands the positive predictive value for the surgical diagnosis of endometriosis is variable: between 25% (to a few studies) reaching 100% with an average of only 63%. Therefore, as in all other fields of surgical gynecology, endometriosis is no exception in the need for histologic confirmation, which can

only be provided by excisional rather than ablative therapy.

The safe use of monopolar diathermy, particularly laparoscopically, is counterintuitive. What is required is a high-wattage cutting current (75–90 W) with a very small electrode producing high power densities, the power being applied for as short a time as possible. The high power density vaporizes the tissue, so there is very little lateral spread. Provided the electrode has a round end, it can also be used for blunt dissection. The authors' personal preference is for 3 mm hooked laparoscopic scissors which can be passed through the operating port and operating laparoscope, or through a trumpet valve washer/sucker. This allows dissection with the blunt end and the gentle grasping of vessels for unipolar coagulation. The relative flexibility of the 3 mm scissors allows for a gentler blunt dissection than using a rigid instrument.

A suitable alternative is a laparoscopic hook, as used by general surgeons for cholecystectomy. This is better than a point electrode as the knee of the hook can be used for blunt dissection (Figure 22.8).

Excision of superficial peritoneal lesions is probably safer than coagulation. Although coagulation is perceived by many to be safer and easier, it is much more prone to allow heat to be applied to underlying structures, which may anyway – in the presence of fibrosis – be obscured, causing their inadvertent injury. The technique is to grasp the peritoneum either above or below the lesion to be excised and retract it medially away from the side wall. The peritoneum is then incised and by means of blunt dissection retracted away from the underlying structures, which can then be observed. Having incised sufficient area anteriorly, the apex of the lesion can be grasped and a

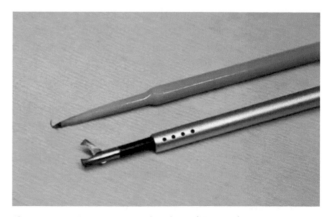

Figure 22.8 Laparoscopic hook and 3 mm laparoscopic hook scissors protruding through a sucker irrigator.

posterior incision made. The peritoneum will then rapidly become looser and excision can occur safely and simply with all the underlying anatomy clearly exposed. Any small underlying vessels can be identified and coagulated before they bleed, producing a bloodless dissection. This method of dissection is safe over the great vessels and the ureter. If there is still concern, dissection can be used prior to starting the excision. A long needle such as a facet block needle or the introducing needle of a Bonanno catheter is useful for infiltrating the side wall. Although infiltration with saline is effective and appears to be safe, there is a theoretical risk of short circuit and a failure of the tissue to cut, so some would prefer to use glycine or sorbitol in these circumstances. Adhesion barriers such as Adept (4% icodextrin, Shire Pharmaceuticals, Basingstoke, UK), although perfectly safe following surgery, are best avoided during the surgical procedure as they contain macrolactates that will carbonize with heat, giving rise to intraperitoneal 'toffee'.

The technique is similar for the excision of nodular or infiltrating endometriosis, which should be grasped and kept under tension. The dissection as far as possible should always be in normal tissue away from the nodule and, if this is achieved, it will be relatively bloodless. A constant ooze of blood suggests that you are in a nodule with its abnormal vasculature: this will be difficult to control, other than by coagulation of the surface, which will also obscure the anatomy. With the excision of uterosacral lesions, the uterosacrals should be transected below the lesion and then grasped and pulled medially. The peritoneum lateral to the lesion should be excised and the underlying fat dissected laterally and away from the lesion. It is important that the dissection is initially as superficial as possible, deepening it only when one becomes aware of the structures underneath. Frequently, the ureter will be displaced medially by the fibrotic lesion and this needs to be identified and dissected laterally away from the lesion, which can usually be achieved bloodlessly by meticulously identifying the small blood vessels and lateral blunt dissection. The excision should be continued up to its insertion in the cervix, as this way it is likely to produce relative denervation to hopefully improve dysmenorrhea. If the lesion is unilateral, the medial aspect is then identified and dissected free. A probe in the rectum is helpful both in identifying this and allowing it to be put under tension and away from the area which is undergoing surgery.

If a block dissection is required, the lateral excision is repeated on the other side, and then the incision line is joined up over the cervix, trying to stay just in the fascia of the peritoneal reflection. By a combination of blunt and sharp dissection, it is then possible to enter the rectovaginal septum. Disease of the uterosacrals may extend some way into the septum and, in this case, the descending cervical branch of the uterine artery will have to be sacrificed. It is important to complete this dissection and ensure that normal extraperitoneal rectum is identified before starting excision of the nodule. Attempts to excise the rectum from the nodule and then remove the nodule are likely to result in inadvertent rectal injury while it is still adherent to the uterosacral ligament and the posterior cervix. Further dissection and retraction will increase the size of the rectal perforation and make it more difficult to repair. Having completed this part of the dissection, both the uterus (which is frequently quite stuck) and the rectum will become more mobile, allowing greater space within the pelvis to complete the operation. With a probe in the rectum to clearly identify it and allow it to be displaced away from the dissection, the peritoneum underneath the lesion can then be excised and, using monopolar cutting diathermy to reduce the thermal spread, the lesion can be excised from the rectum, knowing that the distal margin is free of disease. Furthermore, if the rectum is injured or the lesion is full thickness, disk excision can be carried out and sutured safely, knowing that there is no further disease.

A good clue to the disease being full thickness is the so-called 'rounded rectum', when the rectum is seen to be rounded as it is tethered to the posterior cervix – when the uterus is held in extreme anteversion – and this should alert the surgeon to the need for a full-thickness repair (Figures 22.9 and 22.10).

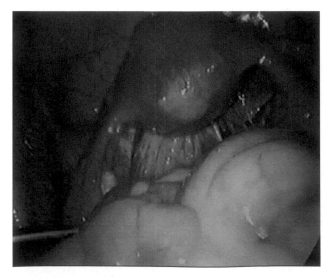

Figure 22.9 Rounded rectum.

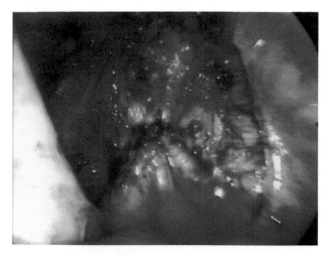

Figure 22.10 Post dissection.

Severe rectal lesions often involve the posterior fornix of the vagina, and this can frequently be indicated by the presence of blue or purple nodules in the posterior fornix. In these circumstances, the vaginal lesion will have to be removed and it is important that the lateral extension of the nodule is dissected out extensively and early before entering the rectovaginal space. At this stage, the vagina will be opened and there may be difficulties in maintaining a pneumoperitoneum, although a wet pack in the posterior fornix will help. Having opened the vagina it is often possible to complete the dissection vaginally, including excision of the rectal nodule and any suturing which may be less time consuming than a laparoscopic repair, particularly if there is leaking from the pneumoperitoneum.

Following surgery, it is important to check the integrity of the rectum. This can best be performed by flooding the pelvis with saline, covering the operative field. The rectum is then instilled with air, either using a sigmoidoscope or, more simply, a bladder syringe. One is looking for extravasation of air into the saline (bubbles). The rapid passage of air, if forced in too quickly, can cause a tear in the mucosa if a musculoserosal stitch has not been placed.

Diathermy can also be used to dissect right around and mobilize the rectum, which can be used to facilitate a laparoscopic segmental resection if required. The diseased section can then be removed through a small Pfannenstiel incision and either an end-to-end or end-to-side staple anastomosis carried out. This procedure, although effective, is likely to cause more bowel disturbance than a disk resection.

These extensive resections will often result in considerable serosanguineous discharge, particularly

over the ensuing 48 hours, so it is sensible to place a soft drain in the pelvis such as a 20 Robinson drain, which can easily pass down a 5 mm port.

Diathermy is also very suitable for the removal of bladder nodules, which are sometimes full thickness and centered on the dome of the bladder and thus well clear of the ureters. Occasionally, these can again be mucosa-sparing; otherwise, the bladder can be closed in either one or two layers laparoscopically and tested for patency by instilling methylene blue through the indwelling Foley catheter. The technique for excision is the same in that one starts in normal tissue and uses cutting diathermy to excise the lesion with a margin of healthy tissue.

Management of ovarian endometriosis by electrosurgery

Ovarian endometriosis is a common site of disease that occurs in 17–44% of patients affected by endometriosis and accounts for 35% of benign ovarian cysts.[22] The left is more frequently affected than the right ovary.[23,24] It is also a marker of the presence of endometriosis elsewhere in the pelvis.[25] Thus, when attempting to treat ovarian endometriosis, the surgeon should also be versed in the surgical management of endometriosis throughout the pelvis in order to gain complete excision and thus the best possible prognosis for patients in the treatment of their chronic pelvic pains.

Although the best management of endometriosis (either medical or surgical) is often disputed, it is clear that the role of medical management for ovarian endometriosis is limited to only endometriomas less than 1 cm in diameter.[26] Above this diameter, the medical treatment of endometriomas results in an almost 100% reoccurrence, with a delaying effect on pregnancy. The management is thus essentially surgical.

The management of ovarian endometriosis by electrosurgery remains controversial, as the histologic basis of ovarian endometriomas is disputed.[27] The standard management of any ovarian cyst is the excision of the cyst with the wall intact. In endometriomas the wall, which is often called a pseudocapsule, is densely adherent to the remaining ovary with no obvious plane of dissection, and removal with the cyst intact is often virtually impossible. This is the most difficult of all the ovarian cystectomies. This may be related to the proposed pathogenesis of endometriomas suggested by Brosens et al,[28] in that these cysts are as a result of the invagination of the endometriosis affecting the ovarian cortex. Proponents of this theory argue that the endometrioma is in fact inverted normal ovarian cortex and that excision of this will reduce the number of primordial follicles and thus fertility. However, other theories include Sampson, who postulated that these cysts are as a result of invasion of endometriosis of the corpus luteal cysts. It was Sampson who first coined the familiar term 'chocolate cysts'.[29]

Although stripping of the cyst is associated with loss of adjacent ovarian tissue, this tissue does not show the morphologic characteristics of normal tissue. As it is usually absent of follicles and therefore may not be of functional value, this is a tissue-sparing technique.[30] Maneschi et al[31] have demonstrated the presence of ovarian tissue when stripping endometriomas in only 19% of specimens compared with up to 80% in cystectomies for other benign ovarian cysts. It can therefore be surmised that any loss of ovarian function in endometriomas that is described in the literature is secondary to the disease rather than the surgical technique.

As cystectomy is challenging, alternative methods of surgical treatment have been used. These include the simple aspiration of the cyst either under transvaginal ultrasound or laparoscopic guidance. These techniques are associated with high recurrence rates (22–100%).[32] To reduce the reoccurrence rate, the use of sclerotherapy using instillation of 50% ethanol[33,34] has been proposed. However, the literature reports concerns with leakage of the cystic contents or, if used, sclerotherapy agents producing at best adhesions and upstaging the disease and at worse peritonitis.[35]

Another proposed technique is the fenestration of the cyst and ablation of the capsule either medically[36] or using the Potassium Titanyl-Phosphate (KTP) laser,[37] bicap bipolar diathermy,[38] or as a two-stage procedure to reduce recurrence rates.[39] It is the authors' belief that these techniques are associated with a higher recurrence rate and have not been proven to reduce the effect on ovarian function compared to the gold standard technique of stripping the cyst wall. There is only one randomized study[40] comparing fenestration and ablation of the capsule. It shows that there is no statistical difference in the recurrence rates of the disease (6.2% vs 18.6%) but a higher pregnancy rate at 24-month follow-up in the excision group. In a retrospective study,[41] it was concluded that at 42 months, excision was associated with a lower reoperation rate (23.6% vs 57.8%). Vercellini et al showed a threefold increased risk of cyst recurrence when comparing the two techniques: odds ratio (OR), 3.09; 95% confidence interval (CI) 1.78–5.36.[42]

Removal of the cyst provides histologic confirmation of the diagnosis and also exclusion of the rare possibility of malignant transformation, which is said to increase in women with endometriomas (standardized incidence ratio 3.1; 95% CI, 1.8–4.9).[43] Such transformation is more common in ovarian compared with nonovarian endometriosis,[44] possibly due to the high local estrogen environment. Such cancers are usually clear cell and endometrioid carcinoma.

Superficial lesions may be treated by electrovaporization or cortical excision. Endometriomas are usually adherent to the pelvic side wall or uterosacral ligament. Dissection often begins with a combination of blunt and electrodissection of the ovary off the side wall. It is imperative to identify the ureter to avoid collateral damage. Often this results in cyst rupture with a stoma that is away from the ipsilateral tube, avoiding damage to the tube. The chocolate contents are intensely irritating to the peritoneum and require suction irrigation for clearance. The cyst is also aspirated and cleaned. The lining may then be examined by extending the ovarian incision and by direct laparoscopic inspection. The cyst wall is identified by its white fibrotic appearance compared to the reddish color of healthy ovarian tissue. Diathermy may be used to make an initial separation between the two layers to provide an initial traction handle. This cut is made a few millimeters from the initial incision site and is only required to be a few millimeters in length and depth. The pseudocapsule is then peeled off the ovary, using two graspers in a stepwise fashion. This is made easy by the fact that the cyst wall is fibrotic and thus able to withstand strong traction. It is important to avoid tearing and excessive bleeding by excessive or too fast traction. This is achieved by always keeping the plane of cleavage in view and by stepping the graspers along the cyst wall and ovarian tissue, so that the graspers are always close to the plane of cleavage, thus improving the effectiveness of the tractional forces exerted. Often, in order to avoid disorientation, it is useful to actually elevate the pseudocapsule and slowly tease off the normal ovarian tissue downwards while elevating the capsule. By careful dissection, bleeding – and thus the use of bipolar cautery – can be minimized in order to minimize damage to normal ovarian tissue. As the cyst is removed, the ovarian cortex often becomes inverted. It is important to remain orientated and maintain the plane of cleavage and to observe and make sure that the ovarian cortex is not being dissected as well. It is important to be aware of the ovarian blood supply and to avoid excessive coagulation near the ovarian hilus. The 3 mm laparoscopic scissors via the operating channel is ideal for this purpose. Close inspection is under high magnification while intermittent irrigation of the cut surface allows identification of fine bleeding sites with precision. This can then be picked up with the fine 3 mm scissors blades in a grasper-like action and a short burst of 60 W coagulation current applied to achieve the desired effect.

It is also important to note that if the uterosacral ligament or side wall is adherent to the cyst, it may harbor residual endometriosis that will need to be excised. Such retroperitoneal fibrosis may overlie the ipsilateral ureter and so difficult ureterolysis is sometimes necessary. To aid such dissection, some authors propose the use of ureteric stents.

The current surgical management in the UK is very variable. In a questionnaire of 651 UK gynecologists by Jones et al, the reported rate of laparotomy was 42.3%.[45] Canis et al[15] suggest that this is secondary to a long learning curve. Therefore, it is imperative before attempting potentially complex surgery that the patient is correctly counseled preoperatively and that the surgeon is aware of the potential problems. It is the authors' routine practice in such patients to administer a bowel preparation preoperatively.

Electrosurgery and adhesions

Widespread destruction of peritoneum will invariably lead to tissue damage, inflammation and subsequent healing. However, this inflammation may lead to the formation of adhesions, particularly ovarian and peritubular adhesions, with a subsequent decrease in fertility, which is of particular concern to young women. It is known that peritoneal regrowth occurs very quickly, but the presence of a coagulum will slow this process, and adhesions are relatively rare after excisional techniques, particularly if all the areas of endometriosis are removed. The presence of residual endometriosis is, however, associated with considerable scarring and adhesion formation, and thus it is very important to excise or treat all the areas of endometriosis that can be seen.

The evidence for the use of adhesion barriers in these circumstances is unknown but there is accruing evidence that low concentration oxygen during intraperitoneal insufflation may significantly reduce this, but the volumes of oxygen being proposed (3%) are not sufficient to increase the risk of explosion with electrosurgery.[46]

Summary

The appropriate application of the correct mode of electrosurgery is predominantly a safe, effective, and cheap way of excising endometriotic lesions that allows histologic confirmation. The methods are as effective as any other modality presently in use, but at considerably less expense.

The use of high power densities allows efficient vaporization of tissue with minimal lateral spread of heat and has the advantage of allowing fine dissection, particularly over bowel and the layers of the rectal wall. However, the safety of these techniques can be increased by a good understanding of the instrumentation, ensuring good maintenance of equipment, particularly the electrodes, and reducing to a minimum the amount of time the current is applied.

REFERENCES

1. Wright JT, Lotfallah H, Jones K, et al. A randomised trial of excision vs ablation for mild (r-AFS 1–2) [revised American Fertility Score] endometriosis. Fertil Steril 2005; 6: 1830–1836.
2. Redwine DB. Laparoscopic excision of endometriosis with 3-mm scissors: comparison of operating times between sharp excision and electro-excision. J Am Assoc Gynecol Laparosc 1993; 1: 24–30.
3. Semm K. Physical and biological considerations militating against the use of endoscopically applied high-frequency current in the abdomen. Endoscopy 1983; 15: 282–288.
4. Soderstrom RM. Electricity inside the uterus. Clin Obstet Gynecol 1992; 35: 262–269.
5. Redwine DB. Monopolar electroexcision of endometriosis. In: Sutton CJG, Diamond MP, eds, Endoscopic surgery for gynaecologists, 2nd edn. London: WB Saunders; 1998: 369–379.

6. Garry R, Clayton R, Hawe J. The effect of endometriosis and its radical laparoscopic excision on quality of life indicators. BJOG 2000; 107(1): 44–54.

7. Sutton CJG, Hodgson R. Endoscopic cutting with lasers. Minim Invasive Therm 1992; 1: 197–205.

8. Sutton C. Power sources in endoscopic surgery. Curr Opin Obstet Gynecol 1995; 7(4): 248–256.

9. Robbins ML. Excision of endometriosis with laparoscopic coagulating shears. J Am Assoc Gynecol Laparosc 1999; 6: 199–203.

10. Redwine DB, Wright JT. Laparoscopic treatment of obliteration of the cul-de-sac associated with endometriosis; long-term follow-up of en bloc resection. Fertil Steril 2001; 76: 358–365

11. Bordelon BM, Hobday KA, Hunter JG. Laser vs electrosurgery in laparoscopic cholecystectomy: a prospective randomised trial. Arch Surg 1993; 128: 233–236.

12. Mayooran Z, Pearce S, Tsaltas J, et al. Ignorance of electrosurgery among obstetricians and gynaecologists. BJOG 2004; 111(12): 1413–1418.

13. Cheng YS. Ureteral injury resulting from laparoscopic fulguration of endometriotic implant. Am J Obstet Gynecol 1976; 126(8): 1045–1046.

14. Kono M, Yahagi N, Kithara M, et al. Cardiac arrest associated with the use of an argon beam coagulator during laparoscopic cholecystectomy. Br J Anaesth 2001; 87: 644–646.

15. Canis M, Mage G, Wattiez A, et al. Laparoscopic treatment of large ovarian endometrioma: why such a long learning curve? Hum Reprod 2003; 18: 5–9.

16. Phipps JH. Thermometry studies with bipolar diathermy during hysterectomy. Gynecol Endoscop 1993; 3: 5–7.

17. Garry R, Fountain J, Mason S, et al. The eVALuate study: two parallel randomised trials, one comparing laparoscopic with abdominal hysterectomy, the other comparing laparoscopic with vaginal hysterectomy. BMJ 2004; 328: 129–133.

18. Control of smoke from laser/electric surgical procedures. National Institute for Occupational Safety and Health (NIOSH), Hazard Controls, US Department of Health and Human Services. Publication No. 96–128, 1996.

19. Recommended practices for endoscopic minimally invasive surgery. AORN standards and recommended practices for perioperative nursing III: Denver, CO: Association of Operating Room Nurses, Inc; 2004: 267–271.

20. Candiani GB, Vercellini P, Fedele L, et al. Mild endometriosis and infertility: a critical review of epidemiologic data, diagnostic pitfalls, and classification limits. Obstet Gynecol Surv 1991; 46(6): 374–382.

21. Wykes CB, Clark TJ, Khan KS. Accuracy of laparoscopy in the diagnosis of endometriosis: a systematic quantitative review. BJOG 2004; 111: 1204–1212.

22. Gruppo italiano per lo studio dell'endometriosi. Prevalence and anatomical distribution of endometriosis in women with selected gynaecological conditions: results from a multicentric Italian study. Hum Reprod 1994; 9(6): 1158–1162

23. Chapron C, Fauconnier A, Dubuisson JB, et al. Does deep endometriosis infiltrating the utero-sacral ligaments present an asymmetric lateral distribution? Br J Obstet Gynaecol 2001; 108: 1021–1024.

24. Al-Fozan H, Tulandi T. Left lateral predisposition of endometriosis and endometrioma. Obstet Gynecol 2003; 101: 164–166.

25. Redwine DB. Ovarian endometriosis: a marker for more extensive pelvic and intestinal disease. Fertil Steril 1999; 72(2): 310–315.

26. Shaw RW. The role of GnRH analogues in the treatment of endometriosis. BJOG 1992; 99: 9–12.

27. Al-Fozan H, Tulandi T. Treatment of ovarian endometrioma: In: Tulandi T, Redwine D, eds. Endometriosis, advances and controversies. New York: Marcel Dekker; 2004: 263–272.

28. Brosens J, Puttemans P, Deprest J. Appearance of endometriosis. Baillière's Clin Obstet Gynecol 1993; 7: 741–757.

29. Sampson JA. Peritoneal endometriosis due to menstrual dissemination of endometrial tissue into the peritoneal cavity. Am J Obstet Gynecol 1927; 14: 422–469.

30. Muzii L, Bianchi A, Croce C, et al. Laparoscopic excision of ovarian cysts: is the stripping technique a tissue-sparing procedure? Fertil Steril 2002; 77: 609–614.

31. Maneschi F, Marasa L, Incandela S, et al. Ovarian cortex surrounding benign neoplasms: a histologic study. Am J Obstet Gynecol 1993; 169: 388–393.

32. Muzii L, Marana R, Caruana P, et al. Laparosopic findings after transvaginal ultrasound-guided aspiration of ovarian endometriomas. Hum Reprod 1995; 10: 2902–2903.

33. Noma J, Youshida N. Efficacy of ethanol sclerotherapy for ovarian endometriomas. Int J Gynecol Obstet 2001; 72: 35–39.

34. Koike T, Minakami H, Motoyama M, et al. Reproductive performance after ultrasound guided transvaginal ethanol sclerotherapy for ovarian endometriotic cysts. Eur J Obstet Gynecol Reprod Biol 2002; 105: 39.

35. Garvey T, Kazer R, Milad M. Severe pelvic adhesions following attempted ultrasound-guided drainage of bilateral ovarian endometriomas; case report. Hum Reprod 1999; 14: 2748–2750.

36. Donnez J, Nisolle M, Gillerot S, et al. Ovarian endometrial cysts: the role of gonadotrophin-releasing hormone agonists and/or drainage. Fertil Steril 1994; 62: 63–66.

37. Jones KD, Sutton CJG. Endometriotic cysts: the case for ablative laparoscopic surgery. Gynecol Endosc 2002; 10: 1–8.

38. Jones KD, Sutton CJG. Recurrence of chocolate cysts after laparoscopic ablation. J Am Assoc Gynecol Laparosc 2002; 9: 315–320.

39. Donnez J, Nisolle M, Gillet N, et al. Large ovarian endometriomas. Hum Reprod 1996; 11: 641–646

40. Beretta P, Franchi M, Ghezzi F, et al. Randomised clinical

trial of two laparoscopic treatments of endometriomas: cystectomy versus drainage and coagulation. Fertil Steril 1998; 70: 1176–1180.

41. Brosens IA, Van Ballaer P, Puttemans P, et al. Reconstruction of the ovary containing large endometriomas by an extra-ovarian endosurgical technique. Fertil Steril 1996; 66: 517–521.

42. Vercellini P, Chapron C, De Giorgi O, et al. Coagulation or excision of ovarian endometriomas? Am J Obstet Gynecol 2003; 188: 606–610.

43. Brinton LA, Grindley G, Persson I, et al. Cancer risk after a hospital discharge diagnosis of endometriosis. Am J Obstet Gynecol 1997; 176: 572–579.

44. Stern RC, Dash R, Bentley RC, et al. Malignancy in endometriosis: frequency and comparison of ovarian and extraovarian types. Int J Gynecol Pathol 2001; 20: 133–139.

45. Jones KD, Fan A, Sutton CJG. The ovarian endometrioma: why is it so poorly managed? Indicators from an anonymous survey. Hum Reprod 2002; 17: 845–849.

46. Elkelani OA, Binda MM, Koninckx PR, et al. Effect of adding more than 3% oxygen to carbon dioxide pneumoperitoneum on adhesions formation in a laparoscopic mouse model. Fertil Steril 2004; 82: 1616–1622.

23 Laser surgery for endometriosis

Philippe R Koninckx and Enda McVeigh

Introduction

Although the definition of endometriosis has not changed over time, our understanding of endometriosis has evolved progressively. It is mandatory therefore to interpret the literature in order to understand which clinical conditions were considered when at a given period the word 'endometriosis' was used. Endometriosis has been defined as endometrial glands and stroma outside the uterus, and this morphologic definition is still the gold standard. At the beginning of the 20th century endometriosis was introduced as severe lesions, i.e. ovarian 'chocolate cysts'[1] and adenomyosis externa.[2–4] In the following years, black puckered lesions in the pelvis found accidentally during surgery were recognized as endometriosis. In the early 1950s, transplantation experiments of endometrium seemed to bring final proof of the pathophysiologic implantation theory of endometriosis, as postulated by Sampson 30 years earlier.[1]

The real history of endometriosis started after the introduction of endoscopy in the 1970s. During diagnostic laparoscopy for pain and infertility, it was suddenly realized that black puckered lesions were frequently observed and a causal relationship to pain and infertility was postulated, i.e. endometriosis, which could be diagnosed only by laparoscopy. Scrutiny for small lesions led in the mid 1980s to the recognition of nonpigmented lesions – i.e. the polipoidal, the vesicular, and later the flame-like lesions – as lesions containing endometrial glands and stroma and thus fitting the definition of endometriosis.[5–8] From that period also originated the terms 'typical lesions' for the black puckered lesions and 'subtle lesions' for the small non-pigmented lesions. It is not surprising that the prevalence of the disease thus increased from initial case reports up to the 1970s, to 5%–20% in women with infertility and/or pelvic pain up to 1985 when only black puckered lesions were considered, and to over 60%–80% when nonpigmented lesions were also recognized.[9–18] In parallel with the changing meaning of the word 'endometriosis' over the decades, our concepts of etiology, pathophysiology, natural history, associated pathology, and therapy have evolved with the increasing awareness and prevalence of endometriosis.

Endometriosis has been considered for decades as the result of the implantation of retrograde menstruated endometrial cells,[1] or as metaplasia[19,20] induced by menstrual debris, or as lymphatic spread.[21,22] The evidence seemed convincing, since transplantation of endometrium could induce endometriosis, since retrograde menstruation occurred in almost all women,[23,24] since this fluid contained viable cells,[25] and since these cells can implant on the peritoneum.[26] The initially nonpigmented or subtle lesions were believed to progress to typical, cystic ovarian endometriosis and/or deep infiltrating endometriosis, and this was assumed to be the natural history of the disease.[27–29] Endometriosis was thus considered as normal endometrial cells in an abnormal location and in an abnormal environment, i.e. the peritoneal fluid.[30]

This hypothesis of implantation/metaplasia and progression to more severe disease, however, has never been proved formally, and has become challenged by new concepts emphasizing cellular differences, e.g. in the endometrial cells and in the endometriotic cells. From 'a normal cell in an abnormal location' endometriosis has become considered as 'abnormal cells in an abnormal location'. This has led to the hypothesis that typical and severe endometriosis should be considered as a benign tumor, whereas subtle endometriosis could become a physiologic condition that occurs intermittently in all women. Only following cellular changes, e.g. a mutation, can these subtle lesions evolve into typical, deep, or cystic ovarian endometriosis. To mark the difference between normal and abnormal cells, subtle endometriosis have been called 'endometriosis', whereas the benign tumours, i.e. typical, cystic, and deep, have been called 'endometriotic disease'.[31]

The definitive treatment of endometriosis has been, from the beginning, surgical destruction or excision. Since the introduction of endoscopic surgery radicality has become questioned, probably more because of the technical difficulty of endoscopic surgery than because of evidence. Theoretical considerations and concepts such as microscopic endometriosis, focal therapy of cystic endometriosis considered as invagination, and debulking of deep endometriosis have questioned the idea that surgery should aim at radical eradication. Even today, the evidence that radical surgery has a better outcome for pain, infertility, recurrence, or progression is scarce. In addition with the availability of synthetic progestagens and oral contraceptives, medical therapy of endometriosis commenced. These therapies were aimed at inactivating endometriosis and proved to be highly effective for pain but ineffective for infertility or preventing recurrence, whereas data on progression are lacking

To evaluate surgery for endometriosis critically we will discuss the differences in surgical techniques with special emphasis on laser endoscopic excision and, subsequently, evaluate indications, techniques, and results of treatment.

History of surgical techniques

Over the last 25 years over 500 articles dealing directly with surgery in the title and over 1800 with surgery in the abstract were published. To interpret these many articles dealing with surgery, and to understand the limited number or overall lack of randomized trials, a clear understanding of the evolution of the various techniques is necessary. Moreover, endoscopic surgery is a relatively young discipline that is characterized by rapid evolvement in techniques and equipment,

whereas the importance of training curves has clearly been shown. Taken together, the absence of randomized controlled trials (RCTs) is not surprising, since the individual endometriosis surgeons have progressively changed/improved their techniques, whereas, to the best of my knowledge, no one endometriosis surgeon can claim to be equally fluent with several techniques. Any RCT thus would evaluate the surgeon rather than the technique.

Up to the end of the 1970s, minimal and mild endometriosis was destroyed endoscopically by heat application (endothermia) and by unipolar or bipolar coagulation. Treatment of more severe endometriotic disease was radically by hysterectomy; in younger women, adnexectomies, rarely cystectomies, and anterior resections of the rectum were performed. This period focused on infertility associated with typical and cystic ovarian endometriosis, whereas deep endometriosis – unless very severe, large, and painful – was not recognized. We may assume that all publications of this period were 'contaminated' by some 5–20% of undiagnosed, and thus untreated, deep endometriosis. Moreover, radical surgery was generally not so radical, often leaving some rectovaginal endometriosis behind, since the importance had not yet been fully recognized, and since incomplete surgery was camouflaged by performing adnexectomies and premature menopause.

In the late 1970s and the early 1980s, microsurgery was introduced, emphasizing gentle tissue handling and careful destruction of superficial endometriosis by bipolar coagulation or resection and removal of cystic ovarian endometriosis followed by reconstruction of the ovary. The stripping technique for ovarian endometriosis was developed during that period and the 60% fertility results achieved can still be considered as a key reference for nondestructive surgery.[32,33]

From 1986–1987 onwards, the concept of minimal and/or nonpigmented endometriosis was introduced.[5] This caused an important shift in the reported incidences of endometriosis, which depend on recognition and awareness. This increasing recognition of endometriosis resulted in a progressive shift of women who were previously classified as 'normal' to women classified as having minimal endometriosis. It is important for the interpretation of results of surgery to recognize this shift, since before 1985 the group of 'normal' women comprised variable numbers of (unrecognized and untreated) women with minimal endometriosis. After 1986, the severity of the disease in the groups of women with minimal/mild disease progressively decreases, since it is diluted with women with subtle endometriosis only. At least until the mid 1990s the bias of nonrecognition of deep endometriotic disease persists.

Since the introduction of endoscopic surgery, several treatments of cystic ovarian endometriosis have been proposed. The removal of the cyst wall by stripping followed by suturing or gluing of the ovary is technically similar to the surgery performed during the microsurgery period. This technique has been challenged by destruction of the cyst wall, by laser vaporization, or by bipolar coagulation. None of these techniques, however, have been clearly defined. Destruction ranges from focal treatment of lesions, to superficial destruction of the whole area, to a much deeper destruction. Stripping can be performed almost without destroying any ovarian stroma, but the result depends to a large extent upon the skill and expertise of the surgeon.[34] It should be recognized that stripping a large endometrioma will necessarily destroy large parts of the ovary, as can be done by misjudging the cleavage planes or by aggressive coagulation of bleeding. These different techniques have been poorly compared, although a lower recurrence rate following stripping seems to be established.

In the 1990s, deep endometriosis was recognized increasingly during laparoscopic surgery,[35,36] or by clinical examination during menstruation.[36] 'Resection of deep endometriosis' comprises techniques which vary from debulking, to complete discoid excision to resection–reanastomosis of the rectum with large margins mimicking oncologic surgery. These differences in technique are rarely stated clearly in the literature, thus making interpretation difficult. Another important and growing bias is the severity of deep endometriosis reported. In some series, deep endometriosis comprises mainly lesions larger than 1 cm^3, whereas in other reports lesions are limited to slightly deeper typical lesions: it is not surprising that in the former series deep lesions are generally unique, whereas in the latter series deep lesions are described as multifocal, especially in the uterosacral ligaments. It is not important to evaluate the enthusiasm of the surgeon to assess or overassess depth, but it seems crucial that all reports on deep endometriosis clearly define the frequency distribution of volume and depth of the lesions operated upon.

In conclusion, in order to interpret correctly the data reported in the literature it is important to be aware of the existing biases:

1. The awareness of subtle endometriosis has increased tremendously the apparent prevalence of endometriosis, thus decreasing the severity of endometriosis in the group with minimal endometriosis.
2. Simultaneously, the group of normal women has changed since the awareness and scrutiny of diagnosis of deep endometriosis will determine the incidence of 'unrecognized' deep endometriosis in the minimal–mild groups.
3. Reporting frequency distributions of depth of penetration and volume of deep disease is necessary to judge whether the series comprise mainly large or mainly small lesions, the smaller ones just fitting the definition of 5 mm.
4. The size of cystic ovarian endometriosis, the presence of adhesions, the pathologic confirmation of the disease to exclude cystic corpora lutea, and the technique used are essential elements to compare series of cystic ovarian endometriosis.

Energy and techniques of CO_2 laser surgery and of electrosurgery

Carbon dioxide laser surgery and electrosurgery differ by the energy characteristics and by the mode of application. The CO_2 laser energy is almost completely absorbed by water. The effect thus is a very superficial heating and, provided sufficient energy is used, instantaneously heating to temperatures inducing a vaporization of tissue, with little thermal spread, i.e. less than 100 μm. To obtain this effect, the laser energy has to be focused on a small area: theoretically, spot diameters of less than 0.5 mm can be achieved, but this requires a perfect lens and working at the exact focal distance. In addition, the CO_2 gas in the laser channel of the laparoscope is heated by adsorption of the laser beam and this results in widening of the spot diameter, an effect known as blooming. Therefore, continuously cooling the CO_2 of the laser channel, e.g. with a high-flow insufflator,[37] or using a CO_2 isotope[38,39] to generate the laser beam are mandatory for a quality cut. The most important difference with electrosurgery is that the energy output is constant over time. The quality of cut is therefore constant, whereas the depth varies with speed of movement of the beam over the tissue. The CO_2 laser has the advantage of coagulating smaller vessels, which provides a rather bloodless cut. Using a defocused beam offers the versatility of vaporizing larger areas, or of applying only superficial heat as in flowering a hydrosalpinx. The major drawbacks of CO_2 laser surgery are the cost of equipment, the smoke production during vaporization, and the blooming in the laparoscope. The direct consequence of these three aspects is that during live surgery, if not performed at home, something is generally missing, giving the audience an undervaluation of the possibilities of laser surgery.

Electrosurgery has the advantage of being more versatile, which results in heating and coagulation below 200 V, sparking with local heating of the air and the adjacent tissue, and thus vaporization above 200 V. In addition, higher voltages will heat the tissue, causing coagulation, i.e. damage. This was known in the past as blended current in electrosurgical units without a voltage stabilizer. The quality of the cut is thus voltage-dependent, and at exactly 200 V, i.e. with minimal sparking, the quality of a CO_2 laser and of an electrosurgical cut is comparable with similar limited tissue damage. The most important difference is that the energy output of electrosurgery is not constant, since it essentially depends on the impedance of the tissues and on the area of contact between the electrode and the tissue. At higher output settings, the intensity of the current will be limited only by the impedance; it is therefore lower or higher according to the area of contact, i.e. the depth of cutting. Thus, electrosurgery easily cuts to a constant depth, notwithstanding an irregular surface. Limiting the energy output is not realistic, unless with a needle electrode in microsurgery, since any increase in contact area results in a drop in voltage and therefore stops cutting and starts coagulation.

Another difference between laser surgery and electrosurgery is the angle of access to the tissues: the laser beam used through the laparoscope will have an almost horizontal access to the rectovaginal septum. Energy used through the secondary ports will have a more vertical line of access, and this difference increases when secondary ports are introduced lower in the abdomen.

Finally almost all laser surgery for endometriosis can be performed with two secondary ports only, placed low in the abdomen, i.e. within bikini limits. For electrosurgery, three secondary ports are generally necessary, which for ergonomic reasons have to be placed higher in the abdomen.

Minimal and mild endometriosis

Diagnosis

Diagnosis of subtle lesions can only be made by laparoscopy. Diagnosis of typical lesions also can only be made by laparoscopy, although larger lesions in the uterosacral ligaments can sometimes be felt as indurations.

Methods of destruction

Ideally, these endometriosis lesions are vaporized or excised with a high-power CO_2 laser. We consider this the method of choice, since this treatment rapidly removes all the endometriosis and not more than the endometriosis, leaving a minimal amount of necrotic tissue. The choice between vaporization and excision depends on the size of the endometriotic lesion, larger lesions being excised more rapidly. This method takes full advantage of the characteristics of a CO_2 laser as a bloodless and precise cutting instrument, with little thermal damage to the surrounding tissue.

Alternative methods of destruction are bipolar coagulation, endothermia, and sharp excision. The first method is less adequate than laser vaporization/excision for typical lesions, since depth of infiltration is difficult to assess by inspection and palpation only. Moreover, the amount of necrotic tissue left behind is more important, which could increase the amount of postoperative adhesions. Sharp excision, together with monopolar or bipolar electrosurgery, is theoretically equivalent to CO_2 laser excision but practically it creates much more tissue damage. Indeed, either extensive prophylactic coagulation is performed before cutting, which results in more tissue damage, or no prophylactic coagulation is done, which is associated with capillary bleeding, poor visualization, and necessitates subsequent coagulation, which cannot achieve the precision of the CO_2 laser beam coagulation for small vessels.

Subtle lesions

If subtle endometriosis is a natural condition occurring intermittently in all women,[29,40] it is logical to postulate that treatment is not necessary since it is not a disease; i.e. it will disappear spontaneously and can reappear later at another localization. Anyway, subtle endometriosis has never been shown to be a cause of infertility or of pain. From a surgical viewpoint, however, this is an academic discussion, since vaporization of these subtle lesions is so easily performed without risks that it might be unwise to leave the possibility that some of these lesions would be or become more invasive or aggressive.

Typical lesions

It is uncertain whether it is useful to treat typical endometriosis to prevent progression. To demonstrate this in RCTs can be argued to be clinically irrelevant since destruction is so easy. Moreover, scientifically, it might be practically impossible to achieve. Considering a 60% prevalence of minimal–mild endometriosis with a progression to severe disease in some 10% after 5 years, it would require an RCT of hundreds of patients over many years, which is unrealistic.

Typical lesions are associated with pain, and in a series of observational studies and in two RCTs it has been shown that destruction of typical lesions results in significantly better pain relief than in a control group. These studies, moreover, confirmed the important placebo effect of some 25% lasting for at least 6 months. The activation of spare nociceptors[41,42] with inflammation and the observation that these lesions are specifically painful when stimulated[43,44] seem important to understand the pathophysiology.

The usefulness as an infertility treatment remains unclear. During the late 1970s an association was shown between endometriosis, luteal phase insufficiency, unexplained infertility, and the luteinized unruptured follicle (LUF) syndrome.[45–48] To understand why this association was questioned later, it is important to realize the shift that took place in the groups of women reported by the recognition of subtle nonpigmented lesions.[49–52] Studies in the baboon confirmed experimentally that endometriosis was associated with the LUF syndrome, that the LUF syndrome was recurrent, and that the LUF syndrome diagnosed by inspection of the ovaries correlated with the absence of ovulation.[53] Recently, the Endocan study showed that treatment improved human fertility.[54] However this study was not blinded, and it can be argued that by telling women that they had endometriosis increased anxiety levels and the LUF syndrome and thus decreased fertility rates. The absence of effect observed in the smaller Italian study[55], and the fact that a 30% cumulative fertility rate in the treated group of the Endocan study was similar to previously reported fertility rates in control groups support this view.

Cystic ovarian endometriosis

Pitfalls of diagnosis

The treatment of cystic ovarian endometriosis remains hampered by misdiagnosing a cystic corpus luteum as a cystic ovarian endometrioma. To the best of our knowledge this problem has not been addressed adequately. Even if only women with pathologically confirmed cystic endometriosis were included, these data do not permit us to

judge to what extent cystic corpora lutea had been operated upon.

A clinical history of the persistence of a cyst under oral contraceptives or luteinizing hormone-releasing hormone (LH-RH) agonists is unreliable for diagnosing cystic ovarian endometriosis: over the years we have operated on several women with a 'chocolate cyst' on ultrasound, persisting for more than 4 months, which turned out to be a cystic corpus luteum. We are fully aware that this clinical observation does not allow any conclusion about prevalence. This is consistent with the observation that ovarian cysts can develop during ovarian down-regulation.[56] Imaging, such as ultrasound and computed tomography (CT) scan has a sensitivity of 70–80% and a specificity of 90–95%.[57–61] This is a valuable method of diagnosis, helping in the clinical management. It will not, however, prevent errors of judgment during surgery. Ovarian flow measurement does not seem to improve specificity or sensitivity substantially.[57] The cancer antigen CA-125 in chocolate fluid has been reported to have a sensitivity and a specificity of nearly 100%.[48,62,63] Unfortunately, until a rapid test becomes available to make the diagnosis during surgery, this remains theoretical.

Our clinical rule of thumb is that, since cystic ovarian endometriosis is so strongly associated with adhesions,[18] a 'chocolate cyst' without adhesions has a high probability of being a cystic corpus luteum, whereas the presence of severe adhesions, especially in the fossa ovarica, enhances the suspicion of endometriosis. This, together with the inspection of the inside lining of the cyst by ovarioscopy[64] or by inspection with the laparoscope,[65] will help us to make a correct judgment in the majority of women. Those with a flattened appearance and red or red and brown mottled ridges were generally endometriosis and those with a dark uniform base, an intracavitary clot, or a yellowish rim were generally corpus lutea or albicans.

Physiopathology

The physiopathology of cystic endometriosis is not entirely understood. It is attractive to consider that many cystic ovarian endometriomas originate from invagination of superficial implants.[66] Especially when the ovary becomes adherent to the pelvic wall by endometriotic implants, it seems logical that a 'pseudocyst' is formed by the accumulation of old blood and debris, thus stretching the ovarian capsule over this cyst.[48,67,68] This phenomenon of invagination and stretching of the ovarian capsule can explain that the inside of the cyst wall is not always entirely covered by endometriosis, which is rather localized as focal endometriotic spots. It thus seems logical to postulate that only these endometriotic spots should be destroyed, and that removing the cyst wall is equivalent to removing the ovarian surface. This mechanism of invagination and stretching of the ovarian capsule does not preclude that some cysts have a different origin. Moreover, a careful histology of the cyst wall reveals that endometriotic glands can be present in the 'so called' cyst wall up to a depth of at least 5–6 mm. Whatever the etiology is, most ovarian cysts are clonal in origin, as repeatedly demonstrated.[69–71]

Surgical pragmatism of size

From a surgical point of view, the size of the ovarian cyst is the most important. For smaller cysts (<5 cm) the cyst wall can generally be stripped easily from the ovary. This process seems to follow a natural plane of cleavage, confirmed indirectly by the fact that it is associated with little bleeding. For cysts larger than 5 cm diameter, the discussion whether the cyst wall should be removed or destroyed, or whether a focal treatment will be sufficient, is purely academic. Indeed, in these women with a large cyst, the remaining ovarian rim will be so thin that resection becomes either technically impossible or practically unrealistic since minimal or no ovarian tissue will be left. Also, the extensive vaporization of these very large areas is unrealistic.

Methods of treatment

Aspiration and rinsing of cystic ovarian endometriosis has been attempted but the recurrence rate is high.[72–74] Ultrasound-guided aspiration moreover resulted the next day in a chocolate cyst in the pelvis when we attempted to do so (unpublished data), which might increase adhesion formation,[75] although it was shown that chocolate cyst fluid does not induce adhesions when injected intraperitoneally in mice.[76]

For smaller cysts, i.e. <5 cm diameter, the method of stripping the cyst from the ovary as initially described by the Clermont-Ferrand group is our method of choice.[34,77,78] It is rapid, technically easy, and complete treatment also when invading glands would be present. Following adhesiolysis, drainage, and rinsing, we incise the ovarian capsule around the cyst opening with the CO_2 laser. Once the plane of cleavage is found, the cyst wall is easily stripped from the ovary. The laser is used to assist cleavage in the right plane and prevents the ovarian capsule being torn in the wrong direction. Closure of the ovary by tissucol or a suture when the remaining ovarian flaps are unequal in size seems logical; it is suggested, although not proven. The cyst wall could be vaporized and some excellent results have been reported.[66] We have stopped using this technique, since it was too difficult to judge the correct depth of vaporization: too superficial destruction resulted in an incomplete treatment and recurrences, whereas a too deep destruction often caused bleeding. The cyst wall could be destroyed by unipolar or semibipolar coagulation. Although attractive, the reported series are too small to compare this technique to vaporization. The third option besides wall excision and wall destruction is focal treatment,[79] but this is overall equivalent to vaporization.

For larger cysts, the pragmatism of size practically excludes excision and/or vaporization. We favor keeping surgery during the first laparoscopy to a minimum, making it a 5–10 minute procedure. We make a large window in the cyst wall, followed by rinsing, some focal treatment, no adhesiolysis, and 3 months of LH-RH agonist treatment is given postoperatively. If, by ultrasound, the cyst is shown to have persisted or reformed, this small cyst is treated during a second surgery with excision; if no cyst is found, it is unclear whether a second intervention is necessary in the absence of pain or infertility. This concept has the indirect advantage that the first operation can always be scheduled as a day case, without bowel preparation, whereas the necessity of a bowel preparation for the second intervention will be known in advance. It remains unclear whether it would be preferable during the first surgery to perform a full adhesiolysis. It is also unclear whether postoperative medical therapy is helpful; it is logical, since it will prevent a corpus luteum developing, whereas a hypoestrogenic milieu could reduce adhesion formation. The number of 'large' endometriomas is insufficient in most centers to perform RCTs, whereas the rapid technical evolution of endoscopic surgery has made RCTs practically impossible until now.

Results

The results of endoscopic and microsurgical treatment are comparable,[80] ranging between 60 and 80% cure of pain, a cumulative pregnancy rate of 60–70% after 6 months to 1 year, and a recurrence rate between 5% and 20%.[81–86] It remains unclear whether preoperative or postoperative medical treatment significantly affects the results.[87]

Stripping is ovarian sparing[88] and clearly has a lower recurrence rate than focal treatment, which in our opinion has been abandoned except for very small lesions. Another argument in favor of stripping is that pathology is obtained which is important considering the 1% unexpected borderline or even malignant cysts.[89]

For larger cysts no clear data are available that favor one technique over another. The pragmatism of size, however, seems to dictate either an ovariectomy in women without a fertility wish or a two-step surgery in women who want to preserve fertility.

Conclusion

Cystic ovarian endometriosis has to be treated, since this condition is associated with pain and infertility and carries the risk of spontaneous rupture. Surgery is the only real treatment, since medical treatment can only inactivate endometriosis without reducing the size of the cyst.[90]

Because of technical and practical surgical considerations, we favor excising smaller cysts by stripping, followed by closure of the remaining flaps if necessary. For larger cysts, a minimal first intervention consisting of marsupialization, rinsing, and focal treatment, followed by LH-RH agonists for 3 months and a second intervention when a cyst persists is proposed.

Results of endoscopic excision of cystic ovarian endometriosis seem not to be totally consistent when listening to the nonreported data. According to Canis et al:[34]

> An anonymous survey conducted among gynaecologists in the UK showed that 50% of ovarian endometrioma are still managed by laparotomy. This surprising result is discussed emphasizing the difficulties of the learning curve, pitfalls in surgical training and mistakes of the pioneers.

And:

> The goal of the endoscopic surgeon should be to achieve adequate surgical treatment. Endoscopic surgery is not a technical gimmick used to avoid laparotomy and to attract patients.

Similarly, we have become convinced that stripping of the ovary for cystic endometriosis still has a long way to go and, considering the difficulty in training and the long learning curve, we should be aware that ovaries can be easily destroyed by making mistakes with cleavage planes, by operating on too large ovaries, and by extensive coagulation at the end of surgery.

Deep endometriosis

Diagnosis, types, and prevalence

Endometriosis can infiltrate the surrounding tissues, resulting in an important sclerotic and inflammatory reaction that can translate clinically into nodularity, bowel stenosis, and ureteral obstruction. The most severe forms of the condition such as rectovaginal endometriosis and endometriosis invading the rectum or the sigmoid have been known since the beginning of the 20th century. These conditions, however, are relatively rare, with an estimated prevalence of less than 1%. This estimation is derived from our observation in Leuven of some 10–20% deep endometriosis in 1988–1991,[18] a period during which endoscopic surgery was not yet well developed and in which deep endometriosis was not yet a well-known entity. Referrals were thus only those for infertility and pain, not for deep endometriosis. Assuming that laparoscopies for infertility are performed in some 10–15% of the population and taking into account that Leuven is a tertiary referral center, the prevalence of deep endometriosis can be estimated to be between 1% (the prevalence is 10% in the younger age group with infertility, which can be estimated at 15% of the population, in a tertiary center, the prevalence is probably slightly overestimated) and 3% (prevalence of 20% of the older age group with infertility). Taking into account the observation that by menstrual clinical examination, deep endometriosis is more frequent, prevalences between 3% and 10% seem a fair estimate.

The endoscopic excision of endometriosis has revealed that endometriosis invading deeper than 5–6 mm is associated with pain and infertility. Three subtypes were described.[91] *Type I* is characterized by a large pelvic area of typical and sometimes some subtle endometriotic lesions surrounded by white sclerotic tissue. Only during excision does it become obvious that the endometriotic lesion infiltrates deeper than 5 mm. Typically, the endometriotic area becomes progressively smaller as it grows deeper; the lesion is thus cone-shaped. *Type II* lesions are characterized by retraction of the bowel. Clinically, they are recognized by the obvious bowel retraction around a small typical lesion. In some women, however, no endometriosis can be seen through the laparoscope, and the bowel retraction is the only clinical sign. Diagnosis is generally not too difficult since during laparoscopy the retraction under which an induration is felt is obvious. In some women, however, the retraction is hardly seen and the induration can be hardly felt. Only during excision the endometriotic nodule becomes apparent, emphasizing the need for a preoperative diagnosis and training in recognizing these lesions. *Type III* lesions are spherical endometriotic nodules in the rectovaginal septum. In their most typical manifestation these lesions are felt as painful nodularities in the rectovaginal septum. At laparoscopy, they generally present as a small typical lesion, and in some women a careful vaginal examination reveals some dark blue cysts (3–4 mm) in the fornix posterior. Type III lesions are the most severe lesions, and they often spread laterally up and around the uterine artery, sometimes causing sclerosis around the ureter. The spread along the uterine artery can be so obvious that this can be considered as an indirect argument for the hypothesis that deep endometriosis has escaped from the inhibitory influence of peritoneal fluid and is mainly under peripheral circulation control. Although they are prominent in most women, these lesions are very often missed, as will be discussed later. Sclerosing endometriosis invading the sigmoid is similar to rectal endometriosis but is situated 10 cm above the rectovaginal septum. This is another form of deep endometriosis, which is fortunately a rare condition and which we could classify as type IV. By pathology, the types II, III, and IV are similar and present as adenomyosis externa, i.e. as glands and stroma in large areas of hyalinous muscular tissue. Since the demonstration of a less-deep pouch of Douglas in women with deep endometriosis, it seems logical to postulate that these three lesions are pathophysiologically similar, type III being situated in the pouch of Douglas on the wall opposing the vaginal wall. Subsequently, the pouch of Douglas is closed by retraction, giving erroneously the impression that these lesions are situated in the rectovaginal septum, which starts lower. It is logical that these lesions are often vaginally visible, since the distance between the vaginal wall and peritoneal cavity is hardly 3–4 mm. The type II lesions are situated higher, generally between the back of the uterus and the rectosigmoid, whereas a lesion at the level of the sigmoid generally is not adherent to the surrounding structures, except occasionally to the ureter under the infundibulopelvic ligament. These concepts seem to constitute another argument to differentiate between slightly larger and deeper typical lesions, the infiltrative type I deep endometriosis, and those with larger nodules, massive retraction, and by pathology adenomyosis externa.

The pathophysiology remains debatable, which for us seems unnecessary. Any review of data will never be able to differentiate between implantation or metaplasia. What for us seems more important is that the clonal origin of these lesions[92,93] strongly suggests a behavior as benign tumors, i.e. the endometriotic disease theory. Alternatively, but equally attractive, is to consider basal endometrium with stem cell characteristics as the origin.[94]

Diagnosis of deep endometriosis should be made before surgery. A retrospective analysis showed that only 50% of the larger lesions are diagnosed by a routine clinical examination. A menstrual clinical examination is the most powerful tool actually available to diagnose deep endometriosis type I, II, and III. By clinical examination during menstruation,[95] painful nodularities are found in some 30% of women with pain or infertility. In the absence of cystic ovarian endometriosis, these nodularities were caused by deep endometriosis in most of the women. The concentrations of CA-125 are increased in women with deep endometriosis and in women with cystic ovarian endometriosis and were proposed as a screening tool. Although specifically increased during menstruation, the variability does not improve the diagnostic accuracy.[96] A late follicular sample has a sensitivity of some 70–90% of endometriotic disease, with a specificity around 95%.[36] Ultrasound and magnetic resonance imaging (MRI) can be used to diagnose deep endometriosis, but their sensitivity is low, especially for the smaller lesions. For type IV lesions, a contrast enema and/or a rectoscopy are necessary. Although hard data are not available, we presume that this diagnosis is easily missed, making prevalence higher than actually believed.

In conclusion, the most powerful tool to diagnose deep endometriosis is a menstrual clinical examination, whereas a routine clinical examination will reveal mainly the very large lesions. A CA-125 assay is a useful screening aid for deep endometriosis, and it might prove to be useful as screening for type IV lesions, which, although severe, are easily missed and cannot be diagnosed by clinical examination. The final diagnosis is the estimation of the depth of infiltration during excisional surgery. The prevalence of the disease increases with age and is estimated at 1–10% in the population and at 10–30% in women with pain and/or infertility. Recently, a series of articles have discussed the usefulness of rectal ultrasound and of MRI for deep endometriosis: until today, this for us remains academically interesting but not really useful. First, mainly the larger lesions are detected; secondly, if severe pain is present, surgery will anyway be necessary and these tests will not influence the type of surgery or the decisions made during surgery. The only clinical usefulness for these investigations could be prediction of the difficulty of surgery, i.e. which endometriosis can be operated by the gynecologist and which should be referred. Today, this is speculation but important given the unpredictability of the surgical difficulty.

Surgical treatment

Surgery for deep endometriosis is unpredictably difficult with the risk of a series of severe complications. Therefore, a preoperative ultrasound, contrast enema, and intravenous pyelography are mandatory, together with a full preoperative bowel preparation. Surgery should be carefully planned. This planning comprises preoperative ureter stenting if gross ureter distortion or hydronephrosis is present, together with the eventual collaboration of an urologist to perform ureter reanastomosis or repair, bladder suturing, ureter reimplantation, e.g. in the case of an aggressive endometriosis deeply infiltrating the bladder and the ureter around the intramural bladder traject of the ureter, or to decide about surgery when the trigonum is invaded. Preoperative planning often requires the collaboration of a colorectal surgeon, since surgery can unpredictably extend from a discoid excision with a muscularis defect, to a resection of the rectum or sigmoid wall necessitating a suture, to a large transmural nodule requiring a resection anastomosis if the defect is too large or, in the case of a combined rectal and sigmoid nodule which cannot be sutured, a pouch anastomosis requiring mobilization of the left hemicolon. The exact borders of competence between disciplines are less important. We want to stress, however, that the preoperative planning should be rigorous; before attempting severe cases it is important to ascertain that the eventual competences which might be required are available and are not accidentally absent. The necessary competences include the anesthetist, since the ventilation capacity, the obesity, and the degree of Trendelenburg can become crucially important to facilitate difficult surgery. The type of lesion will also determine the position of the secondary trocars, which, e.g. for a sigmoid lesion, have to be placed higher than for a rectum lesion. Finally to grasp and summarize the importance of all this, it should be realized that any surgery should be performed within reasonable time limits, even if unforeseen complications happen such as an instrument breakdown together with a pouch anastomosis and a ureter reanastomosis. Prolonging surgery beyond 5–6 hours invariably carries the risk of a severe compartment syndrome of the legs. In conclusion, a careful preoperative planning is mandatory, to predict as precisely as possible what is to be expected, to know which competences should be available, and to judge whether the surgeon's competences make it reasonable to expect that the operation time will not have to be extended beyond some 5 hours. It is without saying that assistants and theater nurses should be trained and experienced. If these conditions are not met, other options should be considered, such as referral of the patient or a laparotomy. Primum non nocere remains the first principle of the surgeon. For this reason, any live surgery performed at congresses should be limited to the expertise of the local situation, and very severe lesions should preferably be operated on away from the cameras, with the full concentration of everybody involved.

The surgical excision of deep endometriosis itself relies upon a combination of visual inspection and tactile information. For the treatment of rectovaginal endometriosis up to the rectosigmoid, we clearly prefer a CO_2 laser (80 W; Sharplan, Needham, MA) together with a high-flow insufflator (Thermoflator, Karl Storz AG, Tuttlingen, Germany)[37] mandatory for smoke evacuation and cooling the laser beam. Guided by visual inspection, together with tactile information of the softness of the tissue, the peritoneum is incised below the lesion at the border between the normal soft tissue and the harder endometriosis. Moreover, endometriosis glows yellowish under the CO_2 laser beam. *First,* the lesion is circumscribed to mark the limits, which are useful during later excision. *Secondly,* the lateral edges of the nodule are dissected to free the nodule if necessary from the ureter, the uterine artery, and from the spinosacral ligament. This is technically the most difficult part of the surgery, since it is very deep and posterior and because of the presence of larger arteries and the nerve. If necessary, the lateral borders of the sigmoid have to be dissected and followed with identification of the ureters. *Thirdly,* the pararectal spaces are identified. This marks the lateral edges of the nodule, and once identified, dissection is bluntly continued downwards. *Finally,* the posterior part of the nodule is dissected from the rectum. We feel that it is important during this dissection that the nodule remains attached to the uterus and cervix or vagina, thus elevating the nodule, whereas the rectum progressively falls down by gravity. This dissection is continued as far as possible, at least until the rectum is completely liberated from the rectovaginal septum. The use of a rectal probe is unclear: it can be useful to identify structures, but it is not always helpful during dissection. Only after the completion of the dissection of the posterior part up to the vaginal wall is the anterior side of the nodule dissected from the cervix and from the vagina. At least in some 20% of women part of the vaginal fornix has to be removed because of endometriotic invasion, whereas we estimate that in some 20% of women the rectum has to be opened to permit a complete resection.[95] In the Leuven series of some 1000 nodules, in the Oxford series of some 160 nodules, and in the Rome series of some 40 nodules, it is noteworthy that resection of the rectum has not been necessary except in 2 women in whom the defect was too large to permit safe suturing. Over the years, excision has evolved and become more radical, but simultaneously as a consequence of referral the severity and size of nodules have increased tremendously. This has resulted in a series of resections necessitating the resection of large areas (5 × 5 cm) of rectum wall with subsequent suture. This I consider today the limit of the technique, and although not yet properly reviewed and audited, the clinical impression of these very large nodules suggests that it may be preferable to have a clean excision of the wall than to leave a very thin and devascularized mucosa. This type of surgery obviously requires preparations for early and late perforations (estimated at 5–10%), with an immediate and early second-look laparoscopy permitting the suturing of these leaks and treating them conservatively without colostomy.

Following 15 years of rectovaginal endometriosis surgery, and following extensive discussions during surgery with my close collaborators, Enda McVeigh, Fiorenzo De Cicco, and Anastasia Ussia, we recently (November 2003) changed the technique of the central dissection of the central part of a large nodule from the rectum slightly. Using sharp dissection, we have the impression that a series of bowel perforations can be avoided and that the planes of cleavage can be more accurately assessed. The drawback is that this dissection takes much more time. For the other parts of the surgery, we definitively prefer to use the CO_2 laser especially for its speed and its hemostatic properties.

A careful description of the excisional technique is mandatory to understand the pros and cons of the reported technique. The advantages of the technique as described are the perfect visualization and the angle of access. Using CO_2 laser excision through the operating laparoscope, excisional surgery is performed with great magnification: excision can be performed with the laparoscope close-in, since the laparoscope carries the 'knife'; excision also has to be performed close-in, since the focal length of the CO_2 laser lens is some 2 cm from the laparoscope. A third advantage is that the direction of access of the rectovaginal septum, and

especially the posterior side of the nodule, is easier through the laparoscope than through a secondary port. Obviously, this technique requires a high-flow insufflator[18] to maintain a clear picture throughout the excision and to permit continuous use of the laser without interruption. Finally, this technique takes maximum advantage of the hemostatic capacity of the laser.

Three other techniques are used for the resection of deep endometriosis:

- sharp dissection, together with electrosurgery through the laparoscope
- sharp dissection, together with electrosurgery through the secondary ports
- a partial rectum resection, followed by reanastomosis, usually with a circular stapler.

It is obvious that each surgeon performs best using the techniques he is most familiar with, and that few endoscopic surgeons are familiar with all techniques. Indeed most surgeons have developed the technique that they started with generally for historical reasons; this, however, should not prevent discussion of the relative advantages of the different approaches, as evaluated by expert surgeons performing surgical procedures often arranged on the basis of friendship. Sharp dissection, together with electrosurgery through the laparoscope, as developed by David Redwine,[97–101] is technically almost identical to the CO_2 laser excision, i.e. permitting a very posterior approach, working-close in with great magnification in a bloodless operating field. The disadvantage is that this technique is physically demanding and less suited for videoendoscopic surgery, thus reducing the possibility of help from an assistant. This technique, however, probably combines the advantage of an improved depth of vision (since a videoscreen is not used) with enhanced tactile information, since sharp dissection is used. Sharp dissection, together with electrosurgery through the secondary ports, is the most widely used technique,[102–113] for several reasons. It is derived from the other endoscopic procedures, it does not require a CO_2 laser, and, possibly even more important, a high-flow insufflator was not available during its development. Because the angle of access is much sharper, surgeons using this technique generally start dissection at the anterior site of the nodule, thus freeing nodule and rectum from the rectovaginal septum. Subsequently, the rectum is dissected from the nodule, which has become freely mobile. Most of these procedures aim at debulking the endometriosis rather than performing a complete resection. The word 'debulking' is chosen when the surgeon prefers not to open the rectum, even if the resection is less complete. It is difficult to estimate whether this 'debulking' attitude is a consequence of the technique used or a consequence of the philosophy often dictated by local and medicolegal considerations. Our experience was that resection of endometriosis using this technique is much more difficult than using the posterior approach, and that the best method to avoid bowel lesions was by avoiding traction and using gravity only.

Resection anastomosis has gained popularity over the last few years.[114,115] The arguments are that a higher recurrence rate in younger women warrants a more radical approach,[116] and that the endometriosis lesion can have focal extensions up to 2 cm from the original lesions, as shown by pathology. This radicality, however, has introduced the complication of bladder dysfunction following surgery, as evidenced by the introduction of the term 'nerve-sparing surgery'.[117] At this moment it is not known whether those performing a complete resection are overtreating their patients or whether those aiming at debulking the lesion are undertreating the endometriosis. Considering a 1% recurrence rate in our series with discoid resection and the pain relief, we still think that a systematic bowel resection for rectovaginal endometriosis is rarely indicated, i.e. only in lesions of more than 4×4 cm.

A few years ago, I wrote that type IV deep endometriosis of the sigmoid requires a resection and subsequent reanastomosis. Since then, I started to do conservative excisional surgery in these patients. This is feasible, but results almost invariably in large wall defects. As discussed for the rectal lesions, these lesions will be reviewed carefully before it is claimed that this is the treatment of choice. Considering, however, the duration of surgery in some patients and some complications in other patients, I am reluctant to propose this as mainstream surgery today. Taking into account only the repair sutures, easily comprising some 25–30 stitches in a difficult angle, it must also be obvious that this will not be mainstream surgery tomorrow.

Complications, treatment, and prevention[117,118]

When part of the rectum wall has to be removed, or when the rectum is accidentally opened, the pelvis is rinsed with a 1% hibitane solution and the wall is sutured endoscopically with two layers of 3–0 Vicryl (Ethicon, Somerville, NJ, USA). A defect in the posterior vaginal fornix is sutured either vaginally or endoscopically. Care is taken to suture these defects watertight. I prefer to suture these defects laparoscopically, for reasons of sterility: during laparoscopic suturing a continuous flow of CO_2 from the abdominal cavity to the vagina prevents contamination.

Surgical excision of deep endometriosis is thus difficult surgery, since it often necessitates dissection far laterally around the ureter and uterine artery. Also, the excision from the bowel wall is difficult, since in 10% of women part of the bowel wall will have to be resected. In 20% of women, especially those with rectovaginal endometriosis, i.e. type III lesions, excision has to be performed up to and including the posterior vaginal fornix. It is important that neither resection of part of the bowel wall nor resection of the vaginal fornix should be considered as complications of surgery, since the postoperative follow-up has been uneventful in a series of over 300 women.

Complications of surgery during the initial series ($n = 225$) have been the transection of the uterine artery in 2 women, necessitating clipping, a ureter lesion in 1 woman, and a late bowel perforation in 6 women. A ureter lesion is a serious complication, and therefore we advocate a preoperative intravenous pyelogram, a careful dissection of the ureter from its landmarks at the pelvic brim, and a liberal preventive stenting if necessary. This is judged even more important, since it became evident that a ureter which is only half cut can rather easily be sutured endoscopically over a double-J stent.[120] A late bowel perforation is an even more serious complication that has occurred in 6 women: 2 women with a type II lesion (1989 and 1991) and 1 woman with a type III lesion (1992) were readmitted after a week with progressively increasing symptoms of peritonitis; 1 woman (1992) with a type I lesion and a history of pouch anastomosis for colitis ulcerosa was observed for 1 week with atypical symptoms that later proved to be a rectum perforation; 2 women (1994) with a type II lesion had acute pelvic pain, 12 hours following surgery and 2 days following surgery, respectively. Although symptoms of peritonitis were minimal, an immediate laparoscopy revealed a bowel perforation in both.

It is important to realize that bowel perforations can occur during the early postoperative days thus necessitating a low-fiber diet and eventual hospitalization. A perforation generally occurs during straining, with acute pelvic pain as the only symptom. Disturbingly, this pain disappears over the subsequent hours, with slight peritoneal irritation as the only symptom. A liberal use of early second-look laparoscopies is advocated in these women before symptoms of peritonitis develop. In some 10 women, we recently demonstrated that even a bowel perforation can be safely sutured endoscopically, thus avoiding a colostomy.

Prevention of a late perforation is even more important. From January 1996, liberal prophylactic suturing of the rectum was introduced whenever the suspicion of a lesion to the muscularis existed. Subsequently, this complication has virtually disappeared. Over the last few years, practice has changed from the traditional resection-anastomosis operation for large lesions to resection of larger portions of the bowel wall with direct repair, this has coincided with complications reappearing in 3 women. It is too early to give a final judgment.

Medical treatment

Medical therapy *before surgery* has been discussed for many years and surgeons have claimed that deep lesions were less vascularized following medical therapy. Recently, it was demonstrated that a pretreatment for 3 months with an LH-RH agonist could shrink the volume of deep lesions.[95] Indeed, in this series, Decapeptyl (triptorelin; 3.75 mg/month) has been given specifically to women with the most severe disease, especially deep lesions. Analysis of data showed that women pretreated with this LH-RH agonist had a higher revised American Fertility Society (r-AFS) score at surgery than those without treatment, confirming the selection bias. Similarly, pretreated women had more and larger cystic ovarian endometriosis that also pointed to the selection bias. As expected, women with pretreatment had a smaller pelvic area of endometriosis. Pretreated women had, however, a smaller volume of deep endometriosis, notwithstanding the fact that because of the selection bias they almost certainly had a much higher volume before treatment. For this reason, we advocate pretreating women with severe deep endometriosis medically for 3 months with a gonadotropin-releasing hormone (GnRH) agonist. We have the impression that danazol might be equally effective, but our series was too small to prove this statistically. Other medical therapies have not been used frequently enough to be evaluated.[121]

Medical treatment *following* excision of deep endometriosis has not been evaluated properly. If excision has been performed completely, medical treatment is probably not necessary. Medical therapy, however, should be considered instead of repeat or more radical surgery for recurring symptoms or failures of excision.

Medical treatment alone has not been addressed specifically in any study because of a lack of a clearcut diagnosis of deep endometriosis without excision. Medical treatment, either by danazol, GnRH agonists, or gestrinone[122–125] does not cure endometriosis; these drugs inactivate the endometriotic lesions, which reappear rapidly after treatment has been stopped.[126] None of these therapies has an important beneficial effect on subsequent fertility.[127] They all improve pelvic pain and the effect persists, often for many months after therapy has been stopped.[128] Since deep endometriosis is strongly associated with pelvic pain, and since cystic ovarian endometriosis does not respond well to medical therapy, it is suggested that the observations and conclusions concerning severe pelvic pain are probably related to deep endometriosis.

Results

Nehzat et al[109] reported 25 pregnancies in 67 women following excision of deep endometriosis. We (P.R.K.) evaluated cumulative pregnancy rate (CPR) in a consecutive series of 900 women with primary or secondary infertility without severe tubal damage and without a severely subfertile husband. Cumulative pregnancy rates were slightly lower in advanced stages of endometriosis, according to the r-AFS classification being 62% and 44% in classes I and IV, respectively. When, however, the duration of infertility was taken into account – which was the strongest predictor of subsequent conception – the differences in CPR between classes I and IV disappeared, suggesting that the differences found between mild and severe endometriosis were mainly a consequence of differences in duration of infertility and possibly in the age of the women.[48]

The only single group with a significantly higher CPR following surgery were women with deep endometriosis. By Cox multivariate regression analysis the following model was established: pregnancy was predicted most strongly by a shorter duration of infertility and by the surgical treatment of cystic ovarian endometriosis and/or of deep endometriosis. From these results it can be concluded that aggressive and complete excision of deep endometriosis can be advocated, with subsequent spontaneous pregnancy rates up to 60%, within 1 year. These results can be considered excellent, taking into account the severity of disease and the large denuded area in the pelvis following excision of deep endometriosis. It remains unclear whether those women who did not conceive after 1 year should be oriented towards in vitro fertilization or to a second-look laparoscopy. As can be derived from indirect evidence, medical treatment alone is probably not the treatment of choice for deep endometriosis and infertility. As suggested, medical pretreatment seems to be useful to facilitate surgery for cystic ovarian endometriosis. Both surgical and medical treatment were reported to be highly successful in treating pelvic pain. Candiani et al[108] reported absence of dyspareunia and dysmenorrhea in 6 and 4 women, respectively, out of 10 after 40 months. Nezhat et al[109] reported moderate to complete pain relief in 162 women out of 175, but in some women two or more interventions had been necessary. Preliminary analysis of our results in 250 women in whom deep endometriosis had been excised with a CO_2 laser, showed a cure rate of pelvic pain in 70% with a recurrence rate of less than 5% with a follow-up period of up to 5 years. These data should be interpreted carefully, since the completeness of excision has steadily increased. The results of recent years strongly suggest an almost complete cure rate without recurrences; this, however, could be an over-optimistic clinical impression that will have to be proven by careful analysis of the data. In addition, medical treatment of pelvic pain is highly efficient, and the effect of treatment often persists after the treatment has been stopped.[128]

essary cannot be excluded but that the probability is probably less than 5%. If a deep endometriotic nodule is found, the necessity of a preoperative medical treatment and of a preoperative contrast enema and intravenous pyelography should be considered. These women always receive a bowel preparation and are admitted to the hospital for at least 48 hours.

This approach has the advantage that the preoperative clinical examination together with the ultrasound scan are used to decide whether the patient will be admitted to the hospital or treated in the 1-day clinic, and whether a bowel preparation will be given. From our experience over the last few years, the accuracy of this procedure is close to 100%, since unexpected deep endometriosis and unnecessary bowel treatments have virtually disappeared from the department.

Surgery remains the cornerstone of the treatment of endometriosis. Medical treatment seems to be indicated, besides pre- and postoperatively as discussed, for women with recurrent pelvic endometriosis and pain or when adequate surgery is not available or is too dangerous.

Discussion and conclusions

We advocate a first-line approach to the diagnosis and treatment of endometriosis that relies on a menstrual clinical examination, an ultrasound scan, and eventually an assay of CA-125. Following these examinations, 4 groups of women can be considered. When the clinical examination during menstruation does not reveal any nodularities, no ovarian cysts are found at ultrasound scan, and the CA-125 concentration is normal, women with infertility and/or pain are scheduled for a day case diagnostic laparoscopy. If an endometrioma is found, larger than 5 cm in diameter, these women are also scheduled as a day case for an initial procedure during which the cyst is opened, rinsed, and focally treated. Postoperatively, these women are treated for 3 months with a GnRH analogue, and eventually scheduled for a second intervention. If a small endometrioma is found on the scan, these women are also scheduled for day case. They are advised that the probability that a bowel preparation would be nec-

Acknowledgments

Mr Stephen Kennedy, and Professor David Barlow from the Department of Obstetrics and Gynaecology, the John Radcliffe Hospital, University of Oxford, UK, Mr Fiorenzo de Cicco, Gemelli Hospital, Università del Sacro Cuore, Rome, Italy, and Mr Anastasia Ussia, Crotone, Italy are thanked for discussions and help during endoscopic surgery for endometriosis. The Departments of Abdominal Surgery at the University Hospital of Gasthuisberg (University of Leuven), with special thanks to Mr Andre D'Hoore of Urology, Mr Ben Van Cleynenbreughel, and Professor Van Acker of Anaesthesiology, for their help and support over the last 10 years. We also wish to thank the theater staff for their dedication and professionalism during surgery and for those staff responsible for postoperative care, who are essential for this type of severe endometriosis surgery. We thank our co-workers and our co-authors of the articles from which data have been reviewed.

REFERENCES

1. Sampson JA. Peritoneal endometriosis due to the menstrual dissemination of endometrial tissue into the peritoneal cavity. Am J Obstet Gynecol 1927; 14: 422–469.

2. Cullen TS. Adeno-myoma of the round ligament. Johns Hopkins Hosp Bull 1896; 7: 112–114.

3. Cullen TS. The distribution of adenomyomata containing uterine mucosa. Am J Obstet Gynecol 1919; 80: 130–138.

4. Cullen TS. Adenoma-myoma uteri diffusum benignum. J Johns Hopkins Hosp Bull 1896; 6: 133–137.

5. Jansen RP, Russell P. Nonpigmented endometriosis: clinical, laparoscopic, and pathologic definition. Am J Obstet Gynecol 1986; 155: 1154–1159.

6. Stripling MC, Martin DC, Chatman DL, et al. Subtle appearance of pelvic endometriosis. Fertil Steril 1988; 49: 427–431.

7. Stripling MC, Martin DC, Poston WM. Does endometriosis have a typical appearance? J Reprod Med Obstet Gynecol 1988; 33: 879–884.

8. Martin DC, Hubert GD, Van der Zwaag R, et al. Laparoscopic appearances of peritoneal endometriosis. Fertil Steril 1989; 51: 63–67.

9. Mahmood TA, Templeton A. Prevalence and genesis of endometriosis. Hum Reprod 1991; 6: 544–549.

10. Rawson JMR. Prevalence of endometriosis in asymptomatic women. J Reprod Med Obstet Gynecol 1991; 36: 513–515.

11. Wheeler JM. Epidemiology of endometriosis-associated infertility. J Reprod Med Obstet Gynecol 1989; 34: 41–46.

12. Houston DE, Noller KL, Melton LJ, et al. Incidence of pelvic endometriosis in Rochester, Minnesota, 1970–1979. Am J Epidemiol 1987; 125: 959–969.

13. Hull MGR, Glazener CMA, Kelly NJ, et al. Population study of causes, treatment, and outcome of infertility. BMJ 1985; 291: 1693–1697.

14. Strathy JH, Molgaard CA, Coulam CB, et al. Endometriosis and infertility: a laparoscopic study of endometriosis among fertile and infertile women. Fertil Steril 1985; 44: 83 88.

15. Moen MH. Endometriosis in women at interval sterilization. Acta Obstet Gynecol Scand 1987; 66: 451–454.

16. Nikanen V, Punnonen R. External endometriosis in 801 operated patients. Acta Obstet Gynecol Scand 1984; 63: 699–701.

17. Bitzer J, Korber HR. [Laparoscopy findings in infertile women]. Geburtshilfe Frauenheilkd 1983; 43: 294–298. [in German]

18. Koninckx PR, Meuleman C, Demeyere S, et al. Suggestive evidence that pelvic endometriosis is a progressive disease, whereas deeply infiltrating endometriosis is associated with pelvic pain. Fertil Steril 1991; 55: 759–765.

19. El Mahgoub S, Yaseen S. A positive proof for the theory of coelomic metaplasia. Am J Obstet Gynecol 1980; 137: 137–140.

20. Suginami H. A reappraisal of the coelomic metaplasia theory by reviewing endometriosis occurring in unusual sites and instances. Am J Obstet Gynecol 1991; 165: 214–218.

21. Moore JG, Binstock MA, Growdon WA. The clinical implications of retroperitoneal endometriosis. Am J Obstet Gynecol 1988; 158: 1291–1298.

22. Ueki M. Histologic study of endometriosis and examination of lymphatic drainage in and from the uterus. Am J Obstet Gynecol 1991; 165: 201–209.

23. Koninckx PR, Ide P, Vandenbroucke W, et al. New aspects of the pathophysiology of endometriosis and associated infertility. J Reprod Med 1980; 24: 257–260.

24. Halme J, Hammond MG, Hulka JF, et al. Retrograde menstruation in healthy women and in patients with endometriosis. Obstet Gynecol 1984; 64: 151–154.

25. Kruitwagen RF. Menstruation as the pelvic aggressor. Baillières Clin Obstet Gynaecol 1993; 7: 687–700.

26. van der Linden PJ, de Goeij AF, Dunselman GA, et al. Amniotic membrane as an in vitro model for endometrium–extracellular matrix interactions. Gynecol Obstet Invest 1998; 45: 7–11.

27. Redwine DB, Koninckx PR, D'Hooghe T, et al. Endometriosis: will the real natural history please stand up? Fertil Steril 1991; 56: 590–591.

28. Koninckx PR, Oosterlynck D, D'Hooghe T, et al. Deeply infiltrating endometriosis is a disease whereas mild endometriosis could be considered a non-disease. Ann NY Acad Sci 1994; 734: 333–341.

29. Vercellini P, Bocciolone L, Crosignani PG. Is mild endometriosis always a disease? Hum Reprod 1992; 7: 627–629.

30. Koninckx PR, Kennedy SH, Barlow DH. Pathogenesis of endometriosis: The role of peritoneal fluid. Gynecol Obstet Invest 1999; 47 (Suppl 1): 23–33.

31. Koninckx PR, Barlow D, Kennedy S. Implantation versus infiltration: the Sampson versus the endometriotic disease theory. Gynecol Obstet Invest 1999; 47 (Suppl 1): 3–9.

32. Gordts S, Boeckx W, Brosens I. Microsurgery of endometriosis in infertile patients. Fertil Steril 1984; 42: 520–525.

33. Brosens I, Gordts S, Boeckx W, et al. Surgical treatment of endometriosis in infertility. Ir J Med Sci 1983; 152 (Suppl 2): 18–21.

34. Canis M, Mage G, Wattiez A, et al. The ovarian endometrioma: why is it so poorly managed? Laparoscopic treatment of large ovarian endometrioma: why such a long learning curve? Hum Reprod 2003; 18: 5–7.

35. Cornillie FJ, Oosterlynck D, Lauweryns JM, et al. Deeply infiltrating pelvic endometriosis: histology and clinical significance. Fertil Steril 1990; 53: 978–983.

36. Koninckx PR, Meuleman C, Oosterlynck D, et al. Diagnosis of deep endometriosis by clinical examination during menstruation and plasma CA-125 concentration. Fertil Steril 1996; 65: 280–287.

37. Koninckx PR, Vandermeersch E. The persufflator: an insufflation device for laparoscopy and especially for CO_2-laser-endoscopic surgery. Hum Reprod 1991; 6: 1288–1290.

38. Nezhat C, Nezhat F. Operative laparoscopy (minimally invasive surgery): state of the art. J Gynecol Surg 1992; 8: 111–142.

39. Adamson GD, Reich H, Trost D. $^{13}CO_2$ isotopic laser used through the operating channel of laser laparoscopes: a comparative study of power and energy density losses. Obstet Gynecol 1994; 83: 717–724.

40. Koninckx PR. Is mild endometriosis a condition occurring intermittently in all women? Hum Reprod 1994; 9: 2202–2205.

41. Cervero F. Visceral pain: mechanisms of peripheral and central sensitization. Ann Med 1995; 27: 235–239.

42. Cervero F, Janig W. Visceral nociceptors: a new world order? [see comments]. Trends Neurosci 1992; 15: 374–378.

43. Koninckx PR, Renaer M. Pain sensitivity of and pain radiation from the internal female genital organs. Hum Reprod 1997; 12: 1785–1788.

44. Demco L. Mapping the source and character of pain due to endometriosis by patient-assisted laparoscopy. J Am Assoc Gynecol Laparosc 1998; 5: 241–245.

45. Brosens IA, Koninckx PR, Corveleyn PA. A study of plasma progesterone, oestradiol-17β, prolactin and LH levels, and of the luteal phase appearance of the ovaries in patients with endometriosis and infertility. Br J Obstet Gynaecol 1978; 85: 246–250.

46. Koninckx PR, Brosens IA. Clinical significance of the luteinized unruptured follicle syndrome as a cause of infertility. Eur J Obstet Gynecol Reprod Biol 1982; 13: 355–368.

47. Koninckx PR, Brosens IA. Diagnosis of the luteinized unruptured follicle syndrome. Proc FIGO, Tokyo, 1977.

48. Koninckx PR, Deprest J, Janssen G, et al. Cumulative pregnancy rates following CO_2-laser endoscopic excision of deeply infiltrating endometriosis. Fertil Steril, Montreal meeting, 1993.

49. Schenken RS, Werlin LB, Williams RF, et al. Histologic and hormonal documentation of the luteinized unruptured follicle syndrome. Am J Obstet Gynecol 1986; 154: 839–847.

50. Haines CJ. Luteinized unruptured follicle syndrome. Clin Reprod Fertil 1987; 5: 321–332.

51. Scheenjes E, te Velde ER, Kremer J. Inspection of the ovaries and steroids in serum and peritoneal fluid at various time intervals after ovulation in fertile women: implications for the luteinized unruptured follicle syndrome. Fertil Steril 1990; 54: 38–41.

52. Mio Y, Toda T, Harada T, et al. Luteinized unruptured follicle in the early stages of endometriosis as a cause of unexplained infertility. Am J Obstet Gynecol 1992; 167: 271–273.

53. D'Hooghe TM, Bambra CS, Raeymaekers BM, et al. Increased incidence and recurrence of recent corpus luteum without ovulation stigma (luteinized unruptured follicle syndrome?) in baboons with endometriosis. J Soc Gynecol Invest 1996; 3: 140–144.

54. Marcoux S, Maheux R, Berube S. Laparoscopic surgery in infertile women with minimal or mild endometriosis. Canadian Collaborative Group on Endometriosis. N Engl J Med 1997; 337: 217–222.

55. Parazzini F. Ablation of lesions or no treatment in minimal-mild endometriosis in infertile woman: a randomized trial. Gruppo Italiano per lo Studio dell'Endometriosis. Hum Reprod 1999; 14: 1332–1334.

56. Jenkins JM, Anthony FW, Wood P, et al. The development of functional ovarian cysts during pituitary down-regulation. Hum Reprod 1993; 8: 1623–1627.

57. Alcazar JL, Laparte C, Jurado M, et al. The role of transvaginal ultrasonography combined with color velocity imaging and pulsed Doppler in the diagnosis of endometrioma. Fertil Steril 1997; 67: 487–491.

58. Mais V, Guerriero S, Ajossa S, et al. The efficiency of transvaginal ultrasonography in the diagnosis of endometrioma. Fertil Steril 1993; 60: 776–780.

59. Outwater EK, Dunton CJ. Imaging of the ovary and adnexa: clinical issues and applications of MR imaging. Radiology 1995; 194: 1–18.

60. Guerriero S, Ajossa S, Paoletti AM, et al. Tumor markers and transvaginal ultrasonography in the diagnosis of endometrioma. Obstet Gynecol 1996; 88: 403–407.

61. Guerriero S, Mais V, Ajossa S, et al. Transvaginal ultrasonography combined with CA-125 plasma levels in the diagnosis of endometrioma. Fertil Steril 1996; 65: 293–298.

62. Koninckx PR, Muyldermans M, Moerman P, et al. CA 125 concentrations in ovarian 'chocolate' cyst fluid can differentiate an endometriotic cyst from a cystic corpus luteum. Hum Reprod 1992; 7: 1314–1317.

63. Koninckx PR. CA 125 in the management of endometriosis. Eur J Obstet Gynecol Reprod Biol 1993; 49: 109–113.

64. Brosens IA, Puttemans PJ, Deprest J. The endoscopic localization of endometrial implants in the ovarian chocolate cyst. Fertil Steril 1994; 61: 1034–1038.

65. Martin DC, Demos Berry J. Histology of chocolate cysts. J Gynecol Surg 1990; 6: 43–46.

66. Donnez J, Nisolle M, Gillet N, et al. Large ovarian endometriomas. Hum Reprod 1996; 11: 641–646.

67. Hughesdon PE. Benign endometrioid tumours of the ovary and the müllerian concept of ovarian epithelial tumours. Histopathology 1984; 8: 977–990.

68. Brosens I, Puttemans P, Deprest J. Appearances of endometriosis. Baillières Clin Obstet Gynaecol 1993; 7: 741–757.

69. Yano T, Jimbo H, Yoshikawa H, et al. Molecular analysis of clonality in ovarian endometrial cysts. Gynecol Obstet Invest 1999; 47 (Suppl 1): 41–45.

70. Tamura M, Fukaya T, Murakami I, et al. Analysis of clonality in human endometriotic cysts based on evaluation of X chromosome inactivation in archival formalin-fixed, paraffin-embedded tissue. Lab Invest 1998; 78: 213–218.

71. Jimbo H, Hitomi Y, Yoshikawa H, et al. Evidence for

monoclonal expansion of epithelial cells in ovarian endometrial cysts. Am J Pathol 1997; 150: 1173–1178.

72. Vercellini P, Vendola N, Bocciolone L, et al. Laparoscopic aspiration of ovarian endometriomas. Effect with postoperative gonadotropin releasing hormone agonist treatment. J Reprod Med 1992; 37: 577–580.

73. Giorlandino C, Taramanni C, Muzii L, et al. Ultrasound-guided aspiration of ovarian endometriotic cysts. Int J Gynaecol Obstet 1993; 43: 41–44.

74. Aboulghar MA, Mansour RT, Serour GI, et al. Ultrasonic transvaginal aspiration of endometriotic cysts: an optional line of treatment in selected cases of endometriosis. Hum Reprod 1991; 6: 1408–1410.

75. Muzii L, Marana R, Caruana P, et al. Laparoscopic findings after transvaginal ultrasound-guided aspiration of ovarian endometriomas. Hum Reprod 1995; 10: 2902–2903.

76. Kennedy SH, Cederholm-Williams SA, Barlow DH. The effect of injecting endometriotic 'chocolate' cyst fluid into the peritoneal cavity of mice. Hum Reprod 1992; 7: 1329.

77. Bruhat MA, Mage G, Chapron C, et al. Present day endoscopic surgery in gynecology. Eur J Obstet Gynecol Reprod Biol 1991; 41: 4–13.

78. Neuhaus SJ, Watson DI, Ellis T, et al. Influence of cytotoxic agents on intraperitoneal tumor implantation after laparoscopy. Dis Colon Rectum 1999; 42: 10–15.

79. Brosens IA, Van Ballaer P, Puttemans P, et al. Reconstruction of the ovary containing large endometriomas by an extraovarian endosurgical technique. Fertil Steril 1996; 66: 517–521.

80. Crosignani PG, Vercellini P. Conservative surgery for severe endometriosis: should laparotomy be abandoned definitively? Hum Reprod 1995; 10: 2412–2418.

81. Adamson GD, Pasta DJ. Surgical treatment of endometriosis-associated infertility: meta-analysis compared with survival analysis. Am J Obstet Gynecol 1994; 171: 1488–1505.

82. Brosens IA. New principles in the management of endometriosis. Acta Obstet Gynecol Scand Suppl 1994; 159: 18–21.

83. Wood C. Endoscopy in the management of endometriosis. Baillières Clin Obstet Gynaecol 1994; 8: 735–757.

84. Canis M, Mage G, Wattiez A, et al. Second-look laparoscopy after laparoscopic cystectomy of large ovarian endometriomas [see comments]. Fertil Steril 1992; 58: 617–619.

85. Fayez JA, Vogel MF. Comparison of different treatment methods of endometriomas by laparoscopy. Obstet Gynecol 1991; 78: 660–665.

86. Busacca M, Marana R, Caruana P, et al. Recurrence of ovarian endometrioma after laparoscopic excision. Am J Obstet Gynecol 1999; 180: 519–523.

87. Muzii L, Marana R, Caruana P, et al. The impact of preoperative gonadotropin-releasing hormone agonist treatment on laparoscopic excision of ovarian endometriotic cysts. Fertil Steril 1996; 65: 1235–1237.

88. Muzii L, Bianchi A, Croce C, et al. Laparoscopic excision of ovarian cysts: is the stripping technique a tissue-sparing procedure? Fertil Steril 2002; 77: 609–614.

89. Marana R, Muzii L, Catalano GF, et al. Laparoscopic excision of adnexal masses. J Am Assoc Gynecol Laparosc 2004; 11: 162–166.

90. Chang SP, Ng HT. A randomized comparative study of the effect of leuprorelin acetate depot and danazol in the treatment of endometriosis. Chung Hua I Hsueh Tsa Chih Taipei 1996; 57: 431–437.

91. Koninckx PR, Martin DC. Deep endometriosis: a consequence of infiltration or retraction or possibly adenomyosis externa? Fertil Steril 1992; 58: 924–928.

92. Nabeshima H, Murakami T, Yoshinaga K, et al. Analysis of the clonality of ectopic glands in peritoneal endometriosis using laser microdissection. Fertil Steril 2003; 80: 1144–1150.

93. Wu Y, Basir Z, Kajdacsy-Balla A, et al. Resolution of clonal origins for endometriotic lesions using laser capture microdissection and the human androgen receptor (HUMARA) assay. Fertil Steril 2003; 79 (Suppl 1): 710–717.

94. Leyendecker G, Herbertz M, Kunz G, et al. Endometriosis results from the dislocation of basal endometrium. Hum Reprod 2002; 17: 2725–2736.

95. Koninckx PR, Timmermans B, Meuleman C, et al. Complications of CO_2-laser endoscopic excision of deep endometriosis. Hum Reprod 1996; 11: 2263–2268.

96. Hompes PG, Koninckx PR, Kennedy S, et al. Serum CA-125 concentrations during midfollicular phase, a clinically useful and reproducible marker in diagnosis of advanced endometriosis. Clin Chem 1996; 42: 1871–1874.

97. Redwine DB. Conservative laparoscopic excision of endometriosis by sharp dissection: life table analysis of reoperation and persistent or recurrent disease. Fertil Steril 1991; 56: 628–634.

98. Redwine DB. Laparoscopic en bloc resection for treatment of the obliterated cul-de-sac in endometriosis. J Reprod Med 1992; 37: 695–698.

99. Sharpe DR, Redwine DB. Laparoscopic segmental resection of the sigmoid and rectosigmoid colon for endometriosis. Surg Laparosc Endosc 1992; 2: 120–124.

100. Redwine DB, Koning M, Sharpe DR. Laparoscopically assisted transvaginal segmental resection of the rectosigmoid colon for endometriosis. Fertil Steril 1996; 65: 193–197.

101. Redwine DB. Severe intestinal (GI) endometriosis (E) and pelvic mapping. Fertil Steril Suppl 1997; S22.

102. Bruhat MA, Mage G, Pouly JL, et al. Advances in pelviscopic surgery. Ann NY Acad Sci. 1991; 626: 367–371.

103. Donnez J, Nisolle M, Gillerot S, et al. Rectovaginal septum adenomyotic nodules: a series of 500 cases. Br J Obstet Gynaecol 1997; 104(9): 1014–1018.

104. Crosignani PG, De CL, Gastaldi A, et al. Leuprolide in a 3-monthly versus a monthly depot formulation for the treatment of symptomatic endometriosis: a pilot study. Hum Reprod 1996; 11: 2732–2735.

105. Vercellini P, Trespidi L, De Giorgi O, et al. Endometriosis

and pelvic pain: relation to disease stage and localization. Fertil Steril 1996; 65: 299–304.

106. Donnez J, Nisolle M, Casanasroux F, et al. Rectovaginal septum, endometriosis or adenomyosis: laparoscopic management in a series of 231 patients. Hum Reprod 1995; 10: 630–635.

107. Martin DC. Pain and infertility – a rationale for different treatment approaches. Br J Obstet Gynaecol 1995; 102 (Suppl 12): 2–3.

108. Candiani GB, Vercellini P, Fedele L, et al. Conservative surgical treatment of rectovaginal septum endometriosis. J Gynecol Surg 1992; 8: 177–182.

109. Nezhat C, Nezhat F, Pennington E. Laparoscopic treatment of infiltrative rectosigmoid colon and rectovaginal septum endometriosis by the technique of videolaparoscopy and the CO_2 laser. Br J Obstet Gynaecol 1992; 99: 664–667.

110. Udagawa Y, Aoki D, Ito K, et al. Clinical characteristics of a newly developed ovarian tumour marker, galactosyltransferase associated with tumour (GAT). Eur J Cancer 1998; 34: 489–495.

111. Ripps BA, Martin DC. Focal pelvic tenderness, pelvic pain and dysmenorrhea in endometriosis. J Reprod Med 1991; 36: 470–472.

112. Reich H, McGlynn F, Salvat J. Laparoscopic treatment of cul-de-sac obliteration secondary to retrocervical deep fibrotic endometriosis. J Reprod Med 1991; 36: 516–522.

113. Martin DC. Medical versus surgical treatment of endometriosis? Fertil Steril 1998; 70: 1183–1184.

114. Possover M, Diebolder H, Plaul K, et al. Laparascopically assisted vaginal resection of rectovaginal endometriosis. Obstet Gynecol 2000; 96: 304–307.

115. Keckstein J, Ulrich U, Kandolf O, et al. [Laparoscopic therapy of intestinal endometriosis and the ranking of drug treatment]. Zentralbl Gynakol 2003; 125: 259–266. [in German]

116. Fedele L, Bianchi S, Zanconato G, et al. Long-term follow-up after conservative surgery for rectovaginal endometriosis. Am J Obstet Gynecol 2004; 190: 1020–1024.

117. Volpi E, Ferrero A, Sismondi P. Laparoscopic identification of pelvic nerves in patients with deep infiltrating endometriosis. Surg Endosc 2004; 18: 1109–1112.

118. Van Rompaey B, Deprest JA, Koninckx PR. Enterocele as a consequence of laparoscopic resection of deeply infiltrating endometriosis. J Am Assoc Gynecol Laparosc 1996; 4: 73–75.

119. Tate JJT, Kwok S, Dawson JW, et al. Prospective comparison of laparoscopic and conventional anterior resection. Br J Surg 1993; 80: 1396–1398.

120. Neven P, van Deursen H, Baert L, et al. Ureteric injury at laparoscopic surgery: the endoscopic management. Case review. Gynaecol Endosc 1993; 2: 45–46.

121. Fedele L, Bianchi S, Zanconato G, et al. Use of a levonorgestrel-releasing intrauterine device in the treatment of rectovaginal endometriosis. Fertil Steril 2001; 75: 485–488.

122. Shaw RW. Endometriosis: current evaluation of management and rationale for medical therapy. In: Brosens IA, Donnez J, eds. The current status of endometriosis. New York: Parthenon; 1993: 371–383.

123. Fedele L, Bianchi S, Bocciolone L, et al. Buserelin acetate in the treatment of pelvic pain associated with minimal and mild endometriosis – a controlled study. Fertil Steril 1993; 59: 516–521.

124. Fedele L, Arcaini L, Bianchi S, et al. Comparison of cyproterone acetate and danazol in the treatment of pelvic pain associated with endometriosis. Obstet Gynecol 1989; 73: 1000–1004.

125. Fedele L, Bianchi S, Arcaini L, et al. Buserelin versus danazol in the treatment of endometriosis-associated infertility. Am J Obstet Gynecol 1989; 161: 871–876.

126. Evers JLH. The second-look laparoscopy for evaluation of the result of medical treatment of endometriosis should not be performed during ovarian suppression. Fertil Steril 1987; 47: 502–504.

127. Hughes EG, Fedorkow DM, Collins JA. A quantitative overview of controlled trials in endometriosis-associated infertility. Fertil Steril 1993; 59: 963–970.

128. Shaw RW. Nafarelin in the treatment of pelvic pain caused by endometriosis. Am J Obstet Gynecol 1990; 162: 574–576.

24 Use of the Harmonic Scalpel* in endometriosis surgery

Charles E Miller

How does the Harmonic Scalpel work?

The three components of the ultrasonic system are a high-frequency, computer-controlled generator, a hand piece that houses the ultrasonic transducer, and a variety of interchangeable blade configurations (Figures 24.1–24.3). The hand piece contains piezoelectric ceramics that look like a stack of 15 nickels piled on top of one another. A computer-controlled electrical signal causes the piezo-electric ceramics in the ultrasonic hand piece to expand and contract (Figure 24.4), converting electrical energy to mechanical motion (ultrasound). The transducer, attached to the mount, transmits the ultrasonic vibration to the attached blade. To simplify, the electric signal sent to the transducer in the ultrasonic hand piece is converted to mechanical motion. The result is vibration of 55 500 cycles/s.

The ultrasonic wave from the hand piece mount is transferred to the laparoscopic blade extender (Figure 24.5). The blade extenders are stabilizing silicon rings positioned equidistant at nodes to

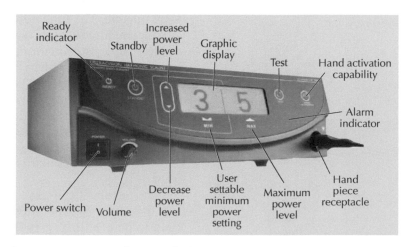

Figure 24.1 Harmonic Generator (GEN04), Ethicon Endo-Surgery, Inc.

* Harmonic Scalpel is a registered trademark of Ethicon Endo-Surgery, Inc.

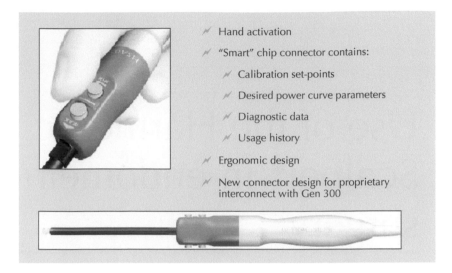

- Hand activation
- "Smart" chip connector contains:
  - Calibration set-points
  - Desired power curve parameters
  - Diagnostic data
  - Usage history
- Ergonomic design
- New connector design for proprietary interconnect with Gen 300

Figure 24.2 Hand piece. Key features and benefits of hand activation. Harmonic, Ethicon Endo-Surgery, Inc.

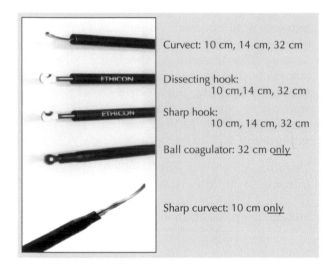

Curvect: 10 cm, 14 cm, 32 cm

Dissecting hook: 10 cm, 14 cm, 32 cm

Sharp hook: 10 cm, 14 cm, 32 cm

Ball coagulator: 32 cm only

Sharp curvect: 10 cm only

Figure 24.3 Interchangeable Harmonic 5 mm blades. Harmonic, Ethicon Endo-Surgery, Inc.

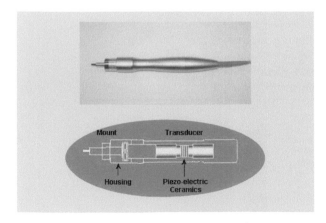

Figure 24.4 The hand piece contains piezoelectric ceramics that look like a stack of 15 nickels piled on top of one another.

direct the flow of energy in a longitudinal direction and to prevent it from being dissipated on the sheath. Motion is again amplified at the tip of the blade.

When the blade comes in contact with tissue, pressure causes coaptation. The hydrogen bonds of the cell's protein moieties are broken. This causes the protein to be denatured and form a sticky coagulum. This coagulum seals coapted vessels. Larger vessels, 3–4 mm, must be desiccated as well as sealed. Desiccation occurs by allowing the temperature of the tissue to be increased. At the same time, the vessel is coapted and sealed.

Figure 24.6 demonstrates the tissue temperature range at which ultrasonic, electrosurgery, and lasers operate. The higher temperatures associated with electrosurgery and lasers result in tissue desiccation and eschar formation. As mentioned, hemostasis is achieved by denaturation of tissue protein and coagulation. These effects occur at the operating tissue temperature of the Harmonic Scalpel; i.e. temperatures less than 100°C. If further desiccation is necessary when using the Harmonic Scalpel, tissue temperatures remain below 150°C; thus, eschar will not form.

The end result of the tissue effect noted above is that there are several advantages of ultrasonic energy over electrosurgery (Figure 24.7). Cutting is precise; there is minimal lateral thermal damage with coagulation. Because tissue temperature remains relatively low even with desiccation, minimal lateral thermal damage is noted. Moreover, there is less tissue sticking and smoke formation. As compared to monopolar electrosurgery,

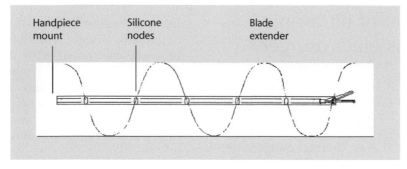

Figure 24.5 Motion through blade extender. The ultrasonic wave from the hand piece mount is transferred to the laparoscopic blade extender. The blade extender is supported by silicone rings positioned at the nodes. The blade vibrates at 55 000 times per second.

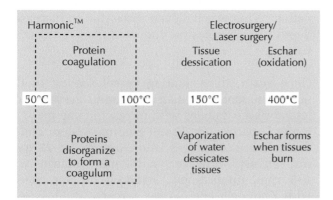

Figure 24.6 Active surgical temperatures. The tissue temperature range at which ultrasonic technology, electrosurgery, and lasers operate.

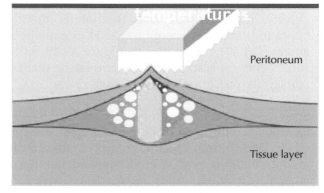

Figure 24.8 Cavitational effect. Motion of the blade creates an area of low pressure, causing fluids to vaporize at low temperatures. Fluid vapor expands, causing the layers to separate, which enhances visualization of a vascular plane of dissection. Harmonic, Ethicon Endo-Surgery, Inc.

- Control and precision over cutting and coagulation
- Minimal lateral thermal tissue damage
- Multifunctional instruments
- Less tissue sticking
- Less smoke formation
- No stray energy
- No neuromuscular stimulation
- No electrical energy to or through patient

Figure 24.7 Advantages of ultrasonic energy over electrosurgery.

- Tissue tension
- Blade sharpness
- Time
- Power level
- Grip force

Figure 24.9 Five factors affecting cutting and coagulation. Harmonic, Ethicon Endo-Surgery, Inc.

there can be no stray energy or electrical energy passing through the patients.

Another advantage of ultrasonic energy is the cavitational effect (Figure 24.8). The motion of the blade and the tissue temperature causes the fluid to vaporize and the pressure to drop. As pressure × volume is a constant, with lowering pressure, volume increases and thus the vapor expands. The end result is that cell layers are separated, which makes dissection easier.

Five factors affect ultrasonic cutting and coagulation (Figure 24.9). They are tissue tension, blade sharpness, time on tissue, power level, and grip force. To enhance cutting, one should keep tissue on tension and use a sharp blade at the highest power level (5) and with the greatest grip force.

Clinical effect of ultrasonic energy versus electrosurgery

In 1988, Hambley et al. studied the depth of thermal injury, utilizing porcine small bowel mesentery.[1] Figure 24.10 shows the results with the various surgical modalities. As can be noted, ultrasonic energy had the least thermal damage: depth was noted to be similar to the CO_2 laser and the Nd:YAG laser and certainly far less than either monopolar or bipolar electrosurgery.

At the 1995 meeting of the Society of American Gastrointestinal Endoscopic Surgeons (SAGES), Dr Joseph Amaral presented a study using the porcine model, comparing the lateral thermal effect of ultrasonic energy (level 3) to monopolar energy (30 W).[2] As noted in Figure 24.10, ultrasonic energy is associated with less lateral thermal spread than monopolar electrosurgery.

The otolaryngology literature also notes an advantage of ultrasonic energy over electrosurgery when performing tonsillectomy. In the canine model, Willging and Wiatrak showed less tissue edema, charring, and desiccation with the Harmonic Scalpel. Moreover, there was decreased weight loss in the Harmonic Scalpel population, indicating faster oral intake.[3]

In a randomized study of pediatric patients undergoing tonsillectomy, performed by Walker and Syed, return to routine activity was faster in the ultrasonic energy population.[4] At 24 hours post-surgery, 27.8% of Harmonic Scalpel-treated patients, as compared to 12% of electrosurgery patients, returned to regular activity. By 72 hours post-surgery, 49.5% of Harmonic Scalpel patients vs 22.7% of electrosurgery patients had returned to routine activity. Furthermore, the ability to sleep was higher post-Harmonic Scalpel vs electrosurgery.

Armstrong et al reported on a prospective study using the Harmonic Scalpel vs electrosurgery for hemorrhoidectomy in *Diseases of the Colon and Rectum* in 2001. The indications were grade III

internal hemorrhoids with external components or grade IV disease.[5] Decreased pain and analgesia required was noted with the Harmonic Scalpel. Whereas 55% of Harmonic Scalpel patients returned to work within 1 week, only 23% of electrosurgery patients could work. The authors hypothesize that the decreased pain is secondary to avoidance of lateral energy.

Tsimoyiannis compared 100 patients undergoing laparoscopic cholecystectomy via electrosurgery to 200 patients treated with the Harmonic Scalpel.[6] While there was no difference in post-operative pain or nausea, subhepatic drainage was longer in the monopolar electrosurgery patient. This was believed to be due to increased depth of tissue destruction secondary to electro-surgery.

Once again, in evaluating vessel sealing in the porcine model, Landman et al found the least collateral tissue damage with ultrasonic energy.[7] The 5 mm Laparoscopic Vessel Sealing System sealed the largest arteries and veins, 6 mm and 12 mm, respectively. However, collateral damage was 1–3 mm. Interestingly, standard bipolar energy with Klepinger and Trimax forceps was less reliable. Collateral damage varied from 1–6 mm. Again, Landman et al found that the Harmonic Scalpel sealed vessels up to 3 mm and collateral damage was 0–1 mm.

The ultrasonic scalpel in endometriosis surgery

As in all surgical procedures, deep endometriosis must be dealt with in a standard fashion. In that way, areas of endometriosis are not missed.

Initially, the surgeon must inspect the abdomen and pelvis. It is especially important to visualize the appendix for endometriosis and adhesions. If endometriosis or adhesions are noted, laparoscopic appendectomy is strongly recommended. Once periappendiceal adhesions have been lysed with the LaparoSonic Coagulating Shears (LCS; Ethicon Endo-Surgery, Inc.) at level 5 (cutting with blade excision of 100 µm), we transect the mesoappendix at the base of the appendix at level 5. The surgeon then transects the appendix at its base, using the linear stapler and cutter. The transected appendix is now placed in a bag and removed.

The next phase of the operation is to perform adhesiolysis. It is imperative that normal anatomy be

Model: Porcine Small Bowel Mesentery	
Harmonic Scalpel	0 mm – 1.5 mm
Monopolar Electrosurgery	0.24 mm – 15.0 mm
Bipolar Electrosurgery	0.12 mm – 9 mm
CO_2 Laser	0.6 mm – 4 mm
Nd: YAG Laser	0.3 mm – 4.2 mm

Figure 24.10 Depth of thermal injury. Data from McCarus SD. JAAGL 1996; 3: 601–668 and Hambley R et al. J Dermatol Surg Oncol 1988; 14: 1213–1217.

restored. This means that adhesions involving the uterus, bowel, and adnexa must be removed. In the process, these organs are completely mobilized. Adhesiolysis is performed utilizing the LCS at level 5. At times, sharp and blunt dissection must be utilized, particularly when dissection is performed next to the bowel or pelvic side wall. Even with the small depth of penetration associated with the LCS, one must be concerned about potential risks to the bowel and ureter. To keep the ureter out of harm's way, when adhesions are dense between the ovary and pelvic side wall, or endometriosis is noted, the surgeon should proceed to ureterolysis. If the ureter cannot be identified through the peritoneum, it is generally recommended to open the peritoneum near the pelvic brim, to initially visualize the ureter. The LCS provides excellent cutting at level 5 with minimal lateral distribution to minimize risk to the uterus on mobilization. Once this is accomplished, further lysis of adhesions or resection of endometriosis over the pelvic side wall and posterior broad ligament can be completed.

Once the adnexa have been completely mobilized, ovarian endometriomata, if present, are removed. The author does not recommend simply creating a fenestration in the endometrium and then desiccating the base. Rather, the author views the endometrioma as a cyst under the capsule of the ovary. An incision is made over the endometrioma at the ovarian capsule's thinnest point. How this incision is made is really of no consequence. Next, the endometrioma fluid is drained. Finally, the cyst capsule is excised. The easiest way to remove the capsule of the endometrioma is to grasp the cyst capsule in the middle of the cyst rather than at the edge. Once the capsule has been removed completely and hemostasis has been achieved, a decision is made whether to close or repair the ovarian capsule. If the pelvic side wall and/or medial posterior broad ligament peritoneum has been resected, or the edges of the ovarian capsule do not come together, it is the author's recommendation to repair the ovarian capsule via a purse-string suture of 4-0 PDS.

Prior to removing deep cul-de-sac endometriosis, remove endometriosis and scar tissue of the cervix vesicouterine peritoneum with the LCS at level 5. If the endometriosis is deep anteriorly, 200–300 ml of normal saline with indigo carmine should be put into the bladder to alert the surgeon to the possibility of bladder perforation if the incision has been too deep.

Finally, our attention is directed to deep cul-de-sac endometriosis. The rectal probe is placed into the rectum. Not only does this allow the surgeon the ability to demarcate the rectum but also the rectum can be mobilized away from the dissection line utilizing the rectal probe. Remember: the position of the uterus must be noted throughout the dissection.

The resection of the endometriosis generally proceeds from the rectovaginal septum toward the rectum, and from the uterosacral ligaments toward the rectum. In order to resect the endometriosis of the rectovaginal septum, or the uterosacral ligaments, grasp the tissue and place it on tension. The LCS at level 5 is used to excise the tissue.

If the resection of endometriosis is so deep that the vagina is entered, repair the area with 3-0 Vicryl or PDS suture. Vicryl can be advantageous as it degrades faster than PDS. PDS, however, is non-filament and not braided; it slides through tissue more easily. Ultimately, the vagina can be repaired via a laparoscopic or vaginal approach.

Superficial endometriosis that is in the serosa or the rectosigmoid, or superficial muscularis, can be resected via sharp dissection with laparoscopic scissors or the LCS. If utilizing the LCS, the tissue must be placed on tension and only small areas resected with each bite. Alternatively, use scissors. Deeper areas of endometriosis that enter deeply into the muscularis must be excised by scissors. Even with little lateral spread of energy, scissors prove to be safer.

Special considerations

In the process of excision of cul-de-sac endometriosis, the rectum may be entered either purposely or inadvertently. In either case, repair of the rectum is necessary. If the rectum is entered with harmonic energy, as with any other form of energy, the desiccated edges of the incision must be trimmed prior to closure. If not, the risk of postoperative perforation is higher. The rectum is repaired in two layers. The first layer includes the full thickness; i.e. rectal mucosa, muscularis, and serosa. The author recommends '0' silk to be used in a continuous fashion. A second layer of '0' silk is then placed in an interrupted fashion. In order to show that the closure is 'air tight', fluid is placed in the cul-de-sac. With the assistant observing via the laparoscope, sigmoidoscopy is performed. If the rectum is properly repaired, no bubbles will be noted in the fluid of the cul-de-sac as the sigmoidoscopy is performed.

Particularly when the cul-de-sac endometriosis is widespread and the resultant dissection is significant, or the uterus is posterior in position, a uterine suspension should be considered. If not, there is greater risk of postsurgical adhesions. In this case, the uterus will become adherent to the cul-de-sac. The author recommends performing the UPLIFT procedure using the Metra PS procedure kit from Inlet Medical.

With the UPLIFT procedure, the round ligaments are invested with permanent or absorbable suture. This suture is used as a conduit to establish a bridge between the lateral abdominal wall and the tissue just proximal to the uterus. In the process, the round ligaments are shortened; as a result, the uterus is repositioned anteriorly away from the dissection.

Under laparoscopic visualization, externally palpate the abdominal wall above the point where the round ligaments insert laterally. A skin nick is made laterally and cephalad to the point of insertion (Figure 24.11). An 18-gauge spinal needle is then placed via the nick and through the length of the round ligament. Then, 10 ml of 1% lidocaine or 0.5% bupivacaine is inserted along the round ligament as the spinal needle is removed. The local anesthetic injection assists with postoperative pain management. It also increases the volume of the round ligament for easier identification and navigation.

The MetraPass suture passer is then inserted through the skin nick, fascia, and muscle, and finally into and down the length of the round ligament to the uterus (Figures 24.12 and 24.13). Permanent or absorbable 'O' suture is then placed into the jaws of the suture passer. The instrument is then removed, taking with it the suture out the skin nick (Figure 24.14). Once through the same nick again, traverse the length of the round

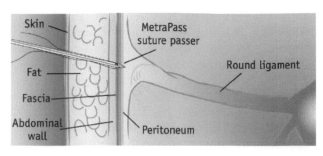

Figure 24.12 The UPLIFT procedure. The MetraPass suture passer is then inserted through the skin nick, fascia, and muscle.

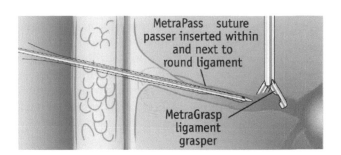

Figure 24.13 The UPLIFT procedure. Then finally into and down the length of the round ligament to the uterus.

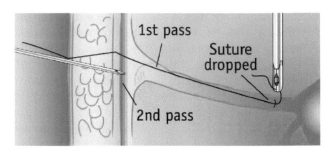

Figure 24.14 The UPLIFT procedure. Permanent or absorbable 'O' suture is then placed into the jaws of the suture passer. The instrument is then removed, taking with it the suture out the skin nick.

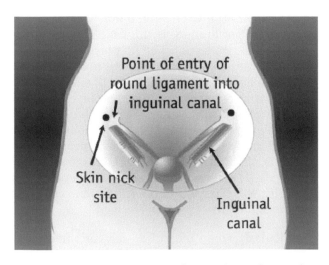

Figure 24.11 The UPLIFT procedure. A skin nick is made laterally and cephalad to the point of insertion.

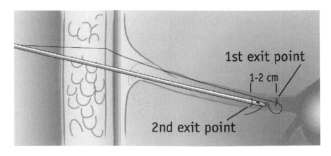

Figure 24.15 The UPLIFT procedure. Once through the same nick again, traverse the length of the round ligament with the suture passer and exit the tip approximately 1 cm away from the original suture passer exit site.

ligament with the suture passer and exit the tip approximately 1 cm away from the original suture passer exit site (Figure 24.15). If the round ligament becomes friable during either excursion of the suture passer, simply weave in and out of the ligament. Grasp the opposite end of the suture and carry it back through the round ligament and out the original skin nick: not only is the round ligament injected with suture but also a fascial bridge is now created between each end of suture.

The procedure is repeated on the opposite side. Once completed, the assistant holding the uterine manipulator anteflexes the uterus. Each suture is then tied, ideally at the same time to keep the uterus midline (Figure 24.16).

At the conclusion, meticulous hemostasis must be noted. Interceed (Johnson & Johnson) or some other antiadhesion agent should then be used in the cul-de-sac.

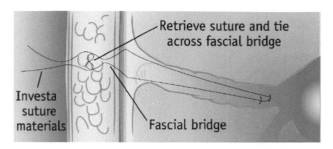

Figure 24.16 The UPLIFT procedure. Each suture is then tied, ideally at the same time to keep the uterus midline.

Acknowledgments

Courtesy, Ethicon Endo-Surgery, Inc. Figures reprinted with permission.

Courtesy, Inlet Medical, Inc. Figures reprinted with permission.

REFERENCES

1. Hambley R, Hebda PA, Abell E, et al. Wound healing of skin incisions produced by ultrasonically vibrating knife, scalpel, electrosurgery, and carbon dioxide laser. J Dermatol Surg Oncol 1988; 14(11): 1213–1217.
2. Amaral JF, Chrostek CA. A comparison of the lateral thermal effect of ultrasonic energy (level 3) to monopolar energy (30 watts) in the porcine model. SAGES (Society of American Gastrointestinal Endoscopic Surgeons) Conference, 1995.
3. Willging JP, Wiatrak BJ. Harmonic scalpel tonsillectomy in children: a randomized prospective study. Otolaryngol Head Neck Surg 2003; 128(3): 318–325.
4. Walker RA, Syed ZA. Harmonic scalpel tonsillectomy versus electrocautery tonsillectomy: a comparative pilot study. Otolaryngol Head Neck Surg 2001; 125(5): 449–455.
5. Armstrong DN, Ambroze WL, Schertzer ME, et al. Harmonic Scalpel vs. electrocautery hemorrhoidectomy: a prospective evaluation. Dis Colon Rectum 2001; 44(4): 558–564.
6. Tsimoyiannis EC, Jabarin M, Giantzounis G. Laparoscopic cholecystectomy using ultrasonically activated coagulating shears. Surg Laparosc Endosc 1998; 8(6): 421–424.
7. Landman J, Kerbl K, Rehman J, et al. Evaluation of a vessel sealing system, bipolar electrosurgery, harmonic scalpel, titanium clips, endoscopic gastrointestinal anastomosis vascular staples and sutures for arterial and venous ligation in a porcine model. J Urol 2003; 169(2): 697–700.

SECTION V
Pain and Infertility

25 Treatment of pain associated with endometriosis

John F Steege, Georgine Lamvu, and Denniz Zolnoun

Introduction

This chapter will review:

- six areas of methodologic concern pertinent to the evaluation of literature dealing with the treatment of pain associated with endometriosis
- clinical evaluation
- medical management

Methodologic concerns

Endometriosis is a chronic illness that has a potentially substantial impact on the individual dealing with the disease, as well as her family. Evaluation and measurement of her pain and its response to treatment is made difficult by:

1. Methodologic difficulties in measuring pain, especially when chronic.
2. Incomplete understanding of the mechanism(s) of pain production from endometriosis.
3. The impact of the hormonal environment upon pain perception itself.
4. Differences in intensity of the placebo effect seen when comparing medical and surgical therapies.
5. The tendency for chronic pain to progressively involve additional surrounding organ systems beyond the reproductive tract.
6. The meaning of the pain in the day-to-day life of the woman with endometriosis.

Pain measurement

As a multidimensional phenomenon, pain has been subjected to attempted measurement from a variety of perspectives. For example, the McGill pain questionnaire[1] has subscales that measure the sensory, affective, and other components of the pain experience with reasonable reliability. Although easier to use, a simple linear scale, such as the visual analog scale (VAS),[2] may combine two or more of these elements of the pain experience to different degrees in different people. This concern and others have led to the recommendation to treat VAS data in nonparametric fashion, rather than assume linearity of the scale and thus treat it in parametric fashion.

Either of these two scales is nevertheless an improvement over earlier scales frequently used in assessment of pain in endometriosis, such as the Biberoglu and Behrman scale.[3] This measure has been used, in various versions, without validation against scales that have been more rigorously tested. Most versions still measure more than one variable within a single scale. There remains a need for a well-validated scale or set of scales to measure pain in women with endometriosis.

Mechanisms of nociception and pain production in endometriosis

In endometriosis, volume of disease does not correlate with clinical pain. A generation ago, clinicians generally taught that pain was inversely proportional to the volume of disease: i.e. those with a little bit of endometriosis had a lot of pain and vice versa. Subsequent studies supported the view that the amount of infiltrative cul-de-sac disease may be proportional to perceived pain,[4–6] whereas some emphasize ovarian disease[7] and others reported that volume of disease has no coherent relationship to pain, being neither directly nor inversely proportional.[8] Our understanding of the mechanisms of nociception in endometriosis remains primitive.

Type of disease, as well as location and volume, may be relevant to pain. Over the last 15 years, many authors have recognized that endometriosis can appear in a variety of different forms in the female pelvis, from clear vesicles, to red flame-like lesions, to dark pigmented lesions with hemosiderin, to white scarring, etc. In earlier gynecologic literature, for example, white scarred endometriosis was described as 'burned out,' implying that it might no longer play a role in symptom production. However, biopsies of such areas often show active endometriosis, and excision often relieves pain.

The three most commonly suggested mechanisms for pain production in endometriosis are:

1. Production of humoral factors such as growth factors and cytokines by activated macrophages and other cells associated with functioning endometriosis implants.[9]
2. The direct and indirect effects of active bleeding from endometrial implants.
3. Irritation of pelvic floor nerves or direct invasion of those nerves by infiltrating endometriosis implants, especially in the cul-de-sac.[10]

It remains plausible, of course, that in any individual more than one or all of these mechanisms may be in operation.

The prostaglandin/other humoral theory is supported by the common clinical experience that many women with endometriosis benefit from analgesics with prostaglandin synthesis inhibiting properties. However, data from clinical examinations and laparoscopic evaluations would suggest in general that when disease is unilateral, pain remains unilateral as well, suggesting that the range of these proposed humoral mechanisms is short.[11]

The localization of pain in its relationship to implants has been explored by the technique of pain mapping under conscious sedation during minilaparoscopy. Demco demonstrated sensitivity in normal-appearing peritoneum in the vicinity of endometriosis implants.[12] On the other hand, Howard et al's detailed study suggests that hemosiderin-laden implants and fibrotic implants are more clearly associated with pain production, with the role of the clear vesicular lesions much less clear.[13] The technique of pain mapping under conscious sedation is a highly operator-dependent clinical art form, the results of which can be profoundly influenced by patient selection, preoperative education, investigator bias, and the nuances of the technique itself. Further work on standardizing this procedure, with calibrated pressure transducers, etc., would be a welcome advance.

Cross-sectional clinical data[14] imply that endometriosis follows a natural progression, from clear vesicles, to red flame-like lesions, to hemosiderin-laden lesions to fibrotic scarred lesions. This generalization seems to apply to those implants located on the peritoneum. Ovarian endometriomas and infiltrative cul-de-sac disease may not follow the same progression. It is also entirely uncertain whether all clear vesicular lesions share the same ultimate destiny of progressing to fibrotic lesions over time, or whether only a subset will follow this path. These questions have profound clinical importance, as we struggle to decide which lesions merit treatment and how aggressive that treatment should be.

In terms of the second commonly voiced hypothetical mechanism for nociception, direct bleeding from endometriosis implants, very little direct evidence exists that this occurs in any great volume. Blood found in the cul-de-sac during laparoscopy is more likely to result from retrograde menstruation rather than direct bleeding from established peritoneal implants. Small amounts of localized bleeding into the peritoneum itself may account for hemosiderin deposition, and the irritation from that bleeding may account for some chronic nociception. If this mechanism were to be important, it would provide an insufficient overall explanatory hypothesis, as pain from this disorder often remains cyclic whereas hemosiderin deposits do not come and go.

The third hypothesis, neural irritation or invasion, has gathered much support over the past decade. The association of infiltrating, nodular endometriosis with pain was noted as early as 1946 by Fallon et al[15] and described in more detail by Sturgis and Call a decade later.[16] More recent clinical series have documented that tender nodularity detected in the cul-de-sac and the uterosacral ligament area is a clinical criterion with approximately 85% sensitivity and 50% specificity for the diagnosis of infiltrative endometriosis.[5] Women with such findings on pelvic examination will very commonly have deep dyspareunia and more severe dysmenorrhea. Those women with infiltration of the uterosacral ligaments and/or diseases directly adjacent to or invading the rectal wall will have dyschezia as well.[4]

Several lines of evidence suggest that the fibrotic infiltrative form of endometriosis is different from the peritoneal disease in several important characteristics:

1. Estrogen and progesterone receptor titers are significantly lower in this form of the disease, suggesting that this form of the disease may respond less well to hormonal manipulation than its counterpart on the peritoneal surface.[16,17]
2. The intensity of pain associated with these lesions has been correlated with the depth of the lesion, with the greatest pain seen when the depth exceeds 6 mm below the peritoneal surface.[5]
3. Both perineural inflammation and direct infiltration of nerves by endometriosis have been observed.[18] This type of histologic change is infrequent in human disease and resembles the type of neural invasion seen in pancreatic cancer, a very painful disease. To date, this neural invasion has been seen only in central pelvic disease, i.e. around the uterosacrals and in the cul-de-sac, and has not been observed in other areas of peritoneal endometriosis or in ovarian disease.

In summary, it would appear that the pain associated with endometriosis may be produced by a variety of mechanisms. The best-elucidated mechanism would appear to be nerve root irritation by the invasive fibrotic posterior cul-de-sac implant. These various sources of nociception that arise from the pelvic tissues may then wend their way toward conscious perception, modulated by the multiple influences described below.

The impact of the hormonal environment on pain perception

It would appear that estrogen levels might play a significant role in modulation of pain perception, at least at a somatic level. A meta-analysis of 16 studies of experimentally induced pain demonstrated that somatic pain sensory pain thresholds were lower (i.e. sensitivity to pain was greater) by about 40% in the immediately premenstrual and menstrual phases of the cycle.[19] Similar exploration of the menstrual cycle's impact upon vis-

ceral pain thresholds, e.g. by rectal manometry, needs to be carried out. This observation is consistent with the well-documented phenomenon of increased symptoms for irritable bowel syndrome (IBS) premenstrually and menstrually, even though bowel motility does not seem to change measurably in women with IBS during these time periods.

In a study of menopausal women with or without estrogen replacement, *somatic* pain thresholds were lowered by half in women on estrogen.[20] The impact of estrogen on visceral pain thresholds would be of obvious interest.

Variations in the placebo effect

The magnitude of the placebo effect may vary with the type of endpoint measured and the type of therapy. Studies monitoring the subjective endpoint of pain often show placebo effects in the range of 40–45%. The same magnitude has been seen in multiple studies of premenstrual syndrome, another disorder with subjective endpoints. Many authors, and the average reader, often assume that a placebo response usually occurs in 30–35% of subjects and may last for 2–3 months. However, two placebo-controlled trials of a surgical intervention (internal mammary artery ligation) for coronary artery disease demonstrated placebo effects of 55 and 100% at 1 year following the procedure.[21] It would appear that surgical therapies for endometriosis may require more long-term evaluation than medical therapies.

Impacts of the chronicity of pain

Pain theory has evolved into ever-more complex models over the past 50 years. The Cartesian theory of pain perception gave way to the gate control theory proposed in 1965 by Melzack and Wall; this was felt to be insufficient to explain many clinical observations of pain and has, in turn, yielded to the neuromatrix theory.[22] In brief, these modifications of earlier pain theories attempt to take into account the complexity of spinal cord mechanisms that may serve a quasi-memory function in chronic pain. More specifically, nociceptive signals emanating from visceral sources may, with time, spread to somatic dermatomes whose nerve supply arises from the same spinal cord segment that supplies a given viscus. In the phenomenon of viscerosomatic convergence, pain may come to emanate from the somatic portion of this mechanism as well as the visceral. Therapies aimed entirely at the visceral origination of the pain may therefore fall short.

Psychologic considerations

By virtue of their own experience, many women with endometriosis soon learn that clinicians lack accurate noninvasive tools for assessing progression of the disease. Pelvic examination is notoriously inaccurate in estimating the volume of endometriosis, and X-ray, ultrasound, and magnetic resonance imaging (MRI) have not improved this overall picture. Laparoscopy remains the gold standard and is sufficiently sensitive to pick up the vast majority of endometriosis lesions. Only one study suggests that, using scanning electron microscopy techniques, microscopic endometriosis may elude detection with laparoscopy in 25% of cases.[23] However, Howard et al's study would suggest that these forms of the disease may play a lesser, if any, role in the pain of endometriosis.[13] This study and others[24] maintain that almost all endometriosis on the peritoneum can be visually detected.

In view of this diagnostic difficulty, the patient with endometriosis often comes to trust her own pain sensations as the best indicator of whether or not the disease is progressing. Fortunately, most endometriosis progresses very slowly, but the informed patient is aware that there are uncommon, but not rare, exceptions to this general rule. When the woman experiences an increase in pain, her understandable conclusion may be that the disease must be rapidly changing, although most often this is not the case. When she also understands the shortcomings of all of the medical and surgical therapies, its impact upon fertility, and the substantial probability of requiring extirpative surgery at some point in her life, the day-to-day stress and anxiety that are part of the disease are understandable. Both anxiety and depression may co-evolve with any chronic pain disorder and may, by spinal cord and central mechanisms, alter pain perception itself, thus contributing to the suffering.

From the above brief review, it is apparent that measuring changes in pain in response to treatments is difficult. Nevertheless, substantial shifts in treatment philosophy need to await the completion of thorough well-designed and replicated treatment trials. The design of such trials should take into account the need to assess pelvic pain using the history and physical examination techniques listed below.

Clinical evaluation of the patient

History

The evolution of pain associated with endometriosis follows a stereotypic pattern in the majority of women with this disorder. A small minority present with patterns and locations of pain that defy understanding. The stereotypic pattern begins with severe dysmenorrhea, often starting soon after menarche. The duration of severe pain, starting with the beginning of menstruation, gradually increases, with the second, third, and fourth days of flow being accompanied by pain just as intense as the first day. As the intensity increases, various (probably prostaglandin-mediated) symptoms may appear, such as nausea, vomiting, and diarrhea. Over years, the pain may start occurring before each menstrual flow begins, and cyclic (later continuous) deep dyspareunia may ensue. As progressively more of the menstrual month becomes involved with pain, dyschezia may begin in those destined to have posterior cul-de-sac involvement close to or in the bowel wall.

Many women note premenstrual alterations of bowel function, being somewhat constipated during the week prior to the onset of menses, then noting looser stools during the menstrual days. In women with endometriosis, this pattern may be accentuated, or symptoms consistent with true IBS may be present. As the duration of pain across the menstrual month increases, so may the IBS symptoms.

Along with associated bowel symptoms, an unknown proportion of women will develop bladder symptoms of frequency, urgency, and nocturia, sometimes reaching the degree seen in interstitial cystitis. The prevalence and the etiology of this association remain unknown.

With time and increasing discomfort often comes symptoms emanating from the musculoskeletal system. Visceral pain may be referred to muscles (adnexa to abdominal wall, vaginal apex to abdominal wall). Decreased physical activity and altered posture may result in 'adaptive shortening' of muscles that may subsequently hurt when pressed or stretched. Painful muscles may then become autonomous pain generators. The levator floor of the pelvis commonly reacts to any chronically painful disorder in the pelvis, regardless of etiology and, likewise, become a self-sustaining source of pain.

Living with symptoms of this magnitude often then becomes a way of life, as opposed to a subtext in an otherwise productive existence. Deconditioning, loss of physical capacity, fatigue, sleep disorder, sexual dysfunction, and disrupted relationships may ensue.

In taking such a history, the clinician is challenged to correlate changes in organic pathology and responses of such pathology to medical and surgical interventions. In many cases, and especially in cases of long-standing, a clear correlation is often either obscure or lacking almost entirely. When one focuses entirely on the disease implants as the culprit, it becomes overwhelmingly tempting, when relief is less than wished, to treat ever more aggressively. In our pelvic pain clinic, we routinely see women in their mid-twenties who have undergone complete hysterectomy and bilateral salpingo-oophorectomy for pain attributed to stage I endometriosis. Thorough evaluation of such women almost always reveals multiple other contributors to their pain that have never been evaluated or treated.

Understanding the multiple factors that may contribute to a person's pain begins with a careful *chronologic* history, as described above. Included in this, of course, is a review of precisely what improvements occurred in response to the treatments undertaken. The assessment continues with a physical examination that looks for multiple components, and looks for them in a manner very different from the routine pelvic examination.

Physical examination

When the history indicates a more complex or long-standing pain problem, the examination begins with the clinician getting ready to make a mental list of components rather than searching for *the* cause of the pain. It works best to let the patient know this is what you are doing, so she does not keep listening for *the* answer.

In addition to a modified pelvic examination, as described below, evaluation of musculoskeletal components is often extremely useful.[25] To begin, attend to the patient's body mechanics from the start. The more that muscular components play a role, the more that the patient may walk stiffly with less arm swing, sit down gingerly, sit with her weight shifted to one buttock, or slump forward in the chair with her weight more squarely on the ischial tuberosities. The last three postural changes are typically seen in a woman with levator spasm: seeing any of these should prompt the examiner to ask the woman if pelvic *pressure* is part of what she feels. The typical response is some version of, 'Yes, it feels as though everything

is going to fall out,' when no deficit of pelvic support is present. This response is virtually *diagnostic* of significant levator spasm.

Before the woman gets undressed for the pelvic examination, ask her to bend forward to touch her toes. If she has weak low back muscles, she will often stop when the fingertips reach the knees, and will complain of pain in the low back when tender sacroiliac joints, arthritis, or soft tissue abnormalities are present.

When you enter the examining room, your patient will typically be sitting up on the end of the examination table. Take this opportunity to palpate the sacroiliac (S-I) joints, ask if they are tender, and ask if any pain felt there travels anywhere else and/or reproduces any of their typical pain. We have seen many women in whom palpation of an S-I joint reproduced *anterior* lower quadrant pain that had been mistakenly attributed to pelvic pathology (Table 25.1).

Then observe how readily the patient goes from the sitting to the supine position. The woman with intrinsic abdominal wall pain, low back pain, or weak abdominal muscles will often rotate to one side, lean on one elbow, and let herself down gradually to the supine position. She will get partially down, then allow herself to drop to the table, once she knows that the distance she drops will be small enough so the landing won't hurt.

When she is supine, ask her to point with one finger to the location of maximum pain, and draw a circle with her finger around the area of the pain. Ask her to point to where the pain may radiate from this main location. Then ask her to press down on the spot of maximal pain, using just enough pressure to elicit the pain. The person with referred pain to the abdominal wall, or in whom the abdominal wall has become a nociception generator in itself, will report pain in response to minimal pressure. Ask her to press down and let go quickly, although true rebound tenderness is rare in the chronic pain patient. Finally, ask her to lift her head slightly off the table so as to tense the abdominal wall and repeat the pressure maneuver. If tenderness to her palpation *decreases* while tensing the abdominal wall, then the source of pain is more likely to be *internal* (visceral) in nature. However, if palpation with the abdominal wall tensed produces *increased* pain, then the abdominal wall itself is part of the problem (Carnett's sign).

Now you're ready to start your part of the examination. You may wish to repeat the above maneuvers with your own hand in order to calibrate how

Table 25.1 Musculoskeletal origins of chronic pelvic pain

Structure	Innervation	Referred pain site(s)	Common disorders
Hip	T12–S1	Lower abdomen; anterior medial thigh; knee	DJD; capsular stiffness or inflammation; bursitis
Lumbar ligaments, facets/disks	T12–S1	Low back; posterior thigh and calf; lower abdomen; lateral trunk; buttock	DJD; capsular entrapments; instability; herniation; capsular stiffness and inflammation
Sacroiliac joints	L4–S3	Posterior thigh; buttock; pelvic floor, anterior lower quadrant	Acute strain; laxity, displacement
Abdominal muscles	T5–L1	Abdomen; anteromedial thigh; sternum	Weakness; strain; diastasis; trigger points
Iliopsoas	L1–L4	Lateral trunk; lower abdomen; low back; anterior thigh	Adaptive shortening; trigger points; protective guarding
Piriformis	L5–S3	Low back; buttock; pelvic floor	Adaptive shortening; trigger points; protective guarding
Pubococcygeus	S1–S4	Pelvic floor; vagina; rectum; buttock	Adaptive shortening; weakness; lengthening strain; trigger points
Obturator internal/external	L3–S2	Pelvic floor; buttock; anterior thigh	Adaptive shortening; protective guarding; weakness
Quadratus lumborum	T12–3	Anterior lateral trunk; anterior thigh; lower abdomen	Adaptive shortening; weakness

DJD = degenerative joint disease

much pressure it took to produce pain. Then examine any tender areas carefully with one fingertip, approaching the tender area slowly from its perimeter, repeating this maneuver by approaching the area slowly from its superior, inferior, medial, and lateral borders. In the course of single-digit palpation of the tender area, note any areas of exquisite tenderness, and mark them with a pen so that you might later return to give a trigger point injection to this spot (Table 25.2).

Some typical referral patterns are worth mentioning at this point. Adnexal pain typically refers to the lower quadrant abdominal wall nearest the adnexum in question. Vaginal apex pain (in someone who has had hysterectomy) will often refer to a small (2 cm diameter or so) area about 5 cm cephalad to the inguinal ligament and 5 cm lateral from the midline. Uterine pain refers to the lower anterior abdominal wall and down the medial aspect of either or both thighs. Uterosacral pain may refer to the mid-sacral area of the low back, in a pattern quite distinct from the S-I joints.

All of these manipulations, with practice, may be accomplished in 3–5 minutes. You are now ready to begin the pelvic examination.

When the history includes complaints of introital pain, careful examination of the vulva is indicated. Make careful note of abnormalities of pigmentation, skin lesions, whitening that may indicate lichen sclerosis, and inflammatory changes. The most common underdiagnosed conditions we see are monilial vulvitis (symmetrical, well-demarcated erythema) and vulvar vestibulitis (focal erythema and sensitivity in the vestibule, especially the posterior half). Some clinicians have speculated that there may be an association between vestibulitis and endometriosis, the common denominator being decreased ability to counteract inflammation.

To detect vestibulitis, separate the labia with two fingers of your nondominant hand, and use a cotton-tipped applicator held in the other hand to gently touch the vestibule. In most circumstances,

Table 25.2 Referred pain: female urogenital system

Structure	Segmental innervation	Potential site for local referred pain
Ovaries	T10–T11	Lower abdomen, low back
Uterus	T10–L1	Lower abdomen, low back
Fallopian tubes	T10–L1	Lower abdomen, low back
Perineum	S2–S4	Sacral apex, suprapubic, rectum
External genitalia	L1–L2, S3–S4	Lower abdomen, medial anterior thigh, sacrum
Kidney	T10–L1	Ipsilateral low back and upper abdominal
Urinary bladder	T11–L2, S2–S4	Thoracolumbar, sacrococcygeal, suprapubic
Ureters	T11–T2, S2–S4	Groin, upper and lower abdomen, suprapubic, anteromedial thigh, thoracolumbar

the most sensitive area is the posterior vestibule, between the 3 and 9 o'clock positions, so it is best to touch starting anteriorly, alternating sides (11, 1, 10, 2, 9, 3 o'clock, etc.).

The speculum examination is next, ideally using a narrow Pederson speculum. If this does not afford an adequate view of the fornices so as to allow inspection of the vaginal mucosa in search of endometriosis implants, then a larger speculum may be needed.

The remainder of the pelvic examination consists of two parts:

- discovering areas of pain
- assessing the size, shape, and mobility of the reproductive organs.

The techniques used for each of these examinations are quite different from each other.

To examine for painful areas, use only the index finger of your dominant hand. Begin by pressing the levators, first at 5 o'clock (left levator), then at 7 o'clock (right levator). Ask if pressure in these areas reproduces the clinical complaint in any way. Ask for contraction/relaxation of the levators to evaluate the patient's control. Asking the patient to 'tighten as if you were holding back a bowel movement' usually results in contraction of the levators. If palpation of the levators reproduces an important part of the pain, but the woman has no success in voluntarily tightening and relaxing them, then pelvic floor physical therapy and/or biofeedback may be needed for her to learn this skill.

Next, supinate the examining hand and palpate the urethra and bladder base. In cases of chronic urethritis or interstitial cystitis, this maneuver usually elicits focal pain. Again, ask if the clinical pain is reproduced. Similarly, in sequence, you should then elicit responses to traction of the cervix in four directions and single-digit palpation of the adnexal areas. When tenderness is elicited, then again examine the abdominal wall for tenderness (with one external hand), repeat the transvaginal single-digit examination, and then finally do your bimanual examination.

The standard bimanual examination is reserved for last, in order to first evaluate the separate contributions of the viscera and the abdominal wall. When both hands are used right from the start, the typical gynecologist interprets any discomfort elicited as due to the pelvic viscera, when this may not be the case.

Several more components need emphasis. A rectovaginal examination is mandatory when examining to evaluate a pain problem. Although this has always been standard teaching, it is surprising how often this is omitted. Focal sensitivity, and certainly nodularity, may betray uterosacral endometriosis. The ability of this examination to detect disease may be increased by exerting anterior traction on the cervix with the vaginal finger while sliding the rectal finger along each uterosacral ligament in turn.

Finally, the piriformis and obturator muscles should be checked. These muscles have the function of externally rotating the leg. Spasm in these muscles can develop as a reaction to other painful stimuli in the pelvis, or may be brought on by exercise trauma and mimic gynecologically derived pain. Both muscles may be palpated trans-vaginally: the obturator, by pressing straight later-ally in the mid-vagina (3 and 9 o'clock); the piriformis, by pressing just posteriorly and cepha-lad to the ischial spines. The muscles should be palpated vaginally while the patient externally rotates each leg in sequence against resistance provided by your other hand.

Whenever tender areas are discovered during the examination, it may be useful to interpret them to the patient, verbally adding to the list of con-tributing factors to be discussed again during your summary.

Laboratory studies

When evaluating acute pain, transvaginal ultra-sound is frequently useful to document ovarian cysts, ectopic pregnancy, and the like. When the pain is chronic, this study and others – MRI and computed tomography (CT) – have far less utility, as the organic disorders that most commonly con-tribute to chronic pain (endometriosis and adhe-sions) are not usually well visualized by these approaches. Certainly, when body habitus or guarding limit the examination, such studies can be helpful. When a good examination has been done but the diagnosis is uncertain, ultrasounds and other imaging techniques have almost no value as a 'fishing expedition'.

Particular mention needs to be made of endometriosis invading the rectosigmoid colon. Dyschezia, often of quite intense degree, often accompanies this problem. The pain may start out associated with menses only, then gradually be present throughout the menstrual month. The bar-ium enema or a transrectal ultrasound are the appropriate studies.[26] Flexible sigmoidoscopy or colonoscopy are most often negative, even in the face of substantial invasion of the colon, since the overlying mucosa is usually intact. The colono-scopist may only see the impression of a slight bulge into the colon, which usually is not sufficient to call pathology.

Laparoscopy

It is our position that laparoscopy should be rou-tinely performed before embarking on more inten-sive medical therapy, such as gonadotropin-releasing hormone (GnRH) agonist injections, for reasons elaborated below. The technique of laparoscopy is extensively described in other chapters of this book. We will only add that we find it most useful to examine the pelvic floor and cul-de-sac tissues by performing rectovaginal examination with one hand, while guiding a 5 mm laparoscopic probe over the pelvic floor with the other. The uterosacral ligaments, cul-de-sac tis-sues, and adjacent rectal wall can be systemati-cally examined by moving probe and fingers together and sweeping from one side to the other. Any retroperitoneal disease present will be readily detected by this method.

The peritoneum should be examined at a close range of 1–2 cm to avoid missing nonpigmented disease. Sufficient still photos are helpful in teaching the patient and her family about the extent of her disease.

Medical management

Endocrine measures

Over the past 5 years, there has been a growing tendency to employ GnRH agonists relatively early in the evaluation and treatment of pelvic pain. We frequently see them used whenever cyclic oral contraceptives do not provide suffi-cient relief. This approach is based on three *erroneous* ideas:

1. If pain goes away when a GnRH agonist is given, then the pain is almost certainly caused by endometriosis (or at least originates from the reproductive organs).
2. GnRH agonists are more effective in treating endometriosis than any other hormonal measures.
3. Even if laparoscopy does not reveal endo-metriosis, it is probably present microscop-ically and is still the culprit.

As described above, when menstrual cyclicity is eliminated, pain may decrease even if the noci-ceptive source is not in the reproductive organs. A randomized, double-blind, controlled trial of estrogen replacement in hysterectomized post-menopausal women showed that estrogen increased pain sensitivity.[20] Eliminating estrogen by means of a GnRH agonist injection may dimin-ish many types of pain that are not emanating from the reproductive organs.

Cochrane reviews of studies comparing GnRH agonists with Danocrine (danazol), progestins, antiprogestins, and oral contraceptives failed to find methodologically acceptable studies that showed GnRH agonists to be superior to any of these other better-tolerated agents.[27–30]

The role of microscopic endometriosis in pain or infertility is unclear at present. A pain-mapping study showed that pain was elicited only from implants that were confirmed to be endometriosis by light microscopic study of biopsies.[13] An often-quoted study showed that in visibly normal pelvic peritoneum taken from women with visible endometriosis in other locations, scanning electron microscopy found endometrial glands in samples taken from visually normal peritoneum in 25% of women sampled.[23] Other studies consistently show that visual detection of endometriosis has very high sensitivity, but only modest specificity when compared to light microscopically documented disease in biopsies.[24] The pelvic floor examination described above as part of diagnostic laparoscopy should most often detect disease hiding beneath a visibly normal peritoneum.[4]

One recent study merits more detailed analysis in view of its potential impact on clinical practice.[31] This study tested the hypothesis that clinical history and physical examination could predict the presence of endometriosis with reasonable accuracy. Participating women had moderate-to-severe chronic pelvic pain that was unrelated to menstruation and incompletely relieved by nonsteroidal anti-inflammatory drugs (NSAIDs). In addition, their pain had failed to respond to a therapeutic trial of doxycycline, 100 mg twice daily for 10 days. The women were randomly allocated to treatment with a placebo injection or depot leuprolide 3.75 mg monthly for 3 months. Laparoscopy was then performed and the pelvic pathology scored using the revised American Fertility Society (r-AFS) score classification system. Of the 95 women, 78 (82.1%) had endometriosis with a mean score slightly above 4 on the rAFS scale. Women given depot leuprolide were amenorrheic. This group clearly had greater relief of dysmenorrhea, pelvic pain, and dyspareunia when evaluated after 3 months of treatment.

While the strict clinical criteria employed in the study were found to predict the presence of endometriosis 82% of the time, the response to depot leuprolide did not accurately diagnose the presence of endometriosis. Of 33 women with endometriosis given depot leuprolide, 27 (81.8%) experienced pain relief. Among 11 women without endometriosis given depot leuprolide, a statistically equivalent 8 (72.7%) noted relief of pain. This nonspecific effect of depot leuprolide on pelvic pain not associated with endometriosis might be accounted for by the impact of estrogen levels on pain threshold discussed above, the

effect of depot leuprolide on irritable bowel symptoms, or to the difficulties in maintaining a truly double-blind study when one treatment produces complete amenorrhea.

Since the publication of this study, depot leuprolide has been advocated as a treatment that should be employed for presumed endometriosis without performing laparoscopy. The arguments in favor of this approach include avoiding the risks and expense of surgery. The arguments against this approach include:

1. The likelihood that in general clinical practice the accuracy of clinical diagnosis will not be as great as that seen in a well-structured study.
2. The cumulative expense of this drug over years.
3. The absence of data supporting the contention that this drug is more effective than other less-expensive and better-tolerated medical therapies.
4. The failure of response to GnRH agonists to diagnose endometriosis (IBS may be improved by these drugs).[32]
5. The considerable probability that pain will recur after the drug is stopped. In this event, laparoscopy is only likely to be delayed (at considerable expense) rather than avoided.

Having stated that relief of pain by GnRH agonists does not diagnose endometriosis, conversely, when pain fails to respond to GnRH agonist therapy, it is unlikely that endometriosis is to blame, unless extensive fibrotic disease is present. The physical examination and laparoscopic techniques described above should detect this type of disease. Removing reproductive organs for minimal disease is unwise, if GnRH agonist therapy has not relieved the pain.

This said, we would recommend a common sense hierarchy for the hormonal management of pain attributed to endometriosis. We start with cyclic oral contraceptives, add NSAIDs, starting 5 days before the onset of menses, and move on to continuous oral contraceptives if these measures fail. Adding continuous progestin (norethindrone 5 mg/day) will provide relief for another large segment of the population. However, in women with this level of symptoms, distress is usually sufficiently high so as to warrant laparoscopy. We routinely employ careful excision techniques for most disease, except for the most superficial (freely mobile) peritoneal lesions.

If pain escapes control by these measures, in the absence of gross infiltrative disease, then we feel we have to be sure we haven't missed other factors.

Reviewing the history again and repeating the careful physical examination described above will usually reveal findings that prompt a broader range of treatments, as described below. We would strongly urge that this approach be employed before extirpative surgery is undertaken, especially if that surgery would close off reproductive options.

If initial evaluation detects contributions by other organ systems in women with endometriosis, it is often helpful to include treatments for these conditions in your therapeutic plan. For instance, physical therapy help for levator spasm, S-I joint pain, or hip muscle pain can often add to the benefits seen with hormonal therapies.

Pain modulators

Analgesics

Nonsteroidal anti-inflammatory drugs. The NSAIDs remain the mainstay of analgesic therapy for endometriosis. If they seem to be having diminishing impact on presumably primary dysmenorrhea, then endometriosis or other organic contributions to the pain should be investigated. At the same time, even when endometriosis is known to be present, these medications often remain at least ameliorative, and should be included along with hormonal or other treatments. The gastrointestinal side effects of the cyclooxygenase-2 (COX-2) inhibitors are less than those of their COX-1 predecessors, but not without increased cost. Insurance reimbursement for the COX-2 inhibitors is usually not provided in the absence of previous endoscopically documented gastric or duodenal ulceration.

Narcotics. Narcotic medications are substantially underutilized in the treatment of endometriosis and menstrually related pain. We find that when pain is limited to the days of menstruation, narcotics may be used quite safely and contribute substantially to improved quality of life. The caveats to this approach are:

- functional musculoskeletal pain does not respond well to narcotics
- some narcotics have mood-elevating effects that may lead to their use for what really is an anxiety or mood disorder
- narcotics should not be used in someone with a prior addiction problem of any type.

When pain is present for more than just the days of menstruation, narcotic management becomes more problematic. At this point, consultation with a pain clinic or a gynecologist skilled in pain management is advisable. By this time, the pain usu-ally requires more than 4–6 tablets of narcotic (e.g. oxycodone), and longer-acting agents warrant consideration. We prefer to use methadone in such situations, as it has no impact on mood, is long acting, very inexpensive, and generally well tolerated (Table 25.3).

When narcotics are given for more than a week out of each month, we present a narcotic contract to the patient. This is a written agreement similar to that used in many pain clinics, which insists that a patient agree to:

- use a set number of pills per day
- always obtain medications from the same pharmacy
- obtain controlled medications only from our clinic.

Further, medications may not be refilled early, and are not refilled if they are lost or stolen. Given these parameters, violations of the contract are relatively uncommon. We find it helps to mail the prescription renewals to the pharmacy rather than to the patient.

Antidepressants

Amitriptyline and nortriptyline have been mainstays of pain management for 50 years.[33] We find them helpful in chronic pelvic pain as well, especially when components of neuropathic pain are present (vulvar vestibulitis, vaginal apex pain after hysterectomy, trigger points, etc). In some patients, they will reduce bladder irritability symptoms. They are often effective in modest doses, between 10 and 75 mg qhs. Constipation is a common side effect that may need supportive care, and vaginal lubrication may diminish on these drugs as well. Dosing should start low (10–25 mg) and increase every 5–7 days, allowing 6 weeks for a full therapeutic trial. These drugs probably modulate pain more by virtue of their impact on the spinal cord and peripheral nerves, and less via central effects on mood.

The selective serotonin uptake inhibitors (SSRIs) provide another useful therapeutic modality for the treatment of mood disorders, although they do not have as clear a salutary effect on pain.

Antiepileptics

In some types of chronic pain, it has become common practice to employ large doses of gabapentin (Neurontin), between 1800 and 3600 mg total daily dose. There are no studies of this drug for treatment of pelvic pain. We find it occasionally quite helpful, but complicated by high cost, fre-

Table 25.3 Narcotics commonly used in chronic pain management

Drug name	Usual dose	Side effects
Hydrocodone bitartrate with acetaminophen: Lortab 2.5/500, 5/500 or 7.5/500 Vicodin 5/750 Lorcet 10/650 Lorcet Plus 7.5/650 (all are scored tablets)	5–10 mg hydrocodone either q6h or q8h Can use additional acetaminophen between doses to potentiate effect	Lightheadedness, dizziness, sedation, nausea and vomiting, and constipation. (These are *common side effects* of all narcotics.)
Oxycodone hydrochloride: Percocet 5 mg with 325mg acetaminaphen Percodan 5 mg with 325 mg aspirin (also contains 0.38 mg oxycodone terephthalate)	1 tablet q6h or q8h Additional acetaminophen between doses may serve to potentiate effect	*Common effects*
Oxycodone controlled-release: OxyContin	10–40 mg q12h	*Common effects*
Methadone hydrochloride: Dolophine 5 or 10 mg scored tablets	2.5 mg q8h to 10 mg q6h Commonly 15–20 mg qd	*Common effects* Lower extremity edema or joint swelling may occur and require discontinuation. Concurrent use of desipramine may increase methadone blood level. Cautious use in patients on monoamine oxidase inhibitors.
Acetaminophen with codeine: Tylenol No. 3, 300 mg acetaminophen with 30 mg codeine	1–2 tablets q6–8h	Common effects Constipation very likely. Nausea and vomiting more common than with other narcotics. More common allergy–rash.
Morphine sulfate: MS Contin or Oramorph	15–60 mg q12h; controlled-release tablets	*Common effects* Higher doses increase risk of respiratory depression.
Fentanyl transdermal system: Duragesic	25 μg patch, 1 q72h Also available in 50 or 75 μg Always start with lowest dose	*Common effects* Patch must be kept from heat sources or dose may be increased. Extreme caution in patients on other central nervous system medications. Respiratory depression can occur.

quent dosing, and substantial side effects. Other drugs in the same class include Lamictal (lamotrigine) and Tegretol (carbamazepine). Lamictal has the added benefit of being a mood-stabilizing medication, and has a more benign side-effect profile than the others in this class. It has a rare, but sometimes serious, side effect of a profuse and highly symptomatic rash. All the drugs in this class require slow up-titration, and take between 2–10 weeks to see therapeutic effect. Regimens this complex require substantial patient education to be effective.

Comorbid diagnoses and therapy

Consistent with the above discussion of history and physical examination, we feel that many women, especially those in whom pain has been present for years, experience symptoms in one or more of the organ systems that surround the reproductive tract. Over time, the neighboring systems seem to talk to each other, sharing conversations not necessarily in the best interest of the host. Although it can be difficult to tell who started the conversation, a careful history can help in this regard. At some point, however, it makes less difference who started it, as it is more productive to simply treat as many of the components as possible.

Bladder symptoms

Symptoms of nocturia (>2 per night), frequency (>8 per day), urgency, and postcoital dysuria are abnormal. The history may be elicited verbally or by questionnaire (e.g. Pelvic Pain and Urgency/Frequency Symptom Scale (PUF)).[34] Symptoms may be primary, as in the case of interstitial cystitis or bacterial urethritis; or secondary to other conditions, such as diminished vaginal lubrication due to hormonal therapies (continuous progestins, GnRH agonists, low-dose oral contraceptives), vaginal pathology (chronic vaginitis, vulvar vestibulitis), musculoskeletal dysfunction (especially levator spasm), or sexual dysfunction (e.g. vaginismus).

The practicing gynecologist can detect urethritis by examination (see above) and can treat it with a 3-month course of antibiotics (such as Macrodantin (nitrofurantoin), sulfonamides), followed by a dose of antibiotic pre- or postcoitally. Careful examination can often distinguish between bladder and urethral tenderness, and hence help the gynecologist determine whether or not a cystoscopy with hydrodistention is needed to look for interstitial cystitis.[35]

Treatment of interstitial cystitis is often best carried out in the hands of a willing and experienced urologist, as it often, as in the case of general pelvic pain, involves adjustment of multiple treatment measures and medications. It is our opinion that treatment with Elmiron should not be initiated on the basis of an elevated PUF scale score alone, as this scale can be high based on genrreral pelvic pain symptoms in the absence of specific bladder symptoms.

Bowel symptoms

Much anecdotal evidence suggests that bowel dysfunction, i.e. IBS, may either begin or be exacerbated in association with gynecologic disease, especially endometriosis. Studies performed in internal medicine settings have documented a higher prevalence of IBS in women undergoing hysterectomy, implying that bowel symptoms may masquerade as gynecologic symptoms, and prompt misguided surgery.[36] What has not yet been well studied is if in fact these bowel symptoms improve after hysterectomy, again suggesting cross-talk between the systems, rather than misdiagnosis or overemphasis of the gynecologic symptoms. Much anecdotal evidence in our pelvic pain clinic suggests that this may be so.

Along with measures aimed at endometriosis, the alert clinician should remain aware of and supportively treat bowel complaints. For example, defecation discomforts associated with cul-de-sac endometriosis may sometimes improve when stool softeners and other treatments for constipation are used.

Further research should be done on the interactions between the gastrointestinal and reproductive systems as they contribute to pelvic pain.

Musculoskeletal symptoms

Perhaps the single greatest contribution to our understanding of chronic pelvic pain in the past 25 years was the recognition by Baker, and Ling that the muscles of the pelvic floor and other muscle groups are frequently major contributors to pelvic pain.[25] The pain seen in women with endometriosis is no exception.

An analogy might be drawn to back pain. Most patients and physicians will recognize that muscle dysfunction can contribute to back pain, and may continue to plague a person when all other mechanical factors have been successfully treated. But few think of muscles as an important part of the pelvis (except, perhaps, our urogynecologic colleagues). In fact, discomforts arising from the levators very commonly join other factors in adding up to a continuous pelvic pain problem. Poorly understood interactions between these muscles and skin areas that may share innervation with them may play a role in many types of pelvic pain (e.g. vestibulitis).

In addition to the levators, the piriformis and obturator muscles may become dysfunctional in response to deconditioning and pain-induced changes in posture and body mechanics. The symptoms emanating from these muscles often include pain while moving the foot from the gas pedal to the brakes (or using the clutch), pain with the first few steps of the day, and pain when climbing stairs.

In the gynecologist's office, the diagnosis of these problems can readily be accomplished by history and physical examination (described above). Pelvic floor relaxation exercises can be taught. If insufficient progress is noted on re-examination, then referral to a qualified physical therapist should be considered.

Dyspareunia

On the list of symptoms that prompt help-seeking in women with endometriosis, painful intercourse is certainly close to the top. In addition to measures already described for treating the endometriosis itself, the suggestions listed here may be of help in overcoming this common and vexing problem. It is evident, in carefully reviewing treatment studies in endometriosis, that dyspareunia is the symptom most refractory to hormonal manipulations alone. We would strongly suspect, although this should be the target of much more research, that much of this pain is the final common pathway for multiple factors not directly related to the endometriosis implants.

Levator spasm, and its cousin, spasm of the introital muscles (vaginismus) are at the top of this list. This spasm may push the erect penis more firmly against the urethra during coitus, thus precipitating bacterial urethritis and cystitis, and perhaps aggravating interstitial cystitis. Exercises similar to the levator exercises may help vaginismus, but in many instances, the accompanying emotional distress makes it difficult for the couple to implement these suggestions. Referral for sexual counseling is indicated in this setting.

Diminished vaginal lubrication may accompany many of the hormonal regimens used to treat endometriosis, including the low-dose oral contraceptives. As a rule of thumb, when menstrual flow is markedly diminished, vaginal lubrication may also be decreased. Suggest supplemental lubrication with vegetable oil or one of the many good commercial lubricants.

In many women with posterior cul-de-sac endometriosis, pain with deep vaginal penetration is common. Two suggestions may help the couple deal with this:

- with sexual arousal, uterine elevation and vaginal lengthening take place, often moving tender spots out of the way
- using the cross-wise position for intercourse helps provide more control over the depth of penetration, thus allowing couples to stay with what is comfortable and pleasurable (Figure 25.1).

Depression

As can be the case with any chronic illness, depression can accompany the symptoms of the disease. In chronic pelvic pain in general, depres-

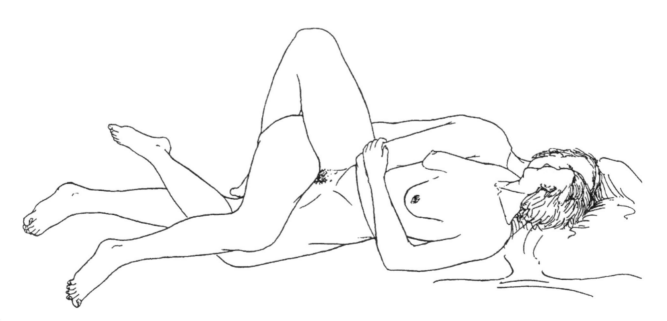

Fig. 25.1 The cross-wise position for intercourse. This position allows ready control over angle and depth of vaginal penetration. Neither partner is supporting his (her) weight, facilitating an unhurried approach.

sion seems most often to co-evolve with the progression of disease, as opposed to preceding it. It appears that depression is less often the 'cause' of the pain, and more often simply a part of the overall distress of the patient. In endometriosis in particular, the uncertainty of its progress and the inherent limitations of our monitoring methods adds to the mental stress of dealing with it.

Nevertheless, when depression symptoms are present, treatment with antidepressants may be helpful. If the tricyclic drugs have already been started for pain management, and the patient has become tolerant of the side effects, then simply increase the dose to the levels commonly used to treat depression (150–200 mg total daily dose). If not, then one of the SSRIs would be a better choice, as their side-effect profiles are superior.

Cognitive-behavioral therapies have gained popularity for the treatment of depression, and may also be helpful in chronic pain. Part and parcel of them are efforts to mobilize the energy a person does have, and engage in more positive and productive activities. This is especially helpful when a person with chronic pelvic pain is treating it as though it were simply acute pain that lasted longer: i.e. hoping that rest will bring about healing. When pain is chronic, rest has limited value, and often serves to further decondition the victim, and remove her from more and more of her usual activities and relationships.

Summary

There are probably at least several mechanisms operating in the nociception associated with endometriosis. Direct mass effect, neural invasion, prostaglandin and cytokine production, inflammation, and neural ingrowth are among the candidates. If one accepts this premise, then multimodal therapy is the logical sequel. Laparoscopic visualization and biopsy remain essential for diagnosis, and laparoscopic treatment performed at the same time makes sense in the hands of those trained to do it. Medication therapy should begin with the simpler endocrine measures, together with NSAIDs. A GnRH agonist should not be used presumptively, as it is very expensive, poorly tolerated, and leads to the wrong diagnostic conclusion in about 25% of cases. Improvement in pain in response to GnRH agonist treatment does not make the diagnosis of endometriosis.

When response to treatment is incomplete, or when pain recurs after initial effective treatment (either pharmacologic or surgical), the clinician must remain alert to the possible development of other contributing factors: symptoms from the gastrointestinal and urologic systems, musculoskeletal factors, neuropathic pain, and affective components. Better management of pain will result from thoughtful attention to all of these factors.

REFERENCES

1. Melzack R. The McGill pain questionnaire: major properties and scoring methods. Pain 1975; 1: 277–299.
2. Jensen MP, Karoly P. Self-report scales and procedures for assessing pain in adults. In Turk DC, Melzack R, eds. Pain measurement and assessment. New York: Raven Press; 1983.
3. Biberoglu KO, Behrman SJ. Dosage aspects of danazol therapy in endometriosis: short-term and long-term effectiveness. Am J Obstet Gynecol 1981; 139: 645–650.
4. Koninckx PR, Lesaffre E, Meuleman C, et al. Suggestive evidence that pelvic endometriosis is a progressive disease, whereas deeply infiltrating endometriosis is associated with pelvic pain. Fertil Steril 1991; 55: 759–765.
5. Ripps BA, Martin DC. Focal pelvic tenderness, pelvic pain and dysmenorrhea in endometriosis. J Reprod Med 1991; 36: 470–472.
6. Fukaya T, Hoshiai H, Yajima A. Is pelvic endometriosis always associated with chronic pain? A retrospective study of 618 cases diagnosed by laparoscopy. Am J Obstet Gynecol 1993; 169: 719–722.
7. Fedele L, Bianchi S, Bocciolone L, et al. Pain symptoms associated with endometriosis. Obstet Gynecol 1992; 79: 767–769.
8. Fedele L, Arcaini L, Parazzini F, et al. Stage and localization of pelvic endometriosis and pain. Fertil Steril 1990; 53: 155–158.
9. Harada T, Iwabe T, Terakawa N. Role of cytokines in endometriosis. Fertil Steril 2001; 76: 1–10.
10. Porpora MG, Koninckx PR, Piazze J, et al. Correlation between endometriosis and pelvic pain. J Am Assoc Gynecol Laparosc 1999; 6: 429–434.
11. Stout AL, Steege JF, Dodson WB, et al. Relationship of laparoscopic findings to self-report of pelvic pain. Am J Obstet Gynecol 1991; 164: 73–79.
12. Demco LA. Pain referral patterns in the pelvis. J Am Assoc Gynecol Laparosc 2000; 7: 181–183.
13. Howard FM, El-Minawi AM, Sanchez RA. Conscious pain

mapping by laparoscopy in women with chronic pelvic pain. Obstet Gynecol 2000; 96: 934–939.

14. Redwine DB. Age-related evolution in color appearance of endometriosis. Fertil Steril 1987; 48: 1062–1063.

15. Fallon J, Brosnan JR, Moran WG. Endometriosis: two hundred cases considered from the viewpoint of the practitioner. N Engl J Med 1946; 235: 669.

16. Sturgis SH, Call BJ. Endometriosis peritonei: relationship of pain to functional activity. Am J Obstet Gynecol 1954; 68: 1421–1431.

17. Donnez J, Gillet N, Nisolle M, et al. Peritoneal endometriosis and 'endometriotic' nodules of the rectovaginal septum are two different entities. Fertil Steril 1996; 66: 362–368.

18. Anaf V, Simon P, El Nakadi L, et al. Relationship between endometriotic foci and nerves in rectovaginal endometriotic nodules. Hum Reprod 2000; 15: 1744–1750.

19. Riley JL, Robinson ME, Wise EA, et al. A meta-analytic review of pain perception across the menstrual cycle. Pain 1999; 81: 225–235.

20. Fillingim RB, Edwards RR. The association of hormone replacement therapy with experimental pain responses in postmenopausal women. Pain 2001; 92(1–2): 229–234.

21. Turner JA, Deyo RA, Loeser JD, et al. The importance of placebo effects in pain treatment and research. JAMA 1994; 271: 1609–1614.

22. Melzack R. From the gate to the neuromatrix. Pain Suppl 1999; 6: S121–126.

23. Murphy AA, Green WR, de la Cruz ZC, et al. Unsuspected endometriosis documented by scanning electron microscopy in visually normal peritoneum. Fertil Steril 1986; 46: 522–524.

24. Balasch J, Creus M, Fabregues F, et al. Visible and non-visible endometriosis at laparoscopy in fertile and infertile women and in patients with chronic pelvic pain: a prospective study. Hum Reprod 1996; 11: 387–391.

25. Baker PT. Musculoskeletal problems. In: Steege JF, Metzger DA, Levy BS, eds. Chronic pelvic pain: an integrated approach. Phildelphia: WB Saunders; 1998: 215–240.

26. Chapron C, Vieira M, Chopin N, et al. Accuracy of rectal endoscopic ultrasonography and magnetic resonance imaging in the diagnosis of rectal involvement for patients presenting with deeply infiltrating endometriosis. Ultrasound Obstet Gynecol 2004; 24(2): 175–179.

27. Prentice A, Deary AJ, Bland E. Progestagens and anti-progestagens for pain associated with endometriosis (Cochrane Review). In: The Cochrane Library, Issue 2, 2001. Oxford: Update Software.

28. Vercellini P, Trespidi L, Colombo A, et al. A gonadotropin-releasing hormone agonist versus a low-dose oral contraceptive for pelvic pain associated with endometriosis. Fertil Steril 1993; 60: 75–79.

29. Selak V, Farquhar C, Prentice A, et al. Danazol for pelvic pain associated with endometriosis (Cochrane Review). In: The Cochrane Library, Issue 2, 2001. Oxford: Update Software.

30. Prentice A, Deary AJ, Goldbeck-Wood S, et al. Gonadotrophin-releasing hormone analogues for pain associated with endometriosis (Cochrane Review). In: The Cochrane Library, Issue 2, 2001. Oxford: Update Software.

31. Ling FW, for the Pelvic Pain Study Group. Randomized controlled trial of depot leuprolide in patients with chronic pelvic pain and clinically suspected endometriosis. Obstet Gynecol 1999; 93: 51–58.

32. Walker JJ, Irvine G. How should we approach the management of pelvic pain? Gynecol Obstet Invest 1998; 45(Suppl 1): 6–11.

33. Goodkin K, Gullion CM. Antidepressants for relief of chronic pain: do they work? Ann Behav Med 1989; 11: 83.

34. Parsons CL, Dell J, Stanford EJ, et al. Increased prevalence of interstitial cystitis: previously unrecognized urologic and gynecologic cases identified using a new symptom questionnaire and intravesical potassium sensitivity. Urology 2002; 60(4): 573–578.

35. Wall LL, Norton PA, DeLancey JOL. Practical urogynecology. Philadelphia: Williams and Wilkins; 1993: 268.

36. Prior A, Whorwell PJ. Gynecologic consultation in patients with the irritable bowel syndrome. Gut 1989; 30: 996.

26 Management of endometriosis and infertility following surgery

David Adamson

Endometriosis

Endometriosis is almost always diagnosed at the time of surgery, usually by laparoscopy or laparotomy. Following surgery, further decisions must be made regarding management of the previously infertile patient who wishes to conceive. Management decisions are complex because of the variability of endometriosis presentation, concomitant disease, outcome of the surgery, other infertility factors, multiple treatment options, and, until recently, a paucity of good studies to inform us of the best treatments. It is not surprising that many clinicians have been confused by the possibilities, resulting in less than optimal care for their patients.[1] However, current concepts increasingly based on reasonable data have resulted in a more evidence-based approach to treatment. Importantly, basic science initiatives should create better understanding and improved future management of this complex medical condition.[2,3] This chapter will present an approach to the post-surgery endometriosis infertility patient.

Evaluation of endometriosis surgery

The first responsibility of the treating physician is to evaluate the surgery that has just been performed. This will include the approach (laparotomy vs laparoscopy vs other), energy sources (e.g. electrosurgery, laser and type, Harmonic Scalpel, or other), techniques (e.g. ablation vs resection,

cystectomy vs coagulation), and skill of the surgeon. If the physician who will be managing the patient was the surgeon, this is much easier. However, this process still requires that the surgeon:

- be honest about the results of his own surgery
- have an objective recording of the findings and results of the surgery by using the American Society for Reproductive Medicine (ASRM) or other documentation forms, operative reports, photographs, and videos
- review any pathology reports.[4]

It is problematic that most surgeons describe the disease at the beginning of surgery in much greater detail than the status of the pelvis after the surgery has been performed. If the managing physician was not the surgeon, it is important to obtain as comprehensive as possible a record of the surgery and also to ask the patient about her understanding of the findings and results of the surgery. The managing physician can then determine the realistic probability of pregnancy with respect to the surgical outcome obtained.

Factors affecting management of infertility following surgery

There are numerous factors in addition to the outcome of surgery that can affect the probability a patient will conceive. Perhaps it is because of this that systems to predict pregnancy rates have been difficult to develop.[5,6] Analyzing varied treatment regimens retrospectively is always complicated.[7] However, recently an endometriosis fertility index (EFI) has been presented that shows promise in helping to evaluate patients' post-surgery probability of pregnancy.[8] In addition to surgical findings and pelvic status following operative intervention, the EFI includes age, duration of infertility, and prior gravidity in assessing the probability of pregnancy following surgery. Younger patients with a history of prior pregnancy and/or short duration of infertility are more likely to conceive with standard types of fertility treatment.[9,10] Other factors to consider include the number of prior operations and other diagnoses. For example, oligo-ovulation and male factor can affect chances for success. Such patients are likely to benefit relatively more from assisted reproductive technologies (ART) than patients with only endometriosis. Additionally, patients with endometriosis-associated pelvic pain are often not prepared to undergo prolonged fertility treatments or those that might exacerbate their pain, leading to alternative treatment choices. Finally, factors that are unrelated to the primary medical condition can have a major effect on management: other fertility and medical conditions, emotional condition of the patient, financial situation if infertility is not covered by health insurance, religious and moral perspectives on different types of treatment, and, finally, the patient's and her partner's wishes. The clinician must evaluate all of these factors in addition to the outcome of surgery before recommending a treatment plan.[11] Then the clinician must communicate effectively with the patient to ensure understanding and appropriate participation in decision-making.[12]

Outcomes of endometriosis surgery

The objective for infertility patients undergoing endometriosis surgery is to have all of the endometriotic disease removed and functionality of the pelvic organs enhanced. The clinician creating the postoperative management plan must have a clear idea of the outcome of the surgery based on the surgeon, extent of disease, surgical approach, surgical techniques, energy sources, and success of the operation. Not surprisingly, the skill and judgment of the surgeon along with the extent of the disease are the most important.

In patients with minimal or mild endometriosis, laparoscopic treatment has been used frequently because treatment can be accomplished easily during diagnostic laparoscopy.[13] However, the ablation or removal of endometriosis implants can increase the risk for post-surgical adhesion formation. Although an association clearly exists between even early stage disease and reproductive dysfunction, it has been unclear whether or not there is a cause–effect relationship between minimal/mild disease and infertility.[14–16] In the past decade, data have been reported that support the surgical approach to infertile patients with minimal or mild endometriosis. A meta-analysis of nonrandomized trials suggested that surgical treatment of early-stage endometriosis-associated infertility might be of value; however, there was sufficient heterogeneity among the studies to diminish confidence in such a conclusion. The average pregnancy rate from several studies evaluating the surgical approach was approximately 58% compared with an average pregnancy rate following expectant management of approximately 45% (Table 26.1).[3,14,17,18] However, the average monthly fecundity rate (in which it could be calculated) for expectant management was 6.8%. This was not significantly different than the monthly fecundity rate following surgery. Thus, the effectiveness of surgery for minimal or mild endometriosis has been difficult to prove.

In a prospective, multicenter, double-blinded, controlled, randomized study by Marcoux and colleagues in a Canadian collaborative trial named ENDOCAN, surgical treatment by laparoscopy resulted in a significantly higher pregnancy rate at 20 weeks than no treatment (29% vs 19%).[19] This study provides convincing evidence that surgery is beneficial in the treatment of minimal or mild endometriosis-associated infertility. Shortly thereafter, however, a second multicenter study demonstrated a live birth rate of 20% in the treatment group and 22% in the controls within 1 year of surgery.[20] When the results were combined, there was no significant statistical heterogeneity and the overall absolute difference was 8.6% in favor of therapy (95% confidence interval (CI), 2.1–15). The number needed to treat (NNT) is 12 (95% CI, 7–49). The Cochrane Review concluded the use of laparoscopic surgery in treatment of minimal and mild endometriosis may improve success rates.[21] Therefore, for every 12 patients found to have stage I/II endometriosis at laparoscopy, there will be 1 additional pregnancy if ablation/resection is performed compared to no treatment. There remain questions as to whether this small benefit is due to removal of adhesions rather than implants.[22]

It is widely accepted that endometriosis of sufficient severity to cause distortion of the pelvis (stages III and IV) impairs fertility by interfering with oocyte pickup and transport. Such anatomic

Table 26.1 Estimated cumulative life table pregnancy rates by treatment group for different stages of endometriosis

| | Entire patient population | | | | | Endometriosis-only subset | | | | |
| | No. | No. pregnant in 3 years | Pregnant (%) | | | No. | No. pregnant in 3 years | Pregnant (%) | | |
			1 year	2 years	3 years			1 year	2 years	3 years
Minimal/mild										
No treatment	15	10	53.3 ± 12.9*	66.7 ± 12.2	66.7 ± 12.2	13	9	61.5 ± 13.5	69.2 ± 12.8	69.2 ± 12.8
Medical treatment	44	20	26.5 ± 7.2	53.0 ± 8.9	62.3 ± 9.3	32	13	25.6 ± 8.4	47.7 ± 10.2	55.2 ± 11.2
Laparoscopy	241	122	43.6 ± 3.5	59.6 ± 3.8	67.8 ± 4.1	134	70	45.5 ± 4.7	60.4 ± 5.1	70.3 ± 5.4
Laparotomy	46	28	55.7 ± 7.9	65.6 ± 7.9	74.3 ± 8.1	13	6	38.0 ± 15.1	50.4 ± 16.4	64.5 ± 16.8
Moderate/severe†										
Laparoscopy	120	52	29.1 ± 4.5	50.8 ± 5.6	62.2 ± 6.2	48	25	32.2 ± 7.5	70.0 ± 9.0	82.0 ± 8.5
Laparotomy	102	37	23.8 ± 4.5	36.7 ± 5.3	44.4 ± 5.6	15	5	20.0 ± 10.3	26.7 ± 11.4	33.3 ± 12.2

* Values are estimates ± SE.

† Eleven patients treated nonsurgically have been excluded from the entire patient population. Three patients treated nonsurgically have been excluded from the endometriosis-only subset.

Source: Reprinted from Fertility and Sterility, 59(1), Adamson et al.[18], *Laparoscopic endometriosis treatment: Is it better?*, 35–44, Copyright 1993, with permission from the American Society for Reproductive Medicine.

distortion is commonly approached via surgery for all types of disease, and endometriosis is no exception. A low background pregnancy rate approaching zero in these women and numerous uncontrolled trials documenting that pregnancies do occur after reparative surgery suggest the value of this approach.[17] As a result, few data exist regarding no treatment or medical treatment and no prospective randomized studies with untreated controls have been reported. The available evidence supports the surgical approach compared with the nonsurgical approach for invasive, adhesive, endometriotic disease.

The laparoscopic approach using excisional techniques has been described in the treatment of infiltrating cul-de-sac endometriosis, often an area of difficult dissection.[23,24] In partial or complete cul-de-sac obliteration, 34 of 46 (74%) infertile couples achieved pregnancy. Of those who conceived, more than one laparoscopy was performed in 13 of 34 women. Comparisons of laparoscopy vs laparotomy in the treatment of complete endometriotic posterior cul-de-sac obliteration and infertility show life table pregnancy rates of approximately 25% at 2 years for either laparoscopy or laparotomy. Other reports support the conclusion that the results obtained by the laparoscopic treatment approach to extensive cul-de-sac and rectovaginal endometriosis are equivalent to the results obtained at laparotomy when performed by experienced laparoscopists.

Patients with endometriosis as the only infertility factor have similar crude pregnancy rates for all stages whether treated with laparoscopy or laparotomy.[17,18] Life table analysis of patients without other infertility factors, however, revealed that laparoscopy was similar to laparotomy for minimal/mild disease and superior to laparotomy for moderate/severe disease. Survival analysis with multiple fixed covariates concurs with these findings in that laparoscopy was significantly better than laparotomy in the endometriosis-only group (87% higher pregnancy rate, $p = 0.031$). In the endometriosis-only group, survival analysis with multiple fixed covariates concurred with the findings that laparoscopy was superior. However, in a meta-analysis of studies comparing laparoscopy to laparotomy, the observed difference in pregnancy rates was not significant.[17] A possible explanation for the differences between these analyses is that meta-analysis does not account for the duration of time to pregnancy, only the final pregnancy rate. Moreover, patients treated by laparotomy generally had longer follow-up, allowing for more time to conceive. Operative laparoscopy may allow for superior results compared to laparotomy with respect to the reformation of adhesions excised at the initial surgery. Although this has yet to be demonstrated conclusively, studies have suggested that de-novo adhesion formation is less frequent following operative laparoscopy.[25] In light of the evidence supporting the equivalent if not better outcome of laparoscopy compared to laparotomy, the laparoscopic approach is preferable in most cases of endometriosis-associated infertility.

In patients with endometriomas who have had cystectomy, normal ovarian function appears to be retained.[26] However, many clinicians are concerned that injury to the ovaries at the time of cystectomy and/or multiple ovarian operations result in reduced ovarian function.

Due to the ineffectiveness of medical treatment in eradicating endometriomas, traditional therapy has required laparotomy.[27] The improvement in laparoscopic technique and technology has allowed the advanced treatment of endometriomas.[28] Pregnancy rates following endometriomectomy at laparoscopy or laparotomy are approximately 50% at 2–3 years by life table analysis; they are not dependent on the number or size of endometriomas but can be affected by the extent of adhesive disease.[28] Ovarian endometriomas have been treated by various surgical techniques, including cyst stripping or ablation, drainage, and wedge excision. The approach of wide excision and drainage has been recommended as an alternative to wedge excision due to less adhesion formation and a recurrence rate of 23%, considered by some to be similar to cyst stripping and ablation. In other studies, resection, stripping, or ablation, perhaps the most widely used techniques, have been shown to have a recurrence rate of less than 10%, with an approximately 20% incidence of de-novo adhesion formation and an approximately 80% incidence of partial dense adhesion recurrence.[29] A recent prospective randomized controlled trial (PRCT) demonstrated higher pregnancy rates, 59% vs 23%, and a lower reoperation rate, 6% vs 23%, in the group with laparoscopic ovarian cystectomy vs fenestration and coagulation.[30]

Adhesions can disrupt normal anatomic relationships and restrict the mobility and distensibility of organs, potentially resulting in decreased fertility. Adhesions are usually removed. However, there are no PRCTs that support an increase in pregnancy rates as a direct result of adhesiolysis in patients with endometriosis. Although often employed, the routine use of pharmacologic agents to prevent postoperative adhesions cannot be recommended on the basis of the available evidence derived from PRCTs.[31–34]

Endometriosis can affect other specific pelvic structures. For tubal endometriosis, CO_2 laser ablation to minimize thermal injury and control depth has been quite effective. Proximal tubal occlusion requires cannulization or resection followed by anastomosis.

Infertility outcomes comparing surgery with other treatments

Results of endometriosis treatment with surgery, and laparoscopy in particular, appear superior to all other types of treatment. This conclusion is based on numerous large studies, including lifetable analysis, survival analysis with fixed covariates, meta-analysis, prospective randomized trials, and summary of all the literature. Each study has its own deficiencies, but all have shown results favoring surgery.[3,14,17–19,35,36] A large study of 579 patients with prospectively recorded data was carried out to evaluate pregnancy rates following laparoscopy for endometriosis and showed that laparoscopy pregnancy rates were equal to or higher than other treatment options for the entire population of 579 patients as well as an endometriosis-only subset consisting of 258 patients with at least one normal tube and fimbria, and normal male factor (see Table 26.1).[18] Laparoscopic treatment of endometriosis was found to result in equivalent or higher pregnancy rates than other treatments, whether or not disease was minimal, mild, moderate, or severe. These differences were up to 101% better than other treatment modalities and, consequently, could be of clinical consequence to the patient. Pregnancy rates at 2 years following surgery were approximately 60% for minimal/mild disease, 50% for moderate disease, and 40% for severe/extensive disease.

Pregnancy rates following medical treatment are usually 5–10% lower at 2 years, and the pregnancies take longer to occur, especially with medical treatment that consumes 6 or more months of time. The pregnancy rate per month is about 4% and stays the same for about 15 months after surgery, and then decreases fairly rapidly to about 2% per month.[18] The difference in rates between surgical and medical therapy for stage I/II disease is primarily due to lost time providing medical treatment. The time savings of up to 6 months is important to women suffering infertility, especially older women, since their fertility may decrease during a half-year of treatment. Meta-analysis of studies comparing surgical treatment with nonsurgical treatment confirms the superiority of surgical treatment, with crude pregnancy rates estimated to be 38% higher than nonsurgical treatment.[17] Meta-analysis comparing laparoscopy to medical or no treatment found strong evidence favoring operative laparoscopy, with the relative risk for pregnancy being 1.47.[17] Meta-analysis also confirms that medical treatment following surgery does not improve pregnancy rates.[17] No data support the use of preoperative ovarian suppression.

Treatment options and outcomes

There are many different ways to manage endometriosis-associated infertility. In order to make rational decisions, the clinician must know each treatment's chance of success for an individual patient and relative to other treatments being considered. Treatment success is conveniently defined as fecundity, which is the probability of a woman achieving a live birth for any given month.[37] Of course, the most important outcome is the birth of a healthy singleton baby. Endometriosis patients appear to have obstetric outcomes not significantly different from infertile controls.[38]

Management of other fertility and medical conditions

Patients may have other fertility and medical conditions that are not related to endometriosis. General medical conditions such as hypertension, diabetes mellitus, or hematologic, renal, or hepatic diseases should be addressed with the appropriate referring physician so that it is possible to treat the patient not only for her fertility problem but also so that it is safe for her to undergo a pregnancy and deliver a healthy baby. Other fertility problems should also be treated. These include ovulatory dysfunction associated with the pituitary, thyroid, adrenal, weight, or other conditions. Pelvic factors such as tubal disease, congenital uterine abnormalities, myomas, intrauterine adhesions, or cervical incompetence need to be managed. Empiric flushing of the fallopian tubes might be indicated.[39] Male factor should be evaluated and treated, if possible, or other options such as donor insemination or ART procedures considered. Repeated pregnancy loss can be an especially difficult challenge that needs consideration and active management. Any of these problems, if left untreated, can render irrelevant any success that might be achieved with endometriosis treatment.

Observation alone following diagnostic laparoscopy

No treatment includes expectant management. In normal young couples, fecundity is 15–20% per month.[40] In untreated women with endometriosis and infertility, monthly fecundity is 2–10%.[41] Given that this chapter is reviewing management following surgery, these data would apply only to women who had a laparoscopy with diagnosis of endometriosis but without surgical treatment at the same time. Most surgeons feel such an approach is inappropriate; if a laparoscopy is performed for suspected endometriosis, the surgeon should have the skills and operating room capability to treat all cases of endometriosis except for possibly the most severe cases. Severe cases should only have surgical intervention by especially skilled surgeons in order to achieve the best outcome with the least risk of complications.

Ovarian suppression

Ovarian suppression can consist of oral contraceptives (OCs), progestins, danazol, gonadotropin-releasing hormone (GnRH) agonists or GnRH antagonists. Four randomized trials have compared ovarian suppression with placebo or no treatment and 8 have compared ovarian suppression medications with danazol.[42] All have been summarized in a meta-analysis by Hughes et al.[41]

The results of our meta-analysis also provide strong evidence that there was no significant difference in crude pregnancy rates between medical treatment and no treatment (Figure 26.1).[17] The combined estimated risk ratio was 0.98, with a 95% CI of 0.81–1.18. No increase in fertility can be demonstrated with these medications when compared with expectant management, nor has any medication proven superior to danazol in this regard. Use of ovarian suppression also delays fertility in that the patient is unable to conceive while being medicated for several months. There are also additional costs and associated side effects, including bone loss. Thus, there appears to be little or no role for primary ovarian suppression in the treatment of minimal or mild endometriosis-associated infertility.[43,44]

Ovarian suppression has been used as an adjunct to surgery in an attempt to improve pregnancy rates. The combined evidence indicates that medical treatment following surgery is not better than surgery alone, whether the surgical approach is via laparoscopy or laparotomy (relative risk, 0.97; 95% CI, 0.87–1.09).[17] Therefore, medical therapy does not have a role in the treatment of endometriosis-associated infertility, either after surgery (laparoscopy or laparotomy) or alone.[45] A summary of the meta-analysis estimates for the various comparisons is presented in Figure 26.1.

Presurgical ovarian suppression has also been suggested to be a beneficial adjunct. Improved pregnancy rates have been reported with presurgical

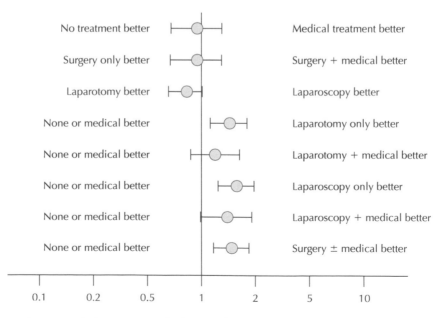

Figure 26.1 Summary of meta-analysis estimates of relative risk of pregnancy (point estimate and 95% confidence interval): comparison of different endometriosis treatments. Reproduced from Adamson and Pasta,[17] with permission from Elsevier.

medical treatment using danazol or GnRH agonists. However, these data and those suggesting improved technical results, reduced adhesions, and reduction in blood flow and inflammation are sufficiently inconclusive so that preoperative ovarian suppression cannot yet be recommended.[45]

Controlled ovarian stimulation

Controlled ovarian stimulation (COS) is the intentional induction of multiple ovulation to increase the number of eggs which are ovulated in an otherwise normally ovulating woman.[46] COS can be performed with either clomiphene citrate (CC) and/or gonadotropins, often in conjunction with intrauterine insemination (IUI) with prepared sperm.[46,47] Sperm processing allows the selection of sperm with the most normal morphology and motility and the absence of white cells and other infectious organisms. IUI avoids cervical problems such as poor mucus, cervical antibodies, and infection.

These treatments are intended to increase the overall fecundity and do not cause regression of endometrial implants (Table 26.2) Randomized trials have addressed the value of controlled ovarian stimulation, and two have combined it with intrauterine insemination.[46,48] These data and review of the literature suggest a control population fecundity of 2–4% per cycle and treated population of 5–18%. From these results, it is apparent that fertility can be hastened in women with unexplained infertility by using COS and IUI. It is not clear that pregnancies occur in women who otherwise never would have conceived.

Many feel that pregnancy rates in stage I/II endometriosis are similar to those for unexplained infertility. Different types of data, including those from prospective randomized studies and large registries, address pregnancy rates with treatment of endometriosis-associated infertility, including expectant, postovarian suppression, surgical, and ART treatment (Table 26.3).[43,49] Since many endometriosis patients are treated with COS, it is important to know baseline endometriosis pregnancy rates when considering the value of adding COS to their treatment. There is a wide range of success reported with cycle fecundity, with CC–IUI increasing the baseline fecundity from 25% to 200%, and with gonadotropins increasing the baseline fecundity from 50% to 400%. The addition of IUI appears to increase pregnancy rates only slightly with clomiphene but possibly double the success with gonadotropins. Baseline cycle fecundity may range from 0–2% per cycle with severe endometriosis to 6–8% per cycle for minimal endometriosis in women less than 30 years of age. In patients without significant anatomic distortion, it could be expected that CC–IUI might create a fecundity rate of 6–8% per cycle or higher, and gonadotropins 12–20% per cycle. Randomized controlled studies of COS–IUI treatment in moderate or severe endometriosis are lacking. The expectation, however, would be for little or no improvement in pregnancy rates because of the high probability of significant anatomic distortion that could interfere with the mechanism of oocyte transport to the fallopian tube.

COS–IUI is probably helpful for women with stage I/II endometriosis. Generally, 3–4 cycles of COS–IUI are clinically appropriate. A maximum number would be 6 cycles of CC and IUI and 6

Table 26.2 Pregnancy rates following treatment for unexplained infertility

Treatment	Monthly fecundity (%)		
	Guzick et al[46]	ASRM[133]	RMN[48]
No treatment	3	3	2*
IUI	4	5	5
Clomiphene	6	5	–
Clomiphene plus IUI	8	8	–
Gonadotropin	8	8	4*
Gonadotropin plus IUI	18	18	9

* Intracervical insemination.
ASRM = American Society for Reproductive Medicine; RMN = Reproductive Medicine Network; IUI = intrauterine insemination.

Table 26.3 Pregnancy rates following treatment of endometriosis-associated infertility

Treatment	Stage/Monthly fecundity (%)		
	Minimal/Mild	Moderate	Severe
Expectant	3	3	0
Ovarian suppression*	3	4	1
Surgical	5	5	3
IVF per cycle (age <35/35–40/>40)	40/30/15	40/30/15	35/25/10

* After discontinuation of ovarian suppression medication
IVF = in vitro fertilization.

cycles of gonadotropin and IUI in selected patients. Some controversy exists as to the optimal number of inseminations per cycle. Data would generally support one well-timed IUI when an adequate number of sperm is present.[50–52] Should timing of insemination be difficult to determine, then two inseminations 2 days apart may be helpful and may improve pregnancy rates.

The quality of sperm prior to sperm wash and following sperm wash will affect the pregnancy rate. IUI is useful for idiopathic male subfertility.[53] In our program, at least 1 million total motile sperm should be available for IUI. Lower numbers than this have resulted in almost no pregnancies. Pregnancy rates have increased somewhat to 5 million total motile sperm per inseminate and increase only gradually after this number.[54] Although it is important to measure sperm parameters, and they do help differentiate fertile from infertile populations, it is difficult to predict outcome for any one couple based on semen analysis parameters or postwash total motile sperm count. Good parameters are not good predictors of success, but very poor count and motility are better predictors of failure.[55–57] It is important that sperm collection processing and insemination be performed according to protocols that minimize the time from collection to insemination.[58] For women younger than 30 years old with short duration of infertility and favorable prognosis, couples with sexual dysfunction, or women using donor sperm, the use of IUI by itself would appear to be beneficial over intercourse or cervical cap insemination (see Table 26.2).[46,48,133] Up to 3–6 cycles of IUI alone would appear appropriate in these selected patients.

Multiple pregnancies with approximately 25% twins, 4% triplets, and 1% quadruplets occur with COS.[59] Severe ovarian hyperstimulation syndrome occurs in approximately 1% of patients, with moderate ovarian hyperstimulation occurring in 5–7% of patients. About 1 patient in 300 requires hospitalization for ovarian hyperstimulation syndrome. Ectopic pregnancy occurs in approximately 5% of patients. The majority of pregnancies occur within 2–4 cycles of treatment. In very young patients with otherwise excellent prognosis up to 6 cycles of ovarian stimulation might occasionally be indicated. Birth defects are slightly increased compared to the general population, but this is widely felt to occur in all infertility patients and is not related to the therapeutic modality, or indeed the absence of it, used to achieve pregnancy.

Ancillary treatments are sometimes utilized with COS. These include progesterone in the luteal phase to support the endometrium, thyroid supplementation for hypothyroidism, low-dose aspirin to improve implantation, dexamethasone to lower androgen levels, and bromocriptine or cabergoline to lower prolactin levels. Letrozole and anastrozole, aromatase inhibitors that block estrogen production, have been used as oral medications in place of CC on days 5–9 and also as co-treatment with gonadotropins.[60,61] Each of these medications has its proponents, and studies in the literature suggesting their benefits. Nevertheless, it is still not clear what role these pharmaceuticals should play in the infertile patient with endometriosis, and their use should be considered on an individual and empiric basis.

Repeat surgery

There are no large randomized studies that support repeat surgery for infertility patients; especially for patients who have stage III/IV endometriosis, in vitro fertilization (IVF) is probably a better option.[43] There are no sufficiently powered prospective randomized trials evaluating the effect on pregnancy outcome of surgical treatment followed by IVF vs IVF alone.[43] In one small retrospective study, the pregnancy rate after 2 cycles of IVF was 70% and within 9 months of repeat surgery it was 24%.[62] Another study showed a 21% pregnancy rate at 1 year following reoperation.[63] Therefore, IVF would seem to be a preferable alternative to repeat surgery for most patients.[43,64]

Assisted reproductive technologies

The assisted reproductive technologies refer to procedures such as IVF, intracytoplasmic sperm injection (ICSI), and assisted hatching (AH). Results for 2002 from the United States IVF Registry gave a live birth per retrieval of 40.7% for women under 35 years old, 35.1% for 35–37 year olds, 24.7% for 38–40 year olds and 13.4% for 41 and 42 year olds.[49] There is only a slight reduction in the success rates with IVF with increasing numbers of cycles, each cycle after the first has approximately 90% the success rate of the first.[65] An increasing duration of infertility also decreases success rates.[66] Previous pregnancy and live birth increases success rates slightly.[66]

Only one RCT looked at IVF vs no treatment for 6 months in endometriosis patients, but the study had only 21 patients in the comparison groups, making conclusions impossible.[67] Another study examined the issue in a retrospective cohort population and was unable to demonstrate a significantly higher cumulative pregnancy rate between women undergoing IVF and untreated women over a 3-year follow-up period.[68] A retrospective study showed IVF to be superior to COS–IUI.[69]

The impact of the diagnosis of endometriosis on outcomes with IVF treatment is not yet clear. There are no large randomized clinical trials to answer several open issues, and cohort trials have been inconclusive.[70] Several studies have shown patients with endometriosis have lower pregnancy rates compared with patients with tubal factor infertility. Further categorization of patients into mild and severe endometriosis groups revealed no difference in outcome in patients with mild disease, with a significantly lower pregnancy rate in patients with severe disease.[70] Some data suggest a deleterious effect on outcome because of difficulty monitoring ovaries, reduced response to gonadotropins, reduced number of oocytes retrieved, reduced fertilization rates, reduced implantation rates, and impaired oocyte or embryo quality. Support for the poor oocyte theory comes from the oocyte donation model where lower pregnancy rates from oocyte donors with endometriosis and no decrease in pregnancy rates in oocyte recipients with endometriosis were observed.[71–72] Other studies, however, have not found any difference in IVF success rates between patients with and without endometriosis and the SART (Society for Assisted Reproductive Technology) data show no difference overall for endometriosis pregnancy rates compared with other diagnostic categories.[73]

With respect to the effect of disease stage on ART outcome, until recently there have only been observational studies.[74] More recently, there has been a case-controlled study and meta-analysis.[75–78] Conclusions have been hampered by the limitations of the classification system and the conflicting and relatively poor-quality data. With laparoscopic oocyte retrieval there may be a reduced pregnancy rate in more severe stages because of difficulty accessing the ovaries. With transvaginal retrieval there is no evidence of a possible decrease in fertility. However, no studies have had the power to evaluate the impact of extensive disease with AFS (American Fertility Society) score of >71, a stage of disease that appears in non-ART treatments to confer a poorer prognosis, or the effect of multiple surgeries on the ovaries.[8]

With respect to endometriomas, there are no randomized trials, and cohort data are conflicting.[77,79–86] Small endometriomas may not matter and large endometriomas may. The most important factor is avoiding damage to the ovary. Pelvic abscess has been reported following egg retrieval in patients with endometriomas, thus providing a potential indication for pre-IVF surgical treatment in some patients, although no PRCTs have shown a benefit of ovarian endometriomectomy before IVF.[87]

The question of whether ovarian suppression prior to IVF is beneficial requires further study. It is clear that down-regulation with GnRH agonists in any patient produces higher pregnancy rates, but it is not known whether 2 weeks or up to 6 months is superior for endometriosis patients. Some data support the use of ovarian suppression for longer periods of time prior to IVF for women with severe endometriosis.[88–91] Other clinicians have not found a difference between endometriosis patients and nonendometriosis patients or stage of disease.[92] Clearly, the amount of time lost during ovarian suppression, especially in older women, reduces at least some of any potential benefit of longer suppression.

In light of the potential adverse effects of endometriosis on the oocyte, consideration of surgical treatment prior to initiating IVF cycles seems reasonable. Improvement in success rates, however, has not been demonstrated using surgical treatment of endometriosis before IVF. Following conservational ovarian surgery, normal ovarian function may be retained in some patients and not in others, and patients' responses to ovarian stimulation may be variable.[82,93–96] There is also controversy over which techniques are most tissue-sparing for follicles.[93,97–99] Moreover, no difference in pregnancy rates or live birth rates was observed between patients who were treated or not treated for endometriosis at the time of gamete intrafallopian transfer (GIFT). Observed reduced pregnancy rates in some studies may also be attributable to reduced ovarian function because of ovarian endometriotic disease and/or prior ovarian surgery, making it mandatory to preserve ovarian volume and function during any surgical procedure. Frequently, surgery has been performed earlier during the course of the infertility work-up and treatment. It is also not clear whether the surgical treatment of endometriosis contemporaneously with GIFT is beneficial, although one randomized study showed that the GIFT pregnancy rate was not affected but following failed GIFT the spontaneous pregnancy rate was higher in the surgically treated group.[100] Another large retrospective study showed no statistical differences.[101]

Although it is probably self-evident that IVF is of value in advanced disease due to the very low background pregnancy rate and the tangible rate of success with the procedure, the value of IVF in early-stage disease is as yet unproven. In other words, whereas pregnancies certainly occur quite rapidly with IVF in women with endometriosis or any other diagnosis, it is unclear whether 1 cycle of IVF is comparable to 1 month, 6 months, 2 years, or longer of attempting conception naturally.[67]

The assisted reproductive technologies of IVF and GIFT can be used effectively to treat infertile patients with endometriosis following failed prior treatment. They are also sometimes appropriate in older women with extensive endometriosis and/or adhesions who do not have pelvic pain or endometriomas and for whom the prognosis following surgery would be limited.

It is important to consider confounding variables when deciding whether to operate on a patient. Patients who are older that 35 years old, have duration of infertility longer than 3 years, have had no prior pregnancy, have known extensive endometriosis lesions, adhesions, or tubal damage, or have had multiple prior operations have a poorer prognosis.

IVF can involve the use of specialized technologies in selected patients, including ICSI, AH, and preimplantation genetic diagnosis (PGD). Endometriosis patients have the same indications for these technologies as nonendometriosis patients. In selected patients, third-party reproduction involving the use of donor sperm, donor oocytes, or a gestational carrier may be indicated. Endometriosis patients also have the same indications for such alternative approaches as nonendometriosis patients.

Overall, although IVF is clearly worthwhile, its degree of value, cost-effectiveness, and optimal method of employment has not yet been satisfactorily answered.

Comprehensive management approach

One way to approach the very complex treatment questions for post-surgical endometriosis patients is to do a cost–benefit approach on all the options that have been described earlier in this chapter. Treatment plans should have an endpoint in mind that is acceptable to the patient, be it IVF, donor oocyte, adoption, or child-free living. It is important that the clinician inform the patient of all these options and what is required to achieve them.

The benefit of any of these choices depends on the value that the patient places on the outcome. Clearly, the outcomes of the choices are not all the same, ranging from the patient's own genetic baby, to an egg donor or sperm donor baby, an adopted baby, or no baby at all. Different patients will view the relative value of these outcomes differently.

In addition to determining the value of various outcomes, patients must know the probability that each outcome may occur. This requires a knowledgeable physician and a comprehensive evaluation of both the male and female. To determine the benefit of any outcome, the relative value of each choice is multiplied by the probability that the outcome will occur:

$$\text{Benefit} = \text{Value} \times \text{Chances of success}$$

Each potential choice is then prioritized according to the one that has the most benefit, the second most, the third most, and so on. The next step will be to evaluate the 'cost' of each choice, since the cost will reduce the benefit and might change the patient's order of priority.

There are four kinds of costs. The first is financial. It is important to determine exactly what is covered by health insurance, so that the amount of personal expense can be determined. The patient decides how much money, if any, she is prepared to spend from medical savings accounts, retirement funds, or savings. Because the cost of care can be such a major stumbling block in some countries, some practices are now beginning to offer treatment packages, affordable financing, and refund guarantees.

The second major cost is time. For younger patients, time is not as critical. Once the woman's age is over 35 years, however, time begins to play a more important role, affecting how quickly she needs to move to intensive treatment such as IVF.

The third major cost is the risk of IVF. Generally, IVF treatment is safe and outcomes for both women and babies are good. But all infertile patients appear to have a slightly higher risk of complications of pregnancy, childbirth, and birth outcome.[102,103] Obtaining high-quality obstetric care and bed rest during the pregnancy can reduce many of these potential problems. Additionally, certain subgroups of IVF patients appear to be at higher risk than others. Further well-designed studies are needed to answer these important issues. However, the risk of death or serious illness from *any* pregnancy, regardless of whether or not IVF is used, is several times higher than the risk of the medications or procedures used in IVF. Physical complications need to be considered, but these are primarily two: ovarian hyperstimulation syndrome (OHSS) and multiple pregnancy.[104] The most important complication of fertility treatment is the risk of multiple pregnancy, twins occurring with about 30% of deliveries and triplets about 3% in the United States.[49,59] However, a healthy baby is the result well over 95% of the time with IVF. In Europe multiple rates are lower, as are pregnancy rates.[105] Other complications are rare.

The final cost is often the most important, and that is the psychologic or emotional cost of infertility. There are ways to help patients deal with the stress, including encouraging communication with their partners, getting them accurate information, answering their questions and providing referral to professional counselors when indicated.

Once patients have determined what is acceptable to them, know their prognosis and planned treatment with timelines, have decided how to afford treatment, and how to manage their personal, family, and work time, they can make a written plan to deal with the many aspects of treatment. Patients should proceed at their own pace, with options acceptable to them, within medically appropriate guidelines.

It is critical that physicians recognize the degree to which endometriosis can physically and emotionally disrupt patients' lives, and provide comprehensive understanding and an empathetic management approach.[106,107] Attention to healthy lifestyle with respect to diet, exercise, sleep, and stress reduction through mind–body techniques can be very helpful. Psychologic support through information can be obtained from organizations such as the Endometriosis Association, RESOLVE, the American Fertility Association, and the ASRM. Personal or group counseling may also be helpful. Some patients may seek nontraditional and unproven approaches to treatment such as acupuncture, herbal medicine, or special diets.[108,109] Management in these chronic, complex situations should focus on an improved quality of life. Treatment of reactive depression is often necessary and often requires a multidisciplinary approach. A comprehensive long-range treatment approach needs to be individualized for each patient. A complete cure can sometimes be achieved only by total hysterectomy and bilateral salpingo-oophorectomy, so family planning should be expedited in endometriosis patients. Patients should be treated with a comprehensive mind–body approach – diet, exercise, sleep, and biofeedback.

Although many patients will conceive with appropriate treatment, and some independent of treatment, some will not. For these patients, the benefits of adoption and child-free living need to be discussed.

Algorithm for management of endometriosis

Endometriosis is obviously an extremely complex medical condition and treatment is similarly complicated.[110] Although the number of good studies is increasing, there are still many unanswered questions regarding endometriosis. Treatment needs to be based on each patient's individual circumstances, objectives, and prognosis (see Table 26.3). However, the algorithm shown in Figure 26.2

is suggested as a possible model that can be modified for individual patients. For patients with suspected endometriosis and infertility, if all other infertility factors are appropriately evaluated and found to be acceptable, it is reasonable in the patient under 37 years old to attempt 3–4 cycles of CC 100 mg/day from cycle day 3 through 7. IUI probably increases pregnancy rates slightly when used in conjunction with CC. Appropriate patients under 32 years old may receive up to 6 cycles.

If the infertility patient fails to conceive on the above regimens, laparoscopy is indicated to confirm the suspected diagnosis of endometriosis. Surgical treatment involving complete laparoscopic resection of the disease should be performed at the time of diagnosis if the surgeon is capable of so doing. The only exception to this approach is the young woman with infertility as her only symptom and extensive superficial peritoneal and/or ovarian disease. Treatment of such lesions may increase pregnancy rates but may also result in pelvic adhesions. For infertility patients, COS and IUI postoperatively for 3–6 months with CC and/or 3–6 months with gonadotropins will increase pregnancy rates.

IVF is usually considered after expectant management and/or COS with IUI has failed following surgery.

For infertile patients who fail to conceive, a second-look laparoscopy at 6–18 months may sometimes be indicated. If extensive endometriosis, adhesions, or tubal abnormalities are found, IVF should be considered within 0–12 months following surgery.

Infertility patients who have not had operative resection or inadequate resection with, minimal and mild disease (no adhesions, no invasive lesions, no endometriomas), need no further treatment. Patients with moderate or advanced disease should be referred for laparoscopy or occasionally laparotomy. Ovarian suppression should not be used.

Infertile patients who do not conceive within approximately 6–15 months should have a repeat laparoscopy for treatment and/or assisted reproductive technologies such as IVF or, rarely, GIFT (see Figure 26.2), depending on the patient's age and other infertility factors. Ovarian suppression with GnRH agonists for 2–6 weeks before COS with gonadotropins increases success rates. IVF is indicated in almost all patients who have failed surgical treatment and/or COS treatment, and occasionally as a first treatment instead of surgery in patients with extensive disease and/or other infertility factors. Adoption or child-free living are also options at this point.

The future

We have much to learn about endometriosis. More detailed evidence-based meta-analysis and prospective randomized studies are being performed to help improve our clinical guidelines. Development of a scoring system that correlates with severity of reproductive dysfunction will be a significant contribution to endometriosis-associated infertility research.[8,74] Accounting for differences among control and treatment groups by using appropriate statistical methods is required given the dearth of prospective randomized trials.[7]

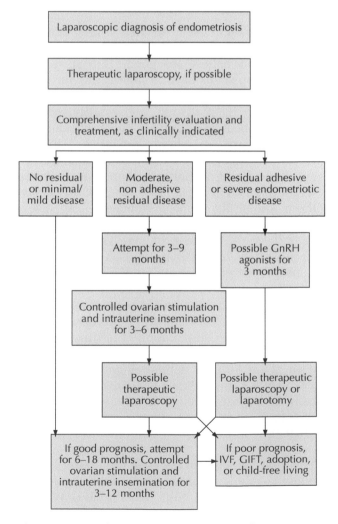

Figure 26.2 Postlaparoscopy management of endometriosis-associated infertility. GIFT = gamete intrafallopian transfer; GnRH = gonadotropin-releasing hormone; IVF = in vitro fertilization. Modified from Adamson.[13]

As more studies are conducted that utilize sophisticated design and statistical methods, more definitive conclusions should be possible regarding the optimal treatment approaches for endometriosis-associated infertility.

The future holds promise for better management of endometriosis. Surgical capabilities will continue to increase, although fewer surgeons will be performing difficult endometriosis operations.[111] IVF results will continue to improve and will be used for many more endometriosis patients.

Basic research currently underway should give us a better understanding of β_3 integrins, haptoglobins, endometrial aromatase P450 expression, tumor necrosis factor alpha (TNF-α), vascular endothelial growth factor (VEGF), cyclooxygenase-2 (COX-2), interleukins, other cytokines, prostaglandins, other hormones, immunology, and the potential role of immunotherapy in new therapeutic approaches.[112–123] Hormones and their interactions with the immune system will be better deciphered.[124] The role of environmental dioxins, matrix metalloproteinases, and cell adhesion molecules will be gradually understood.[125–127] The relationship of endometriosis to uterine and ovarian function, oocyte quality, and embryo implantation will become clearer, as will an improved comprehension of apoptosis and the pathophysiology of endometriosis.[128–130] Studies to determine the genetic basis of endometriosis may lead to much more successful treatment in the years ahead.[131,132] Treatment at the beginning of life will become a reality in this century through the use of PGD. Eventually, all these advances should allow us to markedly improve the management of endometriosis and infertility following surgery.

REFERENCES

1. Gibbons WE. Management of endometriosis in fertility patients. Fertil Steril 2004; 81(5): 1204–1205.
2. Witz CA, Schenken RS. Pathogenesis. In: Speroff L, Adamson GD, eds. Seminars in reproductive endocrinology, endometriosis. New York, NY: Thieme; 1997; 15(3): 199–208.
3. Olive DL, Schwartz LB. Endometriosis. N Engl J Med 1993; 328: 1759–1769.
4. American Society for Reproductive Medicine. Revised American Society for Reproductive Medicine classification of endometriosis: 1996. Fertil Steril 1997; 67: 817–821.
5. Adamson GD, Frison L, Lamb EJ. Endometriosis: studies of a method for design of a surgical staging system. Fertil Steril 1982; 38: 659–666.
6. Guzick DS, Silliman NP, Adamson GD, et al. Prediction of pregnancy in infertile women based on the American Society for Reproductive Medicine's revised classification of endometriosis. Fertil Steril 1997; 67(5): 822–829.
7. Olive DL, Lee KL. Analysis of sequential treatment protocols for endometriosis-associated infertility. Am J Obstet Gynecol 1986; 154(3): 613–619.
8. Adamson GD, Pasta DJ. Pregnancy rates can be predicted by validated endometriosis fertility index (EFI). Fertil Steril 2002; 77(Suppl 1): S48.
9. Practice Committee of the American Society for Reproductive Medicine. Aging and infertility in women. Fertil Steril 2004; 82 (Suppl 1): S102–106.
10. Witt BR, Barad DH. Management of endometriosis in women older than 40 years of age. Obstet Gynecol Clin North Am 1993; 20(2): 349–363.
11. Adamson GD, Baker VL. Subfertility: causes, treatment and outcome. Best Pract Res Clin Obstet Gynaecol 2003; 17: 169–185.
12. Epstein RM, Alper BS, Quill TE. Communicating evidence for participatory decision making. JAMA 2004; 291(19): 2359–2366.
13. Adamson GD. Laparoscopic treatment of endometriosis. In: Adamson GD, Martin DC, eds. Endoscopic management of gynecologic disease. Philadelphia: Lippincott-Raven; 1996: 147–187.
14. Schenken RS, Malinak LR. Conservative surgery versus expectant management for the infertile patient with mild endometriosis. Fertil Steril 1982; 37: 183–186.
15. Akande VA, Hunt LP, Cahill DJ, et al. Differences in time to natural conception between women with unexplained infertility and infertile women with minor endometriosis. Hum Reprod 2004; 19(1): 96–103.
16. D'Hooghe TM, Debrock S, Hill JA, et al. Endometriosis and subfertility: is the relationship resolved? Semin Reprod Med 2003; 21(2): 243–254.
17. Adamson GD, Pasta DJ. Surgical treatment of endometriosis-associated infertility: meta-analysis compared with survival analysis. Am J Obstet Gynecol 1994; 171(6): 1488–1505.
18. Adamson GD, Hurd SJ, Pasta DJ, et al. Laparoscopic endometriosis treatment: Is it better? Fertil Steril 1993; 59(1): 35–44.
19. Marcoux S, Maheux R, Berube S. Laparoscopic surgery in infertile women with minimal or mild endometriosis. N Engl J Med 1997; 337(4): 217–222.
20. Gruppo Italiano per lo Studio dell' Endometriosi. Ablation of lesions or no treatment in minimal-mild endometriosis in infertile women: a randomized trial. Hum Reprod 1999; 14(5): 1332–1334.
21. Jacobson TZ, Barlow DH, Koninckx PR, et al. Laparoscopic surgery for subfertility associated with endometriosis. Cochrane Database Syst Rev 2002; 4: CD001398.

22. Evers JL. Evidence-based reproductive surgery: endometriosis. Int Congr Ser 2004; 1266: 90–95.

23. Donnez J, Nisolle M, Casanas-Roux F, et al. Rectovaginal septum endometriosis or adenomyosis: laparoscopic management in a series of 231 patients. Hum Reprod 1995; 10: 630–635.

24. Reich H, McGlynn F, Salvat J. Laparoscopic treatment of cul-de-sac obliteration secondary to retrocervical deep fibrotic endometriosis. J Reprod Med 1991; 36: 516–522.

25. Diamond MP, Daniell JF, Feste J, et al. Adhesion reformation and de novo adhesion formation following reproductive pelvic surgery. Fertil Steril 1987; 47: 864–866.

26. Marconi G, Vilela M, Quintana R, et al. Laparoscopic ovarian cystectomy of endometriomas does not affect the ovarian response to gonadotropin stimulation. Fertil Steril 2002; 78(4): 876–878.

27. Chapron C, Vercellini P, Barakat H, et al. Management of ovarian endometriomas. Hum Reprod Update 2002; 8(6): 591–597.

28. Adamson GD, Subak LL, Pasta DJ, et al. Comparison of CO_2 laser laparoscopy with laparotomy for treatment of endometriomata. Fertil Steril 1992; 57(5): 965–973.

29. Canis M, Mage G, Wattiez A, et al. Second-look laparoscopy after laparoscopic cystectomy of large ovarian endometriomas. Fertil Steril 1992; 58: 617–619.

30. Alborzi S, Momtahan M, Parsanezhad ME, et al. A prospective, randomized study comparing laparoscopic ovarian cystectomy versus fenestration and coagulation in patients with endometriomas. Fertil Steril 2004; 82(6): 1633–1637.

31. Watson A, Vandekerckhove P, Lilford R. Liquid and fluid agents for preventing adhesions after surgery for subfertility. Cochrane Rev December 30, 1999.

32. Adamson D. Surgical management of endometriosis. Semin Reprod Med 2003; 21(2): 223–234.

33. El-Mowafi DM, Diamond MP. Are pelvic adhesions preventable? Surg Technol Int 2003; 11: 222–235.

34. Watson A, Vandekerckhove P, Lilford R. Liquid and fluid agents for preventing adhesions after surgery for subfertility. Cochrane Database Syst Rev 2000; 2: CD001298.

35. Pierce SJ, Gazvani MR, Farquharson RG. Long-term use of gonadotropin releasing hormone analogs and hormone replacement therapy in the management of endometriosis: a randomized trial with a 6-year follow-up. Fertil Steril 2000; 74: 964–968.

36. Guzick DS, Rock JA. A comparison of danazol and conservative surgery for the treatment of infertility due to mild or moderate endometriosis. Fertil Steril 1983; 40: 580–584.

37. Chandra A, Mosher WD. The demography of infertility and the use of medical care for infertility. Infertil Reprod Med Clin North Am 1994; 5: 283–296.

38. Kortelahti M, Anttila MA, Hippelainen MI, et al. Obstetric outcome in women with endometriosis – a matched case-control study. Gynecol Obstet Invest 2003; 56(4): 207–212.

39. Johnson NP, Farquhar CM, Hadden WE, et al. The FLUSH trial – flushing with lipiodol for unexplained (and endometriosis-related) subfertility by hysterosalpingography: a randomized trial. Hum Reprod 2004; 19(9): 2043–2051.

40. Schwartz D, Mayaux MJ. Female fecundity as a function of age: results of artificial insemination in 2193 nulliparous women with azoospermic husbands. Federation CECOS. N Engl J Med 1982; 306: 404–406.

41. Hughes EG, Fedorkow DM, Collins JA. A quantitative overview of controlled trials in endometriosis-associated fertility. Fertil Steril 1993; 59(5): 963–970.

42. Bayer SR, Seibel MM, Saffan DS, et al. Efficacy of danazol treatment for minimal endometriosis in infertile women. A prospective randomized study. J Reprod Med 1988; 33: 179–183.

43. The Practice Committee of the American Society for Reproductive Medicine. Endometriosis and infertility. Fertil Steril 2004; 81: 1441–1446.

44. Olive DL, Lindheim SR, Pritts EA. Endometriosis and infertility: what do we do for each stage? Curr Womens Health Rep 2003; 3(5): 389–394.

45. Yap C, Furness S, Farquhar C. Pre and post operative medical therapy for endometriosis surgery. Cochrane Database Syst Rev 2004; (3): CD003678.

46. Guzick DS, Sullivan MW, Adamson GD, et al. Efficacy of treatment for unexplained infertility. Fertil Steril 1998; 70(2): 207–213.

47. The Practice Committee of the American Society for Reproductive Medicine. Use of clomiphene citrate in women. Fertil Steril 2004; 82(Suppl 1): 90–96.

48. Guzick DS, Carson SA, Coutifaris C, et al. National Cooperative Reproductive Medicine Network. Efficacy of superovulation and intrauterine insemination in the treatment of infertility. N Engl J Med 1999; 340: 177–183.

49. http://www.cdc.gov/reproductivehealth/ART02/index.htm

50. Osuna C, Matorras R, Pijoan JI, et al. One versus two inseminations per cycle in intrauterine insemination with sperm from patients' husbands: a systematic review of the literature. Fertil Steril 2004; 82: 17–24.

51. Guzick DS. For now, one well-timed intrauterine insemination is the way to go. Fertil Steril 2004; 82: 30–31.

52. Claman P. Simplifying superovulation and intrauterine insemination treatment: evidence and clinical decision making. Fertil Steril 2004; 82: 32–33.

53. Cohlen BJ. Intrauterine insemination for idiopathic male subfertility. Elsevier International Congress Series 1266. 2004; 208–217.

54. Subak LL, Adamson GD, Boltz NL. Therapeutic donor insemination: a prospective randomized trial of fresh versus frozen sperm. Am J Obstet Gynecol 1992; 166: 1597–1604; discussion 1604–1606.

55. Guzick DS, Overstreet JW, Factor-Litvak P, et al. National Cooperative Reproductive Medicine Network. Sperm morphology, motility, and concentration in fertile and infertile men. N Engl J Med 2001; 345: 1388–1393.

56. Iberico G, Vioque J, Ariza N, et al. Analysis of factors influencing pregnancy rates in homologous intrauterine insemination. Fertil Steril 2004; 81: 1308–1313.

57. Van Weert JM, Repping S, Van Voorhis BJ, et al. Performance of the postwash total motile sperm count as a predictor of pregnancy at the time of intrauterine insemination: meta-analysis. Fertil Steril 2004: 82: 612–620.

58. Yavas Y, Selub MR. Intrauterine insemination (IUI) pregnancy outcome is enhanced by shorter intervals from semen collection to sperm wash, from sperm wash to IUI time, and from semen collection to IUI time. Fertil Steril 2004; 82(6): 1638–1647.

59. Practice Committee of the American Society for Reproductive Medicine. Multiple pregnancy associated with infertility therapy. Fertil Steril 2004; 82 (Suppl 1): 153–157.

60. Casper RF. Letrozole: ovulation or superovulation? Fertil Steril 2003; 80(6): 1335–1357; discussion 1339.

61. Karaer O, Oruc S, Koyuncu FM. Aromatase inhibitors: possible future applications. Acta Obstet Gynecol Scand 2004; 83(8): 699–706.

62. Pagidas K, Falcone T, Hemmings R, et al. Comparison of reoperation for moderate (stage III) and severe (stage IV) endometriosis-related infertility with in vitro fertilization-embryo transfer. Fertil Steril 1996; 65(4): 791–795.

63. Cheewadhanaraks S. Comparison of fecundity after second laparotomy for endometriosis to in vitro fertilization and embryo transfer. J Med Assoc Thai 2004; 87(4): 361–366.

64. Pouly JL, Drolet J, Canis M, et al. Laparoscopic treatment of symptomatic endometriosis. Hum Reprod 1996; 11 (Suppl 13): 67–88.

65. Meldrum DR, Silverberg KM, Bustillo M, et al. Success rate with repeated cycles of in vitro fertilization-embryo transfer. Fertil Steril 1998; 69: 1005–1009.

66. Templeton A, Morris JK, Parslow W. Factors that affect outcome of in-vitro fertilisation treatment. Lancet 1996; 348: 1402–1406.

67. Soliman S, Daya S, Collins J, et al. A randomized trial of in vitro fertilization versus conventional treatment for infertility. Fertil Steril 1993; 59: 1239–1244.

68. Kodama H, Fukuda J, Karube H, et al. Benefit of in vitro fertilization treatment for endometriosis-associated infertility. Fertil Steril 1996; 66: 974–979.

69. Dmowski WP, Pry M, Ding J, et al. Cycle-specific and cumulative fecundity in patients with endometriosis who are undergoing controlled ovarian hyperstimulation-intrauterine insemination or in vitro fertilization-embryo transfer. Fertil Steril 2002; 78(4): 750–756.

70. Dokras SA, Olive DL. Endometriosis and assisted reproductive technologies. Clin Obstet Gynecol 1999; 42(3): 687–698.

71. Diaz I, Navarro J, Blasco L, et al. Impact of sibling oocytes: matched case-control study. Fertil Steril 2000; 74(1): 31–34.

72. Simon C, Gutierrez A, Vidal A, et al. Outcome of patients with endometriosis in assisted reproduction: results from in vitro fertilization and oocyte donation. Hum Reprod 1994; 9: 725–729.

73. Sung L, Mukherjee T, Takeshige T, et al. Endometriosis is not detrimental to embryo implantation in oocyte recipients. J Assist Reprod Genet 1997; 14: 152–156.

74. Guzick DS, Silliman NP, Adamson GD, et al. Prediction of pregnancy in infertile women based on the American Society for Reproductive Medicine's revised classification of endometriosis. Fertil Steril 1997; 67: 822–829.

75. Aboulghar MA, Mansour RT, Serour GI, et al. The outcome of in vitro fertilization in advanced endometriosis with previous surgery: a case-controlled study. Am J Obstet Gynecol 2003; 188(2): 371–375.

76. Barnhart K, Dunsmoor-Su R, Coutifaris C. Effect of endometriosis on in vitro fertilization. Fertil Steril 2002; 77: 1148–1155.

77. Spandorfer SD, Rosenwaks Z. Endometriosis. Is IVF the answer for infertility? Stage-related success rates in 1417 consecutive IVF-ET. Available at http://www.obgyn.net/endo/endo.asp?page=/endo/articles/COGI_endo_IVF

78. Azem F, Lessing JB, Geva E, et al. Patients with stages III and IV endometriosis have a poorer outcome of in vitro fertilization-embryo transfer than patients with tubal infertility. Fertil Steril 1999; 72: 1107–1109.

79. Tinkanen H, Kujansuu E. In vitro fertilization in patients with ovarian endometriomas. Acta Obstet Gynecol Scand 2000; 79(2): 119–122.

80. Yanushpolsky EH, Best CL, Jackson KV, et al. Effects of endometriomas on oocyte quality, embryo quality, and pregnancy rates in in vitro fertilization cycles: a prospective, case-controlled study. J Assist Reprod Genet 1998; 15(4): 193–197.

81. Dlugi AM, Loy RA, Dieterle S, et al. The effect of endometriomas on in vitro fertilization outcome. J In Vitro Fert Embryo Transf 1989; 6(6): 338–341.

82. Loh F-H, Tan AT, Kumar J, et al. Ovarian response after laparoscopic ovarian cystectomy for endometriotic cysts in 132 monitored cycles. Fertil Steril 1999; 72: 316–321.

83. Garcia-Velasco JA, Mahutte NG, Corona J, et al. Removal of endometriomas before in vitro fertilization does not improve fertility outcomes: a matched, case-control study. Fertil Steril 2004; 81(5): 1194–1197.

84. Wong BC, Gillman NC, Oehninger S, et al. Results of in vitro fertilization in patients with endometriomas: is surgical removal beneficial? Am J Obstet Gynecol 2004; 191(2): 597–606; discussion 606–607.

85. Suganuma N, Wakahara Y, Ishida D, et al. Pretreatment for ovarian endometrial cyst before in vitro fertilization. Gynecol Obstet Invest 2002; 54 (Suppl 1): 36–40; discussion 41–42.

86. Takuma N, Sengoku K, Pan B, et al. Laparoscopic treatment of endometrioma-associated infertility and pregnancy outcome. Gynecol Obstet Invest 2002; 54 (Suppl 1): 30–34; discussion 34–35.

87. Wei CF, Chen SC. Pelvic abscess after ultrasound-guided aspiration of endometriomas: a case report. Zhonghua Yi Xue Za Zhi (Taipei) 1998; 61: 603–607.

88. Marcus SF, Edwards RG. High rates of pregnancy after long-term down-regulation of women with severe endometriosis. Am J Obstet Gynecol 1994; 171(3): 812–817.

89. Dicker D, Goldman JA, Levy T, et al. The impact of long-term gonadotropin-releasing hormone analogue treatment on preclinical abortions in patients with severe endometriosis undergoing in vitro fertilization-embryo transfer. Fertil Steril 1992; 57: 597–600.

90. Surrey ES, Silverberg KM, Surrey MW, et al. Effect of prolonged gonadotropin-releasing hormone agonist therapy on the outcome of in vitro fertilization-embryo transfer in patients with endometriosis. Fertil Steril 2002; 78: 699–704.

91. Zikopoulos K, Kolibianakis EM, Devroey P. Ovarian stimulation for in vitro fertilization in patients with endometriosis. Acta Obstet Gynecol Scand 2004; 83(7): 651–655.

92. Olivennes F, Feldberg D, Liu HC, et al. Endometriosis: a stage by stage analysis – the role of in vitro fertilization. Fertil Steril 1995; 64: 392–398.

93. Canis M, Pouly JL, Tamburro S, et al. Ovarian response during IVF-embryo transfer cycles after laparoscopic ovarian cystectomy for endometriotic cysts of >3 cm in diameter. Hum Reprod 2001; 16(12): 2583–2586.

94. Sayegh R, Garcia CR. Ovarian function after conservational ovarian surgery: a long-term follow-up study. Int J Gynaecol Obstet 1992; 39: 303–309.

95. Donnez J, Wyns C, Nisolle M. Does ovarian surgery for endometriomas impair the ovarian response to gonadotropin? Fertil Steril 2001; 76: 662–665.

96. Hemmings R, Bissonnette F, Bouzayen R. Results of laparoscopic treatments of ovarian endometriomas: laparoscopic ovarian fenestration and coagulation. Fertil Steril 1998; 70: 527–529.

97. Muzii L, Bianchi A, Croce C, et al. Laparoscopic excision of ovarian cysts: is the stripping technique a tissue-sparing procedure? Fertil Steril 2002; 77: 609–614.

98. Jones KD, Sutton CJG. Pregnancy rates following ablative laparoscopic surgery for endometriomas. Hum Reprod 2002; 17: 782–785.

99. Garry R. The effectiveness of laparoscopic excision of endometriosis. Curr Opin Obstet Gynecol 2004; 16(4): 299–303.

100. Surrey MW, Hill DL. Treatment of endometriosis by carbon dioxide laser during gamete intrafallopian transfer. J Am Coll Surg 1994; 179: 440–442.

101. Corson SL, Batzer FR, Gocial B, et al. Surgical treatment of endometriosis at the time of gamete intrafallopian transfer. J Reprod Med 1991; 36(4): 274–278.

102. Hansen M, Bower C, Milne E, et al. Assisted reproductive technologies and the risk of birth defects – a systematic review. Hum Reprod 2005; 20(5): 328–338.

103. Kallen B, Finnstrom O, Nygren KG, et al. In vitro fertilization in Sweden: risk for congenital malformations after different IVF methods. Birth Defects Res A Clin Mol Teratol January 27, 2005 (Epub ahead of print)

104. Practice Committee of the American Society for Reproductive Medicine. Ovarian hyperstimulation syndrome. Fertil Steril 2004; 82(Suppl 1): S81–S86.

105. Andersen AN, Gianaroli L, Nygren KG. Assisted reproductive technology in Europe, 2000. Results generated from European registers by ESHRE. Hum Reprod 2004; 19(3): 490–503.

106. Clapp DN, Adamson GD. Physicians and nurses: counseling the infertile patient. In: Burns LH, Covington SN, eds. Infertility counseling: a comprehensive handbook for clinicians. New York: Parthenon; 1999: 513–526.

107. ACOG Technical Bulletin #223. Pain management principles. Washington, DC: ACOG; May 1996.

108. Wurn BF, Wurn LJ, King CR, et al. Treating female infertility and improving IVF pregnancy rates with a manual physical therapy technique. MedGenMed 2004; 6(2): 51.

109. Fugh-Berman A, Kronenberg F. Complementary and alternative medicine (CAM) in reproductive-age women: a review of randomized controlled trials. Reprod Toxicol 2003; 17(2): 137–152.

110. Adamson GD. A 36-year-old woman with endometriosis, pelvic pain and infertility. JAMA 1999; 282(4): 2347–2354.

111. Falcone T. Future directions and developments in reproductive surgery. Elsevier International Congress Series 1266. 2004; 107–110.

112. Rier SE, Yeaman G. Immune aspects of endometriosis: relevance of the uterine mucosal immune system. In: Speroff L, Adamson GD, eds. Seminars in reproductive endocrinology, endometriosis. New York: Thieme; 1997; 15(3): 209–220.

113. Sharpe-Timms KL, Young SL. Understanding endometriosis is the key to successful therapeutic management. Fertil Steril 2004; 81(5): 1201–1203.

114. Brosens J, Verhoeven H, Campo R, et al. High endometrial aromatase P450 mRNA expression is associated with poor IVF outcome. Hum Reprod 2004; 19(2): 352–356.

115. Bullimore DW. Endometriosis is sustained by tumour necrosis factor-alpha. Med Hypotheses 2003; 60(1): 84–88.

116. D'Hooghe TM, Debrock S, Meuleman C, et al. Future directions in endometriosis research. Obstet Gynecol Clin North Am 2003; 30(1): 221–244.

117. ESHRE Capri Workshop Group. Diagnosis and management of the infertile couple: missing information. Hum Reprod Update 2004; 10(4): 295–307. Epub June 10, 2004.

118. Fagotti A, Ferrandina G, Fanfani F, et al. Analysis of cyclooxygenase-2 (COX-2) expression in different sites of endometriosis and correlation with clinico-pathological parameters. Hum Reprod 2004; 19(2): 393–397.

119. Giudice LC, Kao LC. Endometriosis. Lancet 2004; 13; 364(9447): 1789–1799.

120. Harada T, Yoshioka H, Yoshida S, et al. Increased interleukin-6 levels in peritoneal fluid of infertile patients with active endometriosis. Am J Obstet Gynecol 1997; 176(3): 593–597.

121. Nothnick WB. Novel targets for the treatment of endometriosis. Expert Opin Ther Targets 2004; 8(5): 459–471.

122. Yamashita Y, Ueda M, Takehara M, et al. Influence of severe endometriosis on gene expression of vascular endothelial growth factor and interleukin-6 in granulosa cells from patients undergoing controlled ovarian hyperstimulation for in vitro fertilization-embryo transfer. Fertil Steril 2002; 78(4): 865–871.

123. Gurates B, Bulun SE. Endometriosis: the ultimate hormonal disease. In: Arici A, ed. Seminars in reproductive medicine, endometriosis. New York: Thieme; 2003; 21(2): 125–134.

124. Seli E, Arici A. Endometriosis: interaction of immune and endocrine systems. In: Arici A, ed. Seminars in reproductive medicine, endometriosis. New York: Thieme; 2003; 21(2): 135–144.

125. Rier S, Foster WG. Environmental dioxins and endometriosis. In: Arici A, ed. Seminars in reproductive medicine, endometriosis. New York: Thieme; 2003; 21(2): 145–154.

126. Osteen KG, Yeaman GR, Bruner-Tran KL. Matrix metalloproteinases and endometriosis. In: Arici A, ed. Seminars in reproductive medicine, endometriosis. New York: Thieme; 2003; 21(2): 155–164.

127. Witz C. Cell adhesion molecules and endometriosis. In: Arici A, ed. Seminars in reproductive medicine, endometriosis. New York: Thieme; 2003; 21(2): 173–182.

128. Garrido N, Pellicer A, Remohi J, et al. Uterine and ovarian function in endometriosis. In: Arici A, ed. Seminars in reproductive medicine, endometriosis. New York: Thieme; 2003; 21(2): 183–192.

129. Hastings JM, Fazleabas AT. Future directions in endometriosis research. In: Arici A, ed. Seminars in reproductive medicine, endometriosis. New York: Thieme; 2003; 21(2): 255–262.

130. Garcia-Velasco JA, Arici A. Apoptosis and the pathogenesis of endometriosis. In: Arici A, ed. Seminars in reproductive medicine, endometriosis. New York: Thieme; 2003; 21(2): 165–172.

131. Guidice LC. Genomics' role in understanding the pathogenesis of endometriosis. In: Arici A, ed. Seminars in reproductive medicine, endometriosis. New York: Thieme; 2003; 21(2): 119–124.

132. Kennedy S. Genetics of endometriosis: a review of the positional cloning approaches. In: Arici A, ed. Seminars in reproductive medicine, endometriosis. New York: Thieme; 2003; 21(2): 125–134.

133. The Practice Committee of the American Society for Reproductive Medicine. Effectiveness and treatment for unexplained infertility. Fertil Steril 2004; 82: 160–163.

27 Endometriosis and assisted reproduction

Jean Luc Pouly, Meenal Kamble, Michel Canis, Laurent Janny,
Revaz Botroschivili, Rusudan Piekrischvili, and Benoît Schubert

Infertility associated with endometriosis accounts for 10–20% of the total infertile number of couples, most cases being resistant to the routine surgical and medical lines of the treatment. Hence, when considering endometriosis-related infertility (ERI), the assisted reproductive technologies (ART) play an important role. However, evidence-based medicine is lacking in this field. In this chapter we look at the role of ART in cases of ERI using our long and wide experience along with the opinions of the other clinicians.

The issue can be divided into several topics:

- What is the place for ART in ERI?
- How do we choose an appropriate type of ART for a particular case?
- Are the results of ART impacted by the endometriosis?
- Is it essential to treat and retreat endometriosis before suggesting ART?
- Are there special endometriosis lesions that require a special type of management?
- What extra management is needed in cases of ART and ERI?
- Is there an impact of ART on the evolution of endometriosis?

What is the place of assisted reproductive technologies in endometriosis-related infertility?

Although it is admitted that laparoscopic surgery is the first choice of therapy for ERI, the results of this surgery remain controversial as they fail to clear certain criticism and issues.

First of all, the remaining overall infertility rate after laparoscopic procedures is unclear. A lot of uncontrolled, selected, partial and nonrandomized series have been published that state that the pregnancy rates range from 30 to 80%. Most of these series report that the vast majority of pregnancies occur rapidly, almost within a year of surgery.[1] On the contrary, randomized controlled trials by Marcoux et al[2] and Parazzini[3] report much lesser pregnancy rates of 34% and 24%, respectively.

In our experience, the delivery rate after first laparoscopic surgery, without exclusion of any cases,[4] was 33% in the older series, being maintained almost constant at 31%, according to the most recent series. The newer controlled study that is in course is expected to give a similar observation. Based on these most recent data, it therefore seems that 65–70% of patients are still infertile after the initial surgery.

Postoperative treatments with progestins, gonadotropin-releasing hormone (GnRH) analogues, and antiaromatase have failed to prove their efficacy in improving the fertility prognosis.[5,6]

The important question arises when considering second-line therapy is the dilemma of selecting between ART and second surgery. To the best of our knowledge, no randomized confirmatory trial has ever been published to focus on this issue. In 1996, Pagidas et al[7] reported a comparative retrospective nonrandomized series that was largely in favor of ART as the second-line therapy when compared with that of second surgery as an alternative. According to these authors, the cumulative pregnancy rate (CPR) for stage III or IV ERI after 3, 7, and 9 months of second surgery were 5.9%, 18.1%, and 24.4%, respectively, whereas the CPR was 33.3% and 69.6%, respectively, after 1 and 2 cycles of in vitro-fertilization (IVF). The most challenging observation was that the cumulative PR after 1 cycle of IVF-ET (in vitro fertilization and embryo transfer) was 33.3%, which is much higher when compared to the CPR of 24.4% after reoperation. Most of the experts have the same opinion.

Hence we arrive at the first conclusion, i.e. 65–70% of ERI patients require a second line of therapy and would benefit more effectively from ART as the treatment option than reoperation.

The second point in support of the place of ART in ERI comes from evidence that the postsurgical prognosis of fertility is not homogeneous. Also, the surgery proves itself to be less efficient in certain circumstances. Again, there is a tremendous lack of evidence to support the following opinions:

- There is no relation between the AFS (American Fertility Society) stage and the fertility prognosis as long as there are no tubal adhesions.
- There is no relation with the presence or absence of endometriomas as long as there are no major adnexal adhesions.[8]
- In case of deep endometriosis (mainly rectovaginal nodules), the fertility results are better than in cases of superficial endometriosis as long as there are no major adnexal adhesions.
- Finally, the crucial point is the presence of adnexal and mainly tubal adhesions. In our experience the pregnancy rate was 52% among patients without adhesions and only 15% in patients with tubal adhesions. These data are classical and are supported by the published data of Kistner and also by Canis et al.[9] The recent report by Aboulghar et al[10] is also confirmatory.

Certain other general factors also play an influence on the CPR:

- After the age of 38 years old, the chance of pregnancy drops dramatically.
- There is a strong correlation between the duration of infertility and the prognosis; in our experience, independent of age, the overall delivery rate was less than 15% when the duration of infertility was longer than 8 years.

- We also found a correlation with sperm quality; in cases of abnormal sperms (mild oligoasthenospermia), the pregnancy rate dropped to 18% from 48% in cases of normal sperm morphology.[4]

Thus, we arrive at the second conclusion of this chapter: it is justifiable to refer patients to ART in whom the estimated prognosis after surgery is very poor. They should be referred immediately after surgery or even instead of surgery. In our experience, we evaluated that 12% of the patients are in this group, but this proportion tends to increase with the age of the patient.

Finally, out of the total ERI patients, 65–70% will be referred to ART. Among them, 10–15% should be referred immediately and the others eventually when they have failed to be pregnant after a 6–12 months delay without conception.

How to choose an appropriate type of assisted reproductive technology for a particular case?

Assisted reproductive technologies include IUI (intrauterine insemination), IVF, ICSI (intracytoplasmic sperm injection), and oocytes donation.

There is no doubt that classical IVF must be preferred in case of tubal pathology or in cases of tubal or ovarian adhesions. ICSI must be reserved for the cases where a patent male factor is associated with ERI. Also, the choice exists only in the cases of nonsevere endometriosis without adhesion, without male factor, in patients less than 38 years old, and with infertility less than 8 years of duration.

Even if the pathophysiology of ERI is controversial,[11,12] there are cogent arguments to think that in cases of mild-to-moderate endometriosis two additional physiologic factors have influence on the CPR:

- There is a disturbance of the physiology of the granulosa under the influence of cytokines. This leads to an alteration of the secretion of inhibin, which induces an impaired secretion of gonadotropins during the late follicular phase. These disturbances lead to poor oocyte and ovulation quality.
- On the other hand, several publications have reported an antispermatozoid effect of the peritoneal fluid. This effect is mainly the immobilization of the spermatozoids and activated phagocytosis by macrophages.

Although IVF will effectively facilitate by-passing these two alterations, IUI with ovarian stimulation (OS) can also achieve these targets.

We tried to evaluate the efficacy of this treatment. For 3 years all the patients with the previous criteria who had failed to be pregnant after laparoscopic surgery were treated by IUI + OS.

Ovarian stimulation was obtained with clomiphene (100 mg/day from day 2 to day 6). Human menopausal gonadotropin (HMG) was added on day 8 (75 IU/day). The monitoring was done with the help of echography, starting on day 10 after menstruation. When the largest follicle reached 20 mm, HCG (5000 IU) was administrered. IUI (with a Percoll separation) was performed 36–38 hours after HCG.

Among 326 patients being treated in this way, the crude delivery rate was 15% per cycle and the cumulative delivery rate after 3 cycles was 41%. Out of the total, 12% of patients had multiple deliveries. Whereas with IVF, in similar cases, the delivery rate was 26% per started cycles (mean transferred embryos: 2.1), a CPR after 2 attempts was 46% and after 3 attempts was 58%. Out of these IVF cases, 23% had multiple deliveries. When a financial comparison was made between the two, there was no doubt concerning the cost–benefit ratio inclining towards IUI. The overall price of an IUI is 500 euros vs 2500 euros for an IVF cycle. Finally, the cost of a delivery was 3518 euros with IUI vs 9586 euros with IVF and the cost of a baby (by addition of the extra cost for the multiple pregnancies and babies) was 4101 euros with IUI vs 9586 euros with IVF. In addition, the psychologic and physical stress was found to be much lower for IUI than for IVF.

Consequently, we suggest that IUI + OS should be considered as second-line therapy after laparoscopic failures provided that there is no absolute indication for IVF or ICSI in the given case (Figure 27.1).

However, two problems are yet to be resolved:

- Can this strategy be proposed even for patients over 38 years old?
- How many IUI attempts should be performed before moving to IVF?

In our study, it was decided to limit the attempts to 3, because the IUI results seem to decline in the higher-range attempts – at least in the case of unexplained infertility.

All authorities do not necessarily agree with this opinion. According to Singh et al[13] the pregnancy rates were as poor as 6% per cycle. Montanaro Gauci et al[14] also claimed that the results were poor, but their study mixed endometriosis and tubal pathologies. For Dmowski et al,[15] IVF must be preferred, as the pregnancy rate after IUI was 11% compared with 47% after IVF (mean transferred embryos: 2.9). But in this series, ART applied only after 3 years of the surgery, probably giving an extra time lag. Some other authors also recommend the use of IUI before IVF.[16–17] Prado-Perez et al[18] have a similar opinion, with excellent results in stage 1 and 2 (>24% pregnancy/cycle) and the lowest result in severe cases (5.6%). This last point is probably related to adhesions, which play an important role in the AFS staging.

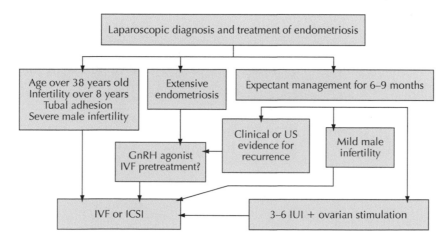

Figure 27.1 Management of endometriosis-related infertility. GnRH = gonadotropin-releasing hormone; ICSI = intracytoplasmic sperm injection; IUI = intrauterine insemination; IVF = in vitro fertilization; US = ultrasound.

What is the impact of endometriosis on the results of assisted reproductive technologies?

A lot of controversial publications have been written on this topic. We have very strong views on this issue, because of studies in the literature being biased or not evidence based. All the studies on this issue until now have made a comparison between reference groups of patients with either tubal infertility, unexplained infertility, or male infertility. All these diagnoses when taken together bias the analysis. The comparison needs to be made between cases of similar groups and performed step by step.

The ovarian reserve in cases of endometriosis-related infertility

There are a large number of publications on this subject. Some authors have reported a decrease in ovarian reserve with less harvested oocytes during IVF attempts or the necessity of increasing the HMG dosage to obtain efficient stimulation. But this opinion of a decreased number of oocytes is generally not admitted by most of the authors.[19]

In our experience among the patients adjusted for age, attempts, range and type of stimulation, the mean number of harvested oocytes were 10.58 ± 7.08 ($n = 593$) in cases of ERI, 9.96 ± 6.77 ($n = 849$) ($p < 0.03$) in tubal infertility, 11.33 ± 6.63 ($n = 506$) ($p = 0.04$) in male infertility, and 10.64 ± 6.68 ($n = 376$) ($p = NS$) in unexplained infertility (Table 27.1). Even if some differences were found, they were minimal, were going in the opposite direction, and did not permit a conclusion of a negative impact on the ovarian reserve.

The fertilization rate

Again, regarding the fertilization rate in ERI patients, the opinions create controversies. For some authors, the fertilization rate is reduced with a negative correlation with the AFS stage, whereas for others there is no difference. These divergences can be explained on the basis of the chosen reference groups.

In Table 27.1 we report our results in terms of fertilization rates, transfer rates, and mean number of embryos in the four previous groups. There is a minimal reduction of the fertilization rate as compared with the fertilization rates of tubal or the unexplained groups that does not seem to have any impact on the transfer rates. The similar observation holds true when the number of the embryos are considered for the above subcategories.

Implantation

When considering implantation, the literature places us in confusion with the divergent data. Some authors report a reduction of the pregnancy rate, and some contradict by reporting an improved rate. But most of them agree on the implantation rate and claim that there is no difference in the implantation rate. Again, the reference groups play an important role in these divergences because it is well known that the implantation rate is reduced in tubal infertility and increased in infertility due to the male factor. In our experience when comparing similar series we were not able to

Table 27.1 Comparison of oocytes collection, fertilization rate, and transfer rate in in vitro fertilization (IVF) among pure endometriosis, pure tubal infertility, pure male infertility or unexplained infertility cases

Indication	Endometriosis	Tubal infertility	Male infertility (IVF)	Unexplained infertility
Number	593	849	506	376
Oocytes	10.58	9.96	11.33	10.64
Fertilization rate (%)	49.0	54.3	29.1	52.9
Transfer rate (%)	85.1	88.2	61.4	84.8
Embryos	5.21	5.47	3.29	5.66

Table 27.2 Comparison of pregnancy rate and delivery rate among pure endometriosis, pure tubal infertility, pure male infertility, or unexplained infertility cases

Indication	Endometriosis	Tubal infertility	Male infertility (IVF)	Unexplained infertility
Number	593	849	506	376
Embryos	5.21	5.47	3.29	5.66
Transferred embryos	2.54	2.68	2.48	2.59
Implantation per transfer	40.1	37.7	34.7	41.0
Clinical pregnancy per transfer (%)	35.4	33.6	32.1	36.3
Delivery per clinical pregnancy (%)	84.9	79.7	84.0	91.3
Delivery per transfer (%)	30.0	26.8	27.0	33.2
Delivery per retrieval (%)	25.6	23.6	16.6	28.1
Implantation rate (%)	15.1	14.4	15.4	16.9

find any difference in either the implantation rate or the pregnancy outcome. Also, the implantation rate calculated by baby per transferred embryo was equivalent in ERI to other groups according to our series (Table 27.2).

The oocytes and embryos quality

The oocyte's quality can be partially evaluated in IVF and more precisely in ICSI, but the evaluation mainly concerns nuclear maturation and it influences the fertilization rate. However, poor cytoplasm maturation can affect the early embryonic development and therefore the embryo's quality and/or development. Many studies have underlined this point. We showed that the blastocyst ratio (ratio of day 2 embryos reaching the blastocyst stage on days 5–6) in late culture was reduced in cases of endometriosis vs tubal or unexplained infertility.[20] Pellicer et al[21] also found a higher rate of arrested embryos on day 3. Simon et al[22] have shown in the oocyte donation model that the chances of pregnancy are reduced when the embryos come from an endometriosis patient but not in the non-endometriosis patient, suggesting a lower embryo quality and not an implantation defect. This seems correlated to an increased apoptosis in the granulosa cells. Nevertheless, this effect is weak, as it generally has a minimal impact on the transfer rate and on the mean number of transferred embryos.

The pregnancy outcome

Endometriosis has also been implicated as a factor responsible for miscarriage. In IVF studies this was recently reported by Yanushpolsky et al.[23] For all the other authors, there does not seem to be any difference.

The overall results

Even if some authors report that the delivery rate is reduced and generally is related to the AFS stage, the general opinion is that there is no impact on this pregnancy rate in cases of ERI when compared with the classical infertility indications such as tubal infertility or unexplained infertility.[24–28]

In cases of ICSI where the cause of the infertility is due to male factor, Minguez et al[29] have shown that the presence of endometriosis has no impact on the delivery rate.

Is it essential to treat and retreat endometriosis before suggesting assisted reproductive technologies?

The lack of valuable data makes it difficult to answer this question.

Practically, the question can be divided into three categories, according to the common clinical situations:

1. After a complete laparoscopic treatment with continued infertility, should endometriosis

be retreated before ART (IVF) in the absence of clinical evidence of recurrence of endometriosis?

It seems evident that a second laparoscopic treatment is not indicated, although there is no data justifying supporting this. The other treatment option would be a medical line of therapy by GnRH agonists. This procedure is also described as 'ultra-long agonist protocol': according to this protocol, depot GnRH analogues are prescribed for a period of 3–6 months and during the last period, ovarian stimulation with follicle-stimulating hormone (FSH) and HMG is started and the IVF procedure performed.

To the best of our knowledge, the work performed by Nakamura et al[30] with a small number of cases is the only randomized study to support this protocol. They found a tremendous difference in the ultra-long protocol vs the standard long protocol, with the results favoring the ultra-long protocol (63% pregnancy rate vs 21%, respectively). Unfortunately, this trial was not confirmed by the case control studies and the study published by Chedid et al[31] found no difference in the treatment protocols in a large nonrandomized trial. In our experience, there is no benefit in retreatment. Moreover this procedure is expensive, time-consuming, and creates a lot of side effects.

2. After a complete laparoscopic treatment and continued infertility, should endometriosis be retreated before ART (IVF) if there is a clinical or echographic diagnostic evidence of recurrence? And if so how?

As previously stated, the general consensus is that a new laparoscopic treatment will offer a minimal chance for a spontaneous conception, and it is better to refer these patients to ART and mainly for IVF.

At this point it is interesting to know whether the new surgical or medical treatment will improve the success rate of IVF. For the medical line of treatment, no scientific data with strict controls are available. For the effect of repeated laparoscopic surgery, there is also no evidence-based answer. The general opinion, based on previous experience, is that there is no necessity to retreat, as it does not seem to change the prognosis. The dilemma for the treatment option mainly arises in recurring endometriomas, which are discussed in detail in the following sections.

3. Is it necessary to treat a clinically evident endometriosis before an IVF that is indicated for other reasons than ERI, such as major male

factor, complete tubal blockage, or repeated tubal pregnancies?

Again there are no randomized controlled trials to answer this question. There are a few series suggesting that endometriosis in such cases, even if left untreated, does not impair the IVF results;[10,32] however, that is an indirect and debatable proof, and needs to be confirmed with direct evidence.

Are there special endometriotic lesions that require a special management?

Endometriosis is a polymorphic disease and all the cases cannot be put in the same clinicopathologic category: the primary lesions can be extremely different and the long-term evolution is highly unpredictable. We would like to focus this section on three different situations (endometriomas, rectovaginal nodules, and extensive endometriosis)

Endometriomas

The management of this lesion has been subject to a large amount of controversy and debate.[33] First, a choice was offered between the surgical techniques of IPC (intraperitoneal cystectomy), as per our group, or ICV (intracystic vaporization), developed by Donnez. Now the debate seems to be closed with two conclusions:

• the IPC offers the better chance of spontaneous pregnancy and the lower risk of recurrence[34,35]
• by contrast, the ICV offers a better chance of preserving the oocyte stock.

The difference between the two techniques during IVF stimulation is 10% in the amount of harvested oocytes in favor of ICV.[36,37] Finally according to current concepts, it is better to perform an IPC when easily feasible and an ICV or an intracystic coagulation (in one step) if IPC appears difficult to perform.

In ART, the occurrence or the recurrence of endometriomas is common. The data are large enough to give the following conclusions:

• presence of an endometrioma has no impact on the result of IVF
• presence of chocolate fluid (hemosiderin) in the follicular puncture does not impair the quality of the oocytes[38]

- it is not necessary to operate and certainly not to reoperate on an endometrioma before an IVF attempt[32,39]
- large endometriomas can be drained (± sclerotherapy)[40] under ultrasound control before beginning an IVF cycle, but the benefits are not clearly established
- the endometriomas do not seem to complicate the pregnancy, the incidence being extremely rare (only 1 reported case of rupture at 3 months of gestation)
- most of the ovarian abscesses occurring after ovum pick-up are among patients with an endometrioma.

In conclusion, the concept is not to reoperate on endometriomas until they are clinically symptomatic (pain). When an endometrioma is found during IVF stimulation, it must be ignored and the cycle continued without special attention. There is limited discussion on the cases of poor response to IVF and they are associated with endometrioma. No controlled data are available to support the concept of a new operation or the opposite. In our opinion, it can be thought of only in the cases of a dramatically poor response and to protect the ovary from adhesions but it must be restricted to a last chance before oocyte donation.

Rectovaginal nodules

Depending upon the adhesion, invasion, and the contraction of the surrounding tissue, this type of lesion can present in extremely variable scenarios. Moreover, severe pain in terms of dysmenorrhea, dyspareunia, cyclical pain, and infertility are frequently associated. The recurrences represent a difficult surgical challenge in terms of conservation and tissue morbidity.

Specially in cases of severe tubal or ovarian adhesions and even in cases of a satisfactory or unsatisfactory surgical procedure, IVF must be considered rapidly after the surgery.

Without tubal or ovarian involvement, the routine general management can be awaited, because of the high possibilities of spontaneous pregnancy.

In cases of recurrence, mainly with severe pain, in an infertile patient, the discussion must be for the choice between a new surgical procedure and IVF. The surgery is not directed towards enhancing fertility, and hence IVF must be preferred to treat infertility in these cases. The patient can be treated with continuous progesterone or estrogen–progesterone while waiting for the IVF. The basic concept is to permit the patient

to get a baby before offering any radical surgical treatment such as a hysterectomy. When the surgery is unavoidable because of the pain, it is mandatory to avoid trauma to the ovaries.

The results of IVF in these cases are similar to the results in standard cases of superficial endometriosis.

Extensive endometriosis

These are cases where the endometriosis can be diagnosed without laparoscopy (perception of rectovaginal nodules, presence of endometriomas at ultrasonographic scan) and with a strong probability of a frozen pelvis. They can also be cases where, during laparoscopy, any operative procedures appear risky in terms of morbidity due to resection-anastomosis of the intestine, colpotomy, ureteric injury, or bladder injury.

In such patients, one of the options is to treat the patient with GnRH analogues before a second operation. The other possibility is to treat the patient with GnRH analogues and to perform an IVF at the end of the medical treatment.

As the surgical treatment offers an extremely low chance of pregnancy, we consider that the second option is more acceptable, even without histologic or visual confirmation of the lesions. IVF offers a much better fertility prognosis. The same principle for the treatment strategy has also been opined by Garcia-Velasco et al[32] and Aboulghar et al.[10]

What extra management is needed in cases of assisted reproductive technologies and endometriosis-related infertility?

There is no particular specific protocol to be followed to achieve ART in cases of ERI, but a few points must be kept in mind:

- Among women with severe tubal blockage and/or endometriomas, it is important and useful to perform a vaginal echographic control before commencing HMG/FSH injections in order to evaluate the periovarian adhesive pouches and the small endometriomas that could be confounded with follicles.
- Among women with clinically evident endometriosis, the ovum pick-up must be

scheduled under general anesthesia because it is often painful under local anesthesia.

- During the ovum pick-up, it is recommended to avoid puncturing through an endometrioma to minimize the risk of abscess; if unavoidable, it should be performed only after the informed and signed consent of the patient for this particular risk. Prophylactic antibiotics do not seem to minimize the risk in these cases and a strict vaginal antisepsis is mandatory.

Is there an the impact of assisted reproductive technologies on endometriosis evolution?

A lot of gynecologists are anxious about the possibility of exacerbating endometriosis because of the high level of estrogens during the stimulation phase. To the best of our knowledge, only 1 anecdotal case was reported that occurred during a pregnancy due to IVF. In our large experience, we have never seen any endometriosis that has flare up after an IVF procedure only. Of course, a recurrence of endometriosis can occur, but that does not seem to be more frequent after ovarian hyperstimulation and/or IVF.

On the other hand, it is generally admitted that a pregnancy improves the fertility prognosis in cases of ERI. The improvement is obviously clear for the pain during the first year but is less evident thereafter. Is it a real effect or a subjective effect in

a patient happy to have a baby? For infertility, the improvement is minimal. We studied the post-IVF fertility among patients that have or have not achieved a pregnancy according to the indications. Among the ERI cases, 7% of the patients became spontaneously pregnant in the following 4 years, vs 3% in cases of tubal infertility, 15% in male infertility, and 25% in unexplained infertility. The natural pregnancy rate was slightly higher among the ERI patients that were pregnant with IVF (10% vs 4%). This is in opposition to the classical idea that these patients are cured from their infertility problems by a pregnancy.

Currently, we are conducting a cohort study to evaluate the long-term evolution of endometriosis and we will be able to answer these questions in the coming years.

Conclusion

The place of ART in the management of ERI is important as it concerns 60–70% of the patients. IUI can be used before IVF in cases without adverse features (adhesion, tubal pathology, long infertility duration, and high maternal age or sperm alteration). There is no necessity to reoperate on endometriosis and even endometriomas before IVF unless indicated or symptomatic. IVF among ERI patients does not justify any specific procedures. The IVF results are good among these patients. Ovarian hyperstimulation for IVF does not significantly expose women to a higher risk of an acute exacerbation of endometriosis.

REFERENCES

1. Nezhat C, Crowgey S, Nezhat F. Videolaseroscopy for the treatment of endometriosis associated with infertility. Fertil Steril 1989; 51(2): 237–240.
2. Marcoux S, Maheux R, Berube S. Laparoscopic surgery in infertile women with minimal or mild endometriosis. Canadian Collaborative Group on Endometriosis. N Engl J Med 1997; 337(4): 217–222.
3. Parazzini F. Ablation of lesions or no treatment in minimal-mild endometriosis in infertile women: a randomized trial. Gruppo Italiano per lo Studio dell'Endometriosi. Hum Reprod 1999; 14(5): 1332–1334.
4. Pouly JL, Drolet J, Canis M, et al. Laparoscopic treatment of symptomatic endometriosis. Hum Reprod 1996; 11 (Suppl 3): 67–88.
5. Adamson GD, Pasta DJ. Surgical treatment of endometriosis-associated infertility: meta-analysis compared with survival analysis. Am J Obstet Gynecol 1994; 171(6): 1488–1504.
6. Yap C, Furness S, Farquhar C. Pre and post operative medical therapy for endometriosis surgery. Cochrane Database Syst Rev 2004; 3: CD003678.
7. Pagidas K, Falcone T, Hemmings R, et al. Comparison of reoperation for moderate (stage III) and severe (stage IV) endometriosis-related infertility with in vitro fertilization-embryo transfer. Fertil Steril 1996; 65(4): 791–795.
8. Canis M, Mage G, Wattiez A, et al. Second-look laparoscopy after laparoscopic cystectomy of large ovarian endometriomas. Fertil Steril 1992; 58(3): 617–619.

9. Canis M, Pouly JL, Wattiez A, et al. Incidence of bilateral adnexal disease in severe endometriosis (revised American Fertility Society [AFS], stage IV): should a stage V be included in the AFS classification? Fertil Steril 1992; 57(3): 691–692.

10. Aboulghar MA, Mansour RT, Serour GI, et al. The outcome of in vitro fertilization in advanced endometriosis with previous surgery: a case-controlled study. Am J Obstet Gynecol 2003; 188(2): 371–375.

11. Navarro J, Garrido N, Remohi J, et al. How does endometriosis affect infertility? Obstet Gynecol Clin North Am 2003; 30(1): 181–192.

12. Pritts EA, Taylor RN. An evidence-based evaluation of endometriosis-associated infertility. Endocrinol Metab Clin North Am 2003; 32(3): 653–667.

13. Singh M, Goldberg J, Falcone T, et al. Superovulation and intrauterine insemination in cases of treated mild pelvic disease. J Assist Reprod Genet 2001; 18(1): 26–29.

14. Montanaro Gauci M, Kruger TF, Coetzee K, et al. Stepwise regression analysis to study male and female factors impacting on pregnancy rate in an intrauterine insemination programme. Andrologia 2001; 33(3): 135–141.

15. Dmowski WP, Pry M, Ding J, et al. Cycle-specific and cumulative fecundity in patients with endometriosis who are undergoing controlled ovarian hyperstimulation-intrauterine insemination or in vitro fertilization-embryo transfer. Fertil Steril 2002; 78(4): 750–756.

16. El Amrani R, Henry-Suchet J, Cornier E, et al. [Comparisons of 2 therapeutic strategies in severe endometriosis, in young women consulting for sterility or pain. II. In the case of infertility, value of ovarian stimulation with intrauterine insemination after surgery]. Gynecol Obstet Fertil 2001; 29(3): 192–199. [in French]

17. Sahakyan M, Harlow BL, Hornstein MD. Influence of age, diagnosis, and cycle number on pregnancy rates with gonadotropin-induced controlled ovarian hyperstimulation and intrauterine insemination. Fertil Steril 1999; 72(3): 500–504.

18. Prado-Perez J, Navarro-Martinez C, Lopez-Rivadeneira E, et al. The impact of endometriosis on the rate of pregnancy of patients submitted to intrauterine insemination. Fertil Steril 2002; 77(Suppl 1): 551.

19. Mahutte NG, Arici A. New advances in the understanding of endometriosis related infertility. J Reprod Immunol 2002; 55(1–2): 73–83.

20. Durruty G, Pouly JL, Janny L. Coculture in endometriosis patients results in less blastocysts (oral presentation). ESHRE, June 1998, Goteborg.

21. Pellicer A, Oliveira N, Ruiz A, et al. Exploring the mechanism(s) of endometriosis-related infertility: an analysis of embryo development and implantation in assisted reproduction. Hum Reprod 1995; 10 (Suppl 2): 91–97.

22. Simon C, Gutierrez A, Vidal A, et al. Outcome of patients with endometriosis in assisted reproduction: results from in-vitro fertilization and oocyte donation. Hum Reprod 1994; 9(4): 725–729.

23. Yanushpolsky EH, Best CL, Jackson KV, et al. Effects of endometriomas on oocyte quality, embryo quality, and pregnancy rates in in vitro fertilization cycles: a prospective, case-controlled study. J Assist Reprod Genet 1998; 15(4): 193–197.

24. Tanbo T, Omland A, Dale PO, et al. In vitro fertilization/embryo transfer in unexplained infertility and minimal peritoneal endometriosis. Acta Obstet Gynecol Scand 1995; 74(7): 539–543.

25. Olivennes F, Feldberg D, Liu HC, et al. Endometriosis: a stage by stage analysis – the role of in vitro fertilization. Fertil Steril 1995; 64(2): 392–398.

26. Tinkanen H, Kujansuu E. In vitro fertilization in patients with ovarian endometriomas. Acta Obstet Gynecol Scand 2000; 79(2): 119–122.

27. Dmowski WP, Pry M, Ding J, et al. Cycle-specific and cumulative fecundity in patients with endometriosis who are undergoing controlled ovarian hyperstimulation-intrauterine insemination or in vitro fertilization-embryo transfer. Fertil Steril 2002; 78(4): 750–756.

28. Barnhart K, Dunsmoor-Su R, Coutifaris C. Effect of endometriosis on in vitro fertilization. Fertil Steril 2002; 77(6): 1148–1155.

29. Minguez Y, Rubio C, Bernal A, et al. The impact of endometriosis in couples undergoing intracytoplasmic sperm injection because of male infertility. Hum Reprod 1997; 12(10): 2282–2285.

30. Nakamura K, Oosawa M, Kondou I, et al. Menotropin stimulation after prolonged gonadotropin releasing hormone agonist pretreatment for in vitro fertilization in patients with endometriosis. J Assist Reprod Genet 1992; 9(2): 113–117.

31. Chedid S, Camus M, Smitz J, et al. Comparison among different ovarian stimulation regimens for assisted procreation procedures in patients with endometriosis. Hum Reprod 1995; 10(9): 2406–2411.

32. Garcia-Velasco JA, Mahutte NG, Corona J, et al. Removal of endometriomas before in vitro fertilization does not improve fertility outcomes: a matched, case-control study. Obstet Gynecol Surv 2004; 59(9): 661–662.

33. Pouly JL. Endometriomas and in vitro fertilization outcomes. J Gynecol Obstet Biol Reprod (Paris). 2003; 32(8 Pt 2): S37–41.

34. Beretta P, Franchi M, Ghezzi F, et al. Randomized clinical trial of two laparoscopic treatments of endometriomas: cystectomy versus drainage and coagulation. Fertil Steril 1998; 70(6): 1176–1180.

35. Saleh A, Tulandi T. Reoperation after laparoscopic treatment of ovarian endometriomas by excision and by fenestration. Fertil Steril 1999; 72(2): 322–324.

36. Canis M, Pouly JL, Tamburro S, et al. Ovarian response during IVF-embryo transfer cycles after laparoscopic ovarian cystectomy for endometriotic cysts of >3 cm in diameter. Hum Reprod 2001; 16(12): 2583–2586.

37. Donnez J, Wyns C, Nisolle M. Does ovarian surgery for endometriomas impair the ovarian response to gonadotropin? Fertil Steril 2001; 76(4): 662–665.

38. Khamsi F, Yavas Y, Lacanna IC, et al. Exposure of human oocytes to endometrioma fluid does not alter fertilization or early embryo development. J Assist Reprod Genet 2001; 18(2): 106–109.

39. Surrey ES, Schoolcraft WB. Does surgical management of endometriosis within 6 months of an in vitro fertilization-embryo transfer cycle improve outcome? J Assist Reprod Genet 2003; 20(9): 365–370.

40. Fisch JD, Sher G. Sclerotherapy with 5% tetracycline is a simple alternative to potentially complex surgical treatment of ovarian endometriomas before in vitro fertilization. Fertil Steril 2004; 82(2): 437–441.

28 An overview of adenomyosis and its surgical management

Ian S Fraser, Rose CY Tse, and Anu Goswami

Introduction

Adenomyosis has long been regarded as a close 'cousin' of endometriosis, although the two conditions behave quite differently. Adenomyosis is a relatively common gynecologic disorder, but has often been described as an elusive disease. Histologically, it is characterized by the extension of endometrial glands and stroma beneath the endometrial–myometrial interface to form nests deep within the myometrium. Subsequent myometrial hyperplasia around the adenomyotic foci is also characteristic. Rokitansky[1] first described the condition in 1860, followed by further descriptions by von Recklinghausen in 1896.[2] In 1908, Cullen[3] classified two histologic types:

- 'adenomyoma,' a tumor-like isolated area of hypertrophic myometrium containing stroma and glandular elements of the endometrium
- 'diffuse adenomyoma,' a distribution of both elements throughout widespread areas of the myometrium.

The term 'adenomyosis uteri' was first used by Frankl in 1925.[4] In 1972, Bird et al[5] stated:

> Adenomyosis may be defined as the benign invasion of endometrium into the myometrium, producing a diffusely enlarged uterus which microscopically exhibits ectopic nonneoplastic, endometrial glands and stroma surrounded by the hypertrophic and hyperplastic myometrium.

Donnez et al[6] described fibrotic nodular 'adenomyosis' invading deep into the rectovaginal space. They make a strong case that this is truly a form of adenomyosis rather than endometriosis. For management, it requires difficult excision of nodular, adherent fibrotic tissue from the posterior vagina, rectum, posterior cervix, and uterosacral ligaments. Koninckx et al[7] described three types of deep-infiltrating 'endometriosis' (which is the same condition described by Donnez):

- Deep-infiltrating disease of type I is a large lesion in the peritoneal cavity, infiltrating conically with the deeper parts becoming progressively smaller. It has been suggested that this type of 'endometriosis/adenomyosis' is caused by infiltration.
- In type II lesions, the main feature is that bowel is retracted over the lesion, which thus becomes deeply situated in the rectovaginal septum although not actually infiltrating it.
- Type III lesions are the deepest and most severe. They are spherically shaped, situated deep in the rectovaginal septum, often only visible as a small typical surface lesion at laparoscopy, or often not visible at all. This lesion is often more palpable than visible, is acutely tender if the patient is examined at the time of menstruation, and gives rise to severe dyspareunia.

Donnez et al[8] have also reported a large series of 405 patients with severe dysmenorrhea or deep dyspareunia due to rectovaginal adenomyotic nodules. Preoperative intravenous pyelography revealed ureteral stenosis with ureterohydro-nephrosis in 18 patients (4.4%). A significantly higher prevalence (11.2%) was observed in nodules ≥3 cm in diameter. Five women (20%) had complete ureteral stenosis and kidney scintigraphy revealed damaged kidney parenchymal function in 18–42%.

Prevalence and incidence

Adenomyosis is said to be commonly found in multiparous women in their forties to fifties.[5] About 80% of cases occur in women at 40–50 years old and 90% in multipara. The incidence reported varies widely in women with menstrual complaints: 5–70%.[5,9] This wide range can be explained by the fact that the diagnosis was mainly obtained on histologic examination of hysterectomy specimens and it tends to include more patients in an older age group. It is doubtful whether the incidence of adenomyosis in younger age groups is similar to that in older age groups when diagnosis is now made more frequently and confidently with modern imaging and hystero-scopic techniques. Besides these factors, the prevalence and incidence also depend on the number of tissue sections taken for histologic examination and the different histologic diagnostic criteria used. Yet, there is no universally agreed 'minimal depth of invasion' criteria for the diagnosis. The normal endometrial–myometrial interface (EMI) is irregular over its entire surface and the normal indentations of the basal endometrium cannot be easily distinguished from an abnormal downgrowth.[10] Ferenczy[11] emphasized the importance of identifying the appearance of myometrial hypertrophy around the foci of adenomyosis.

Pathogenesis

The EMI of the uterus has a unique structure and function. A submucosa is absent and, as a result, the endometrial glands lie in direct contact with the underlying myometrium. The lack of a submucosa renders myometrium vulnerable to invasion by endometrial glands and stroma. The precise etiology and sequence of events leading to adenomyosis are still unknown.[12] The myometrial zonal anatomy was first described with magnetic resonance imaging (MRI) by Hrick et al[13] in 1983.

A junctional zone was described and is a band of low signal intensity on T2-weighted images. It represents the innermost layer of myometrium and forms one side of the EMI. It has been postulated that junctional zone disease, defined as subendometrial smooth muscle hyperplasia with distortion of normal zonal architecture and disturbance of inner myometrial function, predisposes to secondary infiltration by endometrial elements.[10,12] The disturbance of the junctional zone, which could be directly caused by endometrial factors or genetic predisposition, or indirectly by an altered 'immune' response, may be the primary abnormality in the pathogenesis of adenomyosis. It is also possible that certain hormonal conditions, like those found in pregnancy, facilitate the endometrial invasion. The concept of trauma to the deeper endometrium, leading to breakdown of EMI, followed by reactive hyperplasia of the endometrial basalis and its penetration into the myometrium, has been proposed. It was observed that patients with symptomatic adenomyosis have a significantly higher incidence of history of termination of pregnancy or spontaneous abortion. In a mouse model, chronic hyperprolactinemia was shown to have induced the development of adenomyosis. High levels of circulating estrogen and progesterone may also have a synergistic effect. Abnormal immune responses have been demonstrated in adenomyosis and these anecdotal results may suggest the possibility of disturbance of local immune response.[14]

Clinical features

The classical symptoms associated with adenomyosis are excessive menstrual blood loss, accompanied by worsening dysmenorrhea occurring in multiparous women in their forties, usually with an enlarged and tender uterus of less than 12 weeks gravid size. However, about 35% are asymptomatic. Among the rest, 40–50% complain of menorrhagia; 20% have metrorrhagia, and only 15–30% dysmenorrhea.[9,15–17]

Menorrhagia

McCausland[18] has demonstrated a relationship between the depth of adenomyosis and the severity of menorrhagia, although the mechanisms for this association are unclear. During normal menstruation, there are antegrade-propagated sub-endometrial contractions from the fundus to the cervix, and distortion of the junctional zone with adenomyosis may affect these contractions and influence abnormal menstrual loss.[10] Excessive local production of prostaglandins and disturbed estrogen metabolism may also be influences.

Adenomyosis may also be associated with a range of other menstrual symptoms, although the role of coexisting pathologies in symptom generation is unclear (see below).

Dysmenorrhea

Dysmenorrhea was found to be associated with the number of pathologically identified adenomyotic foci as well as with the depth of adenomyosis.[5,15,17] Myometrial penetration to 80% of full depth was found to be a high risk factor for dysmenorrhea.[15,17] The pain could be caused by uterine contractile irritability, pseudodecidual edema, and the local release of pain-stimulating molecules, including prostaglandins, around the adenomyotic foci.

Dyspareunia

Dyspareunia, which is sometimes experienced by patients with adenomyosis, can be due to the enlarged tender uterus. This means the clinical picture of adenomyosis is quite similar to that of endometriosis.

Infertility

Although adenomyosis preferentially affects multiparous women, several reports have shown that patients with adenomyosis have a higher incidence of infertility and early miscarriage.[19] The causality of the relationship is not clear. The subendometrial myometrium or junctional zone has been observed to function distinctly differently from the outer myometrium. There is a defined pattern of contractility that varies with different phases of the menstrual cycle. Contractions are retrograde in all phases of the cycle except during menstruation. It has been speculated that these contractions may be important in sperm transport and conservation of preimplantation blastocysts within the upper part of the uterine cavity. Adenomyosis with disturbance in the junctional zone may impair these contractions and interfere in the sperm transport and blastocyst implantation.

Disturbances of local nitric oxide release and abnormal immune responses have been investigated as possible mechanisms in the causation of infertility or early miscarriages. Optimal levels of nitric oxide are critical for normal sperm function and embryonic development. Ota et al[20] found that the expression of the enzyme endothelial nitric oxide synthase in adenomyosis is persistently high compared with controls throughout the cycle. In adenomyosis sufferers, there is also strong expression of certain cell surface antigens and increase in the number of local macrophages and other immune cells, with local deposition of immunoglobulins (Igs) and complement as well as circulating autoantibodies. Endometrial cells appear to be under 'immunologic stress' and protect themselves by synthesizing heat shock protein, which is strongly expressed in infertile women with adenomyosis. Altered integrin expression may inhibit both embryo implantation and subsequent embryonic development by adversely affecting the microenvironment of the endometrium. In adenomyosis, the most prevalent circulating autoantibodies are antiphosphatidylinositol IgG, antiphosphatidylglycerol IgG, and antiphosphatidylserine IgG. The presence of these antiphospholipid antibodies also suggests a possible correlation with early miscarriages and infertility.

Coexisting pathology

Coexisting pathologies, such as leiomyomata, endometriosis, endometrial hyperplasia, endometrial polyps, salpingitis isthmica nodosa, and even endometrial cancer,[11,12] are commonly reported in women with adenomyosis, and therefore there is often uncertainty about the causal relationship of symptoms with adenomyosis itself. In one pathologic study, 60–80% of adenomyotic uteri contained associated pathology.[21] In 136 patients with histologically proven adenomyosis,[22] it was reported that many symptoms were heterogeneous and nonspecific and could be related to associated pathologies.

Investigation and diagnosis

Traditionally, the diagnosis of adenomyosis was made on histologic examination of hysterectomy specimens; however, recent advances in surgical and nonsurgical diagnostic techniques and the introduction of more conservative treatments have forced a re-evaluation of diagnosis and assessment. Improved accuracy of the preoperative diagnosis and assessment has now become essential in order to improve patient selection for surgery or for other modalities of treatment. A high index of suspicion is necessary in the woman with an enlarged, tender uterus and variations of abnormal uterine bleeding with or without pelvic pain or dysmenorrhea. Such women require specific exclusion of moderate or severe degrees of adenomyosis.

Nonsurgical approaches to diagnosis and assessment

Biochemical

Biochemical testing is of limited value, although serum cancer antigen 125 (CA-125) is frequently elevated and, especially when combined with testing for serum antiphospholipid and other antibodies, may correlate with the presence of adenomyosis in up to 93% of cases.

Hysterosalpingogram

The features on a hysterosalpingogram (HSG) were described by Goldberger et al in 1949[23] (numerous short spicules ending in small sacs extending from the border of the uterine cavity and varying from 1 to 4 mm in length) but are relatively nonspecific. The diagnosis was missed in 75%.

Transabdominal ultrasonogram

Little was studied on a transabdominal ultrasonogram (TAS), as the resolution limits the evaluation for myometrium. Features are nonspecific and include uterine enlargement with posterior wall thickening and a focal honeycomb appearance with irregular 5–7 mm cystic spaces that disrupt the normal echo pattern of the uterus.

Transvaginal ultrasonogram

Transvaginal ultrasonography (TVS) was developed in the 1980s. The higher frequencies which can be used (5–7 MHz) and the proximity of pelvic structures to the transducer improve spatial resolution and reduce imaging artifacts. Myometrium of the normal uterus has three distinct zones of differing echogenicity on TVS:[24] the outer, middle, and inner layers. The inner layer consists of longitudinal and circular smooth muscles and is hypoechoic relative to the middle and outer layers. This is referred to as the subendometrial or myometrial halo. The middle layer is the most echogenic and is separated from the thin outer layer by arcuate venous and arterial plexus. The appearance of the endometrium varies in different phases of the menstrual cycle, but is more echogenic than myometrium.

Uterine enlargement without the presence of leiomyomas and asymmetry of uterine walls are indirect signs for diffuse adenomyosis (Figure 28.1). Brosens et al[25] have emphasized myometrial

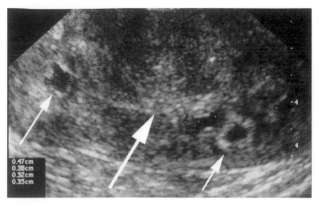

Figure 28.1 Transvaginal ultrasound scan showing a transverse view of the uterine fundus in a woman with severe adenomyosis. There is heterogeneous echotexture of both anterior and posterior myometrium and two small cystic adenomyomas (surrounded by a layer of endometrial-like echotexture) that are identified by the small arrows. The normal endometrium is indicated by the large arrow. Courtesy of Dr Philippa Ramsay.

heterogeneous echogenicity as the best predictor. The most common findings are poorly marginated hypoechoic and heterogeneous areas in myometrium with or without the presence of small myometrial cysts.[26] Discrete adenomyomas may mimic leiomyomas, but the borders are often less distinct.

The overall decreased echogenicity of the adenomyotic myometrium is due to smooth muscle hyperplasia and the heterogeneous appearance is due to the multiple small echogenic islands disrupting the hypoechoic background. These echogenic islands represent the heterotopic endometrial tissue.[26] The presence of dilated cystic glands or hemorrhagic foci within the heterotopic endometrial tissue results in the small myometrial cysts on TVS.

The sensitivity in most studies has been shown to be 76–87%, with specificity of 71–99%. A potential pitfall in the diagnosis is the differentiation of adenomyosis and leiomyomas. The imaging characteristics may overlap, particularly in some adenomyomas that are well-circumscribed and demonstrate a distortion effect on endometrium. In general, features that favor the diagnosis of adenomyosis are a lesion with poorly defined borders, minimal distortion effect on the endometrium or serosa relative to the size of the lesion, elliptical rather than a globular shape, lack of calcification, lack of edge shadowing or whorled appearance of myometrium, small myometrial cysts, and echogenic nodules or linear striations radiating out from the endometrium into the myometrium.

Other conditions that can mimic adenomyosis are endometrial carcinoma, myometrial contraction, myometrial hypertrophy, or vascular calcification. The presence of subendometrial linear striations, subendometrial echogenic nodules, or asymmetric myometrial thickness improves the specificity and positive predictive value of TVS.

Magnetic resonance imaging

The uterus is optimally studied with T-2 weighted sagittal sequences. Three different zones can be seen in the uterus of women at reproductive age.[26] The normal endometrium is represented by a high signal intensity stripe. Immediately below the endometrial stripe is a low signal intensity zone called the junctional zone (JZ), which represents the subendometrial myometrium. It is less vascular than the outer myometrium and consists of compact bundles of longitudinally oriented smooth muscle fibers running parallel to the endometrium. It has a threefold increase in the percentage of nuclear area per unit area of the tissue compared with outer myometrium. The outer layer of myometrium is of intermediate signal intensity. The JZ occupies approximately one-third of the myometrium. Much variation in the normal thickness of the JZ has been reported, with a mean 2–8 mm. There is wide agreement that the normal JZ is regular in thickness and is usually less than 5 mm.

MRI features of adenomyosis (Figure 28.2) include diffuse or focal widening of the low-intensity JZ. Widths between 6 and 12 mm are quoted.[27,28] Reinhold et al[27] and Kang et al[28] found that a maximal JZ thickness ≥12 mm is highly predictive of the presence of adenomyosis, whereas a JZ ≤8 mm usually excludes the disease. With a measurement of 8–12 mm, ancillary findings such as focal and localized thickening of the JZ, poor definition of the JZ borders, or the presence of high signal foci on T2- or T1-weighted sequences can be used to diagnose adenomyosis. High signal foci or linear striations of increased signal may be present within an area of low signal intensity. The areas of low signal intensity have been shown to correspond to the smooth muscle hyperplasia and high signal intensity represents the ectopic endometrium, cystic dilated glands, or hemorrhagic fluid.

MRI was shown to be highly accurate in differentiating adenomyosis from leiomyomas. Although features may overlap, the features that favor the diagnosis of adenomyosis include a lesion with poorly defined borders, minimal mass effect on the endometrium relative to the size of the lesion, linear striations radiating out from the endometrium

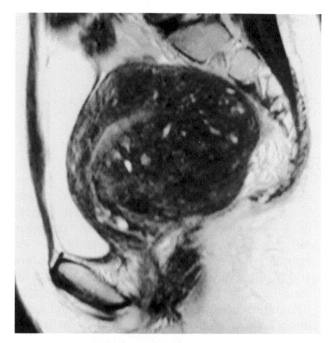

Figure 28.2 Sagittal MRI (magnetic resonance imaging) scan of an enlarged adenomyotic uterus (equivalent to a 6-week gestation). The patient suffered from dysmenorrhea only. Technical details: turbo spin echo (TSE) T2–5 mm sagittal; repetition time (TR) = 4000 ms; echo time (TE) = 99 ms; flip angle = 180°. Courtesy of Dr Kam-wang Siu and Dr CY Tse.

to the myometrium, and absence of large vessels at the margins of lesions.

Sensitivity and specificity as high as 86–88% and 100%, respectively, were reported.[26] Reinhold et al[27] found good correlation between the location of high signal intensity on MRI and echogenic foci on TVS with the depth of the heterotopic glands in histology. However, only 4 cases were studied.

Transvaginal ultrasonography and magnetic resonance imaging

By comparison with TVS, MRI is more expensive and less widely available. However, MRI has the advantage over TVS that it is less operator-dependent and imaging is standard and reproducible. Recent studies by Reinhold et al[27] and others demonstrated comparable accuracy of MRI and TVS, except in the presence of leiomyoma, in which situation MRI is superior to TVS. Hence, TVS and MRI now both play an important role in the diagnosis and assessment of adenomyosis. As TVS is easily accessible, it should usually be the primary tool for the initial work-up for the disease and should be supplemented with MRI when necessary. These imaging procedures will usually both identify adenomyosis, exclude other conditions that give rise to the symptoms, and be suitable for monitoring with conservative management.

Surgical approaches to diagnosis and assessment

Needle biopsy

A small number of studies have assessed myometrial needle biopsy, either transcervical, percutaneous, or by laparoscopic routes. Anecdotal reports have not supported a role for this approach. An early study by Wood et al[29] showed 100% accuracy on using percutaneous ultrasound-guided myometrial biopsy, but the study population comprised just 10 patients and among them only 3 had adenomyosis. Other clinicians have found quite a low sensitivity for a single needle biopsy,[30] in their study, 10 needle specimens were taken from each of 40 adenomyotic uteri and the sensitivity of diagnosis from taking 10 samples from each uterus was 40–67%. However, considering one single biopsy, which should be more practical, the sensitivity ranged from 8 to 18.7% (mean 14%), and depends on the severity of the disease. This low sensitivity in diagnosing adenomyosis was further supported by Brosens and Barker,[31] who found a low sensitivity of 8–19% on single myometrial biopsy. It seems that the sensitivity is too low for clinical practice.

Hysteroscopic endomyometrial biopsy

Whereas severe adenomyosis may have a typical hysteroscopic appearance of surface cavities and trabeculations with areas of neovascularization, milder forms cannot be diagnosed visually. Hysteroscopic diagnostic criteria for adenomyosis have been described by Ota[32] and include the presence of large glandular ostia and networks of irregular, dilated, surface vessels indicating neovascularization. The overall sensitivity for diagnosis of moderate or severe disease was 77.5%. It has been reported that up to 51–66% of women with menorrhagia have hysteroscopically normal uterine cavities in various studies. Therefore, endomyometrial biopsy at the time of hysteroscopy could be valuable. McCausland[18] reported 66% had adenomyosis and it was 60% from Goswami's study.[33] Although the accuracy of the biopsy was not confirmed with a hysterectomy specimen, a single endomyometrial biopsy from the posterior wall of the uterus generally appeared to be representative of the entire surface.[18] Hysteroscopic endomyometrial biopsy is performed with a wire loop. In McCausland's group, a 5 mm loop was used and specimens up to 6 mm deep can be obtained: this has the benefit of allowing examination of the depth of invasion of the heterotopic endometrium into the myometrium, which may help in the planning of treatment. The main drawback is that the procedure has to be carried out under general anesthesia. Patient consent for such a 'deep' biopsy is another concern, particularly in young and infertile women. Selected cases in which medical treatment fails to control the symptoms may merit such biopsy.

Management

Medical management of adenomyosis

There is limited information on the specific effects of different drug treatment for adenomyosis. Based on the principle that endometriosis and adenomyosis are due to ectopic endometrium within myometrium, drugs which have been used for adenomyosis are mostly those applied widely to endometriosis. It is unclear whether possible benefits of these drugs in some cases may be due to the treatment of coexisting endometriosis. It is a commonly held belief that most drug therapies are relatively ineffective in treating adenomyosis; however, there is a real need for effective medical therapies for those women who wish to preserve fertility or avoid surgery and its potential complications.

Conventional medical therapies
Antifibrinolytic agents like tranexamic acid can anecdotally be used for the menorrhagia associated with adenomyosis. Anti-prostaglandin agents also may be anecdotally useful to treat the associated symptoms of pain and heavy bleeding. Combined oral contraceptive pills and oral or intramuscular progestogen therapy have been used to control symptoms associated with adenomyosis, but overall efficacy is uncertain. Breakthrough bleeding is common. The roles of all of these agents require further investigation before any recommendations can be made.

Gonadrotropin-releasing hormone agonists
Gonadotropin-releasing hormone (GnRH) agonists are other well-studied drugs used in the treatment of endometriosis, but again the evidence in favor

of their usefulness in adenomyosis is largely anecdotal. During the course of GnRH agonist treatment of adenomyosis, uterine size decreased and pain was reduced;[34] however, symptoms recurred after treatment stopped. Risks of osteoporosis and hypoestrogenic side effects make GnRH agonists unsuitable for long-term treatment. Although add-back with hormone replacement is proposed nowadays, the effect on adenomyosis is not well studied. Moreover, the cost for the therapy is another concern.

A series of case reports have suggested that fertility may be improved in some adenomyosis patients following a few weeks of GnRH agonist therapy.[34,35] This therapy has sometimes been combined with conservative surgery and sometimes with induction of ovulation or in vitro fertilization (IVF) techniques.

Danazol

Danazol has been shown to be effective in endometriosis in randomized controlled studies; however, apart from anecdotal evidence, direct evidence for a useful clinical effect in adenomyosis is unavailable.

Intrauterine therapies

Local hormones administered in the uterine cavity may be able to exert direct therapeutic effects on adenomyotic tissue. Preliminary clinical experience with intrauterine therapy is promising for adenomyosis, but further clinical trials are necessary. This form of delivery system has the benefits of minimizing systemic side effects and making long-term usage possible.

Levonorgestrel intrauterine system

The levonorgestrel intrauterine system (LNG-IUS; Mirena; Schering AG, Berlin, Germany and Berlex Laboratories, NJ, USA) was initially designed for high contraceptive efficacy but has also proven effective in controlling menorrhagia. It exerts a local effect to cause atrophic endometrium. Fertility is preserved. Side effects are minimal and proven safe for long-term use. Direct data concerning the use of LNG-IUS in adenomyosis patients are very limited. Fedele et al[36] studied treatment with the LNG-IUS in 25 adenomyotic women. One patient experienced IUS expulsion and 1 patient had premature removal of the IUS because of persistent irregular, light blood loss. All the remaining 23 patients had good relief of men-

orrhagia and dysmenorrhea. All of these women were satisfied with the therapy. No other medical therapy has been so promising.

Danazol-loaded intrauterine device

Igarashi M et al[37] in Japan have used a danazol-loaded (300–400 mg) intrauterine device (IUD) in 14 patients with recurrence of adenomyosis. Serum danazol levels were undetectable and side-effects were minimal. Twelve patients had complete remission of menorrhagia and 9 patients had complete remission of dysmenorrhea. After removal of the IUD, 3 out of 4 infertile patients conceived. The result was later confirmed with a larger study of 50 patients by the same authors. This is another interesting approach to therapy which requires further investigation.

Surgical management of adenomyosis

Principles of the surgical approach

Good preoperative assessment is critical to determine the most appropriate surgical approach and to minimize potential surgical complications. Adenomyosis can be a difficult condition to manage surgically when any approach apart from hysterectomy is contemplated because of the loss of surgical planes, difficulty in determining the extent of disease, and because of considerable vascularity of some tumors. Diffuse disease may be particularly difficult to define and excise.

Preoperative assessment should usually include good-quality TVU, or where available, MRI, since these are currently the best techniques for identifying and defining the type and extent of the adenomyosis. Assessment should also include a preoperative complete blood count, blood biochemistry, blood grouping, and blood group antibody check, and saving of serum at the blood bank in case of the small risk of blood transfusion being required. Routine perioperative antibiotics, anesthetic assessment, and thrombosis prophylaxis should be considered according to local protocols.

Women with the deep pelvic adenomyosis described by Donnez et al[6,8] may require more extensive preoperative work-up with intravenous pyelography to exclude ureteral stenosis or occlusion, and sigmoidoscopy or colonoscopy to define rectal involvement.

Potential surgical approaches for management of adenomyosis

1. **Hysterectomy**
   Abdominal
     total
     subtotal
     vaginal
     laparoscopic – laparoscopically assisted vaginal
     total laparoscopic
2. **Laparotomy**
   Adenomyomectomy
   Mass reduction of tumor
3. **Conservative laparoscopy**
   Adenomyomectomy
   Mass reduction of tumor
   Bipolar coagulation
4. **Hysteroscopy**
   Hysteroscopic resection with ultrasound guidance
   Endometrial ablation

Hysterectomy

In the past, hysterectomy was often a choice for those with intractable menorrhagia and dysmenorrhea, and adenomyosis was diagnosed retrospectively. However, with the advent of hysteroscopic means for treating menorrhagia, there is increasing evidence that part of the adenomyosis population can be relieved of symptoms without resorting to hysterectomy. Nevertheless, many will still require this traditional procedure at some stage.

Hysterectomy can be performed by laparotomy, vaginally or laparoscopically, either total or subtotal. Total hysterectomy is a definite cure for adenomyosis. The advantages of subtotal over total hysterectomy include shorter operating time, reduced blood loss, earlier patient discharge, reduced risk of bowel and ureteric injury, and reduced risk of adverse effect on bladder and sexual function. However, there may be residual or recurrent adenomyosis in the cervix that was left behind and subtotal hysterectomy may lead to difficulty in removing associated rectovaginal endometriosis.[38] The techniques used for hysterectomy in adenomyosis do not differ from those used in other straightforward situations. The only difficulties which may be encountered are due to the enlargement of the uterus or to coexisting pathology. However, the adenomyotic uterus is rarely larger than a 12-week pregnancy, and many can be removed safely by the vaginal route – perhaps with bisection or coring in the larger cases. Furuhashi et al[39] reviewed 1246 vaginal hysterectomies in which he divided the patients into 2 groups: those with leiomyomas ($n = 893$) and those with adenomyosis ($n = 353$). There was no difference in operative time and estimated blood loss between the 2 groups when analyzed by uterine weight. However, adenomyosis was associated with an increased risk of bladder injury.

Laparotomy

In general, laparotomy is the preferred approach for localized adenomyoma excision by the relatively inexperienced endoscopist, but it may still require considerable skill and care in planning and executing the best approach to incision and removal.

Successful excision of localized adenomyomas requires precise determination of the extent of the disease, which can be extremely difficult. The disease may be infiltrating close to the fallopian tubes or involve major vessels, and complete excision may not be feasible without proceeding to hysterectomy in the occasional case.

We utilize detailed preoperative transvaginal ultrasound or MRI mapping of the lesion. Preoperative HyCoSy (hysterosalpingo-contrast sonography) with transvaginal ultrasound and intrauterine instillation of galactose microparticles (Levovist; Schering) as a tubal contrast medium may help to define the relationship between the fallopian tubes and the adenomyoma.

These lesions may sometimes be very vascular and we prefer to utilize an effective vasoconstrictor routinely (we use ornipressin, POR 8, 5 U in 60 ml saline; Ferring, Lausanne, Switzerland). This needs to be injected into the myometrium around the periphery of the lesion, paying particular attention to the lateral origin of the major supplying vessels. POR 8 generally acts for about 30 minutes, and, in our experience, is more effective than alternative vasoconstrictors. The anesthetist needs to be warned of the impending myometrial injection, since POR 8 may cause a transient hypertensive effect.

Apart from these precautions, standard surgical techniques are used for excision and repair, bearing in mind that any residual adenomyomatous tissue which could not be removed may be quite friable and does not always hold sutures well.

Endoscopic approaches to adenomyosis

Hysteroscopic endometrial ablation or resection
Endometrial ablation is a highly effective procedure for greatly reducing or eliminating menstrual

blood loss in women with dysfunctional uterine bleeding or bleeding due to systemic coagulo-pathies. However, much anecdotal evidence suggests that a high proportion of the 'failures' can be due to undiagnosed adenomyosis. A number of reports have appeared concerning the response of symptoms in women with adenomyosis following endometrial ablation using the range of hysteroscopic and third-generation procedures. Most of these have focused on the symptom of menorrhagia.

Wortman and Dagget[40] have identified 26 patients who experienced failure after hysteroscopic endomyometrial resection. In 15 (57.7%) patients, the resected specimen was confirmed to contain adenomyosis. McCausland and McCausland[41] reported that 7 out of 8 cases requiring hysterectomy were found to have adenomyosis in the hysterectomy specimen; the 8th patient had no recognized adenomyosis but a hematometra. These reports raise the concern that the presence of adenomyosis, either residual disease or recurrence, could be responsible for many of the failures of endometrial ablation or resection. McCausland and McCausland[41] also found that the likelihood of recurrence of menorrhagia following endometrial ablation, and especially the likelihood of hysterectomy, correlated with the depth of penetration of adenomyotic disease.

There has also been concern about the possible risk of endometrial cancer developing in residual adenomyosis following endometrial ablation. This is theoretically possible, but appears to be very rare. Most cases of malignancy arising in adenomyosis have developed in disease which is deeply sited in the myometrium and well away from the uterine cavity.[42] Hence, endometrial ablation is unlikely to influence such disease.

In spite of these concerns about the relatively lower effectiveness of endometrial ablation in women with adenomyosis, many of these women have great symptomatic improvement. Therefore, endometrial ablation may be an option for some of these women provided that they are aware of the reduced efficacy.

A more controversial approach is the deliberate use of hysteroscopic resection techniques for the removal of deeper diffuse or localized adenomyosis. Wood[38] has reported resection to a depth of 1 cm, which cured the menorrhagia in 12 out of 15 women, but only cured dysmenorrhea in 3 out of 8 women. Five of these 15 women required hysterectomy. Other surgeons have attempted to excise localized areas of adenomyosis using simultaneous rectal ultrasound for guidance. These techniques should only be attempted by hysteroscopic surgeons experienced in the simultaneous use of ultrasound guidance, because of the risks of uterine perforation, bleeding, and fluid absorption.

Laparoscopic management

Laparoscopy in adenomyosis reveals a uterus displaying different levels of congestion, with the area over an adenomyoma appearing more congested. The uterus may have an irregular contour in cases with localized adenomyomas. When an attempt is made to enucleate, it is soon obvious that the lesion lacks the cleavage plane which is found so easily with a leiomyoma. Rectovaginal endometriosis appears on laparoscopy as an obliterated pouch of Douglas, with the lower posterior part of the uterus and the posterior fornix often not being visualized (partial obliteration of the pouch).[1]

Laparoscopic surgical techniques for adenomyosis include adenomyoma resection, bipolar coagulation of adenomyomata, myometrial reduction with electrocautery, and laparoscopic or laparoscopically assisted hysterectomy.

Laparoscopic myometrial excision

Laparoscopic myometrial excision may be considered by experienced surgeons if the adenomyomatous lesions are well circumscribed and accessible from the laparoscopic approach.[38] Hence, careful patient selection is essential. The principles are the same as for adenomyomectomy by the laparotomy approach, but utilizing the principles of advanced laparoscopic surgery. Several case reports have indicated that successful pregnancy may follow,[35,43] but there has been concern about the potential for scar rupture during pregnancy. Hence, great care needs to be taken to ensure a sound uterine repair following the excision procedure.

Laparoscopic adenomyoma resection can be performed with a number of different resection tools depending on the preference of the surgeon and the specifics of the case. Most surgeons will prefer a pure cutting or mixed cutting and coagulating electrical current, and the power will depend on the equipment used. A key issue is hemostasis, but it is also important that the current does not spread too widely and damage large volumes of normal myometrium. Bipolar coagulation may be useful for hemostasis. Resection can be aided by hydroultrasonography monitoring[44] (TVU with peritoneal hydration of physiologic saline) in order to completely resect the affected myometrium.

This can also confirm complete resection. The myometrial defect should be meticulously closed by laparoscopic or minilaparotomy assistance using standard suturing techniques.

Morita et al[45] performed laparoscopic excision of adenomyomas using the same procedure as for laparoscopic myomectomy. They reported no intraoperative or postoperative complications, a hospital stay of only 3 days, and the dysmenorrhea and menorrhagia of their patients disappeared by the end of the first postoperative menses.

Laparoscopic myometrial electrocoagulation

The tissue necrosis produced by this method results in a large area of scar tissue which jeopardizes the strength of myometrium. It also means that there is no tissue sample for pathology. There is a high chance of uterine rupture during subsequent pregnancy.[38] However, a majority of patients may become symptom-free, and hysterectomy may be avoided.[38] Sterilization is recommended together with the laparoscopic surgery.

Wood et al[46] performed laparoscopic myometrial coagulation reduction for localized adenomyomas of less than 4 cm size. They used a 50 W monopolar current with a Corson needle electrode at 1–3 cm depth at about 1 cm intervals until blanching spread 1 cm beyond the needle point. They compared this with myometrial excision performed by minilaparotomy (since one attempted laparoscopic excision of a 7 cm adenomyoma resulted in inability to control bleeding). They reported that myometrial excision cured 7 of 8 patients, and myometrial coagulation reduction in 4 of 7 women. This was in contrast to their hysteroscopic endometrial resection (to a depth of 1 cm), which cured menorrhagia in 12 of 15 patients but only relieved dysmenorrhea in 3 of 8 patients. In their whole series of endoscopic resections, out of 30 patients, 9 required hysterectomy, and 5 of them were from the hysteroscopic endometrial resection group. They concluded that conservative surgical procedures, including hysteroscopic endometrial resection and laparoscopic myometrial coagulation reduction or excision, may reduce the need for hysterectomy in the presence of adenomyosis. Early diagnosis may improve treatment.

Bipolar coagulation of an adenomyoma or an area of adenomyosis has also been performed with the help of bipolar needles in a way similar to myolysis.[47] A 32 cm long myoma bipolar coagulation instrument with two distal, parallel, 5 cm long needles is passed through the lower port and the adenomyoma is systematically perforated at 5–10 mm intervals through the serosal surface to its base, forming parallel cylinders of desiccated and denatured tissue. The endpoint is the paling and blanching of the entire serosal surface. Such techniques appear to have a reasonable clinical effect, but further clinical trials in additional centers are required to determine the final place of such approaches.

Laparoscopic excision of deep pelvic nodules of adenomyosis

Donnez et al[6,8] have described laparoscopic complete dissection of the anterior rectal wall in these difficult patients until loose areolar tissue of the rectovaginal septum was reached. This often requires extensive excision of nodular, adherent fibrotic tissue from the posterior vagina, rectum, posterior cervix, and uterosacral ligaments. In order to define the anatomy, they inserted a sponge on a ring forceps into the posterior fornix, a probe in the rectum, along with a cannula in the uterus for anteversion. Then a careful aqua dissection was done in combination with a CO_2 laser for sharp dissection. Excision of the fibrotic tissue by the side of the rectum was only attempted after rectal dissection was complete. Excision of part of the vagina was usually essential in deep infiltrating adenomyosis, but the rectum did not usually need to be resected. Removal of all visible adenomyotic tissue was performed and also adherent vaginal tissue until a 0.5 cm free margin was obtained. In a series of 500 cases of pelvic pain, 497 underwent laparoscopic excision and 3 underwent a laparotomy excision of adenomyotic nodules and these resulted in a high incidence of good pain relief. Ureteric involvement was not uncommon. Laparoscopic ureterolysis was performed in 16 women; 2 women underwent ureteral resection and ureteroureterostomy. A significant postoperative decrease in ureterohydronephrosis was noted in all patients; however, renal function improved only slightly.

Laparoscopic cul-de-sac dissection, although time-intensive, offers increased fertility potential and significant symptom relief in many of these patients.[48,49] Hysterectomy and rectal resection for such adherent rectovaginal adenomyotic nodules may be associated with a better response and quality of life.[50] However, the surgeon needs to be highly skilled in operative laparoscopy to undertake these procedures, which should usually be performed as part of a multiskilled team that includes a colorectal surgeon.

Uterine artery embolization

Uterine artery embolization (UAE) has recently emerged as an increasingly popular alternative treatment for symptomatic uterine fibroids (leiomyomata). A clinical failure rate of approximately 10% is noted in most reports evaluating its efficacy for myoma treatment. Various investigators have considered adenomyosis as a possible factor contributing to the failure rate. Smith et al[51] reported only 1 out of the 20 cases having UAE for fibroids with menorrhagia had no improvement in her symptoms. Pathologic examination after hysterectomy in that case revealed infarcted fibroids but endometrium, myometrium, and adenomyosis which were unaffected. A selective effect of the embolization was suggested. Goodwin et al[52] also reported adenomyosis in 3 of 6 hysterectomy specimens in women who required surgical treatment after ineffective UAE.

Despite these limited anecdotal reports on adenomyosis-related failure of embolization, there is emerging evidence of an improvement of symptoms in some patients with adenomyosis after UAE. Siskin et al[53] reported a series of 15 cases with diffuse adenomyosis alone or coexisting with fibroids, of whom 14 had improvement of symptoms following UAE. Mean uterine volume was reduced by 42%. Chen et al[54] treated 23 cases of adenomyosis with UAE and in all patients the symptoms were significantly relieved. Dysmenorrhea resolved completely in 19/23 cases. All patients experienced initial reduced menstrual flow after embolization, although 2 recurred in 7–11 months. There was a significant decrease in uterine volume and in blood flow in the uterus and lesions. In the study by Jha et al,[55] 9 cases had adenomyosis-dominant or pure disease and these all experienced clinical improvement after UAE. Eight out of the 9 patients had a decrease in JZ thickness. Mean uterine volume and symptoms were significantly decreased at 3 months and 1 year.

In the initial studies of UAE on uterine leiomyomata, the report of coexisting adenomyosis in those who failed in the treatment with UAE was based ultimately on the pathology of the hysterectomy specimen. High-resolution preoperative imaging with MRI or TVU was not always widely available prior to treatment. Hence, adenomyosis may not always be the dominant cause of failure. Based on the recent literature, the presence of adenomyosis should not be regarded as an absolute contraindication to UAE in women with fibroids. The data to date are limited by the relatively small number of cases treated and the short duration of follow-ups. The long-term efficacy of UAE for treatment of adenomyosis is not known. Larger controlled, and preferably randomized, clinical trials are necessary to determine the value of UAE in patients with different types of adenomyosis and to identify factors which predict good or bad response to embolization. Not until the results of such trials are available should UAE be broadly recommended as a primary treatment of adenomyosis.

Conclusion

Adenomyosis can still be regarded as an elusive disease, because of the need to keep a high index of suspicion about its possible presence in women with variable or vague pelvic symptoms, and its common coexistence with other common pelvic pathologies. Nowadays, diagnosis and preoperative assessment are becoming much more precise with the use of high-resolution TVU and MRI. Precise definition of the extent and site of the disease preoperatively is important in determining the most appropriate medical or surgical approach for management. There are now a number of possible choices for management of most patients with adenomyosis, and the surgeon needs to be aware that medical management with a device such as the LNG-IUS may be a valuable approach for those women who wish to avoid or defer surgery. Hysterectomy may still be the management of choice for many women with adenomyosis, but a variety of other surgical options may also need to be considered. Some patients require complex endoscopic surgery, which should remain the preserve of surgeons with advanced endoscopic skills.

REFERENCES

1. Rokitansky K. Ueber Uterusdruesen-Neubildung. Z Gesell Aerzte Wien 1860; 16: 577–581.
2. Von Recklinghausen F. Die adenomyome und cystadenomyome der uterus. In: Freund AW, ed. Klinische notizen zu den voluminosen adenomyomen des uterus-3. Berlin: Hirschwald; 1896.
3. Cullen TS. Adenomyoma of the uterus. Philadelphia: WB Saunders; 1908.
4. Frank, O. Adenomyosis uteri. Am J Obstet Gynecol 1925; 10: 680–684.
5. Bird CC, McElin TW, Manalo-Estrella P. The elusive adenomyosis of the uterus. Am J Obstet Gynecol 1972; 112: 583–593.
6. Donnez J, Nissole M, Smets M, et al. Rectovaginal septum adenomyotic nodule: a distinct entity: a series of 460 cases. In: Sutton C, Diamond M, eds. Endoscopic surgery for gynecologists, 2nd edn. London: WB Saunders, 1998: 357–362.
7. Koninckx PR, Oosterlynck D, D'Hooghe T, et al. Deeply infiltrating endometriosis is a disease whereas mild endometriosis could be considered a non-disease. Ann N Y Acad Sci 1994; 734: 333–341.
8. Donnez J, Nisolle M, Gillerot S, et al. Rectovaginal septum adenomyotic nodules: a series of 500 cases. Br J Obstet Gynaecol 1997; 104: 1014–1018.
9. Azziz R. Adenomyosis: current perspectives. Obstet Gynecol 1989; 16: 221–235.
10. Brosens JJ, De Souza NM, Barker FG. Uterine junctional zone: function and disease. Lancet 1995; 346: 558–560.
11. Ferenczy A. Pathophysiology of adenomyosis. Hum Reprod Update 1998; 4: 312–322.
12. Uduwela AS, Perera MAK, Li A, et al. Endometrial–myometrial interface: relationship to adenomyosis and changes in pregnancy. Obstet Gynecol Surv 2000; 55: 390–400.
13. Hrick H, Alpers C, Crooks LE, et al. Magnetic resonance imaging of the female pelvis: initial experience. Am J Radiol 1983; 141: 1119–1129.
14. Furuhashi M, Miyabc Y, Katsumata Y, et al. Comparison of complications of vaginal hysterectomy in patients with leiomyomas and in patients with adenomyosis. Arch Gynecol Obstet 1998; 262: 69–73.
15. Levgur M, Abadi A, Tucker A. Adenomyosis: symptoms, histology, and pregnancy terminations. Obstet Gynecol 2000; 95: 688–691.
16. Parazzini F, Vercellini P, Panazza S, et al. Risk factors for adenomyosis. Hum Reprod 1997; 12: 1275–1279.
17. Bensen RC, Sneeded VD. Adenomyosis: a reappraisal of symptomatology. Am J Obstet Gynecol 1958; 76: 1044–1061.
18. McCausland AM. Hysteroscopic myometrial biopsy: its use in diagnosing adenomyosis and its clinical application. Am J Obstet Gynecol 1992; 166: 1619–1628.
19. Olive D L, Franklin RR, Gratkins LV. The association between endometriosis and spontaneous abortion. A retrospective clinical study. J Reprod Med 1982; 27: 333–338.
20. Ota H, Igarashi S, Hatazawa J, et al. Endothelial nitric oxide synthase in the endometrium during the menstrual cycle in patients with endometriosis and adenomyosis. Fertil Steril 1998; 69: 303–308.
21. Vercellini P, Ragni G, Trespidi L, et al. Adenomyosis: a déjà vu? Obstet Gynecol Survey 1993; 48: 789–794.
22. Nikkanen V, Punnonen R. Clinical significance of adenomyosis. Ann Chir Gynaecol 1980; 69: 278–280.
23. Goldberger MA, Marshak RH, Hermel M. Roentgen diagnosis of adenomyosis uteri. Am J Obstet Gynecol 1949, 57: 563–568.
24. Lyons EA, Gratton D, Harington C. Transvaginal sonography of normal pelvic anatomy. Radiol Clin N Am 1992; 30: 663–675.
25. Brosens JJ, De Souza NM, Barker FG, et al. Endovaginal ultrasonography in the diagnosis of adenomyosis uteri: identifying the predictive characteristics. Br J Obstet Gynaecol 1995; 102: 471–474.
26. Reinhold C, Tafazol F, Wang L. Imaging features of adenomyosis. Hum Reprod Update 1998; 4: 337–349.
27. Reinhold C, McCarthy S, Bret PM, et al. Diffuse adenomyosis: comparison of endovaginal US and MR imaging with histopathologic correlation. Radiology 1996; 199: 151–158.
28. Kang S, Turner DA, Foster GS, et al. Adenomyosis: specificity of 5 mm as the maximum normal uterine junctional zone thickness in MR images. AJR Am J Roentgenol 1996; 166: 1145–1150.
29. Wood C, Hurley VA, Fortune DW, et al. Percutaneous ultrasound guided needle biopsy. Med J Aust 1993; 158: 458–460.
30. Popp LW, Schwiedessen JP, Gaetje R. Myometrial biopsy in the diagnosis of adenomyosis uteri. Am J Obstet Gynecol 1993; 169: 546–549.
31. Brosens JJ, Barker FG. The role of myometrial needle biopsies in the diagnosis of adenomyosis. Fertil Steril 1995; 63: 1347–1349.
32. Ota H. Evaluation of hysteroscopy in the diagnosis of adenomyosis. Jap J Fertil Steril 1992; 37: 49–55.
33. Goswami A, Khemani M, Logani KB, et al. Adenomyosis: diagnosis by hysteroscopic endomyometrial biopsy: correlation of incidence and severity with menorrhagia. J Obstet Gynaecol Res 1998; 24: 281–284.
34. Nelson JR, Corson SL. Long-term management of adenomyosis with a gonadotropin-releasing hormone agonist: a case report. Fertil Steril 1993; 59: 441–443.
35. Wang PH, Yang TS, Lee WL, et al. Treatment of infertile women with adenomyosis with a conservative microsurgical technique and a gonadotrophin-releasing hormone agonist. Fertil Steril 2000; 73: 1061–1062.
36. Fedele L, Bianchi S, Raffaelli R, et al. Treatment of

adenomyosis-associated menorrhagia with a levonorgestrel-releasing intrauterine device. Fertil Steril 1997; 68: 426–429.

37. Igarashi M, Abe Y, Fukuda M, et al. Novel conservative medical therapy for uterine adenomyosis with a danazol-loaded intrauterine device. Fertil Steril 2000; 74: 412–413.

38. Wood C. Surgical and medical treatment of adenomyosis. Hum Reprod Update 1998; 4: 323–326.

39. Furuhashi M, Miyabe Y, Katsumata Y, et al. Comparison of complications of vaginal hysterectomy in patients with leiomyomas and in patients with adenomyosis. Arch Gynecol Obstet 1998; 262: 69–73.

40. Wortman M, Dagget A. Reoperative hysteroscopic surgery in the management of patients who fail endometrial ablation and resection. J Am Assoc Gynecol Laparosc 2001; 8: 272–277.

41. McCausland AM, McCausland VM. Depth of endometrial penetration in adenomyosis helps determine outcome of rollerball ablation. Am J Obstet Gynecol 1996; 174: 1786–1794.

42. Colman HI, Rosenthal AH. Carcinoma developing in areas of adenomyosis. Obstet Gynecol 1959; 14: 342–348.

43. Ozaki T, Takahashi K, Okada M, et al. Live birth after conservative surgery for severe adenomyosis following magnetic resonance imaging and gonadotrophin-releasing hormone agonist therapy. Int J Fertil Womens Med 1999; 44: 260–264.

44. Nabeshima H, Murakami T, Terada Y, et al. Total laparoscopic surgery of cystic adenomyoma under hydroultrasonographic monitoring. J Am Assoc Gynecol Laparosc 2003; 10: 195–199.

45. Morita M, Asakawa Y, Nakakuma M, et al. Laparoscopic excision of myometrial adenomyomas in patients with adenomyosis uteri and main symptoms of severe

dysmenorrhea and hypermenorrhea with adenomyosis. J Am Assoc Gynecol Laparosc 2004; 11: 86–89.

46. Wood C, Maher P, Hill D. Biopsy diagnosis and conservative surgical treatment of adenomyosis. J Am Assoc Gynecol Laparosc 1994; 1: 313–316.

47. Phillips DR, Nathanson HG, Milim SJ, et al. Laparoscopic bipolar coagulation for the conservative treatment of adenomyomata. J Am Assoc Gynecol Laparosc 1996; 4: 19–24.

48. Reich H, McGlynn F, Salvat J. Laparoscopic treatment of cul-de-sac obliteration secondary to retrocervical deep fibrotic endometriosis. J Reprod Med 1991; 36: 516–522.

49. Ford J, English J, Miles WA, et al. Pain, quality of life and complications following the radical resection of rectovaginal endometriosis. BJOG 2004; 111: 353–356.

50. Hollett-Caines J, Vilos GA, Penava DA. Laparoscopic mobilization of the rectosigmoid and excision of the obliterated cul-de-sac. J Am Assoc Gynecol Laparosc 2003; 10: 190–194.

51. Smith SJ, Sewall LE, Handelsman A. A clinical failure of uterine fibroid embolization due to adenomyosis. J Vas Interv Radiol 1999; 10: 1171–1174.

52. Goodwin SC, McLucas B, Lee M, et al. Uterine artery embolization for the treatment of uterine leiomyomata midterm results. J Vas Interv Radiol 1999; 10: 1159–1165.

53 Siskin GP, Tublin ME, Stainken KD, et al. Uterine artery embolization for the treatment of adenomyosis: clinical response and evaluation with MR imaging. AJR Am J Roentgenol 2001; 177: 297–302.

54. Chen CL, Liu P, Lu J, et al. Uterine artery embolization in the treatment of adenomyosis. Chung Hua Fu Chan Ko Tsa Chih (Chin J Obstet Gynecol) 2002; 37: 77–79.

55. Jha RC, Takahama J, Imaoka I, et al. Adenomyosis: MRI of the uterus treated with uterine artery embolization. AJR Am J Roentgenol 2003; 181: 851–856.

SECTION VI
Nonsurgical Management of Endometriosis

29 The medical treatment of endometriosis

David L Olive, Elizabeth A Pritts, and Steven R Lindheim

An integral tool in the treatment of endometriosis is the pharmaceutical agent. The use of medications to improve the plight of patients with this disease has allowed millions of women to avoid the pain and complications associated with surgery, as well as frequently providing an adjunctive approach when operative interventions fail. Unfortunately, the medications in use and their nuances of administration are poorly understood by the average clinician.

The original development of medication to treat endometriosis was built upon several observations. First, endometriosis is infrequently encountered in the parous women, but much more often in the nulliparous female, suggesting a protective effect of the hormonal milieu of pregnancy. Secondly, endometrium is known to be estrogen-dependent, with ectopic endometrium presumably behaving in much the same manner. Finally, endometriosis tends to occur nearly exclusively in menstruating, reproductive age women, again suggesting hormonal dependence. These findings suggested the potential benefits of hormonal therapy to alter the normal menstrual cyclicity of the reproductive years, the mainstay of medical treatment for endometriosis.

Recently, however, the approach has changed. We now have a much greater depth of understanding of the pathogenesis, growth, and maintenance of ectopic endometrium, particularly at the molecular level. This has provided drug developers with new, precise molecular targets for treatment of the disease. Currently under development, these newer agents hold the poten-

tial of greater efficacy and flexibility with fewer systemic effects.

This chapter will review those medications currently used as well as those under development for the medical treatment of endometriosis. It will also provide the best available evidence as to the utility of these drugs in combating the many problems associated with this disease.

Established medical treatments of endometriosis

Danazol

The first drug to be approved for the treatment of endometriosis in the United States was danazol, an isoxazol derivative of 17-alpha-ethinyltestosterone. It was originally thought to produce a pseudomenopause, but subsequent studies have revealed the drug to act primarily by diminishing the midcycle luteinizing hormone (LH) surge,[1,2] creating a chronic anovulatory state. Additional actions include inhibitor of multiple enzymes in the steroidogenic pathology[3] and increase in free serum testosterone.[4] The recommended dosage of danazol for the treatment of endometriosis is 600–800 mg/day; however, these doses have substantial androgenic side effects such as increased hair growth, mood changes, adverse serum lipid profiles, deepening of the voice (possibly irreversible), and rarely, liver damage (possibly irreversible and life-threatening) and arterial thrombosis.[5,6] Studies of lower doses as primary treatment for endometriosis-associated pain have been uncontrolled or with small numbers, and thus contain information of limited value.[7] However, due to the many side effects of the drug, alternative routes of administration have been sought. Recently, the use of danazol vaginal suppositories[8] and danazol impregnated vaginal rings[9] have been described in small, uncontrolled trials. Preliminary results suggest side effects may be less severe with the transvaginal approach.

Progestogens

Progestogens are a class of compounds that produce progesterone-like effects upon endometrial tissue. A large number of progestogens exist, ranging from those chemically derived from progesterone (progestins) such as medroxyprogesterone acetate (MPA), to 19-nortestosterone derivatives such as norethindrone and norgestrel. The proposed mechanism of action of these compounds is initial decidualization of endometrial tissue followed by eventual atrophy. This is believed to result from a direct suppressive effect of progestogens upon the estrogen receptors of the endometrium. Recent evidence suggests that another mechanism of action at the molecular level is the suppression of matrix metalloproteinases, enzymes important in the implantation and growth of ectopic endometrium.[10]

The most extensively studied progestational agent for the treatment of endometriosis is medroxyprogesterone. The drug was originally used orally for the treatment of endometriosis, with doses ranging from 20 mg to 100 mg daily; published randomized studies are limited to 100 mg daily. However, the depot formulation has also been used, in a dose of 150 mg every 3 months. Side effects of medroxyprogesterone are multiple and varied, yet even in high doses it seems to be better tolerated metabolically than danazol. A common side effect is transient breakthrough bleeding, which occurs in 38–47% of recipients. This is generally well tolerated and, when necessary, can be adequately treated with supplemental estrogen or an increase in the progestogen dose. Other side effects include nausea (0–80%), breast tenderness (5%), fluid retention (50%), and depression (6%).[11] In published trials, few patients have discontinued the medications secondary to side effects. In contradistinction to danazol, all of the above-mentioned adverse effects resolve upon discontinuation of the drugs.

Norethindrone acetate has also been utilized as a treatment for endometriosis. This 19-nortestosterone derivative has only been analyzed in a retrospective, uncontrolled trial of 52 women.[12] Each patient was treated initially with 5 mg daily, with increases of 2.5 mg increments up to a maximum dose of 20 mg daily, until amenorrhea was achieved. Side effects were similar to those seen with medroxyprogesterone.

Other progestational agents have also been used in the occasional study, including lynestrenol, a gestagen used primarily in Europe. Levonorgestrel, the active ingredient of Norplant, has also been utilized recently, via an intrauterine device delivery system.[13] The drug has been shown to effectively decrease vascular endothelial growth factor (VEGF) and blood vessel proliferation, providing rationale for its use in endometriosis.[14] It has been touted recently as a desirable treatment for rectovaginal endometriosis, although evidence thus far is uncontrolled.[13]

Progestogens may adversely affect serum lipoprotein levels. The 19-nortestosterone derivatives significantly decrease high-density lipoprotein (HDL), a change linked to an increased risk of coronary artery disease.[15] Data on medroxyprogesterone acetate are less clear, with studies demonstrating either no effect[16] or a slight decrease.[17] It is likely that there is a decrement in HDL with all these agents, but the magnitude is related to the specific progestogen and the dose administered. Whether alterations in serum lipoprotein levels for 4–6 months have any clinical significance is unclear.

Oral contraceptives (combination estrogen–progestogen)

The combination of estrogen and progestogen for therapy of endometriosis, the so-called 'pseudopregnancy' regimen, has been utilized for 40 years. Like progestational therapy alone, pseudopregnancy is believed to produce initial decidualization and growth of endometrial tissue, followed in several months by atrophy. This has been observed in women[18] but is in direct conflict with data from the rhesus monkey demonstrating larger implants with considerable local growth following such a therapeutic approach.[19]

Pseudopregnancy regimens have been administered both orally and parenterally. Combination oral contraceptive pills such as norethynodrel and mestranol, norethindrone acetate and ethinyl estradiol, lynestrenol and mestranol, and norgestrel plus ethinyl estradiol have all been tried. Parenteral combinations have included 17-hydroxyprogesterone or depot medroxyprogesterone acetate paired with stilbestrol or conjugated estrogens.

Side effects of pseudopregnancy are often quite impressive, and include those encountered with progestogens alone, as well as estrogenic- and androgenic-related effects. Estrogens may cause nausea, hypertension, thrombophlebitis, and uterine enlargement. The 19-nortestosterone-derived progestogens may cause androgenic effects such as acne, alopecia, increased muscle mass, decreased breast size, and deepening of the voice. Noble and Letchworth, in a comparative trial of norethynodrel and mestranol vs danazol, found that 41% of the pseudopregnancy group failed to complete their course of therapy due to side effects of the medication.[20] However, the medications in this study utilized far higher doses than are found in modern contraceptive preparations. The oral contraceptives commonly prescribed today for combination therapy are most likely to produce a progestogen-dominant picture similar to that of progestogen alone.

Today, oral contraceptives are the most commonly prescribed treatment for endometriosis symptoms. Despite this, there are little data regarding mechanism of action. One recent investigation suggests that oral contraceptives suppress proliferation and enhance programmed cell death (apoptosis) in endometrial tissue, perhaps providing a mechanistic clue for the action of these drugs.[21]

Gonadotropin-releasing hormone agonists

Gonadotropin releasing-hormone (GnRH) agonists are analogues of the hormone GnRH. This hypothalamic hormone is responsible for stimulating the pituitary gland to secrete FSH (follicle-stimulating hormone) and LH, two hormones necessary for normal ovarian function. GnRH is secreted in a pulsatile manner; the correct pulse results in stimulation of FSH and LH release, while too high or too low a pulse rate results in a decrease in pituitary hormone secretion. GnRH agonists are modified forms of GnRH that bind to the pituitary receptors and remain for a lengthy period. Thus, they are identified by the pituitary as rapidly pulsatile GnRH and, after initial stimulation of FSH and LH secretion, result in a shutdown (down-regulation) of the pituitary, and no resulting stimulation of the ovary. The result is a hyoestrogenic state similar to that of the menopause, producing endometrial atrophy and amenorrhea. It is also possible that the drug affects ectopic endometrium via additional mechanisms: animal studies have suggested alterations in plasminogen activators and matrix metalloproteinases, factors important in endometriosis development.[22]

The agonist can be given intranasally, subcutaneously, or intramuscularly, depending upon the specific product, with frequency of administration ranging from twice daily to every 3 months. The side effects are those of hypoestrogenism, such as transient vaginal bleeding, hot flashes, vaginal dryness, decreased libido, breast tenderness, insomnia, depression, irritability and fatigue, headache, osteoporosis and decreased skin elasticity; these are dose-dependent.[23]

A recent modification of GnRH agonist treatment is to 'add back' small amounts of steroid hormone in a manner similar to that used in the treatment of postmenopausal women. The theory is that the requirement for estrogen is greater for endometriosis than is needed by the brain (to prevent hot flashes), the bone (to prevent osteoporosis), and other tissues deprived of this hormone.[24] Interestingly, this 'threshold hypothesis' appears to be true, with estrogen–progestogen, estrogen–progestogen–testosterone, or progestogen only add-back therapy resulting in an equivalent rate of pain relief with far fewer side effects than GnRH agonist alone. Tibolone (Livial, NV Organon, Oss, the Netherlands) is a mixture of estrogen, progesterone, and a weak androgen; it is popular in Europe as hormone replacement therapy in postmenopausal women and is a popular form of 'add-back' therapy which prevents bone loss. It is notable for its low side-effect profile and has been shown to be effective in at least two randomized, controlled trials (RCTs). Estrogen as a solitary add back, however, is less effective and thus is not indicated.[25–27]

Gestrinone

Gestrinone (ethylnorgestrienone, R2323) is an antiprogestational steroid whose effects include androgenic, antiprogestogenic, and antiestrogenic actions, although the latter is not mediated by estrogen receptor binding.

This steroid is believed to act by inducing a progesterone withdrawal effect at the endometrial cellular level, thus enhancing lysosomal degradation of the cellular structure. There is a rapid decrease in estrogen and progesterone receptors in normal endometrium following administration of gestrinone, as well as a sharp increase in 17β-hydroxysteroid dehydrogenase. Interestingly, these cellular effects did not occur in samples of endometriotic tissue.[28]

Gestrinone may also inhibit ovarian steroido-genesis. A 50% decrease in serum estradiol level is noted after administration, perhaps related to the associated significant decline in sex hormone-binding globulin concentration (an androgenic or antiprogestogenic effect).[29] No effect on adrenal function or prolactin secretion has been noted.

Gestrinone is administered orally in doses of 2.5–10 mg weekly, on a daily, twice-weekly, or three-time-weekly schedule. Side effects include androgenic and antiestrogenic sequelae. Although most side effects are mild and transient, several, such as voice changes, hirsutism, and clitoral hypertrophy, are potentially irreversible.

Results of medical treatment

Assessing efficacy

The value of a particular medical treatment upon endometriosis will vary depending upon the thera-peutic goal of the intervention. With regard to endometriosis, there are four outcomes that can be assessed to determine drug efficacy: the anatomic manifestations of the disease, pain symptomatology, infertility status, and quality of life.

The anatomic manifestations of endometriosis, implants and adhesions, can be assessed before and after therapy to determine whether the interven-tion is of value. However, such a simple compari-son makes two assumptions. First, it is assumed that endometriosis is an invariably progressive dis-ease, never to regress on its own; this is unfortu-nately incorrect, as the disease has in fact been noted to regress in both baboons and humans.[30,31] Secondly, the above comparison presupposes that once regression has occurred via medical therapy, it is stable. This, too, is not the case, as implant and adhesion regrowth are both time-dependent phe-nomena. Thus, to address the effect of a medical treatment upon endometriosis lesions adequately, a proper control group for comparison is needed, with longitudinal follow-up.

A second outcome of interest is the effect upon pain. The first requirement of quality pain eval-uation is the need for a valid method of assess-ing pain.[32] A second necessity in pain research is the need for longitudinal evaluation, as pain recurrence is a time-dependent phenomenon. Finally, to determine the efficacy of a drug in relieving pain, a large placebo effect must be accounted for; this phenomenon of relief by an inactive drug may occur in as many as 55% of women with endometriosis-associated pain.[33]

Thus, placebo-controlled trials are needed to determine absolute efficacy; comparative studies between drugs will allow determination of relative efficacy.

The third outcome of interest is fertility enhance-ment. It is rare that the woman with endometrio-sis-associated infertility has absolute infertility due to the disease, as is the case with bilateral tubal blockage or azoospermia. Instead, most women suffering from endometriosis-associated infertility have a relative reduction in fecundity.[31] Thus, they are able to conceive, albeit at a slower rate. To demonstrate improved fertility status after intervention, a comparison group of untreated women is clearly needed. Finally, as fertility is time-dependent, longitudinal assessment is again critical.

A final outcome of interest in the study of endometriosis interventions is quality of life. This outcome parameter is fairly recent in its use as a measure of treatment success, and its application to endometriosis is a particularly recent phenom-enon.[34] A validated quality of life scale has been developed for endometriosis, but to date this tool has been used sparingly.[35]

From the above discussion, it is clear that optimal trials should be properly controlled and random-ized. In addition, it is important to have studies that have a lengthy follow-up, so the long-term course can be determined post-treatment. Studies such as these will be primarily relied upon in the subsequent discussion.

Medical treatment of endometriosis implants

The effect of medications on implant volume, number, and extensiveness has been examined for a number of drugs in a number of ways. Many are poorly controlled or uncontrolled investigations, and often the observations searching for effect are carried out while the patient is on the drug. Thus, what occurs after drug discontinuation is often a mystery.

An effect of danazol upon endometriotic implants has been consistently observed. Uncontrolled trials have demonstrated implant resolution in the vast majority of treated patients.[36,37] Questionable studies have shown a mean decrease of 61–89% of implant volume[38,39] and a 43% decrease in classi-fication score.[40] A single placebo-controlled RCT examined the effect upon implants 6 months fol-lowing completion of drug therapy, with resolu-tion of implants in 18% of the placebo group and 60% of the danazol treatment group.[41]

Although progestogens clearly affect ectopic endometrium, there is limited information of the histologic effect upon endometriosis. In the rhesus monkey, levonorgestrel has been shown to decrease lesion size. In the human, a single randomized prospective trial demonstrated that MPA, 100 mg daily for 6 months, produced complete resolution of implants in 50% of patients and a partial resolution in 13%, whereas corresponding figures for placebo were 12% and 6%, respectively.[41]

Several randomized trials have assessed the ability of gestrinone to decrease anatomic endometriosis. The drug has been shown to lower the amount of disease comparably to danazol,[42] and doses as low as 1.25 mg twice weekly can accomplish this.[43,44]

GnRH agonists have been shown in numerous studies to decrease the classification score of endometriosis in patients on the drug; similar decreases were seen with the complete American Fertility Society (AFS) classification as well as a modified scoring system that excluded points for adhesions[45,46] (Figure 29.1). Thus, the effect is limited to causing a lessening of implant volume. In comparative trials, the decreased AFS score is comparable to that seen with danazol treatment.[47] However no study has evaluated the lingering effect of GnRH on implants after discontinuation of the drug. GnRH agonist plus add-back therapy has also been shown to decrease the AFS classification score, and to a degree similar to that seen with GnRH agonist alone.[48]

Currently, no published data exist for other forms of medical treatment.

Medical treatment of endometriosis-associated pain

Pain relief has also been well demonstrated with danazol, with 84–92% of women responding.[49] A placebo-controlled RCT proved danazol reduced pain significantly better than no treatment for up to 6 months following discontinuation of the drug.[41] No good data exist for longer follow-up periods. Recent evidence suggests the median time to pain recurrence following discontinuation of the medication is 6.1 months.[50]

Few randomized trials exist to evaluate the effects of progestational agents on endometriosis-associated pain. Telimaa and colleagues evaluated the effect of medroxyprogesterone acetate, 100 mg/ day for 6 months. The medication produced a significant and substantial improvement in pain scores while patients received the drug, as well as up to 6 months following discontinuation.[41] In fact, the relative attributable experimental effect (percent decrease in pain severity attributable solely to treatment) was 50–74% at the conclusion of follow-up. Randomized comparative trials suggest medroxyprogesterone to be comparable in efficacy to danazol[51] and GnRH agonists (see Figure 29.1), although lynestrenol performed less well than a GnRH agonist for all aspects of endometriosis-associated pain.[51]

Numerous uncontrolled trials have evaluated pain relief with oral contraceptives, generally demonstrating improvement in 75–89%.[13] A recent randomized clinical trial compared cyclic low-dose oral contraceptives to a GnRH agonist and found no substantial difference in the degree of relief afforded these women by the two drugs,

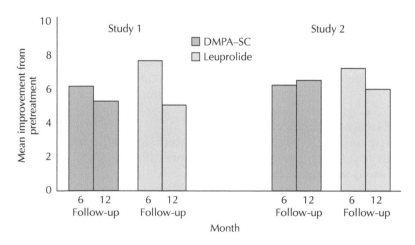

Figure 29.1 Comparison of subcutaneous depot-medroxyprogesterone acetate (DMPA-SC) and leuprolide acetate. Month 6 = end of treatment; 12-month follow-up was an intent-to-treat analysis. Composite scores significantly improved from pretreatment at month 6 and at 12-month follow-up for each treatment group, both studies (p <0.001), within treatment groups.

except that the GnRH agonist provided greater relief of dysmenorrhea.[52] An uncontrolled trial of continuous oral contraceptive pills (OCPs) following failure of cyclic therapy suggested that this regimen may be superior, as 80% responded with pain relief.[53] However, no RCTs have as yet assessed continuous administration.

The effectiveness of GnRH agonists in the treatment of endometriosis-associated pain has been demonstrated in both placebo-controlled and comparative randomized trials. The one placebo-controlled study demonstrated greater effectiveness of the drug at 3 months, at which time those in the placebo group still suffering from pain were allowed to opt out of the study.[54] In comparative trials, GnRH agonists and danazol were equally effective in relieving pain.[47,55–69] A recent RCT comparing subcutaneous depot-medroxyprogesterone acetate to a GnRH agonist showed the two interventions to be comparable in terms of efficacy and side effects.[70] Oral contraceptives have also been compared with GnRH agonists: in a study of 57 women designed to have 80% power to detect a 35% difference in effect, cyclic oral contraceptive treatment was significantly less effective than GnRH agonist treatment for relief of dysmenorrhea, nearly as effective for relief of dyspareunia (statistically significantly different using one of two rating scales, but of questionable clinical importance), and equally efficacious in relieving nonspecific pelvic pain.[52]

Whereas the above studies randomize patients for initial therapy of endometriosis-associated pain, one study has examined the value of GnRH agonists in patients failing primary therapy. Ling and colleagues treated women having failed to obtain relief with OCPs with either GnRH agonist or placebo.[71] Those treated with active drug responded significantly better than those given placebo, with more than 80% experiencing pain relief in 3 months (Figure 29.2). Of interest is the fact that the therapy seemed to be beneficial whether or not endometriosis was seen at laparoscopy.

Several trials have addressed the efficacy of combined add-back therapy and GnRH agonist treatment during 6-month treatment periods.[72–77] In general, pain was relieved as effectively with the combination as with GnRH agonist alone, and it significantly reduced the side effects of the GnRH agonist. The results were similar in three longer trials of approximately 1-year duration.[48,78,79] It seems clear that add-back therapy can be added to GnRH agonist treatment without loss of efficacy but with a substantial amelioration of hypoestrogenic symptoms (Figure 29.3). This seems to be

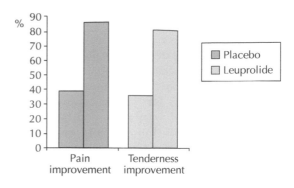

Figure 29.2 Subjective and objective pain relief with empiric treatment of leuprolide, a gonadotropin-releasing hormone (GnRH) agonist, for presumed endometriosis following failure of other medical therapy.

the case even when the add-back therapy is begun during the first month of treatment, suggesting that an 'add-back free' interval at the beginning of a treatment cycle is unnecessary.[77]

Although not approved for use in the United States, gestrinone has been studied reasonably extensively. Comparative trials show gestrinone to be roughly equivalent in pain relief to danazol[42] and GnRH agonists.[80] One study has even shown gestrinone to be slightly more efficacious than GnRH agonist for relief of dysmenorrhea 6 months after discontinuation of medication.[80]

Given the above data, a number of conclusions can be reached regarding treatment of endometriosis symptoms with medical therapy. It appears that most established medical treatments are effective for the primary treatment of endometriosis-associated pain, and all also seem to be roughly equivalent. Thus, for initial treatment the choice should probably be based on the cost and side-effect profile of the drug being considered. However, only GnRH agonists have been proven effective after the failure of a prior medical hormonal therapy. It remains to be seen what the value is for the newer, investigational therapies; the answers will await upcoming efficacy and comparative trials.

Medical treatment of endometriosis-associated infertility

Most of the established medical therapies used to treat endometriosis have been applied to the problem of subfertility in women with endometriosis. These medications inhibit ovulation, and thus are used to treat the disease for a period of time prior to allowing an attempt at conception. Five randomized trials with 6 treatment arms have compared one of these medical treatments

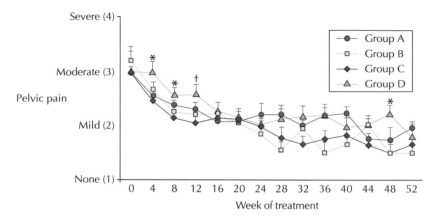

*$p \leq 0.05$ change from baseline compared with Group A
†$p \leq 0.01$ change from baseline compared with Group A

Hornstein MD, et al. *Obstet Gynecol.* 1998;91:16–24.

Figure 29.3 Pain relief with gonadotropin-releasing hormone (GnRH) agonist with and without add-back therapy. Mean pelvic pain score at each visit: Group A = GnRH agonist alone; Group B = GnRH agonist + norethindrone; Group C = GnRH agonist + low-dose conjugated estrogen/norethindrone; Group D = GnRH agonist + high-dose conjugated estrogen/norethindrone. Reproduced with permission from Hornstein et al.[78]

directed at endometriosis to placebo or no treatment with fertility as the outcome measure[81–85] (Table 29.1). Another 8 RCTs compared danazol to a second medication. These latter trials have been summarized recently in a meta-analysis by Hughes et al.[86] Clearly, no increase in fertility can be demonstrated with these medications when compared to expectant management, nor has any medication proven superior to danazol in this regard.

It is important to note, however, that some studies were placebo-controlled, whereas others simply compared medication to no treatment. For this latter study design, follow-up of the patient was begun at the conclusion of therapy; thus, those receiving no treatment began attempting to conceive immediately after the laparoscopy, while those placed on drug therapy were not allowed attempted conception until after the medication

course was completed (generally 6 months). These studies were analyzed as if the time began at the conclusion of 'treatment', but, for the patient, the clock begins ticking at the time of diagnostic laparoscopy. The real question is not who gets pregnant faster after therapy is completed, but rather who gets pregnant faster from the time of diagnosis?

If we reanalyze the above data, with follow-up proceeding from the time of diagnosis instead of conclusion of treatment, a different image emerges (Table 29.2). Now, suppressive medical therapy proves significantly detrimental to fertility. In essence, the interval spent on medical therapy has been wasted time, merely serving to prolong the infertility in a number of couples. Thus, traditional medical therapy for endometriosis has not proven to be of value, and in fact may be counterproductive, to the subfertile patient.

Table 29.1 Meta-analysis of medical therapy for endometriosis-associated infertility

Study (main author)	Medical treatment	Placebo or no treatment	Relative risk	95% confidence limits
Bayer[81]	11/37	17/36	0.63	0.32–1.22
Fedele[84]	17/35	17/36	1.03	0.60–1.76
Telimaa[82]	13/35	6/14	0.87	0.41–2.25
Thomas[85]	5/20	4/17	1.06	0.28–4.29
Harrison[83]	0/50	3/50	0.00	0.00–2.18
Total	46/177	47/153	0.85	0.59–1.22

Table 29.2 Meta-analysis of medical therapy for endometriosis-associated infertility: adjustment for follow-up from time of diagnosis

Study (main author)	Medical treatment	Placebo or no treatment	Relative risk	95% confidence limits
Bayer[81]	11/37	17/36	0.63	0.32–1.22
Fedele[84]	10/35	13/36	0.79	0.36–1.68
Telimaa[82]	4/35	5/14	0.32	0.08–1.24
Thomas[85]	4/20	4/17	0.85	0.20–3.69
Harrison[83]	0/50	3/50	0.00	0.00–2.18
Total	29/177	42/153	0.60	0.38–0.93

This is not to suggest that traditional medical therapy is incapable of playing a role in the treatment of the infertile couple with endometriosis. It is quite possible that a subgroup of infertile women exist who could be helped with drug therapy. However, this subgroup is thus far unidentified; advocates should focus future trials upon somehow stratifying endometriosis patients and then randomizing to drug vs no treatment. Until that time, it is clear that these medications play no role in the treatment of endometriosis-associated infertility.

Experimental medical treatments of endometriosis

RU-486 (mifepristone) and selective progesterone receptor modulators

Progesterone receptor modulators (PRMs) are progesterone receptor ligands that can produce one of three effects.[87] Type I ligands prevent or attenuate PR binding to the progesterone response element;[88] in doing so, they act as pure antagonists of progesterone action. Examples of such ligands include the 13α-configured steroids onapristone and ZK 135,695. Type II progesterone receptor ligands promote progesterone receptor binding to DNA response elements, but their ability to alter gene expression is highly variable and may be site-specific.[89] A number of existing molecules can act in this manner: RU-486, ZK 137,316, and the selective progesterone receptor modulators or SPRMs (J867, J956, J912, J1042; also known as mesoprogestins). Finally, type III ligands promote progesterone receptor binding to the progesterone response element, but transcription does not occur under any circumstances.

Thus, in vivo, type I or type III ligands act as pure antagonists, whereas type II ligands may act as agonists, partial agonists, or antagonists, depending upon the dose, presence or absence of progesterone, and site of action. To date only type II ligands have been used in the treatment of endometriosis.

Progesterone antagonists and agonist–antagonists have been shown in the nonhuman primate model to cause endometrial atrophy, similar to the effect of progesterone. However, the mechanism is completely different. It appears that the primarily antagonistic RU-486 causes a periarteriolar degeneration of endometrial spiral arteries. Partial agonists, such as the SPRMs, also result in a decreased number and size of spiral arteries, but no periarteriolar degeneration is evident.[87] Thus, despite the potential proliferative effect upon endometrium via an antiprogestin effect, the inhibition of vascular supply results in endometrial atrophy.

RU-486 (mifepristone) was the first of this class of drugs to be used to treat endometriosis. The drug is primarily a progesterone antagonist that can inhibit ovulation and disrupt endometrial integrity. Daily doses of this medication range from 50 to 100 mg daily, with side effects ranging from hot flashes to fatigue, nausea, and transient liver transaminase changes. No effects upon lipid profiles or bone mineral density have been reported.

The ability of mifepristone to produce a regression of endometriotic lesions has been variable and apparently dependent upon duration of treatment. Trials of 2 months in the rodent model[90] and 3 months in the human[91] failed to produce regression of disease. However, 6 months of therapy result in less visible disease in women.[92]

Uncontrolled trials suggest possible efficacy for endometriosis-associated pain, although numbers are small.[91] No data have yet been collected regarding fertility enhancement.

The mesoprogestins are partial antagonists of progesterone, but also behave like progesterone in some tissues. This mixed agonist–antagonist effect may prove valuable if an SPRM can inhibit endometrial growth while not producing other systemic effects of progesterone, such as breast tenderness, depression, and fluid retention. The mesoprogestin J867 (asoprisnil) is currently in phase III clinical trials; early studies have suggested efficacy in pain relief with minimal side effects.

Gonadotropin-releasing hormone antagonists

GnRH antagonists, like the long-utilized GnRH agonists, are a group of analogues of the native GnRH molecule. These drugs act by blocking the GnRH receptor directly and preventing it from activating. This results in a down-regulation of the pituitary gland, a reduction of gonadotropin secretion, and suppression of ovarian steroid production. Thus, a hypoestrogenic state ensues, just like with GnRH agonists. Unlike GnRH agonists, however, these drugs do not cause an initial stimulation of gonadotropin and ovarian hormone release.

The GnRH antagonists have multiple changes compared to active GnRH. Substitutions in the first three amino acids result in binding to the GnRH receptor. Position 6 substitution creates a compound with a prolonged half-life, as this is the site generally attacked by degradation enzymes. Finally, early GnRH antagonists produced substantial histamine release, making their use problematic. Substitutions at positions 8 and 10 have eliminated this problem (Figure 29.4).

At the molecular level, the GnRH antagonist interrupts the basic activation process of the GnRH receptor. When GnRH binds to its receptor, the receptor dimerizes and initiates a cascade of events that leads to synthesis and secretion of LH and FSH. With the antagonists, there is competition with the native molecule for the receptor. Given the high binding affinity, relative abundance, and long half-life of the antagonist, these molecules monopolize the GnRH receptors. Thus, dimerization of receptors is prevented (as GnRH cannot bind to them) and gonadotropes do not secrete LH or FSH.

Due to these characteristics of the GnRH antagonists, they offer the theoretical advantage of working faster and more effectively than GnRH agonists, with better patient compliance due to earlier amelioration of symptoms. Studies in animal models of endometriosis have been quite promising,[93] and preliminary clinical trials suggest the drug to be safe and efficacious.[94] A recent investigation in women demonstrated that a GnRH antagonist improved the health-related quality of life of women with endometriosis.[95] Phase III clinical trials are currently ongoing to further validate the use of this medication for endometriosis, as questions regarding relative efficacy and rate of side effects compared to GnRH agonists must be answered.

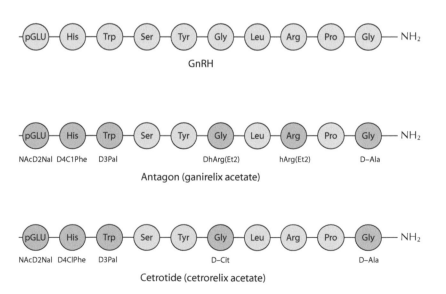

Figure 29.4 Structure of gonadotropin-releasing hormone (GnRH) and GnRH antagonists.

Aromatase inhibitors

It is well recognized that most if not all endometriosis is estrogen-dependent, thus resulting in the effectiveness of medications that interfere with ovarian estrogen production. However, there are two other important sources of estrogen: peripheral tissue and endometriotic cells. Peripheral tissue sites such as adipose tissue and skin fibroblasts are capable of converting androgens to significant amounts of estrogen.[96] Furthermore, large quantities of estrogen can be produced locally within ectopically located endometrium via an intracrine mechanism.[97]

The mechanism by which endometriosis is able to produce its own estrogen is via the expression of the enzyme aromatase.[97] This enzyme, not expressed in normal endometrium, is stimulated by prostaglandin E_2 (PGE_2); the resulting estrogen production then stimulates PGE_2, further enhancing estrogen (Figure 29.5). An obvious therapeutic target would thus be this aromatase enzyme. Aromatase inhibitors have now been tested in the rodent endometriosis model, with good success.[98] In addition, a case report of the use of anastrozole in a postmenopausal woman with severe endometriosis suggests the potential value of this treatment in women.[97] However, substantial bone loss in this woman emphasizes the need for caution with this class of medications, and reinforces the value of larger clinical trials to determine safety and efficacy.

Recently, anastrozole has been combined with a GnRH agonist in the treatment of endometriosis-associated pain. Bone loss was noted to be substantial in the treatment group, but at 2 years post-treatment no difference in bone loss was observed compared to GnRH agonist alone.[99]

Tumor necrosis factor alpha inhibitors

Tumor necrosis factor alpha (TNF-α) is a cytokine that appears to be overproduced in endometriosis patients and may well be at least partially responsible for the influx of peritoneal macrophages known to occur in women with this disease. It has long been believed that this macrophage influx is at least partially responsible for many of the biochemical and symptomatic changes associated with endometriosis. In particular, it has been hypothesized that cytokine attraction of activated macrophages is one of the key initiators of growth factor secretion in the peritoneal cavity, resulting in a favorable environment for endometriosis implantation, growth, and development.

One therapeutic approach that has been considered is some type of blockade of this cytokine. This has been attempted in the baboon, where recombinant human TNF binding protein-1 (TBP-1) was administered to menstrual endometrium prior to seeding the peritoneal cavity with the tissue.[100] In this scenario, endometriosis development was inhibited. Additionally, baboons with

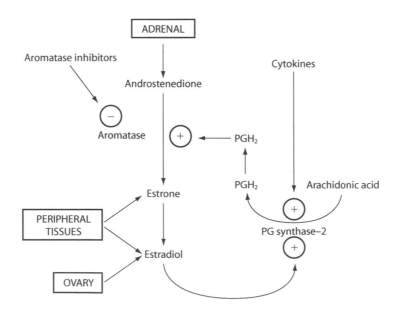

Figure 29.5 The intracellular pathway of aromatase action, and inhibition by aromatase inhibitors. PG = prostaglandin.

endometriosis were treated with TBP-1, GnRH antagonist, or placebo; significantly, less endometriosis was noted with TBP-1 and GnRH antagonist treatment. These studies suggest TBP-1 is effective in treating the physical manifestations of endometriosis in the baboon, and may be of value in the human. Clinical trials, however, have not yet been conducted.

Angiogenesis inhibitors

According to the transplantation theory of endometriosis, when shed endometrium is placed in the peritoneal cavity, the establishment of a new blood supply is essential for the survival of the implant and development of endometriosis. This process, termed angiogenesis, is a complex process involving a number of different but co-ordinated functions. These include proliferation, migration, and extension of endothelial cells, adherence of these cells to the extracellular matrix, remodeling of this matrix, and formation of a lumen.[101]

Several angiogenic factors, i.e. factors that aid in the development of new blood vessels, have been noted as present in endometrium and endometriosis. The most prominently studied of these factors is VEGF, which is responsible for inducing early vascular growth. This molecule has been noted in endometriosis lesions,[102] endometriomas,[103] and the peritoneal fluid[104,105] of endometriosis patients, although in the latter case it is unclear whether levels are the same as or increased over controls. In any event, one logical therapeutic step would be to attempt inhibition of these new vascular structures as a way of deterring the development of endometriosis. This has been attempted in the mouse model, where several angiogenic inhibitors (endostatin, TNP-470, celecoxib, and rosiglitazone) reduced the number and size of lesions.[106] The only human study thus far conducted with an angiogenesis inhibitor was the treatment of endometriosis-associated pain with thalidomide; pain relief was noted in these patients.[107]

Matrix metalloproteinase inhibitors

Matrix metalloproteinases (MMPs) are a family of endopeptidases which play a role in the degradation and turnover of extracellular matrix proteins. Their action is regulated by specific tissue inhibitors called tissue inhibitors of metalloproteinases (TIMPs). The activity of these enzymes in the endometrium is generally regulated by steroid hormones: estrogen is known to increase endometrial MMPs, and progesterone suppresses MMP activity.[108] The mechanisms for these actions, as well as the many additional regulators of the system, are complex and reviewed elsewhere.[108]

Increased matrix metalloproteinase activity has been described in endometriosis, and is believed to be integral in the ability of endometrium to invade tissue and implant successfully. Inhibition of these enzymes might be effective in inhibiting the development of endometriosis. Only one study has been conducted to date: the MMP inhibitor ONO-4817 was used in the mouse model to deter the development of experimental adenomyosis.[109] The value and practicality of this approach in endometriosis remains to be tested.

Pentoxifylline and other immunomodulators

Pentoxifylline is a multisite immunomodulating drug. It inhibits phagocytosis and generation of toxic oxygen species and proteolytic enzymes by macrophages and granulocytes, stifles production of TNF-α, and reduces the inflammatory action of TNF-α and interleukin-1 on granulocytes.[110,111] Thus, this medication influences both the production of inflammatory mediators and the responsiveness of immunocompetent cells to inflammatory stimuli. Given the many immunologic abnormalities described in endometriosis, this medication has some rationale in an attempt to correct immune dysfunction. As it is not an inhibitor of ovulation, pentoxifylline has an advantage over ovulation suppressors when attempting to treat endometriosis-associated infertility: it can be administered throughout the time period of attempting conception. Doses have ranged from 400 to 1200 mg daily. The drug is extremely well tolerated, with the major adverse effects being gastric discomfort and dizziness; both are seen in few patients utilizing the recommended dose, and neither has been shown to occur more often in treated patients than placebo controls when giving commercial preparations of the drug.[112]

Of the experimental treatment for endometriosis, only pentoxifylline has been investigated as a treatment for endometriosis-associated infertility. This drug has the advantage of not inhibiting ovulation and thus can be utilized without delay of attempted conception. A single placebo-controlled RCT with 60 patients resulted in a 12-month pregnancy rate of 31% with pentoxifylline and 18.5% with placebo, a difference not statistically different but intriguing nonetheless.[113] Hopefully, additional, larger trials will further investigate this approach to help clarify the value of this and similar drugs.

Two other immunomodulators have been used experimentally. In the rat model, administration of intraperitoneal loxoribine, an immunomodulator that enhances cytokine activity, results in regression of endometrial explants.[114] Interferon α-2b has been shown to inhibit endometrioma cell growth in culture.[115] No primate studies have been conducted with either drug.

Estrogen receptor beta agonists

It is well established that endometriosis is an estrogen-dependent disease. However, recently it was discovered that estrogen has two receptors: ER-α and ER-β.[116] While ER-α has clearly been related to proliferation of endometrium, the function of ER-β is unclear. This receptor is expressed in a wide variety of tissues, including much of the immune system. However, it is expressed minimally if at all in reproductive tissues. ER-β mRNA has been seen in endometrial stroma, epithelium, and endometrioma,[117,118] but as of yet the actual receptor protein has not been found in these tissues. Nevertheless, utilizing the nude mouse model with explants of human endometriosis, an ER-β agonist was able to produce regression of lesions. Furthermore, this effect was most pronounced when endometrial lesions were originally intraperitoneal. Several possible mechanisms exist. One explanation could be that ER-β agonists are acting as mouse intraperitoneal immunomodulators, enhancing the immunologic response to the explants. A second possible explanation lies in the recognition of ER-β in endothelial cells of endometrial vasculature; an anti-angiogenic effect might also explain the regression of endometrial tissue in the rodent model. Finally, it is as yet possible that improved assays will uncover the presence of ER-β in endometriosis, with the possibility that the receptor acts intracellularly as an ER-α inhibitor by dimerizing with the ER-α molecules to form a faulty product.[119] These possibilities will all be explored in upcoming studies.

Medical therapy following surgery

The use of medical therapy for endometriosis is not restricted to utilization as stand-alone agents. Frequently, clinicians have used drugs in combination with surgical treatment of the disease. When this approach is utilized, the medical therapy may be administered either preoperatively or postoperatively.

Only one randomized trial has evaluated the value of preoperative hormonal therapy.[120] In this study,

women with advanced endometriosis were either treated with 3 months of a GnRH agonist prior to surgery or with surgery alone. Surgery was noted to be easier (but not statistically significantly easier) by the surgeon, but surgical outcome was not assessed in terms of symptomatic relief.

Numerous RCTs have examined the issue of postoperative medical therapy as an effective adjunct for pain. Danazol was found not to enhance the results of surgery when administered for only 3 months,[121] but 6 months of postoperative administration reduced pain vs placebo for at least 6 months following discontinuation of the drug.[122] High-dose medroxyprogesterone behaved similarly.[122] Three RCTs have examined the use of postoperative GnRH agonists: 3 months of treatment was ineffective at enhancing pain relief,[123] but 6 months of postoperative therapy significantly reduced pain scores and delayed recurrence of pain[124,125] (Figure 29.6). The use of oral contraceptives for 6 months following surgery has been shown ineffective in improving the results of surgery.[126] Finally, an RCT comparing postoperative use of a levonorgestrel-containing intrauterine device (IUD) vs surgery alone found that all forms of pelvic pain were significantly reduced postoperatively by the addition of the IUD.[127]

One RCT has examined the use of a single postoperative medical therapy vs two sequential medical treatments following surgery. Morgante and colleagues compared the use of 6 months of postoperative GnRH agonist therapy to 6 months of

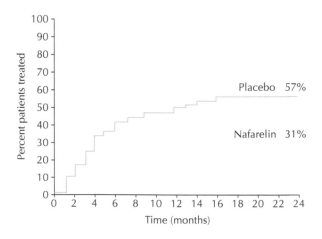

Figure 29.6 Time to symptom recurrence post-ablation. Rate of recurrence of pelvic pain following treatment with surgery alone vs surgery followed by nafarelin, a gonadotropin-releasing hormone (GnRH) agonist, therapy. Reproduced with permission from Hornstein et al.[124]

GnRH agonist followed by 6 months of danazol, 100 mg/day.[128] Twelve months following surgery (at the conclusion of danazol for one group, and after 6 months of no treatment for the other) there was significantly less pain in those treated with the two sequential medical treatments.

The possibility of combining two complimentary medications as a postoperative adjunct has also been tested. A randomized study investigating GnRH agonist plus anastrozole found that the drug combination increased the pain-free interval and decreased symptom recurrence when compared to the postoperative use of GnRH agonist alone.[99] This suggests that such an aggressive polypharmaceutical approach may well prove beneficial in selected instances.

Three studies have investigated the use of postoperative medical therapy for fertility enhancement, utilizing GnRH agonist[124,126] and raloxifene,[129] a selective estrogen receptor modulator. None have demonstrated any enhancement of fertility in women with endometriosis utilizing this approach.

While these studies suggest that postoperative medical therapy is of value when used for 6 months or more, a word of caution must be interjected. As is the case with all surgical trials, the degree of surgical skill and the technique used may be critical in determining the results. At least one retrospective trial has indicated that excision of endometriosis results in greater pain relief than ablation of lesions,[130] yet ablation is generally the treatment of choice with these studies (Figure 29.7). Furthermore, we have no way of ascertaining the degree of surgical skill that was applied in the surgical treatment of these patients. Additional high-quality studies are needed in a variety of settings by a larger number of surgeons to further examine this issue and confirm the above results.

Conclusions

The use of medical therapy for endometriosis is a proven approach to a frequently confounding disease. A wide variety of medications have proven to work in selected patient populations and, in so doing, have enlarged the size of the treatment repertoire available to the clinician combating this disorder. The recent addition of the 'experimental' medications discussed here holds the promise of even more options, perhaps even more effective and with better tolerance.

One clear deficiency in the literature, however, is the lack of a direct comparison between medical and surgical therapy in the treatment of endometriosis-associated pain. Although several randomized trials have been attempted, none has ever been completed. Data from placebo and sham controlled studies suggest similar success rates, but these investigations have been carried out in different patient populations under differing conditions. Until an RCT comparing medicine and surgery is carried out, the relative merits of each is purely speculative.

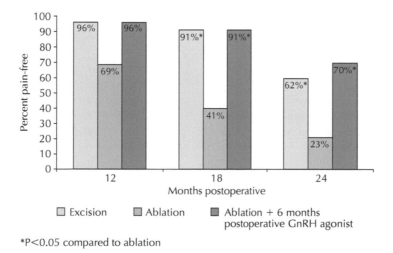

*P<0.05 compared to ablation

Figure 29.7 Endometriosis – postoperative analogue therapy. Pain relief with excision of endometriosis vs ablation of endometriosis versus ablation followed by medical therapy. GnRH = gonadotropin-releasing hormone.

REFERENCES

1. Goebel R, Rjosk HK. Laboratory and clinical studies with the new antigonadotropin, danazol. Acta Endocrinol 1977; 85 (Suppl 212): 134.

2. Floyd WS. Danazol: endocrine and endometrial effects. Int J Fertil 1980; 25: 75–80.

3. Barbieri RL, Canick JA, Makris A, et al. Danazol inhibits steroidogenesis. Fertil Steril 1977; 28: 809–813.

4. McGinley R, Casey JH. Analysis of progesterone in unextracted serum: a method using danazol [17 alpha-pregn-4-en-20-yno(2,3-d) isoxazol-17-ol] a blocker of steroid binding to proteins. Steroids 1979; 33: 127–138.

5. Buttram VC Jr, Belue JB, Reiter R. Interim report of a study of danazol for the treatment of endometriosis. Fertil Steril 1982; 37: 478–483.

6. Alvarado RG, Liu JY, Zwolak RM. Danazol and limb-threatening arterial thrombosis: two case reports. J Vasc Surg 2001; 34: 1123–1126.

7. Vercellini P, Tresid L, Panazza S, et al. Very low dose danazol for relief of endometriosis-associated pelvic pain: a pilot study. Fertil Steril 1994; 62: 1136–1142.

8. Janicki TI. Treatment of the pelvic pain associated with endometriosis using danazol vaginal suppositories. Two year followup. Fertil Steril 2002; 77: S52.

9. Igarashi M, Iizuka M, Abe Y, et al. Novel vaginal danazol ring therapy for pelvic endometriosis, in particular deeply infiltrating endometriosis. Hum Reprod 1998; 13: 1952–1956.

10. Bruner KL, Eisenberg E, Gorstein F, et al. Progesterone and transforming growth factor-beta coordinately regulate suppression of endometrial matrix metalloproteinases in a model of experimental endometriosis. Steroids 1999; 64: 648–653.

11. Olive DL. Medical treatment: alternatives to danazol. In: Schenken RS, ed. Endometriosis: contemporary concepts in clinical management. Philadelphia: JB Lippincott; 1989: 189–211.

12. Muneyyirci-Delale O, Karacan M. Effect of norethindrone acetate in the treatment of symptomatic endometriosis. Int J Fertil Womens Med 1998; 43: 24 27. Erratum in Int J Fertil Womens Med 1999; 44: 215.

13. Fedele L, Bianchi S, Zanconato G, et al. Use of a levonorgestrel-releasing intrauterine device in the treatment of rectovaginal endometriosis. Fertil Steril 2001; 75: 485–488.

14. Lau TM, Affandi B, Rogers PAW. The effects of levonorgestrel implants on vascular endothelial growth factor expression in the endometrium. Mol Hum Reprod 1998; 5: 57–63.

15. Hamblen EC. Androgen treatment of women. South Med J 1957; 50: 743.

16. Hirvonen E, Malkonen M, Manninen V. Effects of different progestogens on lipoproteins during postmenopausal replacement therapy. N Engl J Med 1981; 304: 560–563.

17. Fahraeus L, Sydsjo A, Wallentin L. Lipoprotein changes during treatment of pelvic endometriosis with medroxyprogesterone acetate. Fertil Steril 1986; 45: 503–506.

18. Andrews MC, Andrews WC, Strauss AF. Effects of progestin-induced pseudopregnancy on endometriosis: clinical and microscopic studies. Am J Obstet Gynecol 1959; 78: 776–785.

19. Scott RB, Wharton LR Jr. The effect of estrone and progesterone on the growth of experimental endometriosis in rhesus monkeys. Am J Obstet Gynecol 1957; 74: 852–863.

20. Noble AD, Letchworth AT. Medical treatment of endometriosis: a comparative trial. Postgrad Med J (Suppl 5) 1979; 55: 37.

21. Meresman GF, Auge L, Barano RI, et al. Oral contraceptives treatment suppresses proliferation and enhances apoptosis of eutopic endometrial tissue from patients with endometriosis. Fertil Steril 2001; 76: S47–48.

22. Sharpe-Timms KL, Zimmer RL, Jolliff WJ, et al. Gonadotropin-releasing hormone agonist (GnRH-a) therapy alters activity of plasminogen activators, matrix metalloproteinases and their inhibitors in rat models for adhesion formation and endometriosis: potential GnRH-a-regulated mechanisms reducing adhesion formation. Fertil Steril 1998; 69: 916–923.

23. Dmowski WP. The role of medical management in the treatment of endometriosis. In: Nezhat CR, Berger GS, Nezhat FR, et al. Endometriosis: advanced management and surgical techniques. New York: Springer-Verlag; 1995: 229–240.

24. Barbieri RL. Endometriosis and the estrogen threshold theory. Relation to surgical and medical treatment. J Reprod Med 1998; 43: 287–292.

25. Taskin O, Yalcinoglu AI, Kucuk S, et al. Effectiveness of tibolone on hypoestrogenic symptoms induced by goserelin treatment in patients with endometriosis. Fertil Steril 1997; 67(1): 40–45.

26. Lindsay PC, Shaw RW, Bennink HJ, et al. The effect of add-back treatment with tibolone (Livial) on patients treated with the gonadotropin-releasing hormone agonist triptorelin (Decapeptyl). Fertil Steril 1996; 65(2): 342–348.

27. Hurst BS, Gardner SC, Tucker KE, et al. Delayed oral estradiol combined with leuprolide increases endometriosis-related pain. JSLS 2000; 4: 97–101.

28. Cornillie FJ, Brosens IA, Vasquez G, et al. Histologic and ultrastructural changes in human endometriotic implants treated with the antiprogesterone steroid ethylnorgestienone (gestrinone) during 2 months. Int J Gynecol Pathol 1986; 5: 95–109.

29. Robyn C, Delogne-Desnoeck J, Bourdoux P, et al. Endocrine effects of gestrinone. In: Raynaud J-P, Ojasoo T, Martini L, eds. Medical management of endometriosis. New York: Raven Press; 1984: 207.

30. Cooke ID, Thomas EJ. The medical treatment of mild

endometriosis. Acta Obstet Gynecol Scand 1989; 150 (Suppl): 27.

31. D'Hooghe TM, Bambra CS, Isahakia M, et al. Evolution of spontaneous endometriosis in the baboon (*Papio anubis, Papio cynocephalus*) over a 12-month period. Fertil Steril 1992; 58: 409–412.

32. Williams RC. Toward a set of reliable and valid measurements for chronic pain assessment and outcome research. Pain 1988; 35: 239–251.

33. Kauppila A, Puolakka J, Ylikorkala O. Prostaglandin biosynthesis inhibitors and endometriosis. Prostaglandins 1979; 18: 655–661.

34. Story L, Taylor N, McVeigh E, et al. Assessing health status in endometriosis. In: Olive DL, ed. Endometriosis in clinical practice. London: Martin Dunitz; 2004.

35. Jones G, Kennedy S, Barnard A, et al. Development of an endometriosis quality-of-life instrument: The Endometriosis Health Profile-30. Obstet Gynecol 2001; 98: 258–264.

36. Dmowski WP, Cohen MR. Treatment of endometriosis with an antigonadotropin, danazol. A laparoscopic and histologic evaluation. Obstet Gynecol 1975; 46: 147–154.

37. Barbieri RL, Evans S, Kistner RW. Danazol in the treatment of endometriosis: analysis of 100 cases with a 4-year follow-up. Fertil Steril 1982; 37: 737–746.

38. Doberl A, Jeppsson S, Rannevik G. Effect of danazol on serum concentrations of pituitary gonadotropins in post-menopausal women. Acta Obstet Gynecol Scand 1984; 123(Suppl): 95.

39. Buttram VC Jr, Reiter RC, Ward S. Treatment of endometriosis with danazol: report of a 6-year prospective study. Fertil Steril 1985; 43: 353–360.

40. Henzl MR, Corson SL, Moghissi K, et al. Administration of nasal nafarelin as compared with oral danazol for endometriosis. A multicenter double-blind comparative clinical trial. N Engl J Med 1988; 318: 485–489.

41. Telimaa S, Puolakka J, Ronnberg L, et al. Placebo-controlled comparison of danazol and high-dose medroxyprogesterone acetate in the treatment of endometriosis. Gynecol Endocrinol 1987; 1: 13–23.

42. Fedele L, Bianchi S, Viezzoli T, et al. Gestrinone versus danazol in the treatment of endometriosis. Fertil Steril 1989; 51: 781–785.

43. Worthington M, Irvine LM, Crook D, et al. A randomized comparative study of the metabolic effects of two regimens of gestrinone in the treatment of endometriosis. Fertil Steril 1993; 59: 522–526.

44. Hornstein MD, Gleason RE, Barbieri RL. A randomized double-blind prospective trial of two doses of gestrinone in the treatment of endometriosis. Fertil Steril 1990; 53: 237–241.

45. Cedars MI, Lu JK, Meldrum DR, et al. Treatment of endometriosis with a long-acting gonadotropin-releasing hormone agonist plus medroxyprogesterone acetate. Obstet Gynecol 1990; 75: 641–645.

46. Surrey ES, Gambone JC, Lu JK, et al. The effects of combining norethindrone with a gonadotropin-releasing hormone agonist in the treatment of symptomatic endometriosis. Fertil Steril 1990; 53: 620–626.

47. Henzl MR, Corson SL, Moghissi K, et al. Administration of nasal nafarelin as compared with oral danazol for endometriosis. A multicenter double-blind comparative clinical trial. N Engl J Med 1998; 318: 485–489.

48. Surrey ES, Voigt B, Fournet N, et al. Prolonged gonadotropin-releasing hormone agonist treatment of symptomatic endometriosis: the role of cyclic sodium etidronate and low dose norethindrone 'add-back' therapy. Fertil Steril 1995; 63: 747–755.

49. Bayer SR, Seibel MM. Medical treatment: danazol. In: Schenkel RS, ed. Endometriosis: contemporary concepts in clinical management. Philadelphia: JB Lippincott; 1989: 169–187.

50. Miller JD, Shaw RW, Casper RF, et al. Historical prospective cohort study of the recurrence of pain after discontinuation of treatment with danazol or a gonadotropin-releasing hormone agonist. Fertil Steril 1998; 70: 293–296.

51. Regidor PA, Regidor M, Schmidt M, et al. Prospective randomized study comparing the GnRH-agonist leuprorelin acetate and the gestagen lynestrenol in the treatment of severe endometriosis. Gynecol Endocrinol 2001; 15: 202–209.

52. Vercellini P, Trespidi L, Colombo A, et al. A gonadotropin-releasing hormone agonist versus a low-dose oral contraceptive for pelvic pain associated with endometriosis. Fertil Steril 1993; 60: 75–79.

53. Frontino G, Vercellini P, De Giorgi O, et al. Continuous use of oral contraceptive (OC) for endometriosis-associated recurrent dysmenorrhea not responding to cyclic pill regimen. Fertil Steril 2002; 77: S23–24.

54. Dlugi AM, Miller JD, Knittle J. Lupron depot (leuprolide acetate for depot suspension) in the treatment of endometriosis: a randomized, placebo-controlled, double-blind study. Fertil Steril 1990; 54: 419–427.

55. Anonymous. Goserelin depot versus danazol in the treatment of endometriosis. The Australian/New Zealand experience. Aust N Z J Obstet Gynaecol 1996; 31: 55–60.

56. Chang SP, Ng HT. A randomized comparative study of the effect of leuprorelin acetate depot and danazol in the treatment of endometriosis. Chinese Medical J (Taipei) 1996; 57: 431–437.

57. Cirkel U, Ochs H, Schneider HPG. A randomized, comparative trial of triptorelin depot (D-Trp6-LHRH) and danazol in the treatment of endometriosis. Eur J Obstet Gynecol Reprod Biol 1995; 59: 61–69.

58. Crosignani PG, Gastaldi A, Lombardi PL, et al. Leuprorelin acetate depot versus danazol in the treatment of endometriosis: results of an open multicentre trial. Clin Ther 1992; 14: 29–36(Suppl A).

59. Dmowski WP, Radwanska E, Binor Z, et al. Ovarian suppression induced with Buserelin or danazol in the

management of endometriosis: a randomized, comparative study. Fertil Steril 1989; 51: 395–400.

60. Fraser IS, Shearman RP, Jansen RP, et al. A comparative treatment trial of endometriosis using the gonadotropin-releasing hormone agonist, nafarelin, and the synthetic steroid, danazol. Aust N Z J Obstet Gynaecol 1991; 31: 158–163.

61. Adamson GD, Kwei L, Edgren RA. Pain of endometriosis: effects of nafarelin and danazol therapy. Int J Fertil Med Stud 1994; 39: 215–217.

62. Wheeler JM, Knittle JD, Miller JD. Depot leuprolide versus danazol in treatment of women with symptomatic endometriosis. I. Efficacy results. Am J Obstet Gynecol 1992; 167: 1367–1371.

63. Dawood MY, Ramos J, Khan-Dawood FS. Depot leuprolide acetate versus danazol for treatment of pelvic endometriosis: changes in vertebral bone mass and serum estradiol and calcitonin. Fertil Steril 1995; 63: 1177–1183.

64. The Nafarelin European Endometriosis Trial Group (NEET). Nafarelin for endometriosis: a large-scale, danazol-controlled trial of efficacy and safety, with 1-year follow-up. Fertil Steril 1992; 57: 514–522.

65. Rolland R, van der Heijden PF. Nafarelin versus danazol in the treatment of endometriosis. Am J Obstet Gynecol 1990; 162: 586–588.

66. Kennedy SH, Williams IA, Brodribb J, et al. A comparison of nafarelin acetate and danazol in the treatment of endometriosis. Fertil Steril 1990; 53: 998–1003.

67. Rock JA. A multicenter comparison of GnRH agonist (Zoladex) and danazol in the treatment of endometriosis. Fertil Steril 1991; 56: S49.

68. Shaw RW. An open randomized comparative study of the effect of goserelin depot and danazol in the treatment of endometriosis. Zoladex Endometriosis Study Team. Fertil Steril 1992; 58: 265–272.

69. Prentice A, Deery A, Goldbeck-Wood S, et al. Gonadotropin-releasing hormone analogues for pain associated with endometriosis (Cochrane Review). In: The Cochrane Library, Issue 3. Oxford: Update Software; 1999.

70. Vilos GA, Archer DF, Luciano A, et al. New subcutaneous injection reduces endometriosis-associated pain. Presented at Association of Reproductive Health Professionals 41st Annual Meeting – Reproductive Health 2004. September 8–11, 2004; Washington, DC.

71. Ling FW. Randomized controlled trial of depot leuprolide in patients with chronic pelvic pain and clinically suspected endometriosis. Obstet Gynecol 1999; 93: 51–58.

72. Surrey E, Judd H. Reduction of vasomotor symptoms and bone mineral density loss with combined norethindrone and long-acting gonadotropin-releasing hormone agonist therapy of symptomatic endometriosis: a prospective randomized trial. J Clin Endocrinol Metab 1992; 75: 558–563.

73. Makarainen L, Ronnberg L, Kauppila A. Medroxyprogesterone acetate supplementation diminishes the hypoestrogenic side effects of gonadotropin-releasing

74. Tabkin O, Yakinoghe AH, Kucuk S, et al. Effectiveness of tibolone on hypoestrogenic symptoms induced by goserelin treatment in patients with endometriosis. Fertil Steril 1997; 67: 40–45.

75. Edmonds D, Howell R. Can hormone replacement therapy be used during medical therapy of endometriosis? Br J Obstet Gynaecol 1994 (Suppl 10); 101: 24–26.

76. Kiiholma P, Korhonen M, Tuimala R, et al. Comparison of the gonadotropin-releasing hormone agonist goserelin acetate alone versus goserelin combined with estrogen-progestogens add-back therapy in the treatment of endometriosis. Fertil Steril 1995; 64: 903–908.

77. Moghissi KS, Schlaff WD, Olive DL, et al. Goserelin acetate (Zoladex) with or without hormone replacement therapy for the treatment of endometriosis. Fertil Steril 1998; 69: 1056–1062.

78. Hornstein MD, Surrey ES, Weisberg GW, et al, Lupron Add-Back Study Group. Leuprolide acetate depot and hormonal add-back in endometriosis: a 12-month study. Obstet Gynecol 1998; 91: 16–24.

79. Lee PI, Yoon JB, Joo KY, et al. Gonadotrophin releasing hormone agonist (GnRHa)-Zoladex (Goserelin) and hormonal add-back therapy in endometriosis: a 12-month study. Fertil Steril 2002; 77: S23.

80. The Gestrinone Italian Study Group. Gestrinone versus a gonadotropin-releasing hormone agonist for the treatment of pelvic pain associated with endometriosis: a multicenter randomised, double-blind study. Fertil Steril 1996; 66: 911–919.

81. Bayer SR, Seibel MM, Saffan DS, et al. Efficacy of danazol treatment for minimal endometriosis in infertile women: a prospective, randomized study. J Reprod Med 1988; 33: 179–183.

82. Telimaa S. Danazol and medroxyprogesterone acetate inefficacious in the treatment of infertility in endometriosis. Fertil Steril 1988; 50: 872–875.

83. Harrison RF, Barry-Kinsella C. Efficacy of medroxyprogesterone treatment in infertile women with endometriosis: a prospective, randomized, placebo-controlled study. Fertil Steril 2000; 74: 24–30.

84. Fedele L, Parazzini F, Radici E, et al. Buserelin acetate versus expectant management in the treatment of infertility associated with minimal or mild endometriosis: a randomized clinical trial. Am J Obstet Gynecol 1992; 166: 1345–1350.

85. Thomas E, Cooke I. Successful treatment of asymptomatic endometriosis: Does it benefit infertile women? BMJ 1987; 294: 1117–1119.

86. Hughes E, Ferorkow D, Collins J, et al. Ovulation suppression for endometriosis (Cochrane review). In: The Cochrane Library, Issue 1. Oxford: Update Software; 2000.

87. Chwalisz K, Brenner RM, Fuhrmann UU, et al. Antiproliferative effects of progesterone antagonist and progesterone receptor modulators on the endometrium. Steroids 2000; 65: 741–751.

88. Klein-Hitpass L, Cato ACB, Henderson K, et al. Two types

of antiprogestins identified by their differential action in transcriptionally active extracts from T47D cells. Nucleic Acids Res 1991; 19: 1227–1233.

89. Elger W, Bartley J, Schneider B, et al. Endocrine pharmacological characterization of progesterone antagonists and progesterone receptor modulators with respect to PR-agonist and antagonistic activity. Steroids 2000; 65: 713–723.

90. Tjaden B, Galetto D, Woodruff JD, et al. Time-related effects of RU486 treatment in experimentally induced endometriosis in the rat. Fertil Steril 1993; 59: 437–440.

91. Kettel LM, Murphy AA, Mortola JF, et al. Endocrine responses to long-term administration of the antiprogesterone RU486 in patients with pelvic endometriosis. Fertil Steril 1991; 56: 402–407.

92. Kettel LM, Murphy AA, Morales AJ, et al. Treatment of endometriosis with the antiprogesterone mifepristone (RU486). Unpublished data.

93. Jones RC. The effect of a luteinizing hormone-releasing hormone antagonist on experimental endometriosis in the rat. Acta Endocrinol 1987; 114: 379–382.

94. Martha PM, Gray ME, Campion M, et al. Initial safety profile and hormonal dose response characteristics of the pure GnRH antagonist, Abarelix-depot, in women with endometriosis. Unpublished data.

95. Woolley JM, De Paoli AM, Gray ME, et al. Reductions in health related quality of life in women with endometriosis. Seventh Biennial World Congress of Endometriosis, London, May 14–17, 2000. [Abstract]

96. Bulin SE. Aromatase in aging women. Sem Reprod Endocrinol 1999; 17: 349–358.

97. Bulun SE, Zeitoun KM, Takayama K, et al. Molecular basis for treating endometriosis with aromatase inhibitors. Hum Reprod Update 2000; 6: 413–418.

98. Yano S, Ikegami Y, Nakao K. Studies on the effect of the new non-steroidal aromatase inhibitor fadrozole hydrochloride in an endometriosis model in rats. Arzneimittelforschung 1996; 46: 192–195.

99. Soysal S, Soysal ME, Ozer S, et al. The effects of post-surgical administration of goserelin plus anastrozole compared to goserelin alone in patients with severe endometriosis: a prospective randomized trial. Hum Reprod 2004; 19: 160–167.

100. D'Hooghe TM, Cuneo S, Nugent N, et al. Recombinant human TNF binding protein-1 (r-hTBP-1) inhibits the development of endometriosis in baboons; a prospective, randomized, placebo and drug controlled study. Fertil Steril 2001; 76: S1.

101. Folkman J, Shing Y. Angiogenesis. J Biol Chem 1992; 267: 10931–10934.

102. Donnez J, Smoes P, Gillerot S, et al. Vascular endothelial growth factor (VEGF) in endometriosis. Hum Reprod 1998; 13: 1686–1690.

103. Fasciani A, D'Ambrogio G, Bocci G, et al. High concentrations of the vascular endothelial growth factor and interleukin-8 in ovarian endometriomata. Mol Hum Reprod 2000; 6: 50–54.

104. Mahnke JL, Dawood MY, Huang JC. Vascular endothelial growth factor and interleukin-6 in peritoneal fluid of women with endometriosis. Fertil Steril 2000; 73: 166–170.

105. Barcz E, Kaminski P, Marianowski L. VEGF concentration in peritoneal fluid in patients with endometriosis. Gynekol Pol 2001; 72: 442–448.

106. Levine Z, Efstathiou JA, Sampson DA, et al. Angiogenesis inhibitors suppress endometriosis in a murine model. J Soc Gynecol Invest 2002; 9: 264a.

107. Scarpellini F, Sbracia M, Lecchini S, et al. Anti-angiogenesis treatment with thalidomide in endometriosis: a pilot study. Fertil Steril 2002; 78: S87.

108. Osteen KG, Yeaman GR, Bruner-Tran K. Matrix metalloproteinases and endometriosis. Semin Reprod Med 2003; 21: 155–164.

109. Mori T, Yamasaki S, Masui F, et al. Suppression of the development of experimentally induced uterine adenomyosis by a novel matrix metalloproteinase inhibitor, ONO-4817, in mice. Exp Biol Med 2001; 226: 429–433.

110. Steinleitner A, Lambert H, Roy S. Immunomodulation with pentoxifylline abrogates macrophage-mediated infertility in an in vivo model: a paradigm for a novel approach to the treatment of endometriosis-associated subfertility. Fertil Steril 1991; 55: 26–31.

111. Steinleitner A, Lambert H, Suarez M. Immunomodulation in the treatment of endometriosis-associated subfertility: use of pentoxifylline to reverse the inhibition of fertilization by surgically induced endometriosis in a rodent model. Fertil Steril 1991; 56: 975–979.

112. Physicians' desk reference. Montvale, NJ: Medical Economics Company, Inc; 2002: 784.

113. Balasch J, Creus M, Fabregues F, et al. Pentoxifylline versus placebo in the treatment of infertility associated with minimal or mild endometriosis: a pilot randomized clinical trial. Hum Reprod 1997; 12: 2046–2050.

114. Keenan J, Williams-Boyle P, Massey P, et al. Regression of endometrial explants in a rat model of endometriosis treated with the immune modulators loxoribine and levamisole. Fertil Steril 1999; 721: 135–141.

115. Badawy S, Etman A, Cuenca V, et al. Effect of interferon alpha 2b on endometrioma cells in vitro. Obstet Gynecol 2001; 98: 417–420.

116. Kuiper GGJM, Enmark E, Pelto Huikko M, et al. Cloning of a novel estrogen receptor expressed in rat prostate and ovary. Proc Natl Acad Sci USA 1996; 93: 5925–5930.

117. Lecce G, Meduri G, Ancelin M, et al. Presence of estrogen receptor beta in the human endometrium throughout the cycle: expression in glandular, stromal, and vascular cells. J Clin Endocrinol Metab 2001; 86: 1379–1386.

118. Fujimoto J, Hirose R, Sakaguchi H, et al. Expression of estrogen receptor alpha and beta in ovarian endometriomata. Mol Hum Reprod 1999; 5: 742–747.

119. Pavao M, Traish AM. Estrogen receptor antibodies: specificity and utility in detection, localization and

analyses of estrogen receptor alpha and beta. Steroids 2001; 66: 1–16.

120. Audebert A, Descamps P, Marret H. Pre or post-operative medical treatment with nafarelin in stage III–IV endometriosis: a French multicenter study. Eur J Obstet Gynecol Reprod Biol 1998; 79: 145–148.

121. Bianchi S, Busacca M, Agnoli B. Effects of 3 month therapy with danazol after laparoscopic surgery for stage III/IV endometriosis: a randomized study. Hum Reprod 1999; 14: 1335–1337.

122. Telimaa S, Ronnberg L, Kauppila A. Placebo-controlled comparison of danazol and high-dose medroxyprogesterone acetate in the treatment of endometriosis after conservative surgery. Gynaecol Endocrinol 1987; 1: 363–371.

123. Parazzini F, Fedele L, Busacca M, et al. Postsurgical medical treatment of advanced endometriosis: results of a randomized clinical trial. Am J Obstet Gynecol 1994; 171: 1205–1207.

124. Hornstein MD, Hemmings R, Yuzpe AA, et al. Use of nafarelin versus placebo after reductive laparoscopic surgery for endometriosis. Fertil Steril 1997; 68: 860–864.

125. Vercellini P, Crosignani PG, Fedini R. A gonadotropin-releasing hormone agonist compared with expectant management after conservative surgery for symptomatic endometriosis. Br J Obstet Gynaecol 1999; 106: 672–677.

126. Muzii L, Marana R, Caruana P, et al. Postoperative administration of monophasic combined oral contraceptives after laparoscopic treatment of ovarian endometriomas: a prospective, randomized trial. Am J Obstet Gynecol 2000; 183: 588–592.

127. Frontino G, Vercellini P, De Giorgi O, et al. Levonorgesterel-releasing intrauterine device (Lng-IUD) versus expectant management after conservative surgery for symptomatic endometriosis. A pilot study. Fertil Steril 2002; 77: S25–26.

128. Morgante G, Ditto A, La Marca A, et al. Low dose danazol after combined surgical and medical therapy reduces the incidence of pelvic pain in women with moderate and severe endometriosis. Hum Reprod 1999; 14: 2371–2374.

129. Alvarez-Gil L, Fuentes V. Raloxifene and endometriosis. Fertil Steril 2002; 77: S37.

130. Winkel C. Unpublished data.

30 Treatment of endometriosis with acupuncture and other complementary therapies

Pat Haines

Introduction

Traditional Chinese medicine (TCM) has been used successfully in treating a wide range of conditions, including women's health problems, for around 3500 years. Today, acupuncture as a component of TCM, is increasingly being used in the West. Ahadian[1] has shown that the artificial barriers between the integration of acupuncture and conventional medicine are disappearing and 'acupuncture as a therapy is increasingly being used for gynaecological conditions'.[2]

Treatment

The etiology of endometriosis is still unknown; however, 'new findings on the genetics, possible roles of the environment and immune system and intrinsic abnormalities in the endometrium have given an insight into the pathogenesis of this disorder.'[3] Basic scientific research provides evidence that begins to offer plausible mechanisms for the presumed physiologic effects of acupuncture; 'multiple research approaches have shown that acupuncture activates endogenous opioid mechanisms and may stimulate gene expression of neuropeptides.'[4]

'Modern research reveals that the pain in endometriosis is due to an overabundance of prostaglandins secreted from the nodular masses. Acupuncture has been proved to be active in inhibiting prostaglandin secretion, antagonising

its action and elevating the pain threshold'.[5]

The TCM approach for treatment is based on an holistic history of symptoms or patterns of disharmony in the body, the theory being that it is the imbalances in the flow of Qi or energy, through the meridians or pathways, that is the cause of illness. With the needles inserted at certain acupuncture points (Figure 30.1), the body is stimulated to release its own natural hormones, so improving the functioning of the immune and endocrine systems, reducing pain and restoring the flow of energy.

The diagnosis of endometriosis is arrived at by acquiring a characteristic pattern from all the signs and symptoms presented by the patient. In TCM, the principal pattern that causes painful menstrual periods is blood stasis. However, there are often underlying factors associated with endometriosis, the most common being heat, cold, deficiency or excess patterns. The differentiation has to be assessed before treatment, based on the clinical manifestations of each individual case. The acupuncture points will then be selected.

The aim of the treatment is to remove the blood stasis and invigorate the blood, so increasing the circulation in the pelvic organs, as well as treating the underlying causes. The treatment principle is changed according to the time of the menstrual cycle. During menses, the concentration is on treating the manifestation: i.e. invigorating the blood and stopping pain. At other times in the cycle, the root cause is treated: i.e. the underlying pattern, 'a deficiency pattern in particular, is best

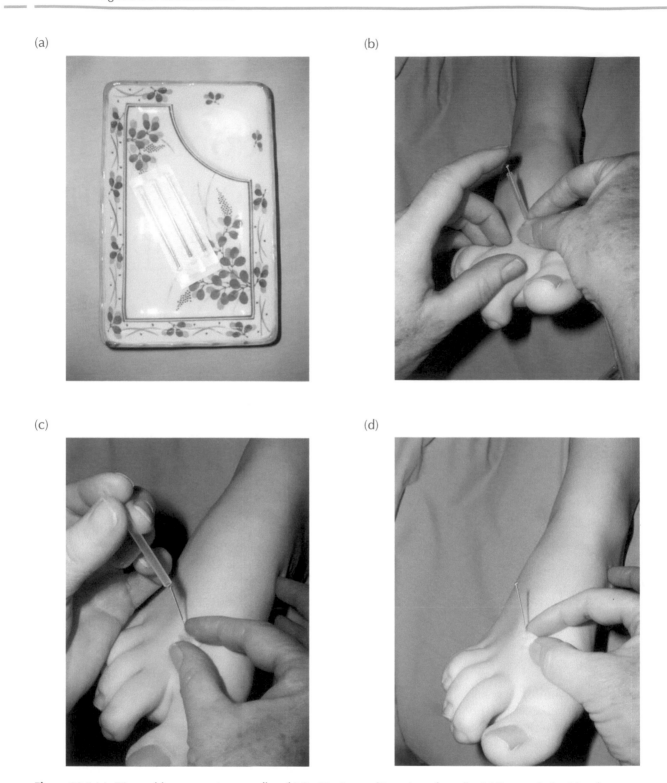

(a)

(b)

(c)

(d)

Figure 30.1 (a) Disposable acupuncture needles. (b) Positioning and insertion of needle. (c) Removal of guide tube. (d) Supporting needle using non-touch technique. (e) Connecting with the channel. (f) Needles left in situ for approx 20 minutes.

(e)

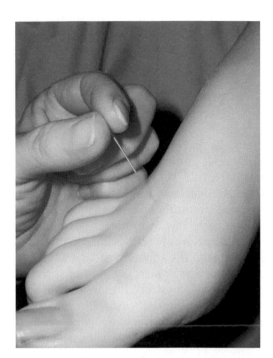

(f)

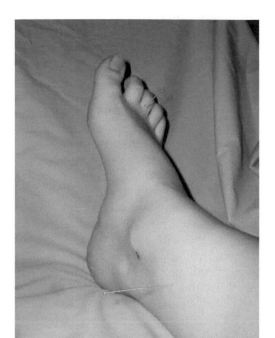

treated during the two weeks or thereabouts, after the period'.[6] In any menstrual problem, Maciocia[6] claims, it takes a minimum of three menstrual cycles to be successful; if dysmenorrhea is due to endometriosis, the treatment may take longer.

Safety

Growing evidence suggests that acupuncture is a safe procedure and serious adverse events are rare amongst trained and regulated practitioners using clean needle techniques.[7,8]

Patients have also reported a wide range of less serious effects, some of which may be seen as an integral part of the healing reaction. This may explain why such adverse events do not appear to dissuade patients from continuing with further treatment.[9]

Clinical trials

Evidence of effectiveness is increasingly being used to determine which health technologies should be incorporated into the public health provision.[10] 'Clinical research on acupuncture poses unique methodological challenges'[4] and some-

times the evidence is either insufficient or negative. 'Misleading results may occur for a number of reasons, false negative results may arise from inadequate treatment schedules and inappropriate control interventions'.[10]

Dincer and Linde[11] showed that randomized trials investigating the specific effects of acupuncture have used a great variety of sham interventions for the control group. However, there is evidence that a sham intervention cannot be considered physiologically inert. Sham interventions can include anything from:

- superficial needling of true points
- needling inappropriate acupuncture points
- needling non-acupuncture points
- using non-skin-penetration devices
- using pseudo-interventions, such as non-penetrating skin probes.

The conclusion was that sham acupuncture could not be considered to be a placebo and therefore great care should be taken in designing and interpreting the results of such trials.

There have been many randomized controlled trials on the effect of acupuncture for the treatment of primary dysmenorrhea. Helms[12] was one of the first to demonstrate that real acupuncture could produce a substantially greater response than a sham intervention and, although small, it was a methodologically sound study. Habek et al[13] showed a 93.3% success rate within 1 year after the treatment of acupuncture for primary dysmenorrhea compared with 3.7% in the placebo group. Acupressure (where pressure is used rather than needles at the acupuncture sites) has also been demonstrated as an effective form of treatment; Chen and Chen[14] recommend its use for self-care of primary dysmenorrhea.

For the management of pain associated with endometriosis, the assessment of acupuncture is more limited. Maciocia[15] claims that 'acupuncture has been reported anecdotally to help control the pain associated with some cases of endometriosis but no controlled studies have confirmed this claim'. Indeed, the supporting studies are small. Tsenov,[16] in his study, showed 24 women with secondary dysmenorrhea to have a satisfactory influence with acupuncture, whereas Liu[17] showed a total effective rate of 91.3%. Wang and Hou[5] showed an overall total success rate of 82.6% in their study, with better results obtained in the mild and moderate cases of endometriosis than in the severe cases: with 97.8%, 83.2% and 63.6% respectively.

'In view of the small number of studies and their variable quality, further studies are justified.'[2] Park et al,'[18] in their studies, demonstrated the efficacy of a sham needle that is designed to telescope instead of penetrating the skin and is therefore a valid control for acupuncture studies. Clinical trials must use an optimal form of treatment and a number of recommendations are being made with 'the aim of improving the design to show the efficacy of these trials in acupuncture in order that they are more conclusive and meaningfully interpreted'.[10]

Chinese herbs

The reputation of Chinese herbs has come under a lot of criticism due to the unregulated distribution and adverse reactions to some of the components. The Register of Chinese Herbal Medicine (RCHM), set up in 1987 to regulate the practice of Chinese herbal medicine in the UK, now represents over 400 fully qualified practitioners. As a result, Chinese herbs are safe when prescribed correctly by a properly trained practitioner.

Chinese herbal medicine usually has good results in the treatment of dysmenorrhea; again effective treatment should be based according to the differentiations. Many acupuncturists are also trained in Chinese herbal medicine and both acupuncture and Chinese herbs, either singly or in combination, give excellent results in painful periods.[6]

Diet and nutritional supplements

Diet may be an important factor in controlling the symptoms of endometriosis, as 'research into the menstrual cycle suggests that, nutritional intake and metabolism may play an important role in the cause and treatment of menstrual disorders'.[19] Although there has been no research investigating the effect of a specific diet in women with endometriosis, the recommendations are to avoid alcohol, caffeine, chocolate, dairy products and the consumption of cold food and iced drinks. Studies by Rossignol and Bonnlander[20] have demonstrated that the severity of menstrual cramping and associated pain can be exacerbated by foods and beverages high in sugar content.

Several studies also demonstrate the benefits of taking nutritional supplements such as vitamins B_1, B_6 and E, evening primrose oil, essential minerals, and fatty acids. Brush[21] demonstrated 61% complete relief of dysmenorrhea and 23% partial relief after 3 months of treatment with evening primrose oil. Some of the alternative treatments have a sound pharmacologic basis and can be very helpful in the management of the symptoms or even of the disease itself. Evening primrose oil, available from health food stores and pharmacists, is a precursor of prostaglandin E_1. Selenium ACE (selenium + vitamins A, C, and E) probably has an anti-inflammatory action and vitamin B_6 acts as a coenzyme in the production of progesterone, which will suppress endometriotic implants.[22]

Sampalis et al[23] concluded that Neptune Krill Oil significantly reduced the symptoms of dysmenorrhea and premenstrual syndrome as well as being more effective than omega-3 fish oil. However, the conclusion of the Cochrane review[19] showed vitamin B_1, taken at 100 mg daily, to be effective for dysmenorrhea. Magnesium was also a promising treatment, although it is unclear as to what dose to recommend. There was insufficient evidence to recommend vitamin B_6, vitamin E, and omega-3 fatty acids due to the fact that the studies were too small.

Lifestyle changes

Early studies have suggested that women who exercise regularly every week decrease their risk of developing endometriosis. Exercise gives a higher muscle to body fat ratio, which means lower levels of estrogen in the body, which may help to suppress the symptoms of endometriosis and so reduce the risk of developing the disease.

However, those benefits are limited to women who exercise more than 4 hours a week,[24] or are involved in aerobics and who began exercising at an early age, in fact before the age of 26. If exercise was started later in life or is done in moderation, the same level of protection may not be reached.[25] Dhillon and Holt[26] showed that women who reported frequent, high-intensity activity during a 2-year period had a 76% reduced endometrioma risk compared with women who engaged in no high-intensity activity.

Support groups

'According to preliminary reports, regular meetings with other endometriosis sufferers may help women with endometriosis learn about the disease and cope better with the many psychological and emotional issues that often accompany this condition.'[27]

One preliminary study found that women who had the opportunity to speak with other women with endometriosis, as well as to meet with their physicians, had a higher satisfaction with their overall care.[28]

Self-help groups include the Simply Holistic Endometriosis (SHE) Trust and the Endometriosis Society, 'where meeting fellow sufferers, can show them that they are not alone with their problems'.[22] The book *Overcoming Endometriosis*[29] provides a well-balanced review of the disease from the patient's point of view.[22]

Conclusion

Many consumers are now seeking alternatives to conventional medicine.[19] My personal preference is with acupuncture and, as a therapy, evidence suggests that it is a safe treatment modality that is effective at the moment, mainly anecdotally, for endometriosis. 'Acupuncture could be indicated as a useful, non-pharmacological alternative'[30] or used as an integrated medical model. It is well suited to deal with many of the functional problems that conventional medicine is not equipped to address.[1] Most importantly, acupuncture and the other therapies provide a mechanism whereby patients regain some control; they offer an alternative for many women, giving them a choice.

Acknowledgments

I would like to thank: Nicola Robinson, Professor of Complementary Medicine at Thames Valley University and Chair of the British Acupuncture Council, and Mark Bovey, Research Co-ordinator at the Acupuncture Research Resource Centre (ARRC), for their kind help and support.

REFERENCES

1. Ahadian FM. Acupuncture in pain medicine: an integrated approach to the management of refractory pain. Curr Pain Headache Rep 2002; 6(6): 444–451.
2. White AR. A review of controlled trials of acupuncture for women's reproductive health care. J Fam Plann Reprod Health Care 2003; 29(4): 233–236.
3. Giudice LC, Kao LC. Endometriosis. Lancet 2004; 364(9447): 1789–1799.
4. Kaptchuk TJ. Acupuncture: theory, efficacy and practice. Ann Intern Med 2002; 136(5): 374–383.
5. Wang H, Hou Q. Acupuncture and moxibustion for treating ectopic endometrium. J Trad Chin Med 2002; 22(3): 203–204.
6. Maciocia G. Obstetrics & gynaecology in Chinese medicine. New York: Churchill Livingstone; 1999: 235–260.
7. Birch S, Hesselink JK, Jonkman FA, et al. Clinical research on acupuncture: part 1. What have reviews of the efficacy and safety of acupuncture told us so far? J Altern Complement Med 2004; 10(3): 468–480.
8. Lao L, Hamilton GR, Fu J, et al. Is acupuncture safe? A systematic review of case reports. Altern Ther Health Med 2003; 9(1): 72–83.
9. Macpherson H, Scullion A, Thomas KJ, et al. Patient reports of adverse events associated with acupuncture treatment: a prospective national survey. Qual Saf Health Care 2004; 13(5): 349–355.

10. White AR, Filshie J, Cummings TM; International Acupuncture Research Forum Clinical trials of acupuncture: consensus recommendations for optimal treatment, sham controls and blinding. Complement Ther Med 2001; 9(4): 237–245.

11. Dincer F, Linde K. Sham interventions in randomized clinical trials of acupuncture – a review. Compliment Ther Med 2003; 11(4): 235–242.

12. Helms JM. Acupuncture for the management of primary dysmenorrhea. Obstet Gynecol 1987 69(1): 51–56.

13. Habek D, Cerkez Habek J, Bobic-Vukovic M, et al. Efficacy of acupuncture for the treatment of primary dysmenorrhea. Gynakol Geburtshilfliche Rundsch 2003; 43(4): 250–253.

14. Chen HM, Chen CH. Effects of acupressure at the Sanyinjiao point on primary dysmenorrhoea. J Adv Nurs 2004; 48(4): 380–387.

15. Maciocia G. Obstetrics & gynaecology in Chinese medicine. New York: Churchill Livingstone; 1998: 691–733.

16. Tsenov D. The effect of acupuncture in dysmenorrhea. Akush Ginekol (Sofiia) 1996; 35(3): 24–25.

17. Liu JX. Clinical study of the treatment of endometriosis with traditional Chinese medicine. Zhongguo Zhong Xi Yi Jie He Za Zhi 1994; 14(6): 337–339.

18. Park J, White A, Stevinson C, et al. Validating a new non-penetrating sham acupuncture device: two randomised controlled trials. Acupunct Med 2002; 20(4): 168–174.

19. Wilson ML, Murphy PA. Herbal and dietary therapies for primary and secondary dysmenorrhoea. Cochrane Database Syst Rev 2001 3: CD002124.

20. Rossignol AM, Bonnlander H. Prevalence and severity of premenstrual syndrome. Effects of food and beverages that are sweet or high in sugar content. J Reprod Med 1991; 36(2): 131–136.

21. Brush MG. Clinical uses of essential fatty acids. New York: Eden Press; 1982: 155–162.

22. Sutton CJG. The treatment of endometriosis. In Studd J, ed. Progress in obstetrics & gynaecology volume 8. Edinburgh: Churchill Livingstone; 1990: 251–272.

23. Sampalis F, Bunea R, Pelland MF, et al. Evaluation of the effects of Neptune Krill Oil on the management of premenstrual syndrome and dysmenorrhoea. Altern Med Rev 2003; 8(2): 171–179.

24. Signorello LB, Harlow BL, Cramer DW, et al. Epidemiologic determinants of endometriosis: a hospital-based case-control study. Ann Epidemiol 1997; 7(4): 267–741.

25. Cramer DW, Wilson E, Stillman RJ, et al. The relation of endometriosis to menstrual characteristics, smoking and exercise. JAMA 1986; 255(14): 1904–1908.

26. Dhillon PK, Holt VL. Recreational physical activity and endometrioma risk. Am J Epidemiol 2003: 158(2): 156–164.

27. Whitney ML. Importance of lay organisations for coping with endometriosis. J Reprod Med 1998; 43(3): 331–334.

28. Wingfield MB, Wood C, Henderson LS, et al. Treatment of endometriosis involving a self-help group positively affects patient's perception of care. J Psychosom Obstet Gynaecol 1997; 18: 255–258.

29. Ballweg ML, Deutsch S. Overcoming endometriosis. London: Arlington Books; 1998.

30. Proctor ML, Smith CA, Farquhar CM, et al. Transcutaneous electrical nerve stimulation and acupuncture for primary dysmenorrhoea. Cochrane Database Syst Rev 2002; 1: CD002123.

SECTION VII

Controversies in Endometriosis Surgery

31 The role of hysterectomy and bilateral salpingo-oophorectomy in the management of endometriosis

Ray Garry and Jason Abbott

Some years ago the senior author (R.G.) published an editorial in which he stated:

> endometriosis is an extra-uterine disease and the aim of treatment should be to remove all this extra-uterine disease while retaining all healthy pelvic tissue including the uterus and ovaries . . . the early resort to hysterectomy is to be deplored'.[1]

This opinion was developed to challenge the then common practice of undertaking hysterectomy and bilateral salpingo-oophorectomy (BSO) whenever common medications and simple surgery had failed to relieve the symptoms of endometriosis.

It remains clear that hysterectomy ± oophorectomy alone is frequently an inadequate treatment for deep invasive endometriosis (Cullen's syndrome[2]). Deposits around and in the rectum frequently progress to produce rectal bleeding and symptoms of partial or complete bowel obstruction, pelvic side-wall lesions can progress to produce ureteric obstruction and renal damage and vaginal vault lesions may cause posthysterectomy cyclical bleeding and persistent deep dyspareunia. In addition, many women continue to have persistent pelvic pain after the removal of their internal genitalia. Thus, the unthinking removal of the uterus cannot be expected to relieve all the protean manifestations of endometriosis. However, are the implications of the editorial true and does hysterectomy have no role in the management of endometriosis? This chapter will review the evidence for and against this concept.

For many women hysterectomy is not an acceptable treatment and particularly for those in whom fertility is a major concern it is clearly an inappropriate approach. This review is directed to those women in whom pelvic pain is the major symptom concern.

To determine the need for hysterectomy in the management of endometriosis the following questions appear pertinent:

1. Does the uterus contribute to the symptoms of endometriosis and does its removal relieve these symptoms?
2. Is the uterus implicated in the causation of endometriotic lesions?
3. Is the uterus involved secondarily by endometrial invasion?
4. What is the role of the ovaries in the production of symptoms and maintenance of endometriotic deposits?

What is the role of the uterus in symptom production?

Redwine was one of the first to point out that endometriosis appears to be associated with several types of pain with a variety of different features.[3] He identified four discrete types of pain:

- dysmenorrhea
- nonmenstrual pelvic pain
- dyspareunia
- dyschezia and bowel dysfunction.

He also demonstrated that careful laparoscopic excision of all extrauterine endometriotic lesions produced prolonged relief of each of these pain elements in many patients. If laparoscopic excision is so effective, what is the role of hysterectomy?

Perhaps the most effective way to establish the role of the uterus in producing the symptoms of endometriosis is to determine the effectiveness of hysterectomy in relieving these symptoms. We have confirmed Redwine's observations that laparoscopic excision can effectively relieve the symptoms associated with endometriosis in the majority of patients, both in a large, long-term prospective study[4] and in a subsequent smaller randomized placebo-controlled trial.[5] In the prospective study, 135 women were followed up for between 2 and 5 years after extensive laparoscopic excision. This approach produced significant reductions in every aspect of pelvic pain and also improved all aspects of the patients health-related quality of life (QoL) and sexual function, as tested by a number of validated instruments.

Redwine hypothesized that the success of this uterine-conserving surgery also indicated that the uterus was not involved in the etiology of endometriotic lesions. He reported that only 19% of patients he treated required further surgery within 5 years of the primary intervention. He took this as evidence to confirm his theory of mulleriosis, in which endometriosis is believed to arise from congenital rests in extrauterine locations.[6] The logic of this theory is that if endometriosis arises from congenital lesions, one

effective attempt at excision should be curative. Moreover, if all lesions do indeed arise outside the uterus, uterine removal should not be necessary.

It could be argued, however, that a 19% recurrence rate in the hands of one of the world's most skilled laparoscopic surgeons is, in fact, quite high for a nonrecurrent condition. Certainly, we were even less successful than this in our attempts to relieve the symptoms of endometriosis by extensive laparoscopic excision: 2–5 years after excision, 76% of our cases reported highly significant improvements, but 8% reported their symptoms were unchanged and 25% reported that they were worse than before index surgery. We calculated, using Kaplan–Meier techniques, that 36% of our group would require repeat surgery within 5 years. Of those not requiring such repeat surgery, some 22% (20/91) required hormonal treatment and 27% (25/91) needed analgesia. Although some patients required multiple interventions, it is evident that a substantial number of our patients were not completely 'cured' by our primary surgery.

The median visual analogue pain score (VAS) for dysmenorrhea was 9 out of 10 (interquartile range (IQR), 7.9). The same score 2–5 years after excisional surgery was 3.3 (IQR, 0–7). This represents a fall from very severe discomfort to levels associated with 'normal' menstruation. Patients with the uterus still in situ however, still sometimes continued to report dysmenorrhea, which in some continued to represent a significant level of discomfort. To further confuse the reader 18% (5/27) of women who had a hysterectomy at some stage during the study also continued to complain of 'dysmenorrhoea' (regular monthly exacerbations of pain indistinguishable to the pain they felt with menstruation prior to hysterectomy) more than 2 years after the hysterectomy. Table 31.1 indicates the relative effectiveness of laparoscopic excision alone compared to such excision combined with hysterectomy in a nonrandomized study.

Table 31.1 Pain scores after excision ± hysterectomy

Type of pain	Hysterectomy		Excision alone		Hysterectomy vs excision alone
	Median	(IQR)	Median	(IQR)	
Pelvic pain	0	(0–20)	34.5	(0–50)	$p < 0.006$
Dyspareunia	0	(0–29)	0	(0–50)	$p = 0.11$
Dyschezia	0	(0–60)	16	(0–57)	$p = 0.97$

IQR = interquartile range.

All patients in this study had the maximal possible amount of endometriotic tissue removed laparoscopically and some also had a hysterectomy performed as an additional procedure. The results suggest that concomitant hysterectomy and excision of endometriosis is more effective than laparoscopic excision alone in relieving the symptoms of dysmenorrhea and pelvic pain. However, hysterectomy adds nothing to the relief of dyspareunia and dyschezia, symptoms that appear to be equally effectively 'cured' by excision alone.

In a 1-year follow-up of the 1380 women entered into the eVAluate study from the authors' group,[7] patients with endometriosis were shown to have significantly greater impairment in various health-related QoL measures than women who were suffering from dysfunctional uterine bleeding (DUB). Hysterectomy, whether or not combined with additional extrauterine excision, produced a marked and highly significant mean improvement in the impaired values of SF-12 PCS and MCS (Short Form-12 Health Survey Physical Component Summary and Mental Component Summary), EQ-5D (EuroQoL), Body Image Questionnaire (BIQ), and Sexual Activity Questionnaire (SAQ) in both groups (Table 31.2).

These data indicate that hysterectomy is as effective in improving all measured aspects of the QoL of patients suffering from endometriosis as in those suffering with DUB, and often returns the values to those obtained from a group of normal women (Table 31.3).

These studies are not comparable, Table 2 is from a large multicenter trial in whom the primary intervention was hysterectomy and the follow-up was

Table 31.2 The effect of hysterectomy on the quality of life of women with endometriosis compared with those with dysfunctional uterine bleeding (DUB) (eVAluate study)

Test*		DUB		Endometriosis	
		Baseline	1 year	Baseline	1 year
SF-12 PCS	(High best)	47.2	54	42.8	52.9
SF-12 MCS	(High best)	46.2	51.4	45.5	51.5
EQ-5D VAS	(High best)	70.4	86.4	67.6	88.1
BIQ	(Low best)	8.3	3.4	8.6	4.0
SAQ Pleasure	(High best)	10.7	13.8	10.3	13.1
SAQ Discomfort	(Low best)	2.0	1.1	2.8	1.4
SAQ Habit	(High best)	0.7	1.0	0.6	1.2

*See text for explanation.

Table 31.3 Effect of laparoscopic excision on quality of life instruments in patients with endometriosis

Test*		Baseline values			2–5 years post-excision		
		Score	Range	NV	Scores	Range	NV
SF-12 PCS	(High best)	43.5	(36–51)	52.8	47.6	(38–54)	52.8
SF-12 MCS	(High best)	47.6	(35–54)	51.9	47.0	(39–55)	51.9
EQ-5D VAS	(High best)	68.8	(19)	86.3	74.9	(21)	86.3
BIQ	(Low best)	NA			NA		
SAQ Pleasure	(High best)	10	(5–12)		12	(9–16)	
SAQ Discomfort	(Low best)	3	(1.5–5)		2	(1.5–3)	
SAQ Habit	(High best)	1	(0–1)		1	(1–1)	

*See text for explanation.

only 1 year and Tables 3 and 4 are from a smaller study in whom the primary indication was laparoscopic excision of endometriosis and who had a longer follow up of 2–5 years. However, the data taken together suggest that hysterectomy with or without laparoscopic excision may still have an important role in improving endometriosis-related symptoms.

Is the uterus implicated in the causation of endometriotic lesions?

We looked carefully at the 33% (44/135) women in our series who required further surgery after primary excision. Of these, 32% (14/44) had no evidence of residual endometriosis and 10% had endometriosis of a lower stage than before surgery, whereas 32% had disease at a similar stage before and after surgery. It was noted that progression to a higher stage after treatment occurred in only 7% (3/44) of the group.[4] In contrast, in a small placebo-controlled trial of laparoscopic excision, progression to a higher stage was observed in 45% of patients in only 6 months, whereas 33% of this group remained at the same stage and the other 22% appeared to improve.[5] Thus, laparoscopic excision appears to favorably alter the natural progression of endometriosis.

These data do not give definite evidence in support of Sampson's theories of transtubal and transuterine spread of endometriosis, nor do they support the various extrauterine metaplasia theories. The relatively high symptom recurrence rate suggests that endometriotic implants have redeveloped or were not completely removed on the first occasion. It is not clear, however, if this is due to inadequate surgery with consequent persistent disease or due to genuine recurrence of 'new lesions'. Therefore, these data do not clarify whether the uterus is involved in the pathogenesis of endometriotic lesions.

There is also confusion about the etiologic link between adenomyosis and endometriosis. It is frequently stated in retrospective pathologic studies that there is no association, but some authorities, including Sampson[8] and Cullen[9] have long considered these to be strongly linked conditions. In our prospective study, 20 of the women had a hysterectomy some time after their primary excisional surgery, 9 (45%) women showed evidence of persistent or recurrent endometriosis alone, and 2 women showed evidence of both endometriosis and adenomyosis, whereas 4 (20%) women contained only adenomyosis. It is impossible to determine if the 30% of cases with classical adenomyosis found in this series suggest an etiologic association between endometriosis and adenomyosis, but it is possible that the observed adenomyosis may be the cause of some of the persistent symptoms. It is important, however, to also note that 4 (20%) of the women with recurrent symptoms sufficiently severe to justify a hysterectomy were found to have no pathology.

These observations suggest that it is important to consider the possibility of coexisting adenomyosis in patients with endometriosis. When suspected by clinical and/or suitable imaging techniques, the presence of coexisting adenomyosis may represent an indication to recommend hysterectomy in addition to excision of extrauterine endometriosis.

Is the uterus involved secondarily by endometriotic invasion?

Those who advocate that hysterectomy is seldom indicated when undertaking extensive excision of extrauterine endometriosis, even when combined with excision of areas of bowel, bladder, or ureter, presumably believe that the uterus is the only organ in the pelvis that is not invaded by aggressive endometriosis. There is abundant evidence that this view is incorrect. The authors have frequently found that attempting to find a plane of dissection between cul-de-sac nodules and the uterus is impossible, because the disease is invading the back of the uterus.

The fact that extrauterine endometriosis may invade the serosal surface of the uterus was very clearly recognized in the 1920s by both Cullen and Sampson. Figures 31.1 and 31.2 are two of Sampson's original drawings very clearly illustrating the penetration of retrocervical endometriosis simultaneously posteriorly into the rectosigmoid colon and anteriorly into the uterine musculature.

The series of colour photographs (Figures 31.3–31.7) show the external and internal features of a case where deep Cullen's syndrome invaded into the posterior aspect of the uterus. In such circumstances, we must consider if it is rational to spend much time and surgical effort removing all possible endometriosis from all parts of the pelvis except the uterus. Obviously when fertility is an issue, uterine removal is not an option, but when pain is the principal symptom and the uterus is clearly involved, it is surely reasonable to con-

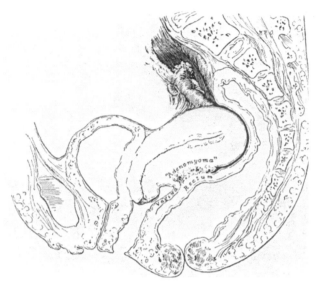

Figure 31.1 Sampson drawing of deep endometriosis invading the uterus.

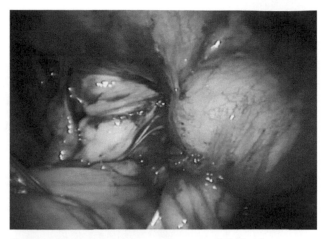

Figure 31.3 Laparoscopic appearance of Cullen's syndrome with deep endometriosis.

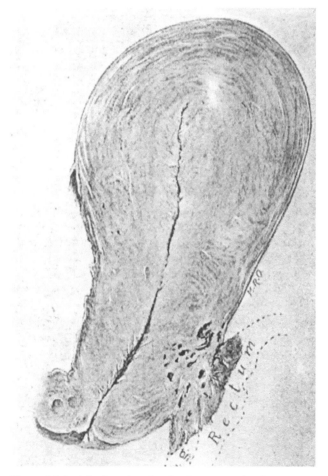

Figure 31.2 A further drawing by Sampson clearly indicating the invasion of both the uterus and the rectum by deep endometriosis.

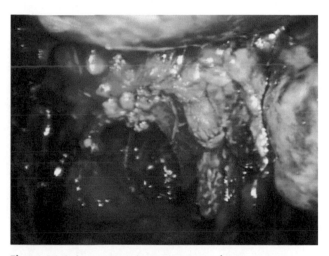

Figure 31.4 Laparoscopic appearance of same case as Figure 31.3 after initial dissection.

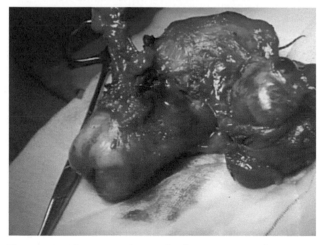

Figure 31.5 Same specimen after hysterectomy, showing cul-de-sac endometriosis still attached to the uterus.

sider adding hysterectomy to the surgical strategy. A large proportion of women do not have endometriotic invasion of the serosal surface of the uterus but preoperative efforts should be made to determine if such uterine involvement is present and, when it is anticipated, concomitant hysterectomy should be actively considered as part of the treatment program.

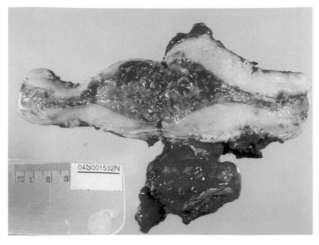

Figure 31.6 Same specimen, showing invasion of uterine wall with Cullen's endometriosis.

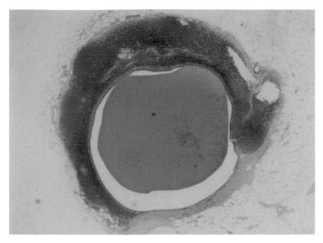

Figure 31.8 Endometriosis in a lymph node.

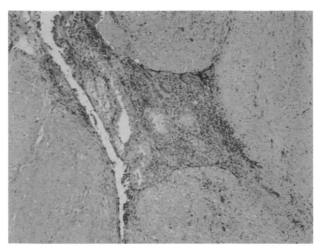

Figure 31.7 Same specimen, showing histology of Cullen's endometriosis invading the posterior uterine wall.

There are classification issues with endometriotic invasion of the serosal surface of the uterus. Is this true Cullen's syndrome type of endometriosis in which a normal uterus is invaded by an aggressive lesion from outside? If so, should the lesion be called uterine endometriosis, or adenomyoma as favored by Cullen and Sampson? Alternatively, are such lesions derived from normal eutopic endometrium and should such lesions be considered a variant of adenomyosis?

The possible relationship between endometriosis and adenomyosis may profoundly influence the gynecologist's approach to management. If endometriosis arises from congenital lesions that undergo some form of metaplasia, the uterus should be irrelevant to the management of all those except patients with obvious direct extension of the disease, as illustrated above, and hysterectomy should play little or no part in the correct management of this disease. If, however, displacement of eutopic endometrium is implicated in the cause of endometriosis, then permanently removing the endometrium may also remove the generative source of the disease. Failure to agree on the origins of endometriosis has resulted in many different and often incompatible therapeutic approaches to this disease. This etiologic confusion has led to a situation of therapeutic anarchy, with surgeons developing treatment management plans based on their individual appreciation of both the cause and possible extent of the disease.

It is well known that Sampson suggested that one method of developing endometriosis was following transtubal migration of viable endometrial tissue in a theory that has now become eponymous with this author. What is less well known is that Sampson also documented other mechanisms for the dissemination of eutopic endometrium, including vascular, lymphatic, and direct transuterine spread. Even in his definitive 1927 paper, almost 50% of the long text was devoted to discussion of vascular and lymphatic spread of endometriotic pieces through the uterus. He documented the relatively frequent occurrence of endometriosis in 'vascular-like' spaces within the uterus. Figure 31.8 illustrates endometriosis in a pelvic lymph node draining the uterus.

All body cavities that communicate with the exterior are lined with mucous membranes, and such membranes contain some of the most rapidly dividing cells in the body. All these membranes except the endometrium are lined on their deepest surface by a basement membrane whose function is to contain the growth of these rapidly dividing cells and ensure that they only proliferate outwards towards the surface of the structure. To facilitate placentation, the endometrium uniquely does not have such a basement membrane and so

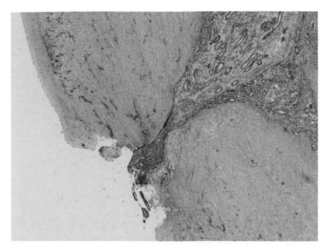

Figure 31.9 Adenomyosis penetrating the myometrium.

penetration into the underlying muscular layers is a very frequent phenomenon. Indeed, unlike other membranes, there is no sharply defined zone between endometrium and myometrium, and irregularities of the inner layer are the normal findings. When penetration of endometrium into the myometrium is excessive, adenomyosis is said to exist. Occasionally, this adenomyosis can spread aggressively through the full thickness of the uterus and erupt through the serosal surface (Figure 31.9). Once the endometrium with its rapid powers of cyclical growth enters the deeper layers of the myometrium it can, and demonstrably does, come into contact with the vascular and lymphatic drainage system of the organ. Spread of malignant endometrium via such routes is well accepted and there appears to be no good reason why benign but invasive endometrium (endometriosis) should not also spread in the same manner.

If the uterus does indeed 'seed' endometriotic implants, whether by the tubes, via direct myometrial penetration, or through lymphatic/vascular embolization, there is a case for prophylactic as well as therapeutic hysterectomy. Such an intervention would, however, be inappropriate if none of these mechanisms were relevant.

What is the role of concomitant oophorectomy?

There is no doubt that many extrauterine endometriotic lesions are estrogen-dependent. Growth of such deposits is encouraged by estrogen stimulation and impaired by estrogen lack. Removal of the ovaries as a source of estrogen production has therefore long been an accepted

adjuvant to hysterectomy in the management of severe endometriosis. Such a policy of concomitant oophorectomy has been shown to be associated with a lower risk of subsequent symptom recurrence and need for repeat, posthysterectomy surgery.

There is also a risk of malignant change occurring in endometriosis; such adverse developments are most likely to occur in ovaries that have been enlarged with endometriotic cysts The risk of this has been estimated as between 0.3% and 0.8%.[10,11] In a long-term national follow-up of 216 851 Swedish women, the risk of women with endometriosis subsequently developing ovarian cancer was found to be 1.92 (standardized incidence ratio (SIR) CI 1.3–2.8) and this risk rose to 4.2 (CI 2.0–7.7) in women with long-standing ovarian disease:[12] 80% of all such malignancies occur in the ovary.[13]

On the basis of these figures, it could be reasonably argued that prophylactic oophorectomy at the time of hysterectomy for endometriosis is prudent surgery that will reduce the risk of symptomatic endometriotic recurrence and lower the chances of subsequent ovarian cancer.

This apparently simple clinical situation is, however, complicated by the age of many of the women requiring this intervention. Almost all are premenopausal and some are still in their relatively early reproductive years. Oophorectomy in such circumstances almost always requires postoperative estrogen replacement therapy. There is abundant evidence that hormone replacement therapy (HRT) in such circumstances may cause persistence/recurrence of endometriotic symptoms. Similarly, some cases of ovarian cancer have been documented as developing in patients receiving HRT after hysterectomy and BSO for the primary treatment of endometriosis.

Oophorectomy therefore, followed by HRT, may not prevent either symptom relapse or the subsequent development of endometriotic-associated malignancy. Moreover, some authorities suggest that symptomatic relapse seldom occurs when preliminary high-quality surgical excision of all endometriotic implants has been undertaken, thereby making oophorectomy unnecessary.[3,14] The experience of the authors does not totally support this view, but these conflicting data must be carefully considered before recommending castration to young patients.

The authors have recently completed a study into the QoL after hysterectomy that casts further doubt about the benefits of simultaneous

Table 31.4 Hysterectomy for endometriosis ± oophorectomy by age			
Age	No oophorectomy	Oophorectomy	Total
Under 45 years old	31 (48%)	35 (52%)	64 (82%)
45 years old +	0	14 (100%)	14 (100%)
Total	31 (40%)	47 (60%)	78 (100%)

oophorectomy and hysterectomy. In a prospective study of 1380 women undergoing hysterectomy, 103 had this procedure performed for endometriosis, of whom 78 of these were available for analysis (Table 31.4).

In a detailed study of the whole group of 1380 women undergoing hysterectomy for a variety of benign indications, we demonstrated that all the indications produced highly significant impairment in the QoL of the women, as judged by SF-12, EQ-5D, BIQ, and SAQ instruments. We also demonstrated that hysterectomy produced large and statistically significant improvements in all these indicators.

We also investigated the effects of concomitant oophorectomy on these outcome measures. The SF-12 and EQ-5D measures were uninfluenced by oophorectomy, but the BIQ and SAQ indicated a marked reduction in the beneficial effects of hysterectomy in women under 45 years old. There was no such adverse effect on women 45 years old and older. The subgroup of women with endometriosis and under 45 years old showed a similar pattern, with impairment of benefit, which again was not found in the older women. The small sample size of this group prevented these differences reaching statistical significance, but the magnitude of the adverse effects suggests a similar clinically important difference. This study indicates that hysterectomy and oophorectomy in younger women is associated with a poorer outcome in terms of some important aspects of QoL than hysterectomy alone. In contrast, in woman over 45 years old, the benefits of concomitant oophorectomy in terms of lower risk of recurrence and possible malignant change can be obtained without obvious deleterious effects on QoL.

Summary

After decades of controversy, there remains strong evidence that the uterus is involved in the pathogenesis of at least some cases of classic endometriosis. Endometriotic implants may arise from retrograde transtubal spread, vascular and/or lymphatic spread, and direct spread from the endometrium through adenomyosis to the serosal surface of the uterus. Endometriosis may also penetrate the uterus from the external serosal surface and invade the myometrium from the 'outside'. If, and when, such etiologic factors are involved, hysterectomy will remove the source of the original and/or secondary manifestations of the disease and may contribute to the prevention of recurrent lesions. Hysterectomy may have a role in preventing disease recurrence

Dysmenorrhea in the form of menstrual-related pelvic pain is the most common and severe component of the endometriosis syndrome complex. Such pain is related to the uterus, and removal of the uterus usually (but not invariably) relieves this most important endometriosis syndrome. The uterus is also clearly sometimes also invaded by aggressive extrinsic endometriotic implants. Hysterectomy may therefore also have a role in immediate relief of endometriosis-related symptoms.

Endometriosis may be found in association with adenomyosis. It is important to diagnosis the coexistence of these two conditions before formulating a treatment plan and in some circumstances hysterectomy combined with surgical removal of extrinsic endometriosis may be required to effectively remove both symptom-producing symptoms.

Concomitant BSO at the time of hysterectomy may reduce the risk of recurrence of lesions and symptoms as well as lowering the theoretical risk of subsequent ovarian cancer. Such potential benefits are offset by an impact on sexual activity and body image when the ovaries are removed in women under 45 years old. The adverse effects on QoL should be balanced against the potential benefits of concomitant oophorectomy, particularly in younger women.

Conclusions

In conclusion, there are a number of reasons why hysterectomy ± oophorectomy should still be actively considered as part of the treatment program for patients with severe endometriosis. Like any other major surgical intervention there are, however, significant risks and potential complications that need to be weighed against this invasive surgical approach. In addition, the effect of hysterectomy on potential fertility obviously means that this approach is frequently contraindicated, even in women with very severe disease. Each patient's symptoms, disease, and needs will require individual assessment, and hysterectomy is certainly not a panacea therapy for every patient. However, some enthusiasts have suggested that hysterectomy has virtually no role in the modern management of endometriosis. The review of the evidence in this paper challenges this view. Oophorectomy also has a role but should not be seen as an inevitable accompaniment to hysterectomy in these cases. It is also important to stress that no discussion on the role of hysterectomy in the surgical management of endometriosis should deflect from the primary need to attempt to completely excise all extrauterine disease. Despite these many caveats, hysterectomy continues to be an important tool in the options available to gynecologists involved in the management of this most troublesome disease.

REFERENCES

1. Garry R. Laparoscopic excision of endometriosis: the treatment of choice? BJOG 1997; 104: 513–515.
2. Garry R. The endometriosis syndromes: a clinical classification in the presence of aetiological confusion and therapeutic anarchy. Hum Reprod 2004; 19: 760–768.
3. Redwine DB. Conservative laparoscopic excision of endometriosis by sharp dissection: life table analysis of re-operation and persistent or recurrent disease. Fertil Steril 1991; 56: 628–634.
4. Abbott JA, Hawe J, Clayton RD, et al. The effects and effectiveness of laparoscopic excision of endometriosis: a prospective study with 2–5 year follow-up. Hum Reprod 2003; 18: 1922–1927.
5. Abbott J, Hawe J, Hunter D, et al. Laparoscopic excision of endometriosis: a randomised, placebo-controlled trial. Fertil Steril 2004; 82: 878–884.
6. Redwine DB. Mulleriosis. The single best-fit model of the origin of endometriosis. J Reprod Med 1988; 33: 915–921.
7. Garry R, Fountain J, Mason S, et al. The eVALuate study: two parallel randomised trials, one comparing laparoscopic with abdominal hysterectomy, the other comparing laparoscopic with vaginal hysterectomy. BMJ 2004; 328: 129–133.
8. Sampson JA. Perforating hemorrhagic (chocolate) cysts of the ovary. Their importance and especially their relation to pelvic adenomas of endometriotic type (adenomyoma of the uterus, rectovaginal septum, sigmoid etc.). Arch Surg 1921; 3: 245–322.
9. Cullen TS. The distribution of adenomyomas containing uterine mucosa. Arch Surg 1920; 1: 215–283.
10. Corner GW, Hu C-Y, Hertig AT. Ovarian carcinoma arising in endometriosis. Am J Obstet Gynecol 1950; 59: 760–766.
11. Mostoufizadeh M, Scully RE. Malignant transformation arising in endometriosis. Clin Obstet Gynecol 1980; 23: 951–963.
12. Brinton LA, Grindley G, Pearson I, et al. Cancer risk after a hospital discharge diagnosis of endometriosis. Am J Obstet Gynecol 1997; 176: 572–579.
13. Heaps JM, Nieberg RK, Berek JS. Malignant neoplasms arising in endometriosis. Obstet Gynecol 1990; 75: 1023–1028.
14. Reich H, McGlynn F, Salvat J. Laparoscopic treatment of cul-de-sac obliteration secondary to retrocervical deep fibrotic endometriosis. J Reprod Med 1991; 36: 516–522.

32 Endometriosis after hysterectomy with and without bilateral oophorectomy

Peter J Maher

Endometriosis, since the first reported case by Von Rokitansky in 1860, is the most enigmatic disease entity in gynecology. The incidence of endometriosis varies between 1 and 10% in women during their reproductive lives. Treatment is modulated according to the woman's desire for fertility together with pain and other symptoms. Treatments range from hormone manipulation, combined with analgesic therapy, to minor and major surgical interventions. In many instances when pain is unable to be controlled or the woman has completed her family, many surgeons advocate definitive therapy in the form of hysterectomy with removal of endometriotic implants with or without bilateral oophorectomy.

Endometriosis is generally considered a disease of women of reproductive age, and implants usually atrophy at the onset of menopause, natural or surgical. The dependence on hormones by extrapelvic disease compared to pelvic endometriosis is poorly understood. In fact, it is not really known whether extrapelvic endometriosis is the same disease pathophysiologically as that which occurs in the pelvic organs. Why some women develop aggressive extrapelvic disease after removal of the reproductive organs is difficult to understand, particularly when these organs are suspected of being the source of retrograde menstruation and continued pelvic seeding of endometrial cells. The probable mechanism rests with transplantation of implants during surgery or activation of latent residual disease. It is also possible that endometriosis outside the pelvis has a totally different origin. Theories such as embryonic rest cells and metaplastic transformation,

although difficult to prove, are appealing. They may also explain why this disease behaves differently from that found in the pelvis.

The ovaries are the major source of sex steroids that affect the functional state of both the intra- and extrauterine endometrium.[1] Therefore, the possibility of an ovarian remnant should be considered as a source of endogenous hormone in a patient who has a recurrence of endometriosis and who has previously undergone hysterectomy and bilateral oophorectomy. Estrogen hypersensitivity and/or progesterone hyposensitivity may be the possible mechanisms for recurrent or persistent disease after definitive surgery.

The role of hysterectomy with or without bilateral salpingo-oophorectomy in the definitive surgical management of endometriosis is, to say the least, controversial. Traditionally, when simple surgical removal of lesions together with adjuvant hormone therapy failed to alleviate the patient's symptoms, the uterus, ovaries, and tubes were removed as 'end stage' treatment. In the 1920s, Sampson and Cullen recognized that the uterus was sometimes invaded from without by endometriosis. In a study by Garry et al,[2] women with endometriosis treated by hysterectomy had most improvement in quality of life after surgery compared with groups treated by hysterectomy for a number of different indications. This study suggests that hysterectomy may still be indicated in some women with endometriosis, although the authors comment that the case for oophorectomy, particularly in women under 45 years old, is less convincing.[3] In patients in whom conservative surgery has been performed, cumulative recurrence rates of 13% at 3 years and 40% at 5 years have been reported.[4]

The ovary

Should a bilateral oophorectomy be performed at the time of hysterectomy based on the assumption that endometriosis is an estrogen-dependent disease? Opinions are divided. Henderson and Studd reported that 45% of patients in whom ovaries were preserved at the time of hysterectomy required further surgery.[5]

Unfortunately, even removal of ovaries at the primary surgery of hysterectomy does not guarantee a disease-free status. There have been several early reports of recurrent endometriosis after total abdominal hysterectomy and bilateral salpingo-oophorectomy.[6,7]

Considerable morbidity has also been reported following removal of residual ovaries due to endometriosis recurrence.[8] In their report, Finan et al reported on 27 patients with a mean interval from index surgery to repeat surgery of 7.8 years. The most common presenting symptom in this group was pain, followed by the objective finding of a pelvic mass: 2 patients sustained an inadvertent enterotomy and 4 patients required a bowel resection. The authors suggest that, in light of readily available estrogen replacement therapy, careful consideration should be given to ovarian removal.

The incidence of symptom recurrence after hysterectomy with ovarian conservation has been reported to be as low as 1% and as high as 85% in different series.[9,10] These variable results may be due to differences in patient selection, severity of disease, or study design. Although most studies indicate the incidence of recurrent symptoms is minimal after hysterectomy with castration, the potential for estrogen replacement therapy to reactivate microscopic or residual endometriotic implants remains unclear.

Some studies suggest delaying the administration of exogenous estrogen therapy for up to 1 year after the primary surgery,[11] whereas other studies indicate that hormone replacement therapy does not stimulate recurrence of symptoms related to endometriosis.[12]

Namnoum et al reported on 138 women who underwent hysterectomy with a diagnosis of endometriosis at Johns Hopkins Hospital over a 13-year period:[13] 109 patients had concomitant oophorectomy and 29 had some ovarian preservation. In this study, patients with ovarian conservation were slightly younger, had more children, and had a lower r-AFS (revised American Fertility Society) score for endometriosis (overall, 59% had severe disease). The mean length of follow-up was 58 months. In the ovarian conservation group, 62% had recurrent symptoms and 31% underwent further surgery, whereas in the castrated group 10% had recurrent symptoms and 4% had further surgery. In this study, the relative risk (RR) for patients with ovarian conservation was 8.1 compared with oophorectomized patients, adjusting for factors such as r-AFS score, previous medical therapy, and age at operation.

The authors acknowledge that, as a referral center, most patients had been referred because of failed medical and surgical therapy previously administered and therefore there is an unavoidable bias toward women who will develop recurrent symptoms. Surgical castration, while appearing to decrease the incidence of recurrent endometriosis, incurs a significant risk of osteoporosis. Estrogen replacement therapy may ameliorate this risk but its long-term use remains questionable.

The intention to remove ovaries at the time of hysterectomy is not always realized. Anatomic distortion can make identification of the whole of the ovary difficult. Identification of the ovarian vessels above the pelvic brim, or as they near the ovary in the infundibulopelvic ligament, is necessary if the adnexum is distorted by disease and previous surgery. The combination of ovarian enlargement, together with post-surgical and endometriosis-induced adhesions, are predisposing factors to the ovarian remnant syndrome (ORS). This ORS can be associated with the recurrence of endometriosis symptoms in patients who have previously undergone total hysterectomy and bilateral salpingo-oophorectomy. Ovarian remnants have even been associated with ureteral obstruction and ovarian adenocarcinoma.[14] It has been suggested that the laparoscopic approach for removal of pelvic contents in the presence of severe ovarian, bowel, and uterine adhesions due to endometriosis may predispose to the ORS due to incomplete excisions at the time of surgery. Fragments of ovarian cortex have been left in situ.[15] Alternatively, cortex may have been dropped during laparoscopic removal and reimplanted into a new location. It has been shown in cats that small ovarian remnants under similar circumstances may implant in the peritoneal cavity and become hormonally active.[16]

Those surgeons skilled in advanced laparoscopy would enthusiastically challenge this assertion, citing the advantages of the endoscopic approach, which include magnification, clear tissue identification (even in difficult circumstances when compared to the open approach), and the use of fine surgical instruments.[17]

The diagnosis of ORS is facilitated by pelvic ultrasound and the measurement of gonadotropins and estradiol. These investigations are often omitted and the recurrence of patient symptoms attributed to disease recurrence or pelvic adhesive disease. Ovulation-inducing drugs, such as clomiphene citrate, are useful in helping to identify the presence of ovarian cortex and may facilitate its visual localization and subsequent removal. Laparoscopic techniques to remove ovaries include staples, electrosurgery, other energy forms, sutures, and endoloop application. In the author's opinion, the use of the endoloop technique increases the possibility of leaving a small remnant of ovary near the hilum due to the imprecise application of the loop suture. Some energy sources, preferably bipolar coagulation, should be used, although this is not always able to eliminate the possibility of ovarian tissue being left behind.[15]

It is important to distinguish ORS from residual ovary syndrome and accessory ovaries. Persistent or recurrent symptoms may be due to the presence of one or both ovaries left at the time of hysterectomy: this is known as residual ovary syndrome, and occurs in 1–3% of such cases.[18] 'Accessory ovaries' is a term used to describe an excess of ovarian tissue, which is attached to an otherwise normal ovary.

A third type of ovary, supernumerary, is described. It has no anatomic connection to the coexistent normally placed ovary and is thought to arise from migrating gonadocytes that contain ovarian follicle tissue during embryogenesis.

The profile for developing ORS includes a history of multiple pelvic surgeries for chronic pain often associated with endometriosis. The clinical features include cyclical pain or even constant pain that is diffuse nonradiating in nature with the presence of a pelvic swelling. Such patients are high risk, and medical treatment has been advocated without tissue diagnosis. Therapies include oral contraceptive pills, medroxyprogesterone, and danazol, but results have been mixed.[19,20]

Pelvic irradiation has been used but carries a significant risk of bowel injury due to bowel immobilization from existing adhesions. Multiple attempts at surgical excision are common and severe complications, including small bowel obstruction, inadvertent enterotomy, prolonged ileus, wound infection, and ureteral injury, may occur.[21] Ovarian ablation after pelvic radiotherapy has been studied extensively, particularly in the context of palliation of advanced breast cancer. The dose of radiotherapy required for ovarian ablation is age-related and is best considered for those women over 48 years old. A total dose of 10–20 Gy is recommended for intact ovaries, the higher dose being reserved for those with a greater bulk of ovarian tissue, i.e. the younger patient.

This treatment rationale is based on the exquisite sensitivity of ovarian germ cells to relatively low doses of radiation, with a subsequent decrease in estrogen and subsequent regression of endometriosis. Although recurrent symptomatic endometriosis is only one of the causes of ORS, some authors believe it to be the only clinical situation in which the use of local irradiation is justified.[22] This situation is adopted only after failed medical and surgical treatment. Prior to the use of irradiation, there should be conclusive proof of well-localized cycling ovarian tissue. The site should be sampled to histologically prove the presence of ovarian tissue.

Hormone replacement therapy and recurrence of endometriosis

The hormone dependence of endometriosis is well known and this is borne out by the fact that the disease is rarely diagnosed before puberty, in the postmenopausal patient, and during pregnancy. Any medication used to produce a state of hypoestrogenicity is also known to be at least temporarily successful in producing a reduction or disappearance of endometriosis deposits. It is for this reason that many physicians advise against the use of hormone replacement therapy in patients with known or treated endometriosis. Most of such advice is based on anecdotal case reports or observational studies. Until recent years, no prospective controlled studies had been performed to confirm this hitherto-held belief.

Matorras et al reported a small prospective randomized trial involving 172 patients.[23] All patients had previously undergone oophorectomy with or without extirpation of the uterus: 150 women were treated with hormone replacement therapy (sequential administration of estrogens and progesterone), and recurrence was diagnosed based on:

- histologic study
- clinical findings (pelvic pain/mass) and ultrasound findings suggestive of endometriosis.

There were 4 cases of recurrence in the HRT group. In 1 case of the recurrence, a large lesion was diagnosed at sigmoidoscopy and was located in the sigmoid colon. However, it is conceivable that this lesion was present at the time of the primary surgery and, in fact, was not a true recurrence but a dormant endometriotic lesion stimulated by the adjuvant hormone therapy.

Two different causes have been proposed for recurrence of endometriosis: first, as previously mentioned, persistence of ovarian tissue; secondly, stimulation of steroid receptors of atrophic tissue by exogenous estrogens. The recurrence rate is known to be much higher in women who undergo ovarian retention at the time of hysterectomy. On the other hand, a study of women with previous hysterectomy and bilateral salpingo-oophorectomy (for other conditions) in whom laparoscopy was later performed for investigation of pelvic pain, endometriosis was found in 34% of cases.[24]

Extrapelvic endometriosis

Pelvic endometriosis continues to be a poorly understood disease entity. Development of many conservative surgical techniques, including local excision, fulguration, and laser vaporization, have provided the long-suffering patient with variably reported relief rates. Adjuvant drug therapies have increased the success of these conservative surgical treatments in some studies. It still remains to be proven that these therapies will truly alter the course of the disease.

Many women still submit to hysterectomy with bilateral gonadectomy after years of progressive pain and failed conservative treatments. Unfortunately, extrapelvic endometriosis is even less well understood than the intrapelvic entity. It is not clear whether it is the same disease or whether it will follow a similar clinical path or can be treated in the same way as pelvic endometriosis. Extrapelvic endometriosis is defined when endometriosis is found outside the pelvic reproductive organs. Sites include the vulva, vagina, urinary tract, intestinal tract, thorax, and abdominal wall. Other sites have been reported, including the extremities and central nervous system, but, as these sites are extremely rare, they will not be further considered.

The true prevalence of pelvic endometriosis at various sites is not precisely known, as the medical literature only contains a variety of case reports, mostly small in number. The American Fertility Society (1985) revised classification is generally used by practitioners to describe the different stages of pelvic endometriosis. This r-AFS scoring system is inadequate when used for disease outside the pelvis. There are no accepted classification systems for extrapelvic disease in general use.

In an excellent review in 1989, Markham et al attempted to categorize extrapelvic endometriosis so as to standardize treatment modalities, treatment outcomes, recurrences, and histopathology.[25] Their system divides extrapelvic endometriosis into four classes:

- Class I involving the intestinal tract
- Class U involving the urinary system,
- Class L involving the lung and thoracic cage
- Class O involving other sites.

They then recommended further subdividing the degree of involvement into extrinsic and intrinsic, with further characterization by size of lesion. As previously mentioned in this chapter, there is a preponderance of anecdotal case reports and management associated with extrapelvic endometriosis, with and without oophorectomy, and therefore conclusions as to the effectiveness of medical and surgical therapies are difficult to analyze.

Endometriosis of the intestinal tract

The intestinal tract is the most common site of extrapelvic endometriosis (Figure 32.1). Symptoms of dysmenorrhea, dyspareunia, and dyschezia should sound warning bells to the gynecologist that bowel involvement is probable. Reports of incidence vary, but most agree that the rectosigmoid region is the most common, followed by the appendix and sometimes cecum. The small bowel is the site least affected. The lower bowel and its relationship to the fallopian tubes combined with the retrograde menstruation hypothesis possibly explains the higher incidence in this area. In many cases of ovarian endometrioma, there is intestinal involvement – a fact often overlooked by the attending gynecologist. In a large review of more than 1900 patients, Redwine reported that ovarian endometriosis appears to be a marker for more extensive intestinal disease when compared to patients without ovarian

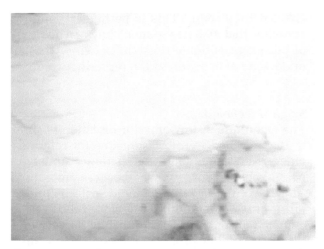

Figure 32.1 Satellite endometriosis in the upper sigmoid colon in a case of persistent rectal nodule following total hysterectomy and bilateral oophorectomy.

involvement.[26] In 482 of his patients who had ovarian endometriosis, 21.7% had complete cul-de-sac obliteration and 2% had partial obliteration. This compared with 5.8% and 1.2%, respectively, in 1303 patients without ovarian endometriosis. This finding has significant implications for those treating patients with ovarian endometriosis.

It is not uncommon for patients who are referred to a tertiary center for definitive treatment of the disease to have undergone multiple laparoscopies and even adnexectomy to relieve their symptoms. Unfortunately, to the untrained eye, cul-de-sac obliteration, partial or complete, may be missed. Even if the entity is recognized, it is essential for the attending surgeon to understand that the simple freeing up of the cul-de-sac will not suffice. There is always endometriosis tissue either attached to the posterior aspect of the vagina, cervix, or the rectum. Tissue attached to the cervix has been named by some authors as adenomyosis. It has even been suggested that rectovaginal endometriosis, aka cul-de-sac obliteration, is an extension of cervical adenomyosis, although there is still much discussion surrounding this theory.

Rectal endometriosis following oophorectomy with or without hysterectomy is probably not a true recurrence but existing disease missed at the time of the definitive surgery. This type of endometriosis is responsible for the most severe and chronic symptoms associated with this disease. Many of these lesions are also not considered active and are thought merely to represent fibrosis, but histologic evaluation reveals a significant level of active disease. These deposits are palpable at both vaginal and rectovaginal examination as

harder, irregular, tender nodules. In the case of disease infiltrating the rectum, edema and lack of mobility can be felt on rectal examination.

In a previous report analyzing rectal surgery in 169 patients, 86% of women who complained of persistent pain had undergone between 1 and 7 surgeries previously.[27] As mentioned, the most likely reason for this rather sad situation is that inadequate surgery had been performed or more likely that the disease was not recognized and therefore no attempt was made to remove it.

In cases of persistent intestinal disease, another explanation may lie in the fact that although the disease was recognized correctly, the lack of proper patient preparation with bowel preparation and lack of the surgical skills to be able to perform 'skinning' of a lesion or discoid resection inhibited appropriate treatment. In such circumstances, these patients are often given medical therapy which is ineffective, particularly in the presence of large fibrotic nodules.

In his series, Varol et al reported 75% 'cure rate' when resection of all disease was performed.[27] Correct diagnosis at laparoscopy of rectal disease with cul-de-sac obliteration requires a sponge forceps placed into the posterior vaginal fornix and the noting of a bulge under the bowel. In a normal pelvis, there is a concave space between the rectum and the uterus. In rectal endometriosis, the rectum becomes attached to the posterior aspect of the vagina and uterus and no posterior vaginal fornix can be seen despite upward movement of the sponge forceps.

Endometriotic nodularity of the bowel and the rectovaginal septum is the most difficult aspect to deal with surgically. It can, however, be managed successfully with low postoperative morbidity.

Similarly, with patients with colon involvement, aggressive surgical management with colonic resection has a high rate of symptom relief, ranging from 91% for rectal pain to 100% for rectal bleeding.[28] Again, evidence shows that failure to remove all the endometriosis, even when the uterus and ovaries are removed, may result in persistent symptoms. These symptoms disappear when all the disease is excised.[29]

A big issue affecting management of these surgically challenging conditions is that endometriosis is usually managed by the gynecologist who has little or no formal training in bowel surgery. On the other hand, the surgeon has little or no knowledge of the management of endometriosis. Close cooperation between these two specialties will give the patient the best chance of a satisfactory outcome.

More than half a century ago, Counsellor stated:

> There is no pelvic operative procedure which at some time is not required for endometriosis or made more difficult by its presence. Future surgeons require more surgical skill and judgment to secure the best way out of an unfortunate situation for the patient.[30]

The principles of treatment for rectovaginal endometriosis remain the same for patients with or without their pelvic reproductive organs. Previous hysterectomy and complete oophorectomy does not necessarily exclude the diagnosis of active endometriosis. In a review of 1000 cases of active disease collaborated by surgery and histopathology, there were 29 patients with surgical menopause and 39 with natural menopause with active endometriosis.[31]

Urbach and colleagues reported on a retrospective review of patients undergoing intestinal resection for endometriosis. The most frequent bowel-related symptoms in this study were pelvic pain, abdominal pain, and rectal pain: 93% of patients underwent low anterior resection of the rectum and distal sigmoid; all patients who were followed up reported subjective improvement; 46% of patients were 'cured', according to the prospectively applied definition (resolution of symptoms without need for further medical or surgical therapy).[32]

It is interesting that in this paper the only variable analyzed that was associated with 'cure' was concomitant hysterectomy and bilateral salpingo-oophorectomy (odds ratio 12) and the authors stated that this association remained significant after correcting for age and the presence of gastrointestinal symptoms. The conclusion drawn by the authors was that total hysterectomy with bilateral salpingo-oophorectomy correlated with improved outcome, a conclusion similar to that drawn by Garry and co-workers.[2] Although this presentation dealt with the small incidence of recurrent endometriosis after pelvic clearance, this and other papers cited provide the gynecologist with the evidence that the best outcome of treatment for severe endometriosis must include removal of the reproductive organs. Although it has been stated that gastrointestinal lesions rarely require surgical intervention, except to exclude malignancy, it is practically very difficult in cases of severe cul-de-sac disease to remove the uterus and appendages and leave the rectum and rectosigmoid that are macroscopically obviously affected by disease. This is particularly relevant, knowing that there is a small but real incidence of persistent endometriosis in patients who have undergone extirpation of the reproductive organs.

Surgical technique

The technique of low anterior resection is similar to that adopted by most surgeons for removal of other rectal pathology. All patients undergoing possible bowel surgery, whether resection or even 'shaving of the rectal or sigmoid surface', undergo full bowel preparation. Only clear fluids are recommended for the 24 hours before surgery and a readily available product, Picoprep® is taken in three doses, two on the day before surgery and one on the morning of the planned event. Antibiotics are not administered until the time of induction of anesthesia. As most patients undergo operative laparoscopy to hopefully treat the disease using minimal access surgery, much of the preliminary dissection is performed in this manner. We have performed more than 50 bowel resections for endometriosis but only 10 have been performed using a total laparoscopic technique.[33]

The decision to abandon total rectosigmoid resection laparoscopically was based purely on the time in the operating theater. In our experience, the procedure was overly lengthy and the postoperative benefits were minimal in terms of patient discharge from hospital and return to normal duties. We have continued to perform much of the mobilization of the sigmoid colon laparoscopically before performing minilaparotomy to complete the anterior resection. When the sigmoid is mobilized, the length of the proximal portion was considered appropriate if it could reach down to the level of the pubic symphysis. If this was achievable, we believe that anastomosis could be performed with minimal amount of tension on the anastomotic site. The presacral space was entered, usually from the right side, and the sigmoid mobilized through to the left side, always paying particular attention to the inferior mesenteric vessels as they become the superior rectal vessels and the left ureter. The main difficulty in dissection encountered in most cases was appropriate definition of the rectovaginal septum in the vicinity of the rectovaginal mass.

In earlier cases, we used a gasless laparoscopic approach that allowed the gynecologist to open the rectovaginal space from a vaginal incision.[34] This shortened the operative time, as normal tissue planes were encountered in the lower portion of the rectovaginal space which were free of disease. The aim of this approach was to ensure that the nodule was mobilized off the vagina and left on the rectal wall. The decision to perform a low anterior resection was often only made at this time of the operation. The advantage of digital examination at the time of gasless laparoscopy was important in the final decision-making as to whether to proceed to bowel resection. With further experience, we feel we are now able to make such decisions at the time of laparoscopy.

When we performed laparoscopic bowel resection, the rectum was divided using a laparoscopic stapling device. The rectal stump was left while a portion of the bowel was resected using another application of a stapling device. The resected portion of bowel was then laid aside for later removal or taken out through the opening in the posterior vagina. The two stumps were then reanastomosed using one of the circular stapling devices passed transanally. It was our experience that placement of the proximal portion of the stapling device was technically difficult and therefore the proximal stump was delivered through a minilaparotomy incision to facilitate precise positioning of the anvil. After we had achieved this in 10 cases, we decided that the time spent did not justify the fact that most patients stayed in hospital for 3–4 days independent of any technique used. We have since limited the total laparoscopic approach to discoid resection only. The colorectal surgeon involved in all our cases often chooses to reinforce the staple anastomosis with interrupted sutures (Figure 32.2). We do not routinely drain the anastomosis and have an aggressive postoperative regimen. We do not routinely wait for the patient to pass flatus

or have open bowels before a full ward diet is resumed. In our reported series of 169 cases, we have had one anastomotic leak following this management plan.[27]

In summary, the treatment of choice in patients with intestinal endometriosis is difficult. There is no doubt that intervention is required when malignancy is a possibility or there is an acute or subacute intestinal obstruction. It is important to remember that, even following such radical therapy, symptoms of endometriosis may persist. In a patient with extensive disease, who still has her reproductive organs, the operation of bowel resection, together with a total hysterectomy and oophorectomy, should be performed if no further childbearing is desired to ensure an optimal outcome.

Urinary tract endometriosis

The finding of endometriosis in the urinary tract organs is a far less common occurrence than that seen in the intestinal tract. Peritoneal implants in the bladder, however, are relatively frequent and easy excision can occur without damage to the muscularis during primary laparoscopy. In general, the superficial implants do not give rise to bladder symptoms and it is only the more infiltrating lesions which give rise to dysuria, frequency, and even hematuria.

The first report of urinary tract involvement was by Judd in 1921.[35] The accepted incidence of urinary tract involvement by endometriosis varies between 1% and 4% in women with pelvic endometriosis. Major morbidity has been reported associated with urinary tract endometriosis. If obstruction occurs, it has been reported to be associated with loss of a functional kidney in up to 30% of cases.[36] Women with a history of caesarean section have also been reported to be at an increased risk of bladder endometriosis in the absence of pelvic endometriosis.[37] It has been hypothesized that this disease entity supports Sampson's theory of histogenesis: endometrial cells may be seeded at the time of delivery under the vesical flap created at the time of caesarean section.[38] It has also been reported in postmenopausal women.[39]

Most urinary tract endometriosis is confined to the bladder, although the ureter has also been implicated. It may be part of the vesical disease but may also occur in relation to ovarian disease, due to its close anatomic relationship with the ureter when adhesive disease occurs on the pelvic wall.[40]

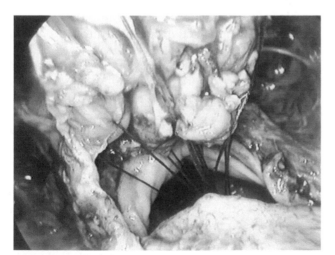

Figure 32.2 Extra sutures, placed transvaginally, to reinforce the anastomosis following the use of a circular stapler.

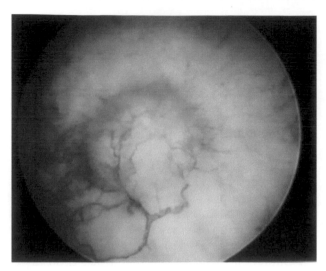

Figure 32.3 Cystoscopic view of near-full-thickness bladder endometriosis.

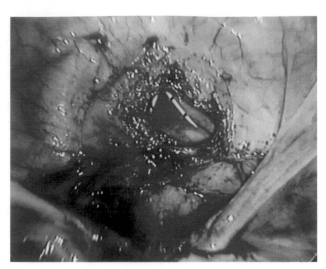

Figure 32.4 Laparoscopic view of resected bladder showing ureteric catheters in place.

As with endometriosis of other anatomic sites, the symptoms are often specific to the organ affected. In patients with known endometriosis, symptoms of dysuria, frequency, suprapubic pain or pressure, and back pain should alert the medical attendant that bladder involvement is a possibility.

Macroscopic hematuria is reported to be relatively uncommon in women with known bladder involvement and probably only occurs in 30% of patients so affected.[41] Endometriosis of the bladder is most commonly seen in the trigone or dorsal wall adjacent to the uterovesical junction (Figure 32.3). Full-thickness disease of the bladder muscle is common here. It possibly results from extension of severe adenomyosis or endometriosis of the anterior wall of the uterus.

Surgical treatment of bladder disease

Endoscopic management of any disease where resection is necessary followed by suturing of a defect requires the skills of an expert laparoscopic surgeon. Bladder disease can be managed by a gynecologist with such skills as long as the trigone and ureters are not involved. It is important before any excisional surgery is undertaken for ureteric catheters to be inserted. This not only identifies the ureteric orifices when the bladder is open but also clearly identifies the intramural portion of the ureter. This allows for palpation identification, thus ensuring that in the case of wide excision of an endometriotic nodule the intramural ureter will not be inadvertently damaged (Figure 32.4).

Preoperative and sometimes intraoperative cystoscopy may be an advantage to identify margins of a lesion and allow precise excision boundaries. Although many surgeons recommend a double-layer closure of the bladder, a single watertight layer of sutures will suffice. It is important to insist that the patient has an indwelling catheter for 7 days after the surgery. A radiographic cystogram should be performed at 7 days prior to removal of the catheter to ensure that there is no leak from the closed defect.

In conclusion, surgical treatment may not always be necessary. The decision to treat should be based on renal function, the severity and extent of the disease, the desire for future fertility, the age of the patient, and, of course, symptoms. There have been reports of success with medical therapy with both gonadotropin-releasing hormone (GnRH) analogues and danazol.[42,43] Again, there are no randomized prospective controlled trials to evaluate which treatment is preferable, but it has been noted that recurrence rates of endometriosis involving the bladder and the ureter are high following the cessation of such treatment.[44,45]

In the author's experience, full-thickness excision through the detrusor muscle and bladder mucosa for endometriosis has a low morbidity as long as the lesion is clear of the ureters and the trigone. If these latter structures are involved, the assistance of the urologic surgeon is always sought. In unsuspected cases of bladder involvement, intraoperative photographs are taken of the lesion and no further surgery is undertaken at that stage. Postoperatively, the patient is fully counseled concerning the need for bladder excision and subsequent postoperative catheter insertion for 7 days. She is also warned of the possibility of an anastomotic leak. Again, it is important to emphasize that if the gynecologist has any doubts about his or her ability to excise the lesion and repair the bladder properly, urologic help must be obtained.

Ureteric endometriosis

Ureteric involvement with endometriosis is one-sixth as common as bladder disease, ocurring in less than 1% of cases in pelvic endometriosis. The incidence of ureteric deformity due to endometriosis correlates with the severity of the endometriosis:[46] deposits on the peritoneum overlying or adjacent to the ureters are the most common and rarely cause distortion or obstruction. Periureteral endometriotic fibrotic reactions represent the 'extrinsic' type of lesion and are capable of causing obstruction and distortion. 'Intrinsic' lesions involving the muscularis or mucosa are much less frequent but do have a greater propensity to cause stricture and subsequent occlusion. The common site of involvement, as expected, is the distal third, usually 3–4 cm above the ureteric orifice.[47] When ureteric obstruction due to endometriosis occurs, an extrinsic lesion should be suspected. A thorough history and strong index of suspicion are required to identify the patient with symptomatic and troublesome ureteric endometriosis. Ultrasound examination may detect hydronephrosis or an intravenous pyelogram may detect the presence of a stricture. It may also have a place in excluding the diagnosis of malignancy. The radiologic features are not specific for endometriosis, and surgical exploration with biopsy will provide a definitive diagnosis.

In all cases where the ureter is involved, a urologic surgeon should be engaged to undertake appropriate surgical management.

Conclusion

Endometriosis, in all its presentations, continues to be the ultimate challenge for the gynecologist. Special surgical skills are required to ensure maximum success rates following excision of the disease. If endometriosis is to be tackled using laparoscopic techniques, the attending surgeon should be skilled in all suturing techniques. Even if open surgery is required, the techniques of bowel and bladder surgery should be familiar to the gynecologist. Resection of bowel and ureteric reimplantation remain the realms of the appropriate surgical specialists and such specialist surgeons should be involved at the earliest possible phase of management when required. Various sites of recurrence of endometriosis, such as the lung, are rarely if ever seen by the gynecologist. The small number of patients with symptoms suggestive of lung disease usually present to the appropriate medical specialist.

In summary, there still remains much to be learned about the etiology and pathophysiology of endometriosis. Despite modern medical management, together with sophisticated minimally invasive surgical therapies, endometriosis continues to be the cause of long-standing pain and subsequent misery for the affected woman. Total pelvic clearance has always been proposed as the definitive surgical treatment for this enigmatic disease – but is it?

REFERENCES

1. Metzger D, Lessey B, Soper J, et al. Hormone resistant endometriosis following total abdominal hysterectomy and bilateral salpingo-oophorectomy: correlation with histology and steroid receptor content. Obstet Gynecol 1991; 78: 946–950.

2. Garry R, Fountain J, Mason S, et al. The effects of hysterectomy, bilateral oophorectomy and benign disorders on the health related quality of life and sexual activity of women (personal communication).

3. Garry R. The effectiveness of laparoscopic excision of endometriosis. Curr Opin Obstet Gynecol 2004; 16: 299–303.

4. Redwine DB. Endometriosis persisting after castration: clinical characteristics and results of surgical management. Obstet Gynecol 1994; 83: 405–413.

5. Henderson AF, Studd JWW. The role of definitive surgery and hormone replacement therapy in the treatment of endometriosis. In: Thomas E, Rock J, eds. Modern approaches to endometriosis. London: Kluwer Academic Publishers; 1991: 275–290.

6. Djursing H, Petersen K, Weberg E. Symptomatic post menopausal endometriosis. Acta Obstet Gynecol Scand 1981; 60: 529–530.

7. Pummonen R, Klemi PJ, Nickkanen V. Post menopausal endometriosis. Eur J Obstet Gynecol Reprod Biol 1980; 11: 195–200.

8. Finan M, Kwark J, Weberg E. Surgical resection of endometriosis after prior hysterectomy. J La State Med Soc 1997; 149: 32–35.

9. Sheets JL, Symmonds RE, Banner EA. Conservative surgical management of endometriosis. Obstet Gynecol 1963; 23: 625–628.

10. Hammond CB, Rock JA, Parker RT. Conservative treatment of endometriosis: the effects of limited surgery and hormonal pseudo pregnancy. Fertil Steril 1976; 27: 756–766.

11. Malinak LR. Proceedings of the ICI Conference on Endometriosis, Cambridge 1989. Carnforth, United Kingdom: Panthenon Press; 1990.

12. Thorn MH, Studd JW. Procedures in practice, hormonal implantation. Br Med J 1980; 280: 848–850.

13. Namnoum A, Hickman T, Goodman S, et al. Incidence of symptom recurrence after hysterectomy for endometriosis. Fertil Steril 1995; 64: 898–902.

14. Fueyo J, Garces J, Soriano JC, et al. Adenocarcinoma of the ovary in the ovarian remnant syndrome. Rev Clin Esp 1990; 186: 415–416.

15. Rana N, Rotman C, Hasson H, et al. Ovarian remnant syndrome after laparoscopic hysterectomy and bilateral salpingo-oophorectomy for severe pelvic endometriosis. J Am Assoc Gynecol Laparosc 1996; 3: 423–426.

16. Shemwell RE, Weed JC. Ovarian remnant syndrome. Obstet Gynecol 1970; 36: 299–303.

17. El-Minawi A, Howard F. Operative laparoscopic treatment of ovarian remnant syndrome. J Am Assoc Gynecol Laparosc 1999; 6: 297–302.

18. Abu-Rafeh B, Vilas G, Misra M. Frequency and laparoscopic management of ovarian remnant syndrome. J Am Assoc Gynecol Laparosc 2003; 10: 33–37.

19. Steege JF. Ovarian remnant syndrome. Obstet Gynecol 1987; 70: 64–67.

20. Koch MO, Coussens D, Burnett L. The ovarian remnant syndrome and ureteral obstruction: medical management. J Urol 1994; 152: 158–160.

21. Pettit PD, Lee RA. Ovarian remnant syndrome: diagnostic dilemma and surgical challenge. Obstet Gynecol 1988; 71: 580–583.

22. Thoms W, Hughes L, Rock J. Palliation of recurrent endometriosis with radiotherapeutic ablation of ovarian remnants. Fertil Steril 1997; 68: 938–940.

23. Matorras R, Elorriaga M, Pijoan J, et al. Recurrence of endometriosis in women with bilateral adenexectomy (with or without total hysterectomy) who received hormone replacement therapy. Fertil Steril 2002; 77: 303–308.

24. Nezhat FR, Admon D, Seidman D, et al. The incidence of endometriosis in post hysterectomy women. J Am Assoc Gynecol Laparosc 1994; 1(part 2): 524–525.

25. Markham SM, Carpenter SE, Rock JA. Extrapelvic endometriosis. Obstet Gynecol Clin North Am 1989; 16: 193–219.

26. Redwine DB. Ovarian endometriosis: a marker for more extensive pelvic and intestinal disease. Fertil Steril 1999; 72: 310–315.

27. Varol N, Maher P, Healey M, et al. Rectal surgery for endometriosis – should we be aggressive? J Am Assoc Gynecol Laparosc 2003; 10: 182–189.

28. Bailey HR, Ott MT, Hastendorp P. Aggressive surgical management for the advanced colorectal endometriosis. Dis Colon Rectum 1994; 37: 747–753.

29. Redwine DB, Perez JJ. Pelvic pain syndrome: endometriosis and midline dysmenorrhoea. In: Arregui ME, Fitzgibbons RJ, Kathouda N, et al, eds. Principles of laparoscopic surgery – basic and advanced techniques. New York: Springer–Verlag; 1995: 545–558.

30. Counsellor VS. Surgical procedures involved in the treatment of endometriosis. Surg Gynecol Obstet 1949; 89: 322–328.

31. Henricksen E. Endometriosis. Am J Surg 1955; 90: 331–334.

32. Urbach DR, Reedijk M, Richard CS, et al. Bowel resection for intestinal endometriosis. Dis Colon Rectum 1998; 49: 1158–1164.

33. Maher P, Wood R. Laparoscopic large and small bowel resection – a critical analysis and review of accepted surgical practice. Presentation at Int Soc Gynec Endosc XIII Annual Meeting, Cape Town, South Africa, 2004.

34. Maher P, Wood C, Hill D. Excision of endometriosis in the pouch of Douglas by combined laparovaginal surgery using the Maher abdominal elevator. J Am Assoc Gynec Laparosc 1995; 2: 199–202.

35. Judd ES. Adenomyomata presenting as a tumour of the bladder. Surg Clin North Am 1921; 1: 1271–1273.

36. Stanley KE, Utz DC, Dockerty MB. Clinically significant endometriosis of the urinary tract. Surg Gynecol Obstet 1965; 120: 492–495.

37. Posner MP, Fowler JE, Meeks GR. Vesical endometriosis 12 years after a caesarean section. Urology 1994; 44: 285–287.

38. Jubanyik KJ, Comite F. Extrapelvic endometriosis. Obstet Gynecol Clin North Am 1997; 24: 411–440.

39. Madgar I, Ziv N, Many M, et al. Ureteral endometriosis in post menopausal women. Urology 1982; 20: 184–187.

40. Wood C, Maher P. Laparoscopic removal of a pelvic endometrioma attached to the ureter. Aust N Z J Surg 1993; 63: 735–736.

41. Sircus SL, Sant GR, Ucci AA. Bladder detrusor endometriosis mimicking interstitial cystitis. Urology 1988; 32: 339–340.

42. Rivlin ME, Krueger RP, Wiser WL. Danazol in the management of ureteral obstruction secondary to endometriosis. Fertil Steril 1985; 44: 274–276.

43. Rivlin ME, Miller JD, Krueger RP, et al. Leuprolide acetate in the management of ureteral obstruction caused by endometriosis. Obstet Gynecol 1990; 75: 532–534.

44. Nezhat CR, Nezhat FR. Laparoscopic segmental bladder

resection for endometriosis: a report of 2 cases. Obstet Gynecol 1993; 81: 882–885.

45. Lam AM, French M, Charnock FM. Bilateral ureteric obstruction due to recurrent endometriosis associated with hormone replacement therapy. Aust N Z J Obstet Gynecol 1992; 32: 83–84.

46. Maxson W. Ureteral abnormalities in women with endometriosis. Fertil Steril 1986; 46: 1159–1161.

47. Brough RJ, O'Flynn K. Recurrent pelvic endometriosis and bilateral ureteric obstruction associated with hormone replacement therapy. BMJ 1996; 312: 1221–1222.

33 Malignancy and endometriosis

Dan C Martin

Introduction

The concerns regarding endometriosis-associated malignancy include endometrioid changes in the ovary and non-ovarian tissue as well as in non-endometrioid malignancies. The risk of malignancy may increase with endometriosis, infertility, adhesions, inflammatory conditions, dysfunction of the apoptotic system, dysfunction of human embryonic stem cells, endocrine dysfunction, and immune dysfunction.

Although ovarian cancer kills more women each year than all other gynecologic malignancies combined, endometriosis-associated ovarian cancers have a better prognosis than non-associated ovarian cancers. Non-ovarian endometrioid malignancy is uncommon but may be an area of increased concern due to a theoretical need of progestins after bilateral salpingo-oophorectomy. Other malignancies such as breast cancer and non-Hodgkin's lymphoma also occur and increase the level of concern.

The term 'atypical endometriosis' has been used to describe both cellular and gross appearances of endometriosis. The use of this term may be confusing. Furthermore, both subtle and dark appearances of endometriosis are anecdotally associated with histologic atypicality as well as low-malignant potential tumor and other cancers. Biopsy of peritoneal lesions is useful for many appearances in order to rule out other pathology

Screening for cancer and endometriosis has much in common. Many of the markers for cancer are similar to the markers for endometriosis. But markers such as cancer antigen 125 (CA-125), may be better for monitoring the course of therapy for cancer and endometriosis than diagnosing these conditions.

Although laparoscopy is a mainstay in the surgical care of cystic pelvic masses and endometriosis, there is concern about the finding of unexpected malignancy. Rupture may mandate the use of chemotherapy in patients who would otherwise be treated by surgery alone. Discussion of the possibility of malignancy and reviewing the surgical options if cancer is found are needed to ascertain the patient's wishes regarding these options.

Epidemiology

The expectancy of finding ovarian cancer in association with endometriosis varies in different populations. Reports in general populations vary from 0.3% to 1.0%.[1,2] At the MD Anderson Cancer Center, 145 of 2200 epithelial ovarian carcinomas were endometrioid. The coexistence of endometriosis and endometrioid carcinoma in those 145 patients was 7.6%.[3]

Vercellini et al found endometriosis was more commonly associated with endometrioid, clear cell, and mixed cancers than with serous, mucinous, or miscellaneous cancers: 26% of endometrioid, 21% of clear cell cancers, and 22% of mixed cell cancers were associated with endometriosis, compared with 4% of serous cancers, 6% of mucinous cancers, and 6% of other cancers.[4]

Takahashi et al studied 324 women with endometriomas or ovarian tumors 5 cm or greater. Laparoscopy was used in 112 patients and laparotomy in 212 patients: at laparoscopy, 76 were endometriomas and 36 were ovarian tumors (all 36 of those were benign); at laparotomy, there were 5 endometriomas, 129 benign tumors, 8 borderline tumors, and 70 malignant tumors. The frequency of endometriosis in benign, borderline, and malignant tumors was 9.7, 12.5, and 11.4%, respectively. This was 30% in women with endometrioid adenocarcinoma.[5]

In 15 publications, the cell types of endometriosis-associated carcinomas were clear cell (39.2%), endometrioid (21.2%), serous (3.3%), and mucinous 3.0%. The incidence of clear cell cancer was higher in Japan and of endometrioid cancer lower in Japan compared with Western countries. The rate of malignancy increases with epithelial atypia.[6]

DePriest et al studied histologic material from 42 patients with endometrioid carcinoma of the ovary. The mean age of the patients was 56 years, and 57% were postmenopausal. Eleven patients (26%) had ovarian endometriosis. Eight patients were postmenopausal and, in 50%, an exact area of histological transition from benign to malignant epithelium was observed. DePriest et al concluded that ovarian endometriosis in postmenopausal women is not an innocuous lesion and should be removed surgically when detected.[7]

Borgfeld and Andolf noted an increased risk of ovarian cancer in women with a hospital discharge diagnosis of endometriosis. Women 15–29 years old discharged with an ovarian cyst or functional cyst had an increased risk of 2.2 and women who had ovarian cysts and had undergone cyst resection or oophorectomy had an increased risk of 8.8. The risk of developing ovarian cancer was inversely related to parity.[8]

Brinton et al found an increase of ovarian cancer after a hospital discharge diagnosis of endometriosis. The majority of ovarian cancers occurred among women with a long-standing history of ovarian endometriosis but without a diagnosis of infertility. In subgroups, there was an increased incidence of breast cancer, ovarian cancer, and non-Hodgkin's lymphoma. Breast and non-Hodgkin's lymphoma were more commonly associated with adenomyosis and non-ovarian endometriosis, whereas ovarian cancer was more commonly associated with ovarian endometrio-sis. Thyroid cancer was associated with adenomyosis but not with endometriosis. The ovarian cancer risk rose with increasing follow-up. Brinton et al concluded that further studies looking at both hormonal and immunologic alterations should be pursued as possible explanations for these excess risks.[9] They subsequently published results of studies showing that patients with primary infertility and endometriosis had an increased risk of cancer. The risk was particularly high for patients who never subsequently conceived.[10]

A collaborative ovarian cancer study showed risks of 0.03% in women with 3 or more term pregnancies or 4 or more years of oral contraception, as opposed to 1.6% in women with no pregnancy and no oral contraception by age 65.[11] Although there is concern that clomiphene increases this risk,[12] the risk associated with resistance to clomiphene is not necessarily a result of using clomiphene. This risk may be from pre-existent factors that were also the indication for clomiphene.

Each childbirth is generally associated with a 15–20% risk reduction for epithelial ovarian malignancy. Women who have used oral contraceptives for 5 years or longer experience about half the risk of ovarian cancer compared with never users. Breast-feeding seems to be protective, whereas ages at menarche and at menopause are less-consistent risk predictors. Tubal ligation and hysterectomy seem to reduce ovarian cancer risk by up to 80%. Although some studies found endometriosis, polycystic ovarian syndrome, and pelvic inflammatory disease to be positively related to ovarian cancer, the role of these factors is not yet established. Most recent studies observed an approximately 50% ovarian cancer risk increase among ever users of hormone replacement therapy (HRT) compared with never users, and the risk increased further with long-term use.[13,14]

Hartge et al noted that the risk varied from 0.3% for those women with 3 or more term pregnancies and 4 or more years of oral contraceptive use to 1.6% for those women with no pregnancies and no oral contraceptives by age 65. A family history of ovarian cancer could increase the risk by age 65 to 4.4% and the lifetime risk to 9.4%. At birth, the cumulative probability of a woman developing ovarian cancer before her 65th birthday is still less than 1% and the probability of ever developing it is less than 2%. By comparison, the lifetime risk is about 13% for breast cancer and about 3% for uterine cancer.[11]

Infertility patients have an increased chance of cancer compared to non-infertility patients. Ovarian malignancy was identified in 1.1% of infertility patients, age 19–37, undergoing microsurgery for tubal disease. This compared with 0.02% seen at appendectomy and/or cholecystectomy in women under 40 and 0.01% during pregnancy.[15]

Parallel to general concerns in infertility and tubal surgery are relationships to psammoma bodies, endosalpingiosis, and *Chlamydia* immunoglobulin G (IgG) titers.[16–20] The *Chlamydia* IgG titers used in this study were not specific for *Chlamydia trachomatis* but also cross-reacted with *Chlamydia pneumoniae*. Studies with titers that are more specific seem indicated, as *C. trachomatis* appears to be associated with factors that are associated with ovarian cancer and, more specifically, with low malignant potential.[21]

Chronic inflammation can result in necrosis and compensatory cell division. This may cause rapid cell division, giving rise to replication errors. A number of inflammatory conditions are associated with ovarian cancer, including asbestos, talc, pelvic inflammatory disease, and endometriosis.[22]

Autoimmune and immune problems are seen with increasing frequency. Sjögren's syndrome is 24 times that of the normal population, systemic lupus erythematosus is 20 times higher, and thyroiditis is 6 times higher. Treatment that shrinks a lesion is associated with a decrease in the elevated levels of auto-antibodies to normal and an increase of the depressed levels of apoptosis to normal. These observations suggest that progressive endometriosis may use the immune system to favor its own growth and invasion by manufacturing cytokines and growth factors and by co-opting the host environment.[22]

Immunologic changes, endometriosis, and cancer are associated with dioxin (2,3,7,8-tetrachlorodibenzo-*p*-dioxin (TCDD). Endometriosis in monkeys had a linear relationship to the exposure levels.[23] Accidental exposure in Italy was associated with an increase in Hodgkin's lymphoma, myeloid leukemia, and thyroid cancer.[24] Further studies on dioxin exposure are needed.

But the incidence of ovarian cancer in infertility patients undergoing ovarian cystectomy is very low. There were no cancers in 377 endometriomas removed at laparoscopy.[25,26] A review of a combined series of 1850 cases noted that 11 (0.6%) of these appeared to be cancer arising within an ovarian endometrioma.[27]

Survival

Heaps et al collected 205 cases of malignancy arising in endometriosis in a review of 43 references. In these studies, 79% of malignancies were ovarian and 21% were extraovarian. These were predominantly low-grade tumors confined to the site of origin. The 5-year survival rate was 77%. When looking at the 11 patients with tumor confined to the extragonadal site of origin, the 57 confined to the ovary, and the 18 who had spread throughout the peritoneal cavity, the 5-year survivals were 100%, 65%, and 10%, respectively. In this study, 14 (7%) of the patients were on estrogen therapy. Many of these tumors were well differentiated and may respond to progestin therapy.[28]

At the MD Anderson Cancer Center, the median survivals were 96 months for stage I endometrioid carcinoma, 52 months for stage II, 34 months for stage III, and 10.5 months for stage IV. Reports of coexistent endometriosis and endometrioid carcinoma in the same patient varied from 1 to 21%.[3]

Pathophysiology

Ovarian cancer is associated with chronic ovulation, endocrine abnormalities, tubal adhesive disease, and positive *C. trachomatis* IgG titers. If chronic peritoneal irritation were the initiating event, patients with increased peritoneal abnormalities could overlap those who fail to respond to ovulation induction.[18,29] The pathophysiology responsible for regression and/or progression of endometriosis may also be responsible for its transformation to endometrioid and clear cell ovarian neoplasia. This may involve alterations in the inflammatory process that have been associated with ovarian cancer.[22] There is an anecdotal relationship of endosalpingiosis with pelvic inflammatory disease, acute salpingitis, and positive *C. trachomatis* IgG titers.[18] But there can be a significant cross-reaction with *C. pneumoniae* titers. Evaluation of *C. trachomatis* IgG titers as a marker in the study of ovarian cancer will require titers that are specific.[20]

A number of inflammatory conditions are associated with ovarian cancer, including asbestos, talc, pelvic inflammatory disease, and endometriosis. Tubal ligation and hysterectomy without oophorectomy are associated with long-term reduction in the risk of ovarian cancer. This may be due to cutting off the pathway from the lower genital tract, and thus blocking environmental inflammants from reaching the pelvis.[22]

Red lesions on the surface of the peritoneum have a rich supply of subperitoneal blood vessels and lymphatics. These lesions can adhere directly to intact mesothelium.[30,31] Vascularization of endometriosis is one of the most important factors in growth and invasion of other tissue by endometriosis.[32]

Donnez and Va Langendonckt concluded that erythrocytes and their pro-oxidant byproducts may be the key to the implantation theory. Erythrocytes, apoptotic endometrial tissue, and cell debris transplanted into the peritoneal cavity have been implicated as potential inducers of oxidative stress. Excessive production of reactive oxygen species may also result from exposure to environmental toxicants and heavy metals. Erythrocytes are likely to reduce pro-oxidant and pro-inflammatory factors into the peritoneal environment. Unless they are appropriately chelated, they may play a key role in the formation of reactive oxygen species. Iron-induced oxidative stress has been implicated in pathologic processes. Macrophages, endometriotic lesions, and peritoneal cells of patients with endometriosis show typical features of iron overloaded tissue. Homeostasis and the peritoneal cavity may be disrupted in women with endometriosis. The presence of retrograde implanted erythrocytes that release pro-oxidant and pro-inflammatory factors into the peritoneal environment may be one of the key factors in the development of peritoneal endometriosis.[32]

Ness has postulated an integrated concept that the same pathophysiology that is responsible for the progression of endometriosis may be responsible for its transformation to endometrioid and clear cell ovarian neoplasia. Two biologic systems may be central to these changes. The first is aberrant inflammation and the second is the hormone balance. Aberrant inflammation may promote the growth and invasion of ectopic endometriosis. Alterations in the inflammatory process have also been associated with ovarian cancer. An excessive estrogen and lack of progesterones may enhance the aggressiveness of endometriosis and may foster malignant transformation.[22]

Cancer initiation, promotion, and progression are kept in check by multiple and redundant intracellular and extracellular controls. These may be overwhelmed by inflammatory cells using toxic oxidants, which may damage the DNA, proteins, and lipids. Chronic inflammation can result in necrosis and compensatory cell division, which may cause rapid cell division and give rise to replication errors. There is an alteration in immune response, including sites of endometriosis surrounded by inflammatory cells and bathed in cytokines. Natural killer (NK) cells have decreased cytoxicity and there is a shift in the ratios of immature and mature encased cells. Peripheral and peritoneal T cells and macrophages are increased and activated. These are associated with a complex mixture of cytokines and growth factors. B-cell function and antibody production also appear abnormal.[22]

Progesterone enhances programmed cell death (apoptosis). Apoptotic cells were found in 1% of the germinal epithelium of the ovary and estradiol-stimulated ovaries. This is compared with 14.5% of the combined estrogen and progestin and 24.9% for progestins alone.[22]

Recent molecular findings in endometriosis include the monoclonality of endometriotic cysts and loss of heterozygosity in the majority of cases associated with adenocarcinoma. Women with a long-standing history of endometriosis have an increased risk of ovarian cancer, most commonly endometrioid and clear cell adenocarcinomas. In these cases, there is a high frequency of atypia in the endometriosis, and the endometriosis and the associated ovarian carcinoma may show identical tumor suppressor gene PTEN mutations.[33] Cell regulation and apoptosis is linked with PTEN located on chromosome 10q23. PTEN is frequently mutated in diverse human cancers and in autosomal dominant cancer predisposition disorders. PTEN is used as a marker in some studies, but it can also be found in healthy tissue.[34]

Human embryonic stem (HES) cells show apparently limitless proliferative potential and differentiation capacity into all tissue types. Adult stem cells are rare cells, that maintain the tissue in which they reside. Adult stem cells have been identified in diverse tissues, including human bone marrow, breast, prostate, brain, and liver. Gargett demonstrated that human endometrium contains a small population of epithelial cells (0.22%) and stromal cells (1.25%) that exhibit stem cell behavior in vitro. These endometrial stem cells may play a role in proliferative disorders of human endometrium, such as endometriosis, adenomyosis, endometrial hyperplasia and endometrial cancer.[35]

Metalloproteinase-9 (MMP9) is critical in breaking down the intracellular matrix and allowing tumor to invade. Host inflammatory macrophages produce MMP9. A central activity of estradiol in promoting endometriosis may be that it promotes MMP expression. Estrogen also induces cyclooxygenase-2 (COX-2), which gives rise to increased concentrations of prostaglandins. Prostaglandins may be responsible for inflammatory changes. In susceptible women, endometriosis may feed upon itself by positively reinforcing the local levels of estradiol and inflammatory mediators. These, in turn, promote angiogenesis, extracellular disintegration, cell proliferation, and abnormal apoptosis, which may enhance the ability of endometriosis to grow and invade. By this mechanism, DNA damage at regulatory sites may initiate, and hormones and cytokines may promote formation of ovarian cancer. This appears particularly true for endometrioid and clear cell carcinomas but not so for serous tumors.[22]

Endometriosis associated ovarian carcinoma

The distinctions of endometriosis associated ovarian carcinoma (EAOC) and endometriosis-associated endometrioid adenocarcinoma (EAEA) have been applied to endometriosis-associated cancers that have a much better prognosis than non-associated ovarian carcinomas. These women are younger, present with earlier disease, and have a longer disease-free interval than those with typical endometrioid adenocarcinoma.[3,36,37] Ezren et al noted that EAOC deviates from non-EAOC in many of its key biologic characteristics. Patients with EAOC:

- have a lower-stage disease
- show a completely different distribution of histologic subtypes
- have predominantly lower grade lesions
- are void of any primary residual tumor
- have demonstrated a significantly better overall survival.[36]

In an MD Anderson Cancer Center series, 11 patients (7.6%) were found to have histologic evidence of endometriosis and endometrioid carcinoma. Grades 1 and 2 accounted for 51% of the patients. This high incidence of grade 1 and 2 histology combined with the knowledge that grades 1 and 2 had a significant improvement in medial survival accounts for the higher overall 5-year survival of 53% of their EOAC.[37]

Endometrioid carcinoma arising in endometriosis

Three criteria for determining the endometriotic origin of a malignant neoplasia were suggested by

Sampson in 1925:[38] the coexistence of benign and malignant tissue within the same organ; demonstration that the cancer is a primary tumor; and the presence of endometrial glands and stroma. A transitional phase between benign endometrium and cancer may also be a requirement.

Malignant transformation in implants of endometriosis is uncommon. When it does occur, the ovary is recognized as the most likely site of such transformation. Addison et al discussed 14 cases of primary adenocarcinoma arising in areas of endometriosis in the rectovaginal area. This is probably the second most common site of malignant transformation in foci of endometriosis.[39]

A case of endometrioid carcinoma arising from endometriosis of the sigmoid colon occurred in a patient treated with unopposed continuous estrogen injection for 20 years after bilateral salpingo-oophorectomy (BSO) because of severe endometriosis. Five similar cases were found in a review of the literature. After BSO, one should add a progestin to estrogen replacement therapy.[40]

Heaps et al reported 10 cases of malignant tumors arising in foci of gonadal and extragonadal endometriosis and discussed 195 previously reported cases. The ovary was the primary site in 165 (78.7%) of the cases, whereas extragonadal sites represented 44 (21.3%). Endometrioid adenocarcinomas accounted for 69% of the lesions, clear cell carcinomas 13.5%, sarcomas 11.6%, and rare cell types 6%. Extragonadal lesions were mostly endometrioid tumors (66%) and sarcomas (25%). Tumors arising in endometriosis were predominantly low grade and confined to the site of origin.[28]

Modesitt et al reported 25 women with ovarian cancer arising in endometriosis, 21 with an extraovarian cancer arising in endometriosis, 33 with endometriosis and ovarian cancer in the same location, and 36 with ovarian cancer and incidental endometriosis. These women were more likely to be premenopausal and to use HRT. The most common histologic types were clear cell (23%) and endometrioid (23%). The most common was stage I (31%) and medial survival was 35 months. Gravidity, grade, stage, histology, and type of chemotherapy correlated with survival.[41]

Role of estrogens and progestins

Just as endometriosis can continue to cause symptoms with no estrogen stimulation,[2,42–44] the development of endometrioid carcinoma in extraovarian sites has occurred after BSO. Four of 28 patients in McMeekin et al's study with EAEA had extraovarian involvement: 3 patients had BSO and 1 patient had paracervical endometriosis.[37]

Brooks' 1977 review demonstrated that only 12% of patients with extragonadal adenocarcinoma were on exogenous estrogen or had estrogen-secreting tumors.[45] Addison et al reported a patient who developed adenocarcinoma in an area of endometriosis in the rectovaginal area during therapy with Depo-Provera (medroxyprogesterone acetate) for 3 months. She was previously treated with Enovid (norethynodrel/mestranol) for 9 months.[39] It is noted that the description of the involvement of the 'septum' in this case may have been more appropriately described as the area of the pouch of Douglas. Most rectovaginal involvement appears to be more rectocervical than rectovaginal.[46]

When patients have incomplete resection of deep involvement, then long-term follow-up with sonography[47,48] as well as the use of progestins as part of replacement therapy appear reasonable.[40] This is similar to the use of progestin to decrease the risk of endometrial cancer.[49] However, these cancers can occur even if progestin is used.[39]

Tamoxifen is a synthetic estrogen agonist/antagonist used in adjuvant therapy as an antiestrogen for breast cancer but with paradoxical estrogenic effects in the endometrial stroma. Tamoxifen can increase the growth or contribute to the development of endometriosis and has been associated with endometrial adenocarcinoma.[50] Due to this risk, there is also concern that it may be related to endometriosis-associated carcinomas. Both the endometrium and endometriosis should be monitored in patients on tamoxifen.

Sonography may reveal tamoxifen-associated focal intracavitary changes in the endometrium that are suggestive of malignancy. These are distinguished from the pseudopolypoid glandulocystic endometrial atrophy that occurs in the myometrium. Sonographic surveillance may be more reasonable than random blind biopsy for monitoring the endometrium and myometrium.[48]

Atypical

The term atypical has been applied to both the histologic appearance of premalignant lesions and the gross appearance of endometriosis.[32,51–53] This can create confusion about whether we are talking about the cellular or the gross appearance of endometriosis. We generally speak of a Pap smear or a biopsy as being atypical rather than saying that a patient has an atypical cervix. In a similar fashion, the use of atypical endometriosis to mean endometriosis with epithelial atypicality can be confusing.[54]

Dark and subtle appearance

'Subtle' or any of the more than 20 descriptive terms in the literature may be more appropriate for the gross appearance,[32,55,56] whereas atypical epithelium may be better applied to transitional or premalignant histologic changes. This is particularly true since subtle lesions have occurred more often (65%) than those which have commonly been called 'typical' (60%).[55] If there is to be a description of 'typical' appearance, then consideration for the age of the patient will be necessary, as the 'typical' appearance varies at different ages.[57–60] Moreover, lesions as small as 180 μm have been recognized and confirmed when looking for peritoneum that did not appear normal rather than looking for a specific appearance.[55] At the other extreme, Myers et al reported 2 patients with endometriosis mimicking stage IV epithelial ovarian cancer.[61] Concepts of 'classical' or 'typical' lesions and lack of careful observation and palpation may interfere with a surgeon's ability to make a proper diagnosis or to provide adequate surgical therapy for these patients.[55]

However, subtle appearances can also be confused with endosalpingiosis, psammoma bodies, and cancer. Subtle appearances are anecdotally associated with atypical histology, low malignant potential tumor, and other cancers.[16–21,54,62] Even dark-appearing endometriosis can be associated with cancer. In one patient, dark implants were noted in association with adhesions that obscured the pelvic side wall. Dissection of the adhesions was needed to reveal a fleshy, gray-tan 1 cm nodule of cancer. Lysis of adhesions to mobilize the ovary, careful examination, and tissue sampling may be necessary to make an accurate diagnosis.[21,63,64]

Two possible high-risk appearances are clustered, clear vesicles and polypoid endometriosis. Clustered, clear vesicles can be subtle in appearance but also associated with cellular atypicality and cancer.[16] Of the 5 patients in my practice with clustered, tightly packed or stacked vesicles, 2 have had low malignant potential tumor and all 5 had endosalpingiosis and/or psammoma bodies.

Polypoid endometriosis is defined as exophytic or polypoid, tumor-like masses that project from a serosal or mucosal surface or from the lining of an endometriotic cyst. Pathologic findings showed macroscopic features, with the tumor appearing as polypoid masses on serosal surfaces or mucosal surfaces. These patients often have surgery with a differential diagnosis including low-grade müllerian neoplasia. This type of endometriosis may form large, often multiple, polypoid masses that 'not only simulate malignant tumors but may also occur after operative removal.' Polypoid endometriosis was associated with dark endometriosis or endometriotic cysts in 18 of the 24 cases.[64]

Histological atypia

Moll et al reported a case with ovarian endometriosis that showed foci of atypia and subsequent development of a large clear cell carcinoma arising in the same ovary 3 years later. In the literature, mild cytologic atypia was common (about 20%) and probably reactive in nature. However, severe atypia was found in 3.6% and was considered potentially malignant. Cellular atypia may define premalignant lesions.[6,51,65]

Cancer screening

Cancer screening is a concern in women at any risk of ovarian cancer. Techniques for screening have varying degrees of accuracy. Deciding who to screen can be difficult. About 25% of cancers develop in women under 50 years old, about 25% in those 50–60 years old and about 50% in those over 60 years old. Picking a specific age group has the risk of missing others. If one looks at familial ovarian carcinoma, the lifetime rate can be high as 7% based on family history and 60% based on screening for *BRCA*-1 gene. However, this group accounts for only about 3% of all cancer victims. A review of studies with 4000 to 22 000 women screened noted significant surgery rates, with cancer being found in 1 of 23–67 patients undergoing surgery. The risk of undergoing nonproductive surgery prompted by the use of routine screening is significant.[66–68]

Although ovarian cancer can be asymptomatic in its early stages, history can be useful.[67] This is particularly true in postmenopausal women. Bloating, fullness, and mid-abdominal distention can be early signs of ovarian cancer and require evaluation. The presence of a pelvic mass increases the chance of cancer. In women with a palpable mass, a combination of examination, tumor marker assessment, and gray-scale ultra-sound has a sensitivity of up to 100% in post-menopausal women and 99% in premenopausal women. When all three indicators are suspicious, 77% of premenopausal women and 83% of postmenopausal women have had malignant tumors.[69]

In addition to ovarian cancer screening, transvaginal sonography can also be used in the evaluation of endometrial hyperplasia and endometrial carcinoma. Sonography is capable of determining the presence of myometrial invasion and endometrial thickness.[47,48] These type of techniques are expected to be useful in monitoring rectovaginal endometriosis. Lateral wall infiltration may be more difficult to follow, as it would be further from the sonographic probe.[21]

In theory, patients with palpable rectovaginal masses which are biopsy-proven to be endometriosis and are not symptomatic can be followed by ongoing examination and vaginal sonography. If growth is noted, resection may become more important. Any growth in the rectovaginal area or rectosigmoid colon should be treated with this in mind.[21]

Cancer antigen 125

Cancer antigen 125 (CA-125) has proven itself to be one of the most useful tumor markers in cancer medicine. The major clinical utility of CA-125 is in monitoring the course of women undergoing treatment or follow-up of ovarian cancer. Other potential uses include the evaluation of the effectiveness of new antineoplastic agents in this malignancy, and in the modification of treatment strategies in individuals whose CA-125 levels fail to decline at an acceptable rate following the institution of therapy.[70]

Cancer antigen 125 for cancer screening

Although CA-125 is not a generally useful test for screening for ovarian cancer,[66–68,70] there are many studies suggesting a role for its use combined with other tests. A multiple logistic regression model was adjusted with endometrial leukocytes, serum CA-125 levels, risk factors, and confounders. The diagnostic performance of this predictive model was defined by a specificity of 95% and a sensitivity of 61%. Furthermore, the positive and negative predictive values were 91% and 75%, respectively. This predictive model represents a novel diagnostic tool to identify women with a high likelihood of suffering from endometriosis.[71]

The inverse relationship between survival and stage at diagnosis of ovarian cancer and lack of early-stage symptoms calls for a cost-effective screening strategy that will facilitate earlier detection and higher cure rates. It is noted that this condition is relatively rare and a positive result requires a surgical procedure for definitive diagnosis. Consequently, a specificity of 99.6% would still result in 10 unnecessary procedures for every case of cancer diagnosed in asymptomatic women. Symptoms include abdominal discomfort or fullness, fatigue, increased urination, and shortness of breath.[72]

Two hundred and twenty-six women underwent pelvic examination, tumor marker assessment, and transvaginal ultrasonography preoperatively. Women whose gray-scale findings were suspicious for malignancy underwent Doppler ultrasonography. Suspicious findings included masses that were fixed or irregular on pelvic examination; CA-125 level greater than 35 U/ml; elevations in serum lactic dehydrogenase, alphafetoprotein, or hCG (human chorionic gonadotropin); and the presence of a substantial solid component on gray-scale ultrasonography. If all three indicators (examination, tumor marker assessment, and gray-scale ultrasound findings) were not suspicious, 99% of premenopausal women and 100% of postmenopausal women had benign masses. If all three indicators were suspicious, 77% of premenopausal women and 83% of postmenopausal women had malignant tumors. Logistic regression identified ultrasound impression and tumor size to be significant predictors of malignancy in premenopausal women, whereas CA-125 level and ultrasound impression were significant in postmenopausal women. Neither color nor spectral Doppler was useful in this setting.[69]

Decision analysis was used to examine the no-screen compared with the screen strategy in a cohort of 40-year-old women of all races and residing in the United States. Screening for ovarian cancer with a combination of CA-125 and transvaginal sonography increases the average life expectancy in the population by less than 1 day. Given the limited effect on overall life expectancy, it is unlikely that mass screening for ovarian cancer with CA-125 and transvaginal sonography would be an effective health policy.[73]

Cancer antigen 125 for endometriosis screening and monitoring

Although CA-125 has been used for cancer screening and monitoring, other diseases, including endometriosis, can have elevated titers. Patients with endometriosis, bilateral pleural effusions, and ascites have had CA-125 titers as high as 440 U/ml.[61]

Bowel preparation for all women undergoing pelvic surgery is associated with nausea, vomiting, dehydration, hypokalemia, and cancellation of surgery. But women with severe adhesions and/or deeply infiltrating endometriosis may need another admission, anesthesia, and surgery if they are not prepared for bowel surgery. Koninckx et al detected pelvic nodularities in 4 women by routine clinical examination but in 22 women by clinical examination during menstruation in a prospective study of 61 women. CA-125 concentrations were higher during menstruation and correlated with deep endometriosis and with deep and cystic ovarian endometriosis. Nodularities at clinical examination or follicular phase CA-125 >35 U/ml were useful to decide that a bowel preparation should be used.[74] Following surgical excision of endometriosis, CA-125 can be used to monitor the completeness of surgery.[75]

Although mean preoperative CA-125 concentrations were not statistically different for women conceiving, mean postoperative CA-125 values were significantly lower for women achieving a pregnancy. Univariate analyses indicated that CA-125 values between 16–25 U/ml preoperatively and <16 U/ml postoperatively were associated with significantly higher pregnancy rates. Multivariate analyses indicated that only postoperative CA-125 concentrations were associated with pregnancy. The findings provide additional support for the clinical use of CA-125 concentrations in selected women with endometriosis. However, no specific treatment was suggested.[76]

Management

In approaching cysts, a decision needs to be made as to whether the ovary will be preserved or removed. If an ovarian cystectomy is to be performed, then preparation for spill of tumor is necessary. Although there is debate about the implications of delay in treatment following inadvertent opening of ovarian cancer,[77] several papers had shown significant ill effect when ovarian cancer was spilled at laparoscopy.[77–79] Of note, in one study, only 7.4% of stage I ovarian cancers were removed using a bag. Spill was common.

Progression was noted in 53% of patients following this type of treatment. Implantation and metastasis were microscopically visible as early as 8 days following the initial surgery.[79] Rupture may increase the stage of the patient's malignancy and mandate the use of chemotherapy in patients otherwise treated with surgery alone.[67] If the ovary is to be removed intact at laparoscopy, bagging is used. The neck or entire bag is exteriorized through a small incision prior to opening the cyst. This problem exists at both laparoscopy and laparotomy. Targarona et al reported that 1 of 11 laparoscopies (9%) and 1 of 12 laparotomies (8%) had tumor implants in the wounds.[80]

The chance that an ovarian cancer will be opened in treating endometriosis is small.[25–27] A larger concern may be identification. The French experience on the other 629 masses in Canis et al study showed that there were 12 tumors of low malignant potential and 7 ovarian cancers.[25] The chance of misidentifying endometriosis has been discussed earlier.[63] The worry is that these more common cancers would be opened in the process of taking care of what is thought to be endometriosis.

Canis et al create a pneumoperitoneum in the left hypochondrium and insert the umbilical trocar toward the left upper quadrant to avoid blind puncture of large cysts. A peritoneal fluid sample is obtained for cytology, and then the cystic ovary, pelvic peritoneum, contralateral ovary, colic gutters, diaphragm, omentum, liver, and bowel are inspected. Adnexal masses that appeared benign are punctured, taking care to minimize spillage. Small cysts (<5 cm) are aspirated with a needle connected to a 20 ml or 50 ml syringe, and large cysts with a 5 mm conical trocar and an aspiration lavage. After careful lavage, the cyst is opened with scissors and the inner wall scrutinized in search of papillary excrescences. If any signs of malignancy are found, laparotomy with a vertical midline incision is performed immediately. Functional cysts have a normal length utero-ovarian, thin cyst wall with some coral-like vessels, saffron-yellow fluid and a retina-like internal wall. In contrast, potentially neoplastic features are a lengthened utero-ovarian ligament, thick cyst wall, and numerous vessels with a comb-like aspect.[25]

Biopsy of any peritoneal component needs to be considered for histology, especially with subtle appearances.[16,19] Morcellation should be avoided. If spill is to be avoided, bagging with exteriorization of the bag prior to opening may be useful. This is accomplished with the bag placed and retrieved through a minilaparotomy, which can be extended if necessary. Allis clamps or temporary sutures can be used to maintain an air seal while the cyst is moved into the bag.[21] Since endometriosis can be transplanted into any incision, bagging may be useful with both endometriosis and malignancy.[21]

Conclusions

Endometriosis, infertility, adhesions, inflammatory conditions, dysfunction of the apoptotic system, dysfunction of hES cells, endocrine dysfunction, and immune dysfunction have been associated with malignancies that include endometrioid cancer, other ovarian cancers, breast cancer, and non-Hodgkin's lymphoma.

Women with EAOC are younger, present with earlier disease, and have a longer disease-free interval than those with typical endometrioid adenocarcinoma. These women appear to have a better prognosis than non-associated ovarian cancers.

The term 'atypical endometriosis' can be confusing and can interfere with the diagnosis of histologic atypicality, low malignant potential tumor, and other cancers. Biopsy of peritoneal lesions is needed for many appearances to rule out other pathology due to this confusion.

Estrogen hormones therapy should be accompanied by progestins, due to concerns about non-ovarian endometrioid malignancy.

There is concern about the finding of unexpected malignancy during treatment of endometriosis and adnexal masses. Discussion, planning, and concern for the possibility of malignancy may be needed with any pelvic surgery.

REFERENCES

1. Taylor PJ. The Canadian Consensus Conference on Endometriosis. J Soc Obstet Gynaecol Canada 1993; 15(3 Suppl): 1–37.

2. Molpus KL. Pathophysiology and management of endometriosis in menopause. Infertil Reprod Med Clin North Am 1995; 6: 805–828.

3. Kline RC, Wharton JT, Atkinson EN, et al. Endometrioid carcinoma of the ovary: retrospective review of 145 cases. Gynecol Oncol 1990; 39: 337–346.

4. Vercellini P, Parazzini F, Bolis G, et al. Endometriosis and ovarian cancer. Am J Obstet Gynecol 1993; 169: 181–182.

5. Takahashi K, Kurioka H, Irikoma M, et al. Benign or malignant ovarian neoplasms and ovarian endometriomas. J Am Assoc Gynecol Laparosc 2001; 8(2): 278–284.

6. Yoshikawa H, Jimbo H, Okada S, et al. Prevalence of endometriosis in ovarian cancer. Gynecol Obstet Invest 2000; 50 (Suppl 1): 11–17.

7. DePriest PD, Banks ER, Powell DE, et al. Endometrioid carcinoma of the ovary and endometriosis: the association in postmenopausal women. Gynecol Oncol 1992; 47: 71–75.

8. Borgfeld C, Andolf E. Cancer risk after hospital discharge diagnosis of benign ovarian cysts and endometriosis. Acta Obstet Gynecol Scand 2004; 83: 395–400.

9. Brinton LA, Gridley G, Persson I, et al. Cancer risk after a hospital discharge diagnosis of endometriosis. Am J Obstet Gynecol 1997; 176: 572–579.

10. Brinton LA, Lamb EJ, Moghissi KS, et al. Ovarian cancer risk associated with varying causes of infertility. Fertil Steril 2004; 82: 405–414.

11. Hartge P, Whittemore AS, Itnyre J, et al. Rates and risks of ovarian cancer in subgroups of white women in the United States. Obstet Gynecol 1994; 84(5): 760–764.

12. Whittemore AS, Harris R, Itnyre J, et al. Characteristics relating to ovarian cancer risk: collaborative analysis of 12 US case-control studies. II. Invasive epithelial ovarian cancer in white women. Collaborative Ovarian Cancer Group. Am J Epidemiol 1992; 136: 1184–1203.

13. Parazzini F, Negri E, La Vecchia C, et al. Hysterectomy, oophorectomy, and subsequent ovarian cancer risk. Obstet Gynecol 1993; 81(3): 363–366.

14. Riman T, Nilsson S, Persson I. Review of epidemiological evidence for reproductive and hormonal factors in relation to the risk of epithelial ovarian malignancies. Acta Obstet Gynecol Scand 2004; 83(9): 783–795.

15. Lais CW, Williams TJ, Gaffey TA. Prevalence of ovarian cancer found at the time of infertility microsurgery. Fertil Steril 1988; 49(3): 551–553.

16. Martin D, Khare V, Parker L. Clear and opaque vesicles: endometriosis, psammoma bodies, endosalpingiosis or cancer. In: Coutinho EM, Spinola P, de Moura LH, eds. Progress in the management of endometriosis. New York: Parthenon Publishing; 1994.

17. Wesche A, Khare VK, McCartney J, et al. Lymphoma and a serous tumor of low malignant potential in the same ovary. J Gynecol Surg 1994; 10: 189–192.

18. Khare VK, Martin DC. Anecdotal association of endosalpingiosis with *Chlamydia trachomatis* IgG titers and Fitz-Hugh–Curtis adhesions. J Am Assoc Gynecol Laparoscopists 1995; 2: 143–145.

19. Martin DC, Khare VK, Miller BE. Association of *Chlamydia trachomatis* immunoglobulin gamma titers with dystrophic peritoneal calcification, psammoma bodies, adhesions, and hydrosalpinges. Fertil Steril 1995; 63: 39–44.

20. Martin DC, Khare VK, Miller BE, et al. Association of positive *Chlamydia trachomatis* and *Chlamydia pneumoniae* immunoglobulin-gamma titers with increasing age. J Am Assoc Gynecol Laparosc 1997; 4: 583–586.

21. Martin DC. Cancer and endometriosis: do we need to be concerned? Semin Reprod Endocrinol 1997; 15: 319–324.

22. Ness RB. Endometriosis and ovarian cancer: thoughts on shared pathophysiology. Am J Obstet Gynecol 2003; 189: 280–294.

23. Rier S, Martin DC, Bowman RE, et al. Endometriosis in rhesus monkeys (*Macaca mulatta*) following chronic exposure to 2,3,7,8-tetrachlorodibenzo-*p*-dioxin. Fundam Appl Toxicol 1993; 21: 433–441.

24. Pesatori A, Consonni D, Tironi A, et al. Cancer in a young population in a dioxin-contaminated area. Int J Epidemiol 1993; 22(6): 1010–1013.

25. Canis M, Mage G, Pouly JL, et al. Laparoscopic diagnosis of adnexal cystic masses: a 12-year experience with long-term follow-up. Obstet Gynecol 1994; 83: 707–712.

26. Nezhat F, Nezhat C, Allan CJ, et al. Clinical and histologic classification of endometriomas. Implications for a mechanism of pathogenesis. J Reprod Med 1992; 37: 771–776.

27. Mostoufizadeh M, Scully RE. Malignant tumors arising in endometriosis. Clin Obstet Gynecol 1980; 23: 951–963.

28. Heaps JM, Nieberg RK, Berek JS. Malignant neoplasms arising in endometriosis. Obstet Gynecol 1990; 75: 1023–1028.

29. Rossing MA, Daling JR, Weiss NS, et al. Ovarian tumors in a cohort of infertile women. N Engl J Med 1994; 331(12): 771–776.

30. Nisolle M, Casanas-Roux F, Donnez J. Early-stage endometriosis: adhesion and growth of human menstrual endometrium in nude mice. Fertil Steril 2000; 74: 306–312.

31. Witz CA, Cho S, Centonze VE, et al. Time series analysis of transmesothelial invasion by endometrial stromal and epithelial cells using three-dimensional confocal microscopy. Fertil Steril 2003; 79(Suppl 1): 770–778.

32. Donnez J, Van Langendonckt A. Typical and subtle atypical presentations of endometriosis. Curr Opinion Obstet Gynecol 2004; 16(5): 431–437.

33. Wells M. Recent advances in endometriosis with emphasis on pathogenesis, molecular pathology, and neoplastic transformation. Int J Gynecol Pathol 2004; 230(4): 316–320.

34. Wang N, Chang J. Are aberrant transcripts of FHIT, TSG101, and PTEN/MMAC1 oncogenesis related? Int J Mol Med 1999; 3(5): 491–495.

35. Gargett C. Stem cells in gynaecology. Aust N Z J Obstet Gynaecol 2004; 44(5): 380–386.

36. Erzen M, Rakar S, Klancar B, et al. Endometriosis-associated ovarian carcinoma (EAOC): an entity distinct from other ovarian carcinomas as suggested by a nested case-control study. Gynecol Oncol 2001; 83: 100–108.

37. McMeekin DS, Burger RA, Manetta A, et al. Endometrioid adenocarcinoma of the ovary and its relationship to endometriosis. Gynecol Oncol 1995; 59: 81–86.

38. Sampson J. Endometrial carcinoma of the ovary arising in endometrial tissue of that organ. Arch Surg 1925; 10: 1–72.

39. Addison WA, Hammond CB, Parker TT. The occurrence of adenocarcinoma in endometriosis of the rectovaginal septum during progestational therapy. Gynecol Oncol 1979; 8: 193–197.

40. Duun S, Roed-Petersen K, Michelsen JW. Endometrioid carcinoma arising from endometriosis of the sigmoid colon during estrogenic treatment. Acta Obstet Gynecol Scand 1993; 72: 676–678.

41. Modesitt SC, Tortolero-Luna G, Robinson JB, et al. Ovarian and extraovarian endometriosis-associated cancer. Obstet Gynecol 2002; 100: 788–795.

42. O'Connor DT. Endometriosis. Edinburgh: Churchill Livingstone; 1987.

43. Redwine DB. Endometriosis persisting after castration: clinical characteristics and results of surgical management. Obstet Gynecol 1994; 83: 405–413.

44. Metzger DA, Lessey BA, Soper JT, et al. Hormone-resistant endometriosis following total abdominal hysterectomy and bilateral salpingo-oophorectomy: correlation with histology and steroid receptor content. Obstet Gynecol 1991; 78: 946–950.

45. Brooks JJ. Malignancy arising in extragonadal endometriosis. Cancer 1977; 40: 3065–3073.

46. Martin DC, Batt RE. Retrocervical, rectovaginal pouch, and rectovaginal septum endometriosis. J Am Assoc Gynecol Laparosc 2001; 8(1): 12–17.

47. Lerner JP, Timor-Tritsch IE, Montegudo A. Use of transvaginal sonography in the evaluation of endometrial hyperplasia and carcinoma. Obstet Gynecol Surv 1996; 51: 718–725.

48. Parsons AK, Fleischer AC, Londono JL. Sonohysterography and sonohysterosalpingography. In: Fleischer AC, Manning FA, Jeanty P, et al, eds. Sonography in obstetrics and gynecology, 6th edn. New York: McGraw-Hill; 2001.

49. Gambrell RD Jr. Combined continuous hormone replacement therapy: a critical review. Obstet Gynecol 1995; 86: 869–870.

50. Hajjar L, WooShin K, Nolan GH, et al. Intestinal and pelvic endometriosis presenting as a tumor and associated with tamoxifen therapy: report of a case. Obstet Gynecol 1993; 82: 642–644.

51. Moll UM, Chumas JC, Chalas E, et al. Ovarian carcinoma arising in atypical endometriosis. Obstet Gynecol 1990; 75: 537–539.

52. Rock JA. Endometriosis and pelvic pain. Fertil Steril 1993; 60: 950–951.

53. Bergqvist A, Melin A, Sparen P. Endometriosis and the risk of malignancy. WES E-Newsletter 2004.

54. Martin DC. Research aspects of endometriosis surgery. Ann N Y Acad Sci 2002; 955: 353–359.

55. Martin DC, Hubert GD, Vander Zwaag R, et al. Laparoscopic appearances of peritoneal endometriosis. Fertil Steril 1989; 51: 63–67.

56. American Society for Reproductive Medicine. Revised American Society for Reproductive Medicine classification of endometriosis: 1996. Fertil Steril 1997; 67: 817–821.

57. Goldstein DP, De Cholnoky C, Emans SJ. Adolescent endometriosis. J Adolesc Health Care 1980; 1: 37–41.

58. Redwine DB. Age-related evolution in color appearance of endometriosis. Fertil Steril 1987; 48: 1062–1063.

59. Koninckx PR, Meuleman C, Demeyere S, et al. Suggestive evidence that pelvic endometriosis is a progressive disease, whereas deeply infiltrating endometriosis is associated with pelvic pain. Fertil Steril 1991; 55: 759–765.

60. Davis GD, Thillet E, Lindemann J. Clinical characteristics of adolescent endometriosis. J Adolesc Health 1993; 14: 362–368.

61. Myers TJ, Arena B, Granai CO. Pelvic endometriosis mimicking advanced ovarian cancer: presentation with pleural effusion, ascites, and elevated serum CA 125 level. Am J Obstet Gynecol 1995; 173: 966–967.

62. Martin DC. Laparoscopic appearance of endometriosis. First revision. Color atlas. 2nd edn. Memphis: Resurge Press; 1991.

63. Hunt RB. Laparoscopic management of adnexal masses. Presented at Gynecologic Surgery for Clinicians, Chicago, Illinois, May 14, 1997.

64. Parker RL, Dadmanesh F, Young RH, et al. Polypoid endometriosis – a clinicopathologic analysis of 24 cases and a review of the literature. Am J Surg Pathol 2004; 28(3): 285–297.

65. Steed H, Chapman W, Laframboise S. Endometriosis-associated ovarian cancer: a clinicopathologic review. J Obstet Gynaecol Can 2004; 26(8): 709–715.

66. ACOG Committee Opinion #128: routine cancer screening. Washington: American College of Obstetricians and Gynecologists; 1993.

67. Rubin SC, Lewis JL. Surgery for cancer of the ovary. In: Nichols DH, ed. Gynecologic and obstetric surgery. St. Louis: Mosby–Year Book; 1993: 664–680.

68. Creasman WT. Ovarian cancer screening. ACOG Clin Rev 1997; 2(2): 1, 2, 14, 15.

69. Roman LD, Muderspach LI, Stein SM, et al. Pelvic examination, tumor marker level, and gray-scale and Doppler sonography in the prediction of pelvic cancer. Obstet Gynecol 1997; 89: 493–500.

70. Markman M. The role of CA-125 in the management of ovarian cancer. Oncologist 1997; 2: 6–9.

71. Gagne D, Rivard M, Pagé M, et al. Development of a nonsurgical diagnostic tool for endometriosis based on the detection of endometrial leukocyte subsets and serum CA-125 levels. Fertil Steril 2003; 80(4): 876–885.

72. Rollins G. Developments in cervical and ovarian cancer screening: implications for current practice. Ann Int Med 2000; 133: 1021–1024.

73. Schapira MM, Matchar DB, Young MJ. The effectiveness of ovarian cancer screening: a decision analysis model. Ann Int Med 1993; 118: 838–843.

74. Koninckx PR, Meuleman C, Oosterlynck D, et al. Diagnosis of deep endometriosis by clinical examination during menstruation and plasma CA-125 concentrations. Fertil Steril 1996; 65: 280–287.

75. Koninckx PR, Muyldermans M, Meuleman C, et al. CA 125 in the management of endometriosis. Eur J Obstet Gynecol Reprod Biol 1993; 49: 109–113.

76. Pittaway DE, Rondinone D, Miller KA, et al. Clinical evaluation of CA-125 concentrations as a prognostic factor for pregnancy in infertile women with surgically treated endometriosis. Fertil Steril 1995; 64: 321–324.

77. Maiman M, Seltzer V, Boyce J. Laparoscopic excision of ovarian neoplasms subsequently found to be malignant. Obstet Gynecol 1991; 77: 563–565.

78. Hsiu J, Given F, Kemp G. Tumor implantation after diagnostic laparoscopy biopsy of serous ovarian tumors of low malignant potential. Obstet Gynecol 1986; 68: 905–935.

79. Kindermann G, Maassen V, Kuhn W. Laparoscopic management of ovarian tumors subsequently diagnosed as malignant. J Pelvic Surg 1996; 2: 245–251.

80. Targarona EM, Martinezx J, Nadal A, et al. Cancer dissemination during laparoscopic surgery: tubes, gas, and cells. World J Surg 1998; 22: 55–61.

34 Complications of surgery for endometriosis

B Victor Lewis

Surgery for endometriosis is technically demanding. Minor degrees of endometriosis are best treated by laparoscopic surgery, but advanced disease is also suitable for treatment by minimal access surgery. In deep infiltrative disease the surgeon must eradicate all endometriotic deposits to prevent recurrence of the disease, but laparoscopic surgery for advanced disease should only be carried out by experienced surgeons who operate on a regular basis. However, even if laparotomy is the preferred surgical technique, the technical demands of advanced infiltrative disease still present the surgeon with potentially formidable problems.

Apart from the general complications of any operation, laparoscopic surgery has specific risks, some of which may be unavoidable. The risk of anesthesia, sepsis, and venous thrombosis are common to all surgical procedures and will not be further considered. However, strict adherence to basic principles and good technique can eliminate many potential problems and significantly reduce the risk of others. The greatest risk is during the initial insertion of the Veres needle, trocar, and cannula. Each surgeon has his own technique and it is impossible to recommend one method. However, whichever entry technique is preferred, there are basic principles which are well documented and must be strictly adhered to if risks are to be minimized. The specific structures at risk during entry to the abdomen are the inferior epigastric vessels, the whole length of the intestine, the aorta, and the common iliac and external iliac vessels. The structures at risk during laparoscopic surgery are the intestine, the bladder, the ureters, and branches of the internal iliac artery.

Prior to induction of anesthesia, informed consent is necessary and must be documented. Ideally, consent for surgery should be obtained by the surgeon performing the procedure, although it is acceptable to delegate consent to an assistant provided the assistant is himself fully cognizant of the proposed procedure and potential complications.

Bladder injuries during insertion of the Veres needle can be eliminated by preoperative catheterization. An empty bladder lies behind the symphysis pubis and cannot be injured by the Veres needle or trocar. Alternatively, women can be asked to void prior to transport to the operating theater.

The open or closed technique for laparoscopic entry

It is claimed by Hasson,[1,2] that visual insertion of the trocar and cannula eliminates the risk of bowel injury during entry and this technique is preferred by most general surgeons performing laparoscopic cholecystectomy. Open laparoscopy is a surgical procedure that utilizes a small abdominal incision to advance a blunt-tipped laparoscopy cannula into the peritoneal cavity under continuous visual control. It has never been popular amongst gynecologic surgeons, who prefer a closed technique, but may be appropriate when there is a high risk of adhesions in women who have had previous midline laparotomies. There is little evidence that the open technique is safer with regard to bowel injury, although it almost completely eliminates major vessel injury, and the overall view – expressed in the consensus document published in 1999[3] – was that there was little advantage in the Hasson technique. Other techniques of visual insertion of the laparoscope using optical trocar systems, or the Ternamian screw, which pushes the abdominal wall tissues out of the way under continual upward traction rather than divide them as the trocar is pushed down,[4] have been tried but are not widely used.

The commonest site of insertion of the Veres needle is the lower end of the umbilical scar. Suprapubic insertion of the needle may be useful in obese women, because the abdominal wall is thinner immediately above the pubic symphysis where the superficial fascia adheres to the rectus sheath. Palmer's point,[5] in the left hypochondrium below the costal margin in the midclavicular line, is almost always free of adhesions and is a safer point of entry when laparoscopic surgery is carried out on women with previous midline laparotomy incisions, provided splenomegaly can be excluded. Other than Palmer's point, the surgeon should insert the instruments strictly in the midline to eliminate the risk of damage to the inferior epigastric artery. There is no unanimity of opinion as to whether a patient should be fully supine or in the Trendelenburg position when the Veres needle is inserted. Nor is there unanimity of opinion as to whether the Veres needle should be inserted at 90° to the abdominal wall or at 45° to the horizontal with the point of the Veres needle directed into the pelvis. In modern practice it is almost universal for disposable Veres needles to be used. However, if reusable needles are preferred, the point must be sharp.

Most right-handed surgeons grasp the abdominal wall with their left hand, lifting up the abdomen, thereby increasing the distance between the front and back of the peritoneal cavity, which protects the great vessels on the posterior abdominal wall and the intestine. The surgeon should estimate the thickness of the abdominal wall and insert the Veres needle so that only 1 or 2 cm enter the abdomen. In the absence of adhesions from previous surgery, old pelvic inflammatory disease, or advanced endometriosis, adherence to the above principles almost eliminates bowel injury. Although the extent of endometriosis cannot be assessed with certainty until the laparoscope is inserted, the presence of a fixed enlarged tender mass on bimanual examination, prior to surgery, together with preliminary transvaginal ultrasound scans and possible computed tomography (CT) scans should indicate advanced disease and warn the surgeon of possible problems with entry into the abdomen.

When the point of the Veres needle enters the peritoneal cavity, the surgeon should hear an audible click as the sheath covering the point slips into place. However, a guarded needle does not protect the intestine from puncture. The reservoir of carbon dioxide gas is connected to the Veres needle and when the valve is opened the gas should flow freely at a pressure which does not exceed 10 mmHg. If the flow is low and the pressure is high, either the point of the Veres needle is in the muscle or fascia of the abdominal wall or the needle is blocked.

In most cases the surgeon will know the point of the Veres needle protrudes into the abdominal cavity because of lack of resistance, coupled with the free flow of gas, the low pressure, and the audible click when the guard over the point of the Veres needle returns to its original position. If the surgeon is uncertain if the point of the needle is in the abdominal cavity, or in a woman who has had previous abdominal surgery with the probability of bowel adhesions, a valuable supplementary test is the saline test. The surgeon injects 5–10 ml of saline through the Veres needle. If the point of the needle is in the abdominal cavity, there will be minimal resistance to flow of the saline and, because fluid dissipates among loops of small bowel, saline cannot be withdrawn. If the point of the needle is in the abdominal wall, there will be resistance to saline injection. If the point of needle is inside the intestine lumen, the surgeon will withdraw dark fluid, in which case the Veres needle should be withdrawn and the laparoscopy either abandoned or the needle should be inserted at an alternative point on the abdominal wall.

The Veres needle (Figure 34.1) must not be inserted to its full depth, especially in thin women, because this increases the risk of bowel

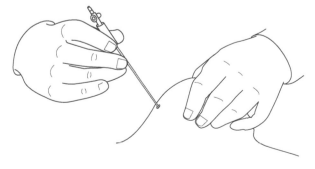

Figure 34.1 Insertion of Veres needle. Redrawn with permission from Gordon et al.[11]

perforation. In obese women with a thick abdominal wall, it is necessary to insert the Veres needle deeper, but the surgeon should always lift up the abdominal wall with his left hand. In very fat women, a long Veres needle should be used. The short 7 cm needle may not penetrate the abdominal wall, whereas a 15 cm needle has a higher success rate.

When the surgeon is confident that the point of the Veres needle lies freely in the abdominal cavity, the carbon dioxide gas should be allowed to flow. It is recommended that between 2 and 4 L of carbon dioxide gas should flow into the abdomen, depending upon the stature of the patient. During the flow of gas, the surgeon should regularly percuss the abdomen to ensure it is resonant. When the intra-abdominal pressure begins to rise, the abdomen should be symmetrically distended, producing a large bubble of carbon dioxide gas into which the trocar and cannula can be safely inserted. The bowel, being heavier than carbon dioxide, sinks to the back of the abdominal wall unless there are adhesions, and it follows that the bowel cannot be injured.

The Veres needle is withdrawn and the trocar and cannula inserted, usually at an angle of 45°, with the point directed into the pelvis. The abdominal wall causes resistance to insertion, particularly with the larger 10 mm trocars, but the resistance is less if a smaller 5 mm trocar is preferred. Pressure on the abdominal wall during insertion of the trocar causes the abdominal wall to indent, which reduces the size of the carbon dioxide gas bubble and increases the risk of the trocar perforating the bowel. It is essential therefore that the surgeon uses a technique to limit the depth of insertion, ensuring the point of the trocar only protrudes 2–3 cm into the abdominal wall. There are several techniques available to prevent unexpected deep insertion following the sudden loss of resistance, but the most common method is to use the index finger of the surgeon's right hand along the barrel of the trocar (Figure 34.2).[6,7]

The risk of indentation of the abdominal wall reducing the distance between the front and back of the abdomen can be eliminated using the technique recommended by Garry et al in which the volume of carbon dioxide gas inflated into the abdomen is increased until the intra-abdominal pressure rises to 25 mmHg. The trocar can then be safely inserted vertically into a large bubble of gas without the risk of reducing the distance between the front and back of the abdomen by pressure. When the trocar is safely in place, excess carbon dioxide should be released to prevent anesthetic and ventilation complications.

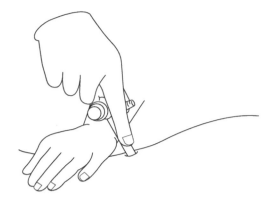

Figure 34.2 Insertion of the primary trocar and cannula.

It has been shown high intra-abdominal pressures up to 25 mmHg at the time of insertion of the trocar are associated with an increased depth of the gas bubble and an increased splinting effect of the abdominal wall. This technique has been shown to be associated with a lower risk of bowel injury.[7] If such high pressure is used it should be maintained only until the trocars are inserted, following which the pressures should be reduced to the normal working pressure of 12–15 mmHg.

Modern textbooks do not emphasize the safety precautions required to reduce the risk of intestinal and vascular injury during insertion of the Veres needle and the trocar, but the early pioneers were insistent that security steps should be undertaken. Kurt Semm,[8,9] writing in 1976, 1977, and 1984, emphasized the need for palpation of the aorta, a needle test, an aspiration test, a needle insufflation pressure test, and a sounding test during creation of the pneumoperitoneum. Semm also emphasized that the great vessels on the back of the abdominal wall may be only 1–2 cm behind the umbilicus when patients are slim.

Gasless laparoscopy

Although nearly all gynecologists create a pneumoperitoneum with a Veres needle before inserting the trocar, a small number of surgeons simply rely on manual elevation of the abdominal wall and strict attention to the depth of insertion of the trocar. The small number of surgeons using the gasless technique do not report an increase in bowel injury, which emphasizes the fundamental principles of increasing the distance between the front and back of the abdominal wall and only inserting the point of the trocar into the abdominal cavity.

Insertion of the laparoscope

Following the successful introduction of the trocar and cannula, a warmed laparoscope is inserted and the pelvis and abdomen carefully examined. It is good practice to look into the upper abdomen to exclude perihepatic adhesions often seen in old chlamydial infections. The surgeon should also ensure that, so far as possible, the bowel is free from adhesions to the abdominal wall. The head of the operating table is depressed to remove loops of small bowel from the pelvis and the pelvis examined to assess the extent of endometriosis and to stage the disease. Included in the assessment is the size of the endometrioma, the extent of bowel adhesions, and whether the bladder is adherent to the endometrioma. The surgeon then has three options:

1. to proceed to laparoscopic surgery
2. to delay laparoscopic surgery for several months until pretreatment with gonadotropin-releasing hormone (GnRH) analogues is completed
3. to abandon laparoscopy and proceed to laparotomy.

Even if the surgeon decides on laparoscopic surgery, he should always be prepared to convert to laparotomy if insuperable technical difficulties occur. It is therefore mandatory that all patients are advised of this before operating and that the appropriate consent form is signed to avoid potential medicolegal problems if a laparotomy has to performed.

Insertion of secondary ports

Laparoscopic surgery involves at least two additional ports in the right and left lower abdomen and possibly a third port in the midline. These must be inserted under direct vision to reduce the risk of injury to the external iliac and common iliac arteries. The main risk of inserting secondary trocars is injury to the inferior epigastric artery. This major vessel arises from the external iliac artery just above the inguinal ligament and runs upwards in the rectus sheath to anastomose with branches from the superior epigastric artery in the upper abdomen. Injury to the vessel results in arterial bleeding that will cause a large hematoma in the abdominal wall. Continued arterial bleeding into the abdominal cavity will lead to hypovolemic shock.

There are three methods of identifying and avoiding injury to the vessel.[6] First, in a thin woman the outline of the artery can be visualized by trans-illuminating the interior of the abdomen with the laparoscope. Secondly, the surgeon can insert the secondary trocar in the safety triangle outlined by the obliterated umbilical vessels, which can be identified through the laparoscope. However, probably the best method of avoiding injury to the inferior epigastric artery is to insert the trocar lateral to the rectus sheath with the point directed into the midline under direct vision to protect the external iliac artery.

If the epigastric artery is injured, bleeding can be arrested using a mattress suture inserted from the outside of the abdomen. However, because of the anastomotic connections to other vessels, both ends of the transected artery must be ligated. An alternative method is to remove the trocar, insert a Foley catheter through the small incision so that the balloon is inside the abdomen, inflate the balloon, and apply pressure. Finally, the bleeding can be stopped by enlarging the small incision, dissecting down to the bleeding artery, and clamping and ligating the vessel.

Precautions during lararoscopic surgery for extensive endometriosis

It is almost inevitable that loops of small bowel, sigmoid colon, and rectum are adherent to a large endometrioma and are at risk during mobilization of the endometrioma and pelvic dissection. Adequate preoperative bowel preparation is therefore important and the bowel should be emptied by enemas or suppository prior to surgery. A blunt probe inserted into the rectum through the anus helps the surgeon to identify the correct plane of cleavage. When surgery is completed, sterile water or saline infused into the pelvis enables the surgeon to identify gas bubbles indicative of bowel injury. The indications to convert to a laparotomy are poor vision and uncontrolled bleeding. Most bowel injuries are best treated at open surgery, although a skilled surgeon can repair the bowel with laparoscopic suturing, but this should not be attempted if there has been a leak of fecal material into the abdomen.

Advanced infiltrative disease is a relative indication for a laparotomy. A highly skilled surgeon, operating on a regular basis, can use minimal access surgery even in the most advanced endometriosis and this approach is acceptable so long as the general principle of total eradication of all the disease is accepted.[10,11]

Finally, the operative findings and the procedure should be recorded with either multiple still color photographs or on video. Many surgeons record their findings on CD, which acts as a permanent record.

Adhesions

Adhesions between loops of bowel and the abdominal wall cause significant technical problems during laparoscopic surgery. Adhesions obscure the surgeon's view into the pelvis and significantly increase the risk of bowel injury during blind insertion of the Veres needle, trocar, and cannula. Adhesions between the intestine and an endometrioma increase the risk of bowel injury during dissection. The commonest causes of adhesions are endometriosis itself, chronic pelvic inflammatory disease, previous abdominal surgery (especially midline incisions), inflammatory bowel disease (including Crohn's disease or diverticulitis), and abdominal tuberculosis commonly seen in developing countries but increasingly common in Western society with increased immigration.

A previous laparoscopy or low transverse incision, particularly for caesarean section, increases the risk of bowel adhesions slightly, but the main risk is with women who have had previous midline incisions, especially if they extend into the upper abdomen. The frequency of bowel adhesions leading to injury during blind insertion of the trocar and cannula has been documented by Audebert using a microlaparoscope passed through a Veres needle inserted at Palmer's point to identify adhesions in a series of 900 women.[12] In 519 patients with no previous surgical history,

the risk of severe adhesions was only 0.38%. In 140 women with a history of previous laparoscopy, the risk of severe adhesions was 0.71%. In women with a history of a low transverse Pfannenstiel incision, the risk of potential severe adhesions was 6.89%; however, in 96 women who had a previous laparotomy with a midline incision, the risk of severe adhesions was 25.31%, indicating the danger of a laparoscopy in these women (Table 34.1). This is the group of patients where a saline test is valuable and in whom Palmer's point should be considered as an alternative site of entry. Many of these women will have had previous laparoscopies, but a history of a successful laparoscopy in the past does not mean the risk is eliminated for repeat procedures.

Bowel injury

All parts of the intestine are susceptible to injury from the stomach, jejunum, ileum, cecum, ascending transverse and descending colon, sigmoid colon, and rectum. The stomach is at particular risk of perforation by the trocar if it is distended by the anesthetist or by carbon dioxide gas insufflated through a misplaced Veres needle. The transverse colon is mobile but may lie underneath the umbilicus, and again is susceptible to injury if the abdominal wall is not elevated prior to insertion of the Veres needle, or if it is distended by carbon dioxide gas from a misplaced Veres needle. Loops of bowel are frequently hidden in or behind adhesions, which should never be divided unless the surgeon can see both sides or unless the adhesion is transparent. Adhesiolysis should be performed using a minimum of two secondary ports, so that the adhesion can be grasped and put on tension before being cut.

Table 34.1 Frequency of umbilical adhesions according to previous surgical history

Patient group*	Number	Adhesions (%)	Severe adhesion with potential risk (%)
Group I	519	0.77	0.38
Group II	140	1.42	0.71
Group III	145	21.37	6.89
Group IV	96	53.12	25.31
Total	900	9.77	4.77

* Group I = no surgery; Group II = previous operative laparoscopy; Group III = previous low transverse incision; Group IV = previous midline incision.

Bowel injury recognized at surgery

Only 40–50% of bowel injuries are recognized at surgery because of fecal leakage into the peritoneal cavity, fecal contamination of the trocar point, or an offensive odor.[13] If a hole in the intestine is recognized, it can be sutured laparoscopically, providing the surgeon is experienced in laparoscopic suturing and tying knots in the abdomen. In accordance with standard surgical principles, the incision should be closed in two layers and the patient prescribed broad-spectrum antibiotics, nil by mouth for 48 hours, and a nasogastric tube inserted. If there is fecal contamination, a laparotomy should be performed and most gynecologists should seek assistance from a general surgeon.

If a laparotomy is performed, the abdominal incision should be relatively small at first and the injured loop of small bowel exteriorized and repaired in two layers. If the sigmoid colon and rectum are injured, the incision must be larger because the large intestine cannot be exteriorized. The peritoneal cavity should be washed out with large quantities of fluid and the abdomen closed with drainage. Again, the patient should be prescribed intravenous antibiotics and a nasogastric tube should be inserted to keep the upper gastrointestinal tract empty.

The main reason for a defunctioning ileostomy, or colostomy, proximal to the bowel injury, is fecal peritonitis, but such radical surgery can almost always be avoided if the intestinal injury is treated immediately before fecal peritonitis has developed.

Bowel injury not recognized at surgery

Regrettably, approximately 50% of bowel injuries are not recognized at the time of surgery. The most important symptom of possible bowel injury is postoperative pain. Even women undergoing extensive surgery for endometriosis should have minimal postoperative pain, which is easily controlled with small doses of analgesic drugs. Occasionally, women may need opium alkaloids for postoperative pain, but almost never more than a single dose. A woman who has had uncomplicated laparoscopic surgery should improve hourly. Persistent pain should always lead to review by a senior gynecologist because of the high likelihood of bowel injury and the necessity for an early laparotomy. No patient should be discharged from hospital until they are fully recovered from anesthesia, have minimal pain, and are able to walk by themselves.

Regrettably, many patients with bowel injuries are discharged from hospital but readmitted within a few hours to the Accident & Emergency Department where they may be seen by relatively junior casualty doctors, untrained in laparoscopic surgery. The possibility of a bowel injury may not be considered and patients will be wrongly diagnosed as having pain due to residual carbon dioxide gas in the abdominal cavity and treated conservatively. Carbon dioxide is absorbed rapidly and never causes pain or prolonged abdominal distention. The physical signs for the first few hours after laparoscopic bowel injury may be minimal until peritonitis occurs. Apart from pain, the physical symptoms consistent with a bowel injury are abdominal distention, local tenderness, rebound tenderness, vomiting, and diarrhea, with absent bowel sounds indicating an ileus. An offensive umbilical discharge may indicate a fistula. The patient will be 'unwell', anxious, with a tachycardia and a pyrexia. These physical signs are almost diagnostic of peritonitis caused by fecal contamination, or intra-abdominal bleeding.

Investigations include a hemoglobin and complete blood count, C-reactive protein levels together with blood urea, electrolytes, and liver function tests. An abdominal X-ray may show gas under the diaphragm from the leaking bowel and an ultrasound scan may show echoes in the abdomen or pelvis indicative of a hematoma. However, radiography and ultrasonography are less important than the physical signs.

The most senior resident gynecologist should be called to assess the patient's condition and in turn notify the consultant on call and an early general surgical opinion should be obtained. Problems arise when the gynecologist called to review the patient is not the operating surgeon. Further problems can arise if a woman is admitted as an emergency to another hospital because no operative notes will be available. However, the patient, or her relatives, should give a clear history of a recent laparoscopy and will almost certainly know the provisional diagnosis of endometriosis. The most common mistake in dealing with late bowel injuries is delay in performing a laparotomy. The patient should be given large doses of intravenous antibiotics and dehydration corrected with intravenous fluids. An early laparotomy is much safer than delay. The abdominal incision should be midline subumbilical, but may need to be extended upwards. A wide exploration of the abdominal cavity and the whole of the gastrointestinal tract should be undertaken and the injury identified. It is essential that the surgeon excludes multiple injuries, because a second small injury can be missed.

Having explored the abdominal cavity, assessed the degree of fecal contamination, and separated adherent loops of intestine, the surgeon must then decide whether to resect the bowel with end-to-end or end-to-side anastomosis, suture the hole in the intestine in two layers, or perform an ileostomy or colostomy. The decision should be made by a senior gynecologist and a surgeon, and should not be delegated to resident staff, because these women are extremely ill and are likely to have a prolonged postoperative stay with multiple late complications.

Following surgery for a laparoscopic bowel injury, women should be nursed in an intensive care unit where their electrolytes, liver function tests, and hemoglobin and white cell count can be carefully monitored. They will need intravenous fluids monitored via a jugular venous pressure line and large intravenous doses of broad-spectrum antibiotics. Many women need respiratory support with a ventilator before they can be transferred to a general ward.

Long-term sequelae of laparoscopic bowel injury

Wound sepsis and dehiscence

Following extensive peritonitis, there is a high risk of wound sepsis causing dehiscence of the abdominal scar, which necessitates a second laparotomy. In many women, the skin edges separate but the deeper tissues remain intact. The surgeon then has a choice of resuturing the abdominal wall under local or general anesthetic, but surgery should be delayed and the wound allowed to granulate if there is extensive infection. Delayed surgery may be necessary to debride the abdominal wound prior to secondary suture. Many of the women undergoing laparoscopic surgery for endometriosis are young and may need later reconstructive or cosmetic surgery to improve the ugly appearance of an abdominal scar which has become infected.

Fertility

Although dysmenorrhea and dyspareunia are the main reasons for laparoscopic surgery in endometriosis, a significant proportion of women will undergo surgery because of subfertility. If the bowel is injured and the trauma recognized and immediately repaired, it is probable that fertility will not be affected. However, if there is peritoni-

tis, a pelvic abscess is likely, which in turn causes peritubal adhesions or a pyosalpinx, leading to permanent sterility and necessitating in vitro fertilization. If long-term fertility is compromised, damages awarded by a court will be significantly higher.

Gastrointestinal symptoms

If a large segment of small bowel is resected, the patient may develop chronic diarrhea, steatorrhea, weight loss, and the malabsorption syndrome. Although malabsorption is uncommon, chronic diarrhea and attacks of colic are more frequent and should be treated symptomatically.

Adhesions

Adhesion formation is inevitable following reconstructive surgery for a bowel injury and dense adhesions almost inevitably result from fecal peritonitis. Most adhesions are silent but there is a small risk of late intestinal obstruction, the incidence being approximately 5%. Subacute intestinal obstruction necessitates admission to hospital but most cases settle with conservative treatment, including analgesic drugs and intravenous fluids. Acute intestinal obstruction is less common and necessitates urgent emergency surgery that can be technically demanding. Even opening the abdomen and manual separation of adherent loops of intestine are hazardous.

Complications of fecal peritonitis

Even fit young women become dangerously ill if the treatment of fecal peritonitis is delayed. The longer the interval between bowel injury and diagnosis, the greater the risk of death. Even those women who recover may have long-term complications, which include septic emboli in the lungs or brain; the adult respiratory distress syndrome, necessitating respiratory support; coagulation abnormalities, including disseminated intravascular coagulation; and a subphrenic abscess, necessitating drainage.

A small proportion of women will have residual multiple intraperitoneal abscesses or a pelvic abscess. The diagnosis of an abscess is made by ultrasound scans and treatment is usually carried out by interventional radiologists with drainage of the abscess under ultrasound control. However, if the abscess cannot be effectively treated by drainage, a laparotomy may be necessary.

Laparoscopic bowel injuries causing fecal peritonitis almost inevitably cause long-term chronic ill health for many years after the initial trauma. These major complications will prevent women returning to work for months or years following the laparoscopy, will disrupt home life and cause major economic hardship to the family, and may result in multiple hospital admissions over a long period of time. The earlier the diagnosis, the less serious the long-term complications.

Bowel herniation

Herniation of a loop of bowel or omentum through the primary subumbilical trocar incision, or through the site of a secondary port, is uncommon with 5 mm instruments but is more likely to occur when a 10 mm trocar and cannula are used, or larger instruments are inserted through the right and left lower abdomen. Herniation usually occurs within the first 48 hours and necessitates readmission to hospital with colic and vomiting. The pain is localized and bowel sounds will be present, which helps to distinguish a herniation of a loop of bowel from bowel injury and fecal peritonitis. An immediate laparotomy is needed.

The surgeon first releases the herniated bowel and then assesses the viability of the intestine. In most women the bowel is healthy and can simply be replaced into the abdominal cavity and the incision closed. However, if the surgeon thinks bowel viability is doubtful, because the dark color of the bowel does not recover, it is safer to resect the injured segment with an end-to-end anastomosis. Bowel herniation can almost always be avoided if the surgeon makes small secondary incisions and repairs the rectus sheath, or the external oblique aponeurosis, using a J-shaped needle upon completion of surgery.

Bowel injury during surgery to resect endometriosis

The majority of bowel injuries occur during entry, but a significant proportion of immediate and late bowel complications occur as a result of laparoscopic surgery to eradicate endometriosis. The bowel is at significant risk of injury because it is almost inevitable that a large endometrioma will be surrounded by adherent bowel and may be buried beneath the mesentery or adherent to the pelvic side wall close to the ureter, the external iliac artery, and branches of the internal iliac artery. These adhesions must be mobilized and divided before the endometriosis can be resected.[10] Preoperative enemas are essential to ensure the bowel is empty; blunt probes in the vagina and rectum will help the surgeon to identify planes of cleavage and blunt dissection or hydrodissection carries less risk of injury. Most adhesions are better cut when they are on tension from a pair of grasping forceps and the rotating scissors are helpful. No adhesion should be cut unless the surgeon can be certain a loop of bowel is not adherent.

Power sources include bipolar electrocautery, unipolar electrocautery, carbon dioxide diode or KTP laser energy, the harmonic scalpel, and helium plasma energy.

The carbon dioxide laser is a highly effective method of eradicating superficial localized deposits of endometriosis. The neodymium:YAG (Nd:YAG) laser is less commonly used but allows precise destruction of individual endometriotic foci and, unlike the carbon dioxide laser, can penetrate deeply into tissues.[7] Great care must be taken to ensure the energy source is directed accurately and always applied under direct vision. The main risk is injury to deeper tissue, including branches of the internal iliac artery and the ureter. Endometriotic deposits on the surface of the bowel or bladder can be vaporized by laser energy, but care must be taken to ensure the depth of destruction is limited to the superficial layer. Bipolar electrical energy is localized with minimal spread and is probably safer than unipolar energy, although unipolar is acceptable provided the surgeon has a clear view of the area surrounding the endometriotic deposit because of the risk of spread of energy outside the field of vision. Unipolar electrocautery close to or on the surface of the bowel carries a significant risk of delayed injury due to avascular necrosis. The spread of energy into the muscularis of the bowel may be invisible and may only present several days later with fecal peritonitis from a hole in the intestine. Electrical energy causing a burn to the bowel is more difficult to treat by resection and will probably need a defunctioning colostomy rather than simple suturing of the defect, because the surrounding tissue may be injured and heal poorly. Other less commonly used power sources include the KTP–argon lasers, or the harmonic scalpel, which cause less smoke or char.

At the completion of surgery, it is important to visualize the bowel and fill the pelvis with sterile water or saline, which will immediately identify any opening into the mucosa.

Injury to the ureter and bladder

The bladder is at risk of direct injury from the Veres needle or trocar unless it is empty prior to surgery. A woman who develops urgency or hematuria following surgery should be suspected of bladder injury and should have an early cystoscopy, an intravenous pyelogram, or a cystogram. A small injury can be treated conservatively with a Foley catheter or suprapubic drainage, but it is safer to suture a larger injury rather than to manage such trauma conservatively. The ureter is at risk when it crosses the pelvic brim and the common iliac artery into the pelvis. A large endometrioma will be adherent to the medial side of the ureter, which should always be identified at an early stage in laparoscopic surgery. The ureter can be identified by its characteristic peristaltic movement.

Some surgeons perform a preliminary cystoscopy and retrograde catheterization, leaving a ureteric catheter in place. Such a maneuver may help to identify the ureter during laparoscopy but many gynecologists find ureteric stenting unhelpful. Illuminated ureteric stents are available, the principle being that the laparoscopic surgeon can identify when he is dissecting close to the ureter because the light from the illuminated stent becomes visible.[14] However, only a minority of surgeons find these stents are helpful in reducing the risk of ureteric injury. The fundamental principle is to identify the whole length of the pelvic ureter before an endometrioma is resected. The ureter is at special risk when the endometriosis infiltrates the pelvic side wall and is active on the lateral side of the ureter. It is then technically more difficult to separate the endometrioma from the ureter. Isolated spots of endometriosis overlying the ureter, or close to the ureter, can be destroyed with great precision using a KTP or carbon dioxide laser beam, but the energy should only be applied for a short time to the surface of the ureter. If a ureteric injury is identified during laparoscopic surgery, a urologist should be consulted with immediate retrograde catheterization and ureteric stenting. This may be all that is necessary, whereas if a ureter is inadvertently severed, a laparotomy is almost inevitable with either an end-to-end anastomosis or a ureteric reimplantation into the bladder.

If a ureteric injury is unrecognized during surgery, there will be a leak of urine into the peritoneal cavity causing postoperative pain, abdominal distention, and dysuria. The intra-abdominal collection of urine can be identified by an ultrasound scan and should be recognized as urine by measuring the urea content when the collection is drained. An immediate laparotomy by a urologist is required.

Conclusion

The major complications of laparoscopic surgery most commonly occur during insertion of the trocar and cannula. These complications are almost always avoidable in a woman who has had no previous surgery or who does not have a history of pelvic inflammatory disease or chronic bowel disease.[15,16] It is essential to use a simple repeatable insertion technique, ensuring the point of the trocar only penetrates the abdominal cavity a short distance and an adequate bubble of carbon dioxide gas will provide a high degree of safety. It is unacceptable to argue that bowel injury is an inevitable complication of laparoscopic surgery in a small percentage of women and cannot be avoided because the entry technique is blind unless Hasson's method is utilized, but even an open technique does not provide full protection. The literature shows the risk of bowel injury during laparoscopic entry varies between 1 and 3 per 1000, but these figures are probably an underestimate because many complications are not reported. Few countries require notification of all laparoscopic complications, but in Finland a comprehensive report of every complication is required.[17] The Finnish Hospital Discharge Register, maintained by the National Board of Health, collect data of every inpatient in all Finnish Hospitals.[18] The incidence of bowel injury during laparoscopic entry procedures was very low, at 0.3 per 1000, but the complication rate was higher with difficult operative laparoscopies in women with severe endometriosis and adhesions; 22% of all major injuries, including vessel injuries, were entry-related and the authors emphasize 'safety guidelines should be followed during every step of laparoscopy'.

In a more recent publication from Finland, the incidence of all major complications decreased significantly between 1993 and 1998, when the figure was 1.4%.[18] These authors found ureteric injuries were the most serious but most of the operative laparoscopies were laparoscopic hysterectomies rather than for ablation of endometriosis. However, because of the large numbers of patients on the register the authors were able to identify individual complications. The incidence of bowel injury during diagnostic laparoscopy was very low, at 0.2 per 1000, but this increased during operative laparoscopy, to 1.8 per 1000. Only 21% of all the injuries were diagnosed and managed during the primary operation, which emphasizes that the diagnosis of bowel damage may be delayed.

The risk of major complications occurring during entry was chronicled by Chapron and his colleagues,[19] who reviewed 17 patients with major vascular complications, of which 76.5% occurred during entry and only 23.5% occurred during the laparoscopic surgery. The French authors confirmed that the most important risk factors in major vascular injury are the surgeon's lack of experience and lack of care in very thin or very obese women. The French Special Interest Group on Reproductive Surgery emphasized the need for graduated in-depth training in laparoscopic surgery, which should include didactic courses, lectures, videotapes, computer-generated programs, hands-on activity (including experience with pelvic trainers and/or animal models), assistance in the operating room, and supervised surgery.[20]

A note of caution is necessary when interpreting some of these multicenter studies: they usually come from centers of excellence, which are usually tertiary referral hospitals where most of the surgery is performed by experienced surgeons. It is more realistic to look at prospective studies that look at all operations performed in a single hospital by all levels of staff, including those in training: for example, the studies by Jones et al[21] looked at all laparoscopies over the course of a year at the Royal Surrey County Hospital (a district general hospital), Guildford, UK, and another study by Richardson and Sutton[22] at the Chelsea and Westminster Hospital (a teaching hospital), London, UK. All data were collected prospectively and major complications rates were much higher than in the studies quoted above. At the Chelsea and Westminster Hospital, the bowel was damaged three times in 836 laparoscopies; none of the women had previous surgery or were in the high-risk category. This is a rate in excess of 3/1000, or 10 times that reported in large multicenter studies, but the fact that the data were collected prospectively means that it is likely to be a more realistic

reflection of the actual morbidity of first entry for laparoscopy. The rate was similar at the Royal Surrey County Hospital except that 1 of the 3 cases of bowel injury had previously had a panproctocolectomy; the bowel injury was caused by an experienced bowel surgeon employing the Hassan 'open' entry technique advocated by the Royal College of Surgeons as being safer than the closed Veres needle technique usually employed by gynecologists.

Although laparoscopic bowel injuries at entry are recognized as the main cause of bowel trauma, attempts to reduce the risk with the Hassan open technique, large-diameter optical trocars, or the Ternamian endoscopic threaded imaging port, manufactured by Stortz, do not eliminate the risk.[4] The Ternamian threaded trocar is rotated under laparoscopic vision and enters the abdominal cavity by displacing fascia and muscle laterally. Theoretically, the risk of bowel injury should be reduced because the trocar is inserted under direct laparoscopic vision.

It is commonly claimed that in a small number of women there is an inevitable and unavoidable risk of bowel injury because of the blind-entry technique. However, in women without previous abdominal surgery, the risk of major bowel and vascular injury during closed insertion of the Veres needle, trocar, and cannula can almost always be avoided by stringent adherence to the basic techniques described in the early literature published by Palmer in France[5] and Kurt Semm in Germany,[8,9] and more recently by Chapron et al.[23]

In spite of the complexity of laparoscopic total excision of pelvic endometriosis, the incidence of major complications is surprisingly low, presumably because only highly experienced laparoscopic surgeons will embark upon such advanced surgery. Strict adherence to basic principles will reduce the incidence of major complications to an absolute minimum in spite of increasingly sophisticated and complex surgery.

REFERENCES

1. Hasson HM, A nodified instrument & method for laparoscopy. Am J Obstet Gynaecol 1971; 110: 886–887.

2. Hasson HM, Open laparoscopy as a method of access in laparoscopic surgery. Gynaecol Endosc 1999; 8: 353–361.

3. A consensus document concerning laparoscopic entry techniques. Gynaecol Endosc 1999; 8: 403–406.

4. Ternamian AM. A second generation laparoscopic port system. Gynaecol Endosc 1999; 8: 397–401.

5. Palmer R. Safety in laparoscopy. J Reprod Med 1974; 13: 1–5.

6. Gordon AG, Taylor PJ. Practical laparoscopy. London: Blackwell Scientific Publications; 1993: 18–25.

7. Garry R. Laparoscopy, In: Shaw RW, Soutter WP, Stanton SL, eds. Gynaecology 2nd edn, Churchill Livingstone, Edinburgh, 1997, Chapter 4, 53–70.

8. Semm K. Endoscopic intra-abdominal surgery, 2nd edn. Kiel: Christian-Albrechts University; 1984: 8–12.

9. Semm K. Atlas of gynaecologic laparoscopy and hysteroscopy. Philadelphia: WB Saunders; 1977.

10. Redwine DB. Monopolar electroexcision of endometriosis. In: Sutton C, Diamond M, eds. Endoscopic surgery for gynaecologists, 2nd edn. Philadelphia: WB Saunders; 1988: 369–389.

11. Rock JA, Hurst BS. Laparoscopic surgery for endometriosis. In: Gordon AG, Lewis BV, De Cherney AH, eds. Atlas of gynaecological endoscopy, 2nd edn. London: Mosby-Wolfe; 1995: 86–90.

12. Audebert AJM. The role of microlaparoscopy for safer wall entry. Gynaecol Endosc 1999; 8: 363–367.

13. Schrenk P, Woisetschlager R, Rieger R, et al. Mechanism management & prevention of laparoscopic bowel injuries. Gastrointest Endosc 1996; 43: 572–574.

14. Phipps JH. Laparoscopic hysterectomy. In: Gordon AC, Lewis BV, DeCherney AH, eds. Atlas of gynaecological endoscopy, 2nd edn. London: Mosby-Wolfe; 1995: 118–124.

15. Bayer SR. Trocar injuries to the large intestine. In: Corfman RS, Diamond MP, DeCherney AH, eds. Complications of laparoscopy & hysteroscopy, 2nd edn. Oxford: Blackwell; 1997: 35–37.

16. Metzger D. Trocar injuries to the small intestine. In: Corfman RS, Diamond MP, DeCherney AH, eds. Complications of laparoscopy & hysteroscopy, 2nd edn. Oxford: Blackwell; 1997: 38–42.

17. Harkki-Siren P. The incidence of entry related laparoscopic injuries in Finland. Gynaecol Endosc 1999; 8: 335–338.

18. Harkki-Siren P, Kurki T, Sjoberg J, et al. Contemporary reviews. Obstet Gynaecol 2000; 12: 67–74.

19. Chapron CM, Pierre F, Lacroix S, et al. Major vascular injuries during gynaecological laparoscopy. J Am Coll Surg 1997; 185: 461–465.

20. Chapron C, Devroey P, Dubuisson JB, et al. ESHRE European Society for Human Reproduction and Embryology. Committee of Special Interest Group on Reproductive Surgery guidelines for training, accreditation and monitoring in gynaecological endoscopy. Hum Reprod 1997; 12: 867–868.

21. Jones KD, Fan A, Sutton CJG. Safe entry during laparoscopy: a prospective audit in a district general hospital. Gynaecol Endosc 2002; 11(2–3). 85–88.

22. Richardson RE, Sutton CJG. Complications of first entry: a prospective laparoscopy audit. Gynaecol Endosc 1999; 8: 327–334.

23. Chapron C, Querleu D, Bruhat MA, et al. Surgical complications of diagnostic and operative gynaecological laparoscopy: a series of 29,966 cases. Hum Reprod 1998; 13: 867–872.

35 Distant endometriosis

Agneta Bergqvist

Introduction

Extragenital endometriosis is rare in any population, and almost all publications are case reports or retrospective reviews. In 1990 all publications that could be identified in English, German, French, Spanish, Italian, Dutch, Polish as well as the five Scandinavian languages were reviewed and resulted in a Swedish monograph, based on 954 publications.[1] Since then, several more cases have been published, but no epidemiologic study has been performed, showing the incidence of different types of extragenital endometriosis. As each type of extragenital endometriosis is rare, except bowel and urinary tract endometriosis, no center and no specialist will ever collect large series of any specific type. Thus, no evidence-based data are available and there is no consensus concerning the treatment of these forms of endometriosis.

Endometriotic tissue has been found almost anywhere in the body and can be localized to nearly any tissue structure besides the spleen. Even if the most common localization is the pelvis, cases with more remote localizations, such as the extremities, spine, meninges, and brain, have been reported.

Endometriotic lesions are often located in muscles – both skeletal and smooth muscles – and both in muscles that are frequently active and in muscles that are usually relaxed. Endometriotic lesions are also often located in connective tissue, such as fascias and scars, but seldom in mucosa, lymph nodules, and lungs, and they are rare in other parenchyma tissues such as liver, kidney, or brain. The tissue environment has a great impact on how the lesions develop as well as on how the lesions respond to hormones. Lesions localized to connective tissue, i.e. sparsely vascularized, usually develop a large volume of hard fibrosis. Lesions localized to muscles that are well vascularized more often cause a hyperplasia of the surrounding muscle cells.

Women with distant endometriosis often have had symptoms for several years, and have consulted different doctors before the correct diagnosis finally has been made (Figure 35.1). The main symptoms are pain and local bleeding that usually, at least initially, is cyclical. Some cases have symptoms of genital endometriosis as well, like dysmenorrhea and dyspareunia. The symptoms are related to the affected organ and the

---

Varying signs and symptoms during the menstrual cycle
Increasing signs by time
Pain the most common symptom
Pronounced tenderness at palpation
Other symptoms depending on the organ/tissue involved

Figure 35.1 Common symptoms characteristic for extragenital endometriosis.

women not always spontaneously notice the connection to their periods. Furthermore, organ specialists other than gynecologists often forget to consider a possible relationship to menstruation, which is why they fail to identify the diagnosis. An endometriotic lump is often taken for a malignancy until the histopathologic pattern is shown.

This chapter will cover all types of extragenital endometriosis reported in the literature, besides bowel and urinary tract endometriosis, which are dealt with in detail elsewhere in this book. Many of the distant localizations described below are very rare but are included just to make the list complete and to remind the reader of endometriosis as a differential diagnosis in many areas. The chapter will also, as far as possible, illustrate the results of the treatment alternatives published so far. Diagnostic investigations and treatment has to be performed in proper collaboration between the relevant specialist and a gynecologist.

Principles for treatment of distant endometriosis

Several aspects have to be taken into consideration when treatment of distant endometriosis is planned. It is extremely important to discuss the therapeutic alternatives with the patient and to consider her priorities, but also to a relevant organ specialist in cases of non-gynecologic endometriosis. Is a local extirpation possible or is generalized hormonal treatment to be preferred? Some guidelines are helpful for this decision. Endometriotic lesions localized to muscles or parenchyma tissue such as lungs, kidneys, or liver in general respond well to hormones, i.e. to reduced estradiol exposure by ovarian down-regulation or gestagen treatment. The choice of drug is based on the patient's preference with regard to future fertility and previous experiences of the effect and side effects of different hormones, but also a possible need of rapid regression in order to avoid serious organ destruction. Healing of endometriotic lesions often takes a long time and 6 months of ovarian down-regulation is sometimes not sufficient. Lesions localized to connective tissue or lesions that have developed a large volume of dense fibrosis are usually less sensitive to hormonal changes and, if they do respond, the regression is often slow and takes a long time. These cases often require surgical extirpation. Distant endometriosis seldom recurs if the surgical extirpation has been complete.

Malignant transformation has been reported in most types of extragenital endometriosis: besides the bowel and urinary tract endometriosis, it also occurs in endometriosis in scars, the umbilicus, and the lung.

Endometriosis in the abdominal wall, umbilicus, skin or subcutaneous tissue

Incidence and sites

Endometriosis in or under the skin
These lesions occur mainly in the scars after gynecologic surgery or at the site of another trauma, often minor[1–3] (Figure 35.2). Scar endometriosis has been reported after 1–2% of abdominal hysterotomies, but also after laparotomies for other indications, mainly gynecologic. The symptoms usually start 0.5–3 years after the surgery. The incidence is higher after hysterotomy for termination of pregnancy in the second trimester (3.5%) than after caesarean section in the third trimester (0.5%). Endometriosis may also appear in scars after a perineotomy, above all if curettage has been done at the time of delivery, and also in scars after operations of Bartholin's cysts. Some rare cases of endometriosis in penetration canals through the abdominal wall after amniocentesis, laparoscopy, or sutures from the uterus have been reported.[4,5]

Umbilical endometriosis
Endometriosis causes 25% of umbilical tumors. It is usually located in the lower part of the umbilicus, extends all through the abdominal wall, and is sometimes connected to an umbilical hernia.[6] (Figure 35.3).

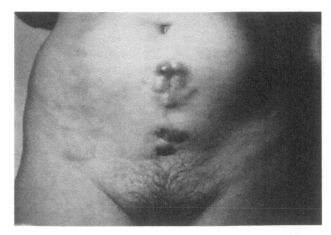

Figure 35.2 Endometriosis in a lower abdominal middle line scar after hysterectomy.

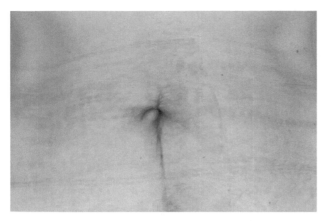

Figure 35.3 Umbilical endometriosis in the lower part of the umbilicus.

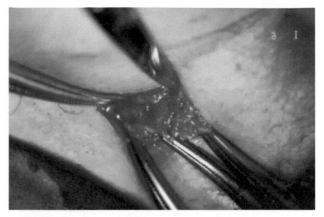

Figure 35.4 A subcutaneous endometriotic nodule in the abdominal wall, attached to the underlying fascia, independent of any scars.

Symptoms

The nodules are usually solitary. The size may vary from a few millimeters up to 4–8 cm, and the varying size during the menstrual cycle may be easily recognized. The nodule is usually densely fixed to muscles, fascia, or scar tissue, less often to the skin, and almost never extends through the peritoneum. It may be hard or cystic and fairly well demarcated, blue-red, blue-brown or light red, depending on age, depth under the skin, and the quantity of blood included in the tissue. The nodule is sometimes tender, particularly before and during bleeding episodes, when blood in rare cases appears through a fistula in the skin.

Diagnosis

The palpable identification of the nodule is, together with the history, usually enough indication for extirpation, but if further diagnostic examination has to be performed, ultrasound with or without fine-needle biopsy or magnetic resonance imaging (MRI) are to be preferred rather than computed tomography (CT).[7,8]

Treatment

Cutaneous, subcutaneous, umbilical, and scar endometriosis are usually easy to extirpate, and surgery should be preferred (Figure 35.4). However, it is of the utmost important to extirpate the nodule completely, otherwise the risk of recurrence is high. Extensive resections of endometriosis in the fascia sometimes have to be strengthened by patch grafting.[9] Cases less available for extirpation may be treated hormonally if malignancy can be excluded.[10]

Case history 1

A 40-year-old woman had developed an endometriotic nodule in a perineotomy scar 3 years after her third delivery. The lesion had been incompletely extirpated twice, and each recurrence resulted in a larger nodule extending more dorsal towards the sphincter muscle. Finally, the endometriosis nodule extended into the anal sphincter muscle and involved about 50% of the sphincter muscle circumference, extending into the surroundings like a sun fan. The lesion was extremely tender at palpation and terribly painful at defecation, sitting, and for most kinds of body movement. It was judged as not available for further surgery because of a high risk of fecal incontinence. Hormonal treatment was introduced. She has now been symptom-free on almost continuous gonadotropin-releasing hormone (GnRH) agonist treatment for 9 years without adverse events, and the nodule has diminished to the size of a grain of rice. Two trials to stop treatment have resulted in a recurrent painful growth within a few months and she now refuses to interrupt the treatment once more before she becomes menopausal.

Endometriosis in the inguinal region or the major nerves

Incidence and sites

Inguinal endometriosis

Inguinal endometriosis is usually localized to the inguinal canal, often close to the inguinal part of the round ligament or an inguinal hernia, but sometimes to a femoral hernia or medially towards the labium major or the pubic bone. The lesion is usually localized outside the peritoneal sac, covered by an intact peritoneum, not invaded by endometriosis[11] (Figure 35.5). Other localizations of endometriotic lesions causing catamenial inguinal pain are the extraperitoneal and the intra-abdominal parts of the round ligament as well as endometriosis in lymph glands, the groin, or the sacrococcygeal region.[12] Right-sided cases are more common (87%) than left-sided cases,[1] but also bilateral cases exist. Lesions up to 10 cm have been reported.

Endometriosis in major nerves

Histologically verified endometriosis in the sciatic nerve is rare and 70% are right-sided.[1,13] Two cases of bilateral involvement have been reported. A 'pocket sign', which means an evagination of the peritoneum towards the sciatic spine, has been reported in some cases.[14] The endometriotic lesion has been localized to the sciatic spine or where the nerve appears under the piriform muscle.[2,15] Rare cases of endometriosis in the uterosacral ligament have involved the obturator nerve, and lesions in the groin have involved the inguinal or the ileo-inguinal nerve, all of which gave rise to pain in the groin or over the adductor muscle. Lesions in the uterosacral ligaments may also lead to severe pain that simulates sciatica. A remnant ovary with endometriosis tightly adherent laterally in the pouch of Douglas has also been reported to involve the obturator nerve.[16]

Symptoms

The most common symptom is pain localized to the groin or thigh, or, in case of nerve involvement, to the innervated area. The pain can appear independent of menstrual periods and worsens on physical activities such as jumping. Some

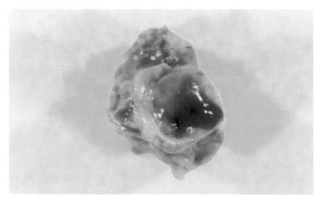

Figure 35.5 An endometriotic nodule extirpated from the bottom of an inguinal hernia sac. The peritoneal surface covering the lesion is intact but has a bluish discoloration.

cases are, however, pain-free. Other symptoms from involved major nerves are neurologic defects, muscle weakness, muscle atrophy, and desensitization.

Diagnosis

On examination, a nodule may be palpable, which may be exquisitely tender, mostly during menstruation when it may expand. The lesion may be mistaken for an incarcerated hernia or lymphadenitis. Endometriosis affecting the sciatic nerve may cause distinct tenderness at the sciatic spine. If the lesion is not palpable, a neurologic examination, CT, MRI, myelography, or electromyelography might be helpful.[15,17] A final diagnosis is usually not made until after exploration and histologic verification. Involvement of one of the big nerves has to be considered in cases of extensive hard fibrotic endometriosis extending from the uterosacral ligament towards the pelvic wall and the patient has pain radiating down the leg.

Treatment

Inguinal endometriosis

The inguinal lesions are sometimes easy to extirpate and, if so, surgery is to be preferred, but sometimes the lesions are very delicately localized close to the big vessels or in muscles, when hormonal treatment should be the first choice of treatment.

Endometriosis in big nerves

Although endometriosis sometimes invades the big nerves, splitting the nerve bundles[13] and causing bleeding and even nerve degeneration, resection of the nerve is not possible. If the nerve is involved mechanically, decompression and neurolysis is usually recommended and the endometriotic tissue and fibrosis should be excised as radically as possible to restrict further damage to the nerve.[18,19] However, successful hormonal treatment without surgery has been reported.[20] Postoperative ovarian down-regulation treatment is needed, usually for a long time.

Case history 2

In a 35-year-old nulliparous woman with severe right-sided sciatic pain, orthopedic surgery was unsuccessful. The woman had had pelvic endometriosis previously treated, and a new visit to her gynecologist revealed a tense and tender nodule, about 2 × 3 cm, above and lateral to the sciatic spine. Deep pelvic endometriosis was suspected and surgery was performed by an extraperitoneal approach.[21] The extensive lesion, localized in the uterosacral ligament, dorsal cervix, and dorsal vaginal pouch, reaching the right pelvic wall and ending up in a 3 × 3 cm endometriotic cyst in the obturator membrane, was completely removed, keeping the pelvic organs intact. The lesion obstructed the sciatic nerve, which was decompressed. Pain disappeared completely. Nineteen months after surgery, the woman became pregnant.

Case history 3

A 39-year-old woman with severe endometriosis for the past 10 years had had extensive pelvic surgery for endometriosis on 5 occasions, including left-sided nephrectomy because of a completely obstructed left ureter causing silent renal failure and later a total hysterectomy and bilateral oophorectomy. The last laparotomy was performed because of a 10 cm large endometriotic cyst between the rectum and the sacral bone, with hard fibrosis extending along the left vaginal wall to the sciatic spine. The cyst and extensive fibrosis were extirpated, but the distal part towards the sciatic spine was impossible to remove surgically. Histology revealed extensive endometriosis in the extirpated tissue. She did not tolerate hormonal treatment, as gestagens made her suicidal. Two years after the fifth operation, severe pain recurred in her left pelvis, radiating towards the rectum; it required opiates and repeated hospitalization for pain relief. Vaginal palpation revealed, at a depth of 10 cm, an intensely tender 2 cm long, rounded nodule tightly fixed medially to the sciatic bone. Diagnostic MRI showed a lesion 27 × 23 mm, obviously adherent to the levator ani muscle, the left part of the vaginal apex, the left rectal wall, and the left pelvic wall (Figure 35.6). The nodule was evaluated by an expert team – consisting of orthopedic surgeons, rectal surgeons, vascular surgeons, neurosurgeons, and a gynaecologic surgeon – and all the experts judged the lesion to be impossible for surgical extirpation. A decision was made to instill methotrexate into the lesion. After two injections, the lesion regressed and pain decreased. Two years later, the woman has only slight pain intermittently, when she needs some pain killers, and she can perform her daily activities and her job without limitations.

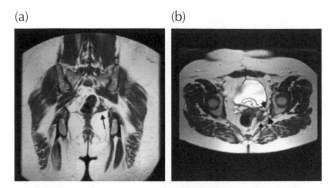

Figure 35.6 Coronal (a) and transverse (b) MRI showing a fibrous lesion (which is probably a complication of deep endometriosis) adherent to the left levator ani muscle (arrow), the left part of the vaginal top and the left rectal wall (open arrow), and the left pelvic wall (arrowheads).

Endometriosis in the extremities or neck

Incidence and sites

Endometriosis has been reported to occur anywhere in the thigh (Figure 35.7), often in direct connection to one of the big muscles but in some cases fixed to the skeleton.[18,22,23] In some, but not all cases, the skin covering the nodule has a slight bluish discoloration. Very rare cases of endometriosis have been reported in the elbow, the forearm, and neck.[24] In some cases, the nodule has appeared after local trauma, usually blunt.

Symptoms

These lesions are tender more or less continuously, but the pain may increase during menstruation.

Diagnosis

In some, but not all, cases a nodule can be palpated. When needed, a further investigation using fine-needle biopsy, ultrasound, MRI, or CT is useful before a decision is made concerning the therapeutic mode.[22]

Treatment

When exploration has been performed, the lesions have been found to be less well circumscribed and without a capsule. Such lesions localized to muscles may be difficult to extirpate completely without excessive destruction of the muscle, and hormonal treatment should be preferred.

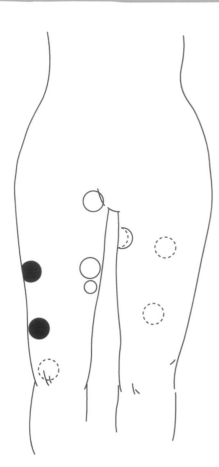

Figure 35.7 An illustration of the distribution of the published endometriotic lesions in the thigh region.

Case History 4

A 37-year-old healthy woman had noticed a reddish tumor under her right index fingernail that did not disappear for some months. The hand surgeon removed the lesion, believing that it was a tumor (Figure 35.8). Histology revealed endometriosis.

Thoracic endometriosis

Incidence and sites

Pleural endometriosis
Endometriosis in the lungs and pleura has been reported in about 150 cases, pleural endometriosis being by far the commonest type.[18] The lesions are usually solitary, but miliary spread exists. Right-sided involvement is more common, both in cases with pleural and lung lesions.[1,25] All cases of catamenial hemothorax as well as 90% of all cases of catamenial pneumothorax have been right sided,[1] in comparison to pneumothorax caused by congenital defects, which are usually left sided.

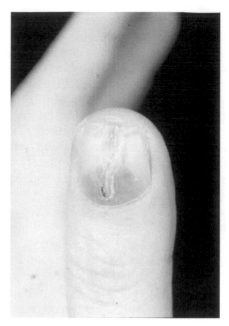

Figure 35.8 Endometriosis under the nail in the right index finger.

Pleural endometriosis is often restricted to the diaphragm; endometriosis extending all through the diaphragm has been reported. The degree of pneumothorax varies from sparse in some cases to complete in other cases.

Pulmonary endometriosis
Pulmonary lesions may appear anywhere in the lungs (Figure 35.9). An interesting comparison can be made between endometriosis in the lungs and endometriosis in the pleura. Women with pleural endometriosis often have a history of pelvic endometriosis, which is rare in cases with pulmonary endometriosis.[26] On the other hand, women with endometriosis in the lung often have a history of surgery of the uterus, which is much less common in cases with pleural endometriosis.[18] Thus, the pathogenesis of the two types might be different and coexistence of the two is extremely rare.

Symptoms

Pleural endometriosis
Recurrent pneumothorax at menstruation, 'catamenial pneumothorax', is pathognomonic for pleural endometriosis,[27] Hemothorax is less strictly related to the menstrual cycle.[18] The chest pain is usually one sided. Dyspnea and coughing depend on whether there is pneumothorax or hemothorax. The median age for the onset of symptoms is 35 years old, which differs from cases with idiopathic

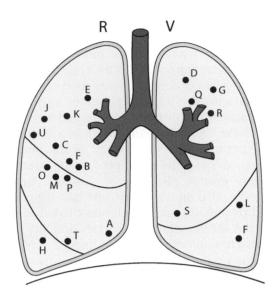

Figure 35.9 An illustration of the distribution of pulmonary endometriosis, published up to 1991.

pneumothorax. The mean number of pneumothoraces before diagnosis is 5, but there are case reports of more than 40 episodes of pneumothorax until the diagnosis was reached and proper hormonal treatment was introduced. Catamenial pneumothorax may recur also during menses induced by oral contraceptives or pregnancy.

Pulmonary endometriosis

Hemoptysis, usually cyclical, may occur when the lesion in the lung tissue is connected to the bronchial tree. The hemoptysis is usually sparse but more profuse coughing of blood has been reported. Between the menstrual bleeding periods, the patient is symptom-free. Patients without symptoms have been reported.[18]

Diagnosis

The history is important, recognizing the time relationship to the menstrual cycle.

Pleural endometriosis

Chest X-ray, CT or MRI visualize a pneumothorax or hemothorax usually as a narrow cleft, but pleural lesions can seldom be identified because of their small size, even when a pleuroscopy is performed. Pleural endometriosis might rarely be visualized as minor bluish-, reddish-, or brownish spots like typical peritoneal lesions, but sometimes only hemosiderin-loaded inclusions or fibrotic spots are identified. Fine-needle biopsy

and cytologic examination of pleural exudates are seldom diagnostic and even bronchoscopy during an active hemoptysis.[28] Endometriosis has been histologically verified in about one-third of the reported cases with catamenial pneumothorax. Most of the reported cases, and even those with pleural endometriosis which could not be histologically verified, have had endometriosis at other sites. Symptoms have disappeared during ovarian inactivation treatment, indicating that the pneumothorax is associated with the endometriotic disease.[29]

Pulmonary endometriosis

Pulmonary lesions appear as small cystic defects or irregular condensations, which may simulate a malignant process as well as tuberculosis.[30] Typically, the lesions will vary in size during the menstrual cycle and sometimes disappear between the menstrual bleeding episodes. Thus, it is important to perform the imaging strictly during the time of menstrual bleeding or the symptomatic period. Endobronchial lesions with a connection to the bronchial tree might be identified as solitary or multiple cystic lesions or only sparse blood in a bronchus when a bronchoscopy is performed. However, other endometriotic nodules in the lung tissue cannot be revealed by bronchoscopy.[26] In cases with endobronchial endometriosis, cytology of brushings from the lesion might show clusters of cells resembling endometrium.

Treatment

Women with thoracic symptoms, whether or not caused by endometriosis, have to be handled by thoracic/lung specialists initially. A pneumothorax often requires hospitalization. If the air cleft is large, as well as in cases of hemothorax, a thoracocentesis and active thoracic drainage, respectively, has to be performed. When the acute situation is under control, a more sustained treatment has to be introduced.

Pleural endometriosis

Drainage combined with hormonal treatment is preferred in cases with pleural endometriosis. The minimal duration of hormonal ovarian inactivation is 6 months, but if recurrence appears, a more durable hormonal treatment has to be initiated.[31] If the patient cannot tolerate the hormonal treatment or if the pneumothorax or hemothorax recur in spite of ongoing hormonal treatment, a surgical approach has to be considered. Local excision of pleural lesions is not sufficient and usually there is not even anything to see. A pleurodesis, or pleurectomy, has to be performed, although not even this technique completely prevents recurrences. Diaphragmatic defects are not uncommon and a systematic coverage of the diaphragm surface by a mesh has been recommended.[32]

Pulmonary endometriosis

Also, in cases of pulmonary lesions, hormones should be the first line of treatment if a malignancy can be excluded. A proper response can often be noticed. If not, or in cases of recurrent symptoms in spite of ongoing anovulatory treatment, a wedge or segmental resection might have to be done, if possible by a video-assisted thoracoscopy.[33,34]

However, usually these patients first end up in a chest or lung clinic with severe acute chest pain or coughing blood and, as most specialists in those fields are seldom aware of thoracic endometriosis, the patients often go to primary surgery. Unfortunately, recurrences after surgery are very common. An increased awareness about endometriosis as a cause of catamenial pneumothorax, hemothorax, or hemoptysis should result in a higher frequency of primary hormonal treatment in cases where a malignancy can be excluded.

The attacks of thoracic pain and dyspnea are usually highly terrifying and long-time chronic anovulatory treatment to prevent recurrences is crucial. Regular controls for years are important, as progress may occur in spite of treatment, either surgical or hormonal. Women who wish to be pregnant of course have to interrupt the treatment, but because of the high risk of recurrences they might need assisted reproduction to reduce the treatment-free period.

Case history 5

A previously healthy woman had her first right-sided pneumothorax at the age of 26. She had a pleural drainage. Two months later she had a right-sided pneumothorax again, treated conservatively with drainage. After another two monthly catamenial pneumothoraces, she had a thoracotomy with resection of the apical lesions in the right lung. Histology verified endometriosis. The month after surgery she had a left-sided pneumothorax and a thoracotomy and pleurectomy was performed. Histology verified endometriosis also in the left pleura. During 8 months of post-operative treatment with gestagens she was symptom-free, which is why she then stopped treatment as she wanted to become pregnant. This occurred 2 months later. The pregnancy and 10 months of breast-feeding were uneventful, and 3 months later she became pregnant again. During the 3rd month of pregnancy she had a recurrence of a 3 cm left-sided pneumothorax, which was treated conservatively. The rest of the pregnancy, as well as 5 months of breast-feeding, went without any events. She entered gestagen treatment again but, still on treatment, she had a 3 cm right-sided pneumothorax, which was treated conservatively. A CT revealed small cysts apically in both lungs. Three months later she had an almost total left-sided pneumothorax again, now treated with Metacrine instillation. Two weeks later she had an extensive left-sided pneumothorax, which was treated with Metacrine again. Since then, she has been on continuous treatment with a GnRH agonist and has not had any recurrences for 2.5 years. Vaginal estrogen application resulted in pleural pain that disappeared when the estrogen was omitted. She is now 33 years old, symptom-free, and repeated DEXA examinations have shown a stable osteopenia. However, the woman insists on continuing the GnRH agonist treatment because of fear of more pleural incidences. She has never had any indications of pelvic endometriosis and has never had a laparoscopy.

Endometriosis in the liver, gall bladder, pancreas, or diaphragm

Hepatic endometriosis

At least 6 cases of hepatic endometriosis have been published.[35–37] Not all of the women had a history of endometriosis or of concomitant pelvic endometriosis. No typical symptom pattern can be distinguished; the women have had cyclic or acyclic abdominal pain or been asymptomatic. The lesions revealed by MRI, ultrasound, and/or CT have been cystic, in some cases multicystic, measuring 6–12 cm (Figure 35.10). Lesions have been localized to either the right or the left liver lobe. In at least two of the cases, the nodule was adhesive to the diaphragm.

At laparotomy a hard elastic mass has been noted and a resection was performed. At least one case was treated with a GnRH agonist before surgery, resulting in a prompt reduction of the nodule size.

(a)

(b)

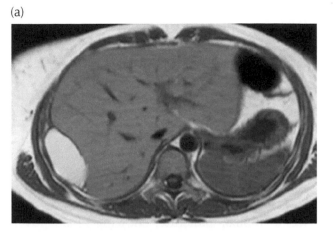
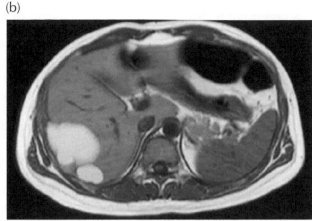

Figure 35.10 (a–b) MRI showing endometriotic cysts in the liver. For explanation of figure parts see the text.

Endometriosis in the pancreas

In the literature three histologically verified cases of endometriotic cyst in the pancreatic tail have been reported.[38]

Diaphragmatic endometriosis

Some cases of diaphragmatic endometriosis have been reported, all causing chronic pain in the right shoulder region. Most cases showed implants of a few millimeters, but in one case a 4 cm diaphragmatic cyst compressed the liver surface. Usually, the lesions have been described as superficial, but cases with endometriotic growth all through the diaphragm have been reported. The lesions are usually multiple and may be localized anywhere in the diaphragm, and also in the posterior part, covered by the liver.[39] Successful laparoscopic vaporization after hydrodissection has been performed,[40] but in some cases open resection of the diaphragm had been preferred.[39]

Endometriosis in the diaphragm has to be remembered at diagnostic laparoscopy when the laparoscope can easily be turned upwards to allow inspection of the diaphragm.

Case History 6

A woman who has never been pregnant had problems with dysmenorrhea and heavy bleedings for 2 weeks of every 4 all the time from menarche at the age of 9. Although treated with oral conraceptives from the age of 13 she had pronounced menstrual pain and had to stay home from school several days every month. At the age of 21 she had a left-sided oophorectomy because of a large endometrioma that had destroyed her ovary. No hormonal treatment was given afterwards. An 8 cm right-sided ovarian endometriotic cyst had to be removed 5 years later. As she wanted to become pregnant, no hormonal treatment was introduced, but after a recurrence of a right-sided endometrioma, she started with oral contraceptives. Because of increasing pain she turned to gestagen treatment. The pain disappeared with the bleedings. Four years later she stopped the treatment for pregnancy plans. When the menses reappeared, they were followed by fever up to 39°C and a high C-reactive protein (CRP) up to 306 mg/L. One year after she had stopped with gestagens, pain started in the right flank and back. Appendectomy was performed, showing a normal appendix but endometriosis in the sigmoid colon. The pain was severe and required morphine. A CT showed cysts in the liver and MRI confirmed two well-limited cysts dorsolaterally in the right liver lobe measuring 26 × 60 mm and 48 × 73 mm, respectively, as well as a smaller one 16 × 26 mm. Further ventrally subcapsularly in the right liver lobe, a fourth cyst, 8 × 12 mm, was identified. The cysts were identical with endometriosis cysts (Figure 35.10a). The liver function tests were normal. The patient had a continuous painful pressure under the right costal arch and down to the pelvis. Ultrasound examination showed that the cysts had increased in size; under anesthesia, the largest cyst was punctured and 90 ml of mucous dark red fluid was aspirated. During aspiration, the other three cysts collapsed as well, indicating a communication between them. No biopsy could be obtained from the inside of the cyst walls when they had collapsed. The fluid contained only regressively changed cells. The pain disappeared for about 1 month after puncture. Although the gestagen treatment continued and she was bleeding-free, the pain came back and 1 year later an ultrasound examination identified the two largest cysts again, although now smaller, measuring 30 × 15 mm and 20 × 10 mm, respectively. Instillation of alcohol in the cysts was discussed, but declined. Now she had also developed a palpable endometriotic nodule in the rectovaginal septum, protruding into the vagina. Surgery was discussed, but first the gestagen dose was increased. She was still bleeding-free but the pain sustained. A new MRI 1 year ago, 3 years after the first one, showed that the cysts in the liver as well as in the right ovary had disappeared (Figure 35.10b). Very slowly the pain has reduced, but still she requires high doses of pain killers.

Case History 7

A 35-year-old women had pelvic endometriosis diagnosed at the age of 21, mainly localized to the point of attachment of the uterosacral ligaments to the cervix. She had been more or less symptom-free on gestagens, and later continuous oral contraceptives through the years. The treatment was interrupted four times, but the pelvic pain recurred within 1–2 years. During the 5th cessation of treatment, she began to develop diffuse epigastric pain radiating to the back and, because of suspected cholecystitis, a laparoscopic cholecystectomy was planned. At the laparoscopy, disseminated endometriosis was recognized covering the complete abdominal surface of the diaphragm like a blueberry hill. A biopsy verified endometriosis. Gestagen treatment was introduced again and the pain disappeared; she has now been symptom-free on continuous treatment for 6 years.

Endometriosis in the spine or brain

Endometriosis in the spine

At least two cases with histologically verified vertebral endometriosis have been reported.[41] One woman had pain in the lower back for half a year. X-ray showed a bone destructive process in LI-LIV. The endometriosis was surgically removed. The other 26-year-old woman had a back trauma at the age of 14. From the age of 25 she had back pain, and an acute exacerbation during menstruation led to lumbar puncture, showing blood. Myelography showed a 1–1.5 cm tumour on the inside of the dural sac, adherent to the nerve roots in the cauda equina. Histology after extirpation showed endometriosis. A few more cases have been reported but the data are sparse.

Cerebral endometriosis

Two cases of histologically verified cerebral endometriosis have been reported.[42] One woman had catamenial seizures and the other woman had episodic headache unrelated to the menstrual cycle. In both cases CT revealed ring-enhanced foci surrounded with brain edema and in one case MRI elucidated a hyperintense focus with a capsule and old bleeding. In both cases the lesions, extirpated by open neurosurgery, were localized to the gray-white junction.

Acknowledgments

Dr Viggo Blomlie, Department of Radiology, Sabbatsbergs Hospital, and Dr Eva, Department of Radiology, Ersta Hospital, Stockholm, Sweden are highly acknowledged for contributing the MRI pictures of my patients.

REFERENCES

1. Bergqvist A. Extragenital endometrios. Sweden: Organon; 1990.
2. Bergqvist A. Extragenital endometriosis. A review. Eur J Surg 1992; 158: 7–12.
3. Dwivedi AJ, Agrawal SN, Silva YJ. Abdominal wall endometriosis. Dig Dis Sci 2002; 47: 456–461
4. Kaunitz A, DiSant'Agnese PA. Needle tract endometriosis: an unusual complication of amniocentesis. Obstet Gynecol 1979; 54: 753–755
5. Martinez-Serna T, Stalter KD, Filipi CJ et al. An unusual case of endometrial trocar site implantation. Surg Endosc 1998; 12: 992–994

6. Michowitz M, Baratz M, Stavorovsky M. Edometriosis of the umbilicus. Dermatologia 1983; 167: 326–330

7. Yu CY, Perez-Reyes M, Brown JJ, et al. MR appearance of umbilical endometriosis. J Comput Assist Tomogr 1994; 18: 269–271

8. Liary CC, Liou B, Tsai CC, et al. Scar endometriosis. Int Surg 1998; 83: 69–71.

9. Blanco RG, Parithivel VS, Shah AK, et al. Abdominal wall endometriomas. Am J Surg 2003; 185: 596–598.

10. Purvis RS, Tyring SK. Cutaneous and subcutaneous endometriosis. Surgical and hormonal therapy. J Dermatol Surg Oncol 1994; 20: 693–695.

11. Sataloff DM, LaVorgna KA, McFarland MM. Extrapelvic endometriosis presenting as a hernia: clinical reports and review of the literature. Surgery 1989; 105: 109–112

12. Felding C, Nyrnberg LE, Moesgaard J. Endometriosis of the round ligament. Ann Chir Gynaecol 1989; 78: 327–328

13. Vercellini P, Chapron C, Fedele L, et al. Evidence for asymmetric distribution of sciatic nerve endometriosis. Obstet Gynecol 2003; 102: 383–387.

14. Binkovitz LA, King BF, Ehman RL. Sciatic endometriosis: MR appearance. J Comput Assist Tomog 1991; 15: 508–510.

15. Descamps P, Cottier JP, Barre I, et al. Endometriosis of the sciatic nerve: case report demonstrating the value of MR imaging. Eur J Obstet Gynecol Reprod Biol 1995; 58: 199–202.

16. Scully RE, Galdabini JJ, McNeely BU. Case 23–1980. Presentation of a case. N Engl J Med 1980; 302: 1354–1358.

17. Fedele L, Bianchi S, Raffaelli R, et al. Phantom endometriosis of the sciatic nerve. Fertil Steril 1999; 72: 727–729.

18. Bergqvist A. Different types of extragenital endometriosis: a review. Gynecol Endocrinol 1993; 7: 207–221.

19. Papapietro N, Gulino G, Zobel BB, et al. Cyclic sciatica related to an extrapelvic endometriosis of the sciatic nerve: new concepts in surgical therapy. J Spinal Disord Tech 2002; 15: 436–439.

20. DeCesare SL, Yeko TR. Sciatic nerve endometriosis treated with a gonadotropin releasing hormone agonist. A case report. J Reprod Med 1995; 40: 226–228.

21. Bergqvist A, Bergqvist D, Lindholm K, et al. Endometriosis in the uterosacral ligament giving orthopedic symptoms through compression of the sciatic nerve and surgically treated via an extraperitoneal approach keeping the pelvic organs intact. Case report. Acta Obstet Gynecol Scand 1987; 66: 93–94.

22. Gitelis S, Petasnick JP, Turner DA, et al. Endometriosis simulating a soft tissue tumor of the thigh: CT and MR evaluation. J Comput Assist Tomogr 1985; 9: 573–576.

23. Giangarra C, Gallo G, Newman R, et al. Endometriosis in the biceps femoris. J Bone Joint Surg 1987; 69: 290–292.

24. Navratil E, Kramer A. Endometriose in der Armmuskulatur. Klin Wschr 1936; 15: 1765–1770.

25. Joseph J, Sahn SA. Thoracic endometriosis syndrome: new observations from an analysis of 110 cases. Am J Med 1996; 100: 164–170.

26. Bateman ED, Morrison SC. Catamenial haemoptysis from endobronchial endometriosis – a case report and review of previously reported cases. Respir Med 1990; 84: 157–161.

27. Davies R, Kalinowski S. Recurring spontaneous pneumothorax and its association with endometriosis. Br J Dis Chest 1971; 65: 222–224.

28. Lolis D, Adonakis G, Kontostolis E, et al. Successful conservative treatment of catamenial pneumothorax with GnRH agonist. Arch Gynecol Obstet 1995; 256: 163–166.

29. Espaulella J, Armengol J, Bella F, et al. Pulmonary endometriosis: conservative treatment with GnRH agonists. Obstet Gynecol 1991; 78: 535–537.

30. Flieder DB, Moran CA, Travis WD, et al. Pleuro-pulmonary endometriosis and pulmonary ectopic deciduosis: a clinicopathologic and immunohistochemical study of 10 cases with emphasis on diagnostic pitfalls. Hum Pathol 1998; 29: 1495–1503.

31. Seltzer VL, Benjamin F. Treatment of pulmonary endometriosis with a long-acting GnRH agonist. Obstet Gynecol 1990; 76: 929–931.

32. Bagan P, Le Pimpec Barthes F, Assouad J, et al. Catamenial pneumothorax: retrospective study of surgical treatment. Ann Thorac Surg 2003; 75: 378–381.

33. Cassina PC, Hauser M, Kacl G, et al. Catamenial hemoptysis. Diagnosis with MRI. Chest 1997; 111: 1447–1450.

34. Roberts LM, Redan J, Reich H. Extraperitoneal endometriosis with catamenial pneumothoraces: a review of the literature. JSLS 2003; 7: 371–375.

35. Markham SM, Carpenter SE, Rock JA. Extrapelvic endometriosis. Obstet Gynecol Clin North Am 1989; 16: 193–219.

36. Cravello L, D'Ercole C, Le Treut YP, et al. Hepatic endometriosis: a case report. Fertil Steril 1996; 66: 657–659.

37. Bohra AK, Diamond T. Endometrioma of the liver. Int J Clin Pract 2001; 55: 286–287.

38. Lee DS, Baek JT, Ahn BM, et al. A case of pancreatic endometrial cyst. Korean J Intern Med 2002; 17: 266–269.

39. Redwine DB. Diaphragmatic endometriosis: diagnosis, surgical management and long-term results of treatment. Fertil Steril 2002; 77: 288–296.

40. Nezhat F, Nezhat C, Levy JS. Laparoscopic treatment of symptomatic diaphragmatic endometriosis: a case report. Fertil Steril 1992; 58: 614–616.

41. Carta F, Guiducci G, Fulcheri E, et al. Radicular compression by extradural spinal endometriosis. Case report. Acta Neurochir (Wien) 1992; 114: 68–71.

42. Ichida M, Gomi A, Hiranouchi N, et al. A case of cerebral endometriosis causing catamenial epilepsy. Neurology 1993; 43: 2708–2709.

36 Conclusions and the future

Christopher Sutton

It is always difficult to gaze into the crystal ball and try to predict the future: this can be difficult enough in any situation, but is even more difficult with a disease such as endometriosis. In just about every article one reads about endometriosis the word 'enigmatic' appears at some stage – usually in the introductory paragraph. According to the *Oxford English Dictionary* the word enigma basically means a riddle and enigmatic suggests something that is ambiguous, obscure, or perplexing; this is a very apt description of endometriosis. Having read this book from cover to cover, the reader will see that it does not obey any firm rules: the etiology is still perplexing, and treatment and outcomes can be very variable. In many of our surgical studies we get excited about success rates in terms of pain relief of the order of 70%, but the patients who make our clinics something of a misery usually belong to the other 30% who fail to respond to the prescribed treatment, be it medical or surgical.

Nevertheless, there are grounds for optimism and the chapters on etiology by Stephen Kennedy and his colleagues from Oxford and on pathogenesis by Michelle Nisolle and her team from Liege clearly indicate that research has progressed very rapidly in the past decade. With each new discovery we are one step nearer to understanding the cascade of events at a molecular level that contribute towards the implantation of endometrial cells in ectopic situations and their further proliferation, and the reasons that they cause pain and infertility.

Some 20 years ago, when laparoscopic surgery was developing at a furious pace, each conference saw some new exciting technique or development in instrumentation and surgical skill which resulted in considerable polarization between surgical and medical treatment of this disease. Looking back on those days, it seems to me that we were all a little shortsighted. Surgeons seriously thought that surgery was the only answer and I remember making some deprecating remarks about medical therapy being outmoded and outdated, based on the number of unpleasant side effects, the problems associated with long-term use, and the well-known fact that the disease appeared to recur in many patients after medication was discontinued. By contrast, many of our colleagues who favored medical treatment tended to sneer at the fact that much of our evidence was anecdotal or based on retrospective trials which could easily be biased by the strength of personality of the surgeon, the faith of the patient, and the belief in the increasingly sophisticated technology used during laparoscopic surgery. Clearly, unless a study is prospective and double-blind, it is always open to serious misinterpretation; yet such studies are very difficult to perform, especially if they involve a placebo arm when no surgical treatment has taken place and yet neither the patient nor the person involved in the follow-up are aware of this.

In our department we played a major role in conducting the first of these studies and the evolution and problems encountered are documented in chapters in this book dealing with the treatment of superficial peritoneal endometriosis and the history of the disease. Clearly, there were criticisms of our study, in that stage IV disease was not included and also we used a laparoscopic uterine nerve ablation as part of the treatment protocol. Subsequent studies have shown that the uterine nerve ablation procedure does not add to the already beneficial effects of ablating the endometriotic implants, and this has been confirmed in another study from Professor Vercellini's unit in Milan. Professor Garry, when he was working in Middlesborough, conducted a trial very similar to ours but included stage IV disease and also various quality of life and sexual health outcome measurements and it was remarkable how similar the results were to our original study. In both these studies there was a huge placebo effect at 3 months, which was not present at 6 months, underlying the difficulty in interpreting such studies and also emphasizing that it is useless to review patients until at least a 6-month interval has elapsed between the surgical procedure and the follow-up visit.

Although these various studies have improved our status in the eyes of our academic colleagues, there was nevertheless a significant number of patients who do not seem to benefit, either because the diagnosis is wrong and endometriosis was not the cause of the pain in the first place (the pain of irritable bowel syndrome and the symptoms can be remarkably similar to those of endometriosis) or because psychologic, psychosomatic, and marital problems play an enormous role in the response to treatment. We are becoming uncomfortably aware that many of these patients have a history of sexual abuse in childhood and yet gynecologists often feel uncomfortable in asking the relevant questions to uncover this.

In the future I think surgical treatment will become more specialized and centers of excellence in the treatment of endometriosis will be established. There will be considerably more collaboration between gynecologists and our colleagues in other specialties, particularly urology and coloproctology. Along with the amazing progress that surgeons have made in operative laparoscopy in recent years, I suspect that the new generation of laparoscopic colorectal surgeons will increasingly take over the management of deep infiltrating endometriosis (adenomyosis) in the rectovaginal septum but that gynecologists will still need to be present at the operation and use their skills in dealing with the disease in the pelvic side walls and adhesive disease between the tubes and the ovaries.

I think we have reached a stage where we should stop quibbling about the superiority of one energy source over another. It is increasingly obvious that the well-known findings of Professor Tulandi from Montreal, who many years ago pointed out that it is

the skill of the surgeon and careful patient selection that are the important factors rather than that one energy source is better than another. Clearly, electrocoagulation is too imprecise to be used for deep infiltrating disease but surgeons who are skilled in the use of the CO_2 laser or electrosurgery will get very similar results; nevertheless, considerable work needs to be done in the future on the collection of follow-up statistics and audit of the various procedures as well as to avoid serious complications. The availability of the internet to voice one's opinions to potential patients without any censorship or peer review has created a dangerous opportunity for some self-promoting specialists to advertise their skills and to deprecate the work of others. I hope in the future that this practice will be viewed with the contempt that it deserves, because I think we are tired of seeing inane remarks on our computer screens, such as 'laser treatment should be banned' or 'shining light at the lesion is useless', because often the purveyors of this misinformation have never done a double-blind, prospective, randomized trial in their lives and it is unlikely that they will ever do so.

As the main editor of this volume with its international cast of authors, it has been both interesting and frustrating although very hard work. Nevertheless, it has been extremely educational and, although I would like to mention the efforts of many of the contributors, I would like particularly to bring the attention of the reader to two chapters. In Chapter 5 on outcome measures, Ray Garry draws attention to his suggestion of a new classification of endometriosis, which is essentially based on the clinical examination and relies entirely on the presence or absence of painful nodular disease on initial pelvic examination. This would be a much more realistic approach than the various classifications we have had in the past, because it would ensure that those conditions without nodules, which he classifies as Sampson's syndrome, would be referred to normal jobbing gynecologists at district hospitals who can perform easy laparoscopic surgery on superficial peritoneal endometriosis. The other group with obvious nodules, which he classifies as Cullen's syndrome, requires much more intensive investigation and referral to tertiary centers of excellence where there is a team of highly experienced laparoscopic surgeons with no constraints on the time taken for the surgery or financial constraints on the sophistication of the equipment used. In the future this would help us considerably and would probably allow this type of laparoscopic surgery for deep infiltrating disease, which can be as difficult as any cancer surgery, to be sufficiently skilled that it would be recognized as a subspecialty in its own right and would ensure that patients with the most severe disease would get the best possible treatment.

The other exciting chapter is the one by David Olive (Chapter 29), who draws attention to the way that basic research, in particular molecular biology and phenomena such as neo-angiogenesis, which have parallels in cancer research, is slowly leading the way to the development of a whole series of exciting therapies, such as immune modulators and antiangiogenesis drugs, which I think will take the treatment of endometriosis forward into this new millennium.

My vision of the future is one where medical treatment and surgical treatment are not at opposite poles but can be integrated. Along with the increasing skill and sophistication of laparoscopic surgery for the primary eradication of disease, we can rely on increasingly sophisticated medical therapy to prevent relapse or recurrence, all of which would be to the benefit of our patients.

Index

421

T - #0555 - 071024 - C444 - 279/216/21 - PB - 9780367391669 - Gloss Lamination